Herbal Medicines

Herbal Medicines

A guide for healthcare professionals

SECOND EDITION

Joanne Barnes
BPharm, PhD, MRPharmS

Research Fellow
Centre for Pharmacognosy & Phytotherapy
The School of Pharmacy
University of London, UK

Linda A Anderson
BPharm, PhD, FRPharmS

Principal Pharmaceutical Officer
Medicines Control Agency
London, UK

J David Phillipson
DSc, PhD, MSc, BSc(Pharm), FRPharmS, FLS

Emeritus Professor, Centre for Pharmacognosy & Phytotherapy
The School of Pharmacy
University of London, UK

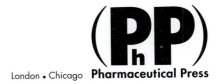

London • Chicago

Published by the Pharmaceutical Press

Publications division of the Royal Pharmaceutical Society of Great Britain

1 Lambeth High Street, London SE1 7JN, UK
100 South Atkinson Road, Suite 206, Grayslake, IL 60030-7820, USA

First published 1996
© Pharmaceutical Press 2002

Text design by Barker/Hilsdon, Lyme Regis, Dorset
Typeset by Bibliocraft Ltd, Dundee
Printed in Great Britain by The Bath Press, Bath

ISBN 0 85369 474 5

A catalogue record for this book is available from the British Library

Front cover images: *Zingiber officinale, Allium sativum, Panax pseudoginseng, Trifolium pratense, Capsicum frutescens.*
© The Natural History Museum, London

This book is dedicated to the memory of the late Dr W Gwynne Thomas, former Director of Pharmaceutical Sciences at the Royal Pharmaceutical Society of Great Britain. The inspiration for the book came from him and it is due to his efforts that the necessary funding was obtained.

Contents

Preface to the Second Edition

INTEREST IN HERBAL MEDICINES has continued to grow since publication of the first edition of this book. This is shown in several ways, for example, by increased retail sales of herbal medicinal products in Europe and the USA, as well as the greater awareness among the public and healthcare professionals about natural health products and complementary therapies. Industrially produced new herbal products, mainly based on single-herb extracts standardised for a specific active ingredient, continue to be developed. Good-quality clinical research to support the reputed effects of many herbs is lacking. Nevertheless, several herbal medicines have been investigated in well-designed clinical trials and, for a small number of herbs, systematic reviews and meta-analyses of randomised controlled trials have been published.

The safety of herbal products continues to be a matter of concern, even though toxic herbs have been eliminated from products manufactured in developed countries. There is, for example, a growing appreciation that herbal medicines may interact with concurrently used pharmaceutical medicines. The potential for herb–drug interactions has been highlighted by the recognition that St. John's wort (*Hypericum perforatum*) may interact with certain prescription medicines, including HIV protease inhibitors, oral contraceptives, selective serotonin reuptake inhibitors (SSRIs), theophylline, ciclosporin and warfarin. The havoc that may be caused by the use of a toxic herb, either for perceived medicinal purposes, or through inadvertent or deliberate substitution of a medicinal herb, is well illustrated by species of *Aristolochia* used in traditional Chinese medicine. Nephrotoxic and carcinogenic effects of *Aristolochia* in humans have been reported in Europe, China, Japan and the USA. Disquiet over the safety of herbs used in herbal products, whether licensed as medicines or sold as unlicensed products, is reflected by medicines regulatory authorities world-wide, highlighting the need for healthcare professionals to be aware of such problems.

The rationale for this book, and an explanation on how to use it, are covered in the preface for the first edition. In the intervening years, it has become apparent that the text is a valuable source of information for all groups of healthcare professionals, and that it is used throughout Europe, North America and Australasia. The chapter 'Introduction to the Monographs' has been completely revised for the second edition, and includes a summary of the current position of herbal medicines, mainly in Europe, as well as commenting on the possible future regulation of herbal medicinal products in the European Union.

Seven new herbal monographs have been added to the second edition so that 148 herbs are now included. Furthermore, 10 of the previous monographs have been extensively revised and rewritten, and a further 33 have been updated. There have been a number of significant publications on herbal medicines since the first edition was prepared, not least the monographs produced by the European Scientific Cooperative on Phytotherapy (ESCOP). At the time of the first edition, three volumes of ESCOP monographs had been published, and there are now a further three volumes, providing a total of 60 monographs on medicinal plant drugs.

The preparation of the monographs for the first edition of this book involved the use of 35 general references, in addition to specific references pertinent to each monograph. For this second edition, 65 general references are included, reflecting the growth in the literature on medicinal herbs. This increase in the literature, together with additional knowledge on the quality, safety, efficacy and legal requirements for herbal medicinal products, has led to a clear need to update this book for healthcare professionals.

The views expressed in this book are those of the authors and do not represent those of the Medicines Control Agency or European Medicines Evaluation Agency or European Medicines Evaluation Agency.

Acknowledgements

We are grateful to Paul Weller, Linda Horrell and Louise Wykes of the Pharmaceutical Press for their active help and encouragement with this work. Our thanks also go to Pepi Hurtado-Lopez and Suzannah Harris for their assistance in preparation of the manuscript.

Preface to the First Edition

Not so many years ago the advances being made in medicine and the innovations of the pharmaceutical industry made it seem inevitable that the use of herbal remedies in developed countries would decline to insignificance. It is somewhat of a paradox, therefore, that at a time when there is such an unprecedented number of therapeutic drugs available for the treatment of all forms of disease, that herbal remedies continue to be demanded by the general public. In fact, this demand has steadily increased over the past decade and as a result of enquiries from practising pharmacists, the Royal Pharmaceutical Society of Great Britain commissioned this volume in order to provide factual information on medicinal herbs.

The chapter 'Introduction to the Monographs' sets the herbal scene in the light of complementary therapies and goes on to consider UK and European legislation. The control of herbal remedies is a matter of concern to the Royal Pharmaceutical Society who have pointed out that the public may be at risk due to the sale of herbal products which are not licensed as medicines. All medicines are assessed for their quality, safety and efficacy and these parameters should be used to assess all herbs and herbal products which are intended for medical use.

The majority of herbal products sold in the UK are not licensed as medicines and because herbs are 'natural' some people consider that they must be safe. This is simply not true and some herbs are capable of causing adverse effects. With herbs, as with all medicines, it is necessary to consider precautions for specific patient groups, contra-indications, warnings and the potential for interaction with other medicines. Summary tables giving examples of herbal ingredients with potential adverse reactions, or those which are best avoided during pregnancy, are included in the chapter 'Introduction to the Monographs'.

Sensitive scientific methods for investigating the chemical constituents of herbs and for determining their biological activities are now available and a number of herbs are currently being subjected to detailed scientific scrutiny. A short account of such work and some relevant examples are given.

The major part of the text deals with 141 herbs which have been selected on the basis that they are ingredients of herbal remedies which are on sale in UK pharmacies. There is a brief section on 'How to Use this Handbook' on p. 1. The purpose and scope of the handbook, and a background on the standard monograph sections is given. The reader is advised to consult this section before referring to specific monographs.

Each herb is the subject of a monograph which is in a datasheet-type format. In addition to the names, synonyms and plant part used, each monograph indicates whether the herb is, or has been, the subject of a monograph in the European or a national pharmacopoeia. The legal category, food use and herbal doses are given where known, the constituents are listed briefly together with any documented pharmacology and human use. For some herbs, little pharmacology and particularly clinical information is available, and the reader may need to ascertain the current state of medical and scientific evidence. Any side-effects and toxicity are listed together with contra-indications and warnings. Each monograph carries a section on 'Pharmaceutical Comment' in which there is a brief comment on the advisability of using the particular herb for medicinal purposes. In some instances, the literature clearly indicates that the risk to benefit ratio precludes the use of the herb and if this is the case then it is clearly stated in the monograph.

A set of literature references is included with each monograph but some judgement has had to be exercised in the extent to which references are cited. In an attempt to overcome the vast numbers of references which could be included for some of the monographs, the references have been divided into two categories, general and specific. There are some 35 general references which include review books of herbal use, pharmacopoeial descriptions, chemistry, pharmacology and toxicology. For well-known medicinal herbs such as cascara, only general references are cited, whereas for lesser known herbs or for herbs undergoing recent investigation, every attempt has been made to cite original literature references in order to help those readers wishing to delve more deeply into the subject.

As the book has developed, it has become obvious that it would be of wider use to healthcare professionals other than pharmacists. It is our hope that this text will prove to be of benefit to all who deal with herbs which are used for medical treatment.

The views expressed in this book are those of the authors and do not represent those of the Medicines Control Agency or European Medicines Evaluation Agency.

About the Authors

Dr Joanne Barnes
BPharm, PhD, MRPharmS

Jo Barnes is a pharmacist and has been a research fellow in the Centre for Pharmacognosy & Phytotherapy at the School of Pharmacy, University of London since 1999. Her main research interests are the clinical efficacy and safety of herbal products (phytomedicines), the role of the pharmacist in ensuring the safe and effective use of complementary medicines, and the implications of complementary medicine use for pharmaceutical care.

Dr Barnes holds a PhD from the University of London and a postgraduate certificate in pharmacovigilance and pharmacoepidemiology from the London School of Hygiene and Tropical Medicine.

Dr Barnes was previously a research fellow in the Department of Complementary Medicine at the University of Exeter, where she was also Senior Editor of the review journal *Focus on Alternative and Complementary Therapies (FACT)*. She is a member of the editorial board or editorial advisory committee of several journals, including *Complementary Therapies in Medicine*, the *International Journal of Pharmacy Practice*, *Phytotherapy Research*, *FACT* and *Drug Safety*. She is a member of the Royal Pharmaceutical Society's Science Committee's working group on complementary/alternative medicine, and the Independent Review Panel on Borderline Products.

Her career has included employment as a clinical pharmacist at Queen's Medical Centre in Nottingham, a medical information pharmacist at Fisons Pharmaceuticals, and a period as a pharmacist at the Royal London Homoeopathic Hospital. She has also worked in pharmaceutical publishing, as a features editor for Adis International Ltd in Auckland, New Zealand, before returning to the UK to begin an academic career. Dr Barnes is a regular contributor to the *Pharmaceutical Journal*.

Dr Linda A Anderson
BPharm, PhD, FRPharmS

Linda Anderson obtained her first degree in Pharmacy and her PhD in Pharmacognosy at the Welsh School of Pharmacy in Cardiff. She was a postdoctoral research and teaching fellow at the School of Pharmacy, University of London from 1981 to 1987.

Dr Anderson joined the Medicines Control Agency (Department of Health, UK) in 1987.

Within the MCA, she was initially involved in the assessment of new chemical entities and is now mainly involved with abridged applications and has specific responsibility for herbal products. She is Principal Assessor to the Committee on Safety of Medicine's (CSM) Sub-Committee on Chemistry, Pharmacy and Standards (CPS) and is UK delegate to the European Committee on Proprietary Medicinal Products (CPMP) Quality Working Party. Dr Anderson is also UK Delegate to the European Medicines Evaluation Agency (EMEA) Working Group on Herbal Medicinal Products and is Vice-Chair of the British Pharmacopoeia Committee on Crude Drugs and Galenicals. She is a member of the Royal Pharmaceutical Society's Science Committee's working group on complementary/alternative medicine.

Linda Anderson has been awarded a Fellowship of the Royal Pharmaceutical Society of Great Britain (2001).

Professor J David Phillipson
DSc, PhD, MSc, BSc(Pharm), FRPharmS, FLS

David Phillipson graduated BSc in Pharmacy (1956), MSc (1959), and DSc (1979) from the University of Manchester, and PhD (1965) from the University of London. He was Lecturer in Pharmacognosy (1961–1972) at the Department of Pharmacy, Chelsea College, London, and Senior Lecturer (1973–1979), Reader in Phytochemistry (1979–1981), and Professor and Head of the Department of Pharmacognosy (1981–1994) at the School of Pharmacy, University of London. On retirement he became Emeritus Professor of Pharmacognosy. In 1995 he was appointed as Wilson T S Wang Distinguished International Visiting Professor at the Chinese University of Hong Kong from January to June. His research included investigations of the chemistry and biological activities of natural products from higher plants with special interests in indole and isoquinoline alkaloids, and plants used in traditional medicines for the treatment of malaria and other protozoal diseases. Collaboration with the pharmaceutical industry included the application of radioligand–receptor binding assays in the search for natural products with activity in the central nervous system.

David Phillipson has received awards from the Phytochemical Society of Europe including the Tate and Lyle Award (1982), Medal (1994), and the Pergamon Prize for Creativity in Plant Biochemistry (1996). He was awarded the Korber Foundation Prize for Achievement in European Science (1989) in collaboration with Professor M.H. Zenk of the University of Munich and four other European colleagues, was presented with the Harrison Memorial Medal of the Royal Pharmaceutical Society of Great Britain (1999), and with the Sir Hans Sloane Medal of the Faculty of the History and Philosophy of Medicine and Pharmacy, Society of Apothecaries (2001). In 1985 he was Science Chairman of the British Pharmaceutical Conference and has been Secretary (1977–1982), Vice-Chairman (1982–1984, 1986–1988) and Chairman (1984–1986) of the Phytochemical Society of Europe. He has been awarded Fellowships of the Royal Pharmaceutical Society of Great Britain (1980) and of the School of Pharmacy, University of London (1998).

He has supervised 33 PhD students and 11 post-doctoral researchers, publishing some 210 full research papers, 150 short communications, 42 review articles, and has edited six books on natural products. Collaborative research was established with scientists in many countries world-wide and in 1989 he was appointed Honorary Professor of the Chinese Academy of Medical Sciences at the Institute of Medicinal Plant Research and Development, Beijing, China. For 19 years he was a member of the Natural Products Group of the International Foundation for Science, Sweden, helping to award research grants to individual young scientists in developing countries. He has been a member of a number of national and international committees.

How to Use this Book

Purpose and Scope

This handbook is intended to serve as a reference work for pharmacists, doctors and other healthcare professionals, assisting in their provision of advice on the use of herbal medicines to members of the public. The book is not intended to represent a guide to self-diagnosis and self-treatment with herbal medicines, and should not be used as such.

The term 'herbal medicine' (or 'herbal remedy') is used to describe a marketed product, whereas 'herbal ingredient' refers to an individual herb that is present in a herbal medicine. 'Herbal constituent' is used to describe a specific chemical constituent of a herbal ingredient. Thus, as examples, Valerian Tablets are a herbal product, valerian is a herbal ingredient, and valtrate is a herbal constituent of valerian.

The main criterion for inclusion of a herbal ingredient in the text is its presence in herbal medicines that are used in the UK, particularly those which are sold through pharmacies. In addition, herbs which have recently been the subject of media or scientific interest have also been included. The aim of the handbook is to draw the attention of the reader to the reputed actions and uses of herbal ingredients, and to whether or not these have been substantiated by *in vitro* animal or human studies. In addition, any known or potential toxicities of herbal ingredients, and how these may influence the suitability for inclusion in herbal medicines or for use with conventional medicines, are also discussed.

Introduction to the Monographs

The introductory section to the 148 monographs on the individual herbal ingredients contained in this handbook discusses the legal aspects of herbal medicines including licensed medicines and non-licensed products in the UK and within the European Union (EU). All medicines are assessed for their quality, safety and efficacy and, in the context of herbal medicines, there are often specific criteria which are not encountered in the assessment of other medicines. As a first line in ensuring the safety and efficacy of herbal medicines there is a series of guidelines for quality assessment and this is briefly discussed. In terms of safety, it is a popular conception that just because herbs are 'natural' then they must also be safe. This is a misconception, and it is emphasised that some herbal ingredients have the capability to cause adverse effects, whilst some are decidedly toxic. Within the context of the 148 monographs on herbal ingredients, most have documented adverse effects, or the potential to interact with other medication, and few can be recommended for use during pregnancy.

Three tables in the Introduction and 22 appendices after the monographs summarise the safety aspects of these herbal ingredients and give information on biologically active herbal ingredients and their active principles. Clinical efficacy has not been established for the majority of the herbal ingredients described in this handbook and, in some instances, there is a lack of documentation for chemical constituents and for pharmacological actions.

The Herbal Monographs

Some 148 monographs on individual herbal ingredients found in herbal products comprise the bulk of this handbook. They are presented in alphabetical order with respect to their preferred common name. The index includes preferred common names, other synonyms and the Latin binomial names, and should be used to assist in the location of a particular monograph. A data sheet-type format was chosen for the monographs because it was felt important to arrange the relevant information in a format familiar to pharmacists and doctors. Although conventional data sheets are written for products, it was decided to draw up the data sheets for herbal ingredients and not for products.

The headings used in the herbal monographs are listed on the next page with a brief explanation of the information held under them.

Monograph title	Common name for the herbal ingredient; if more than one common name exists, this is the chosen preferred name.
Species (Family)	Preferred botanical name with authority, together with the plant family.
Synonym(s)	Other common or botanical names.
Part(s) Used	Plant part(s) traditionally used in herbal medicine.
Pharmacopoeial and Other Monographs	Key pharmacopoeial monographs and texts on herbal medicines.
Legal Category	Legal category of the herb with respect to licensed products. For the majority of herbal ingredients this will be the General Sales List (GSL).
Constituents	Main documented chemical constituents grouped into categories such as alkaloids (type specified), flavonoids, iridoid glycosides, saponins, tannins, triterpenes, volatile oil and other constituents for miscellaneous and minor chemical components.
Food Use	Provides an indication as to whether the herbal ingredient is used in foods. The Council of Europe (COE) category, which reflects the opinion of the COE on the suitability of the herbal ingredient for use as a food flavouring, is quoted where applicable. Also where applicable, the Food and Drugs Administration (FDA) listing is stated, e.g. Generally Regarded as Safe (GRAS), and Herb of Undefined Safety.
Herbal Use	States the reputed actions and uses of the herbal ingredients, based on information from several sources. In some instances, current investigations of particular interest are included.
Dosage	States the traditional dose of the herbal ingredient, mainly from the British Herbal Pharmacopoeia (BHP) and German Commission E monographs, giving doses for plant part used (herb, rhizome, leaf), liquid extract and infusion. Where possible, dosages used in clinical trials are included.
Pharmacological Actions	Describes any documented pharmacological actions for the herbal ingredient. This is further divided into a section on *In vitro and animal studies* and a *Clinical studies* section, which describes studies involving humans.
Side-effects, Toxicity	Details documented side-effects to the herbal ingredient and toxicological studies. If side-effects or toxicity are generally associated with any of the constituents in the herbal ingredient, or with its plant family, then these are mentioned here. *See also* Table 1 (p. 15) and Table 2 (p. 16) in the Introduction to the Monographs.
Contra-indications, Warnings	Describes potential contra-indications and potential side-effects, and individuals who may be more susceptible to a particular side-effect. This section should be used in conjunction with Appendices 1–23, which are placed after the monographs (p. 496). Comments on Pregnancy and lactation are included; a summary is provided in Table 3 of the Introduction to the Monographs (p. 18).
Pharmaceutical Comment	This section is designed to give the reader an overall summary of the monograph contents, indicating the extent of phytochemical, pharmacological and clinical data available for the herbal ingredient, whether or not proposed herbal uses are justified, concerns over safety and, based on this information, whether or not the herbal ingredient is considered suitable for use as a herbal medicine
References	References are included at the end of the text on each monograph. There is considerable literature on herbal plants and general references have been selected for use with the handbook. These General References, referred to as G1, to G65, are listed after the Introduction (p. 28). For some well-known herbal ingredients only general references are cited. The majority of the monographs also contain specific references which are cited at the end of each monograph.

Introduction to the Monographs

A general disillusionment with conventional medicines, coupled with the desire for a 'natural' lifestyle has resulted in an increasing utilisation of complementary and alternative medicine (CAM) across the developed world.

A study of long-term trends in the use of CAM therapies in the United States of America reported that the use of CAM therapies has increased steadily since the 1950s.[1] Use of CAM has increased independent of gender, ethnicity and level of education, but is more common in younger people. The use of herbal medicine increased particularly in the 1970s and then again in the 1990s. The report concluded that the continuing demand for CAM will affect delivery of healthcare for the foreseeable future. Several other studies have documented the growing use of CAM in the United Kingdom, with the most common complementary therapies reported as acupuncture, homeopathy, herbal medicine and manipulative therapies, chiropractic and osteopathy.[2]

In their report on complementary and alternative medicine, the House of Lords Select Committee on Science and Technology's Subcommittee on Complementary and Alternative Medicine highlighted the lack of comprehensive information on the use of herbal medicines in the UK.[3] Estimates of herbal medicine use are available, but it is difficult to gauge usage accurately as many products are considered to be food supplements. Nevertheless, a national telephone survey of a nationally representative sample of 1204 British adults found that around 7% of those contacted had used herbal medicines in the previous year.[4] In another survey, over 5000 randomly selected adults in England (not the UK) were sent a postal questionnaire on their use of CAM.[5] Around 20% of the respondents had bought an over-the-counter herbal remedy in the previous 12 months.

Estimates of expenditure on herbal medicines vary, but data generally show that the global market for herbal products has grown rapidly in the past decade. In the USA, annual retail sales of herbal medicines were estimated to be US$ 1.6 billion in 1994,[6] and almost US$ 4 billion in 1998.[7] Retail sales of herbal products in the European Union (EU) were estimated to be US$ 7000 million in 1996.[8] A detailed analysis of the European herbal medicines market reported that Germany and France make up more than 70% of the market

share.[9] In 1997, total sales of herbal products (using wholesale prices) were US$1.8 billion in Germany and US$1.1 billion in France. In the UK, retail sales of herbal products are reported to have increased by 43% in the period from 1994 to 1998, with retail sales of licensed herbal medicinal products reported to be £50 million in 1998.[3]

These figures demonstrate that herbal medicinal products are being used increasingly by the general public on a self-selection basis to either replace or complement conventional medicines. Against this background of increasing usage of herbal medicines by the public, several major public health issues have raised concerns about these products. The substitution of toxic *Aristolochia* species in traditional Chinese medicines (TCM) has resulted in cases of serious renal toxicity and renal cancer in Europe, China and America.[10] The emergence of interactions between St. John's wort (*Hypericum perforatum*) and certain prescription medicines has necessitated regulatory action world-wide and has highlighted the need for healthcare professionals to have up-to-date scientific information on the quality, safety and efficacy of these products.[11]

Pharmacists need to be able to advise the consumer on the rational and safe use of all medicines. To fulfil this role with respect to herbal medicines, a pharmacist should be reliably informed of their quality, safety and efficacy. Also, many other healthcare professionals are becoming increasingly aware of their patients' use of herbal medicines and need to be informed of the suitability of these products for use as medicines.

This handbook brings together in one text a series of monographs on 148 herbs commonly present in herbal medicinal products sold through pharmacies in the UK. Various appendices are also presented, grouping together herbs with specific actions, and highlighting potential interactions with conventional medicines.

As a preface to the monographs, an overview of UK and European legislation concerning herbal products is provided, together with issues pertaining to their quality, safety and efficacy. In addition to retail purchase, herbs can be obtained by picking the wild plant or from a herbal practitioner. This handbook does not discuss the self-collection of plant material for use as a herbal remedy or the prescribing of herbal medicines by herbal practitioners.

Herbal Medicines and Phytotherapy

Herbal medicines are also referred to as herbal remedies, herbal products, herbal medicinal products, phytomedicines, phytotherapeutic agents and phytopharmaceuticals. The use of herbal medicines in an evidence- or science-based approach for the treatment and prevention of disease is known as (rational) phytotherapy. This approach to the use of herbal medicines contrasts with traditional medical herbalism in the UK, which uses herbal medicines in a holistic manner and mainly on the basis of their empirical and traditional uses. Plants have been used medicinally for thousands of years by cultures all over the world. According to the World Health Organization, 80% of the world's population uses plant-based remedies as their primary form of healthcare;[12] in some countries, herbal medicines are still a central part of the medical system, such as Ayurvedic medicine in India and traditional Chinese medicine. Herbal medicine has a long history and tradition in Europe.

Although these two approaches – traditional/holistic and rational/evidence-based – are entirely different, in some instances they use the same terminology. For example, traditional herbalism is also described as 'phytotherapy' and refers to preparations of plant material as 'herbal medicines'.

Furthermore, herbal medicines and homeopathic remedies are often mistaken by the layperson to be similar. However, homeopathy is based on the principle of 'like should be treated by like', and involves the administration of minute doses of remedies that, in larger doses, produce symptoms in a healthy person mimicking those expressed by people who are ill. Many, but not all, homeopathic remedies originate from plants. By contrast, herbal medicine (phytotherapy) involves the use of dried plant material or extracts of plant parts in therapeutic doses to treat the symptoms exhibited. In this respect, it is similar to conventional medicine.

Regulatory Controls on Herbal Medicines

Herbal medicinal products in Europe

Herbal products are available in all Member States of the European Union (EU), although the relative size of their markets varies between countries. Since the late 1980s, the regulation of herbal products has been a major issue within the EU because of the differences between Member States in the way herbal products are classified and the difficulties this might present in the completion of the single market for pharmaceuticals.

According to Council Directive 65/65/EEC, a medicinal product is defined as 'any substance or combination of substances presented for treating, or preventing disease in human beings or animals' or 'any substance or combination of substances which may be administered to human beings or animals with a view to making diagnosis or to restoring, correcting or modifying physiological functions in human beings or animals is likewise considered a medicinal product'.[13]

Herbal products are considered as medicinal products if they fall within the definition of the Directive. However, the legal classification is complicated by the fact that in most Member States herbal products are available both as medicinal products with therapeutic claims and also as food/dietary supplements without medicinal claims. The situation is further complicated in that some Member States, including the UK (*see below*), have national provisions which permit certain herbal medicinal products to be exempt from the licensing provisions under specific conditions. In general, in all Member States, herbal products are classified as medicinal products if they claim therapeutic or prophylactic indications.

The advent of the new pan-European marketing authorisation system raised questions with regard to herbal products and, in particular, concerns that major differences in their classification/assessment would hinder free circulation within the EU. The new systems for marketing authorisations involve three procedures: centralised, decentralised (mutual recognition) and national.[14] The centralised procedure is mandatory for biotechnology products, and optional for high-technology products and medicinal products containing new active substances. The decentralised procedure or mutual recognition system involves agreement of assessment between the member states involved; this procedure became compulsory from 1 January 1998, for products requesting authorisation in more than one member state. Since then, simultaneous national applications have been possible, but the mutual recognition system automatically becomes involved once an authorisation has been granted in the first Member State. The original intention was to retain existing national procedures for medicinal products requesting authorisation in a single Member State only. However, in view of the difficulties posed by lack of harmonisation, the European Commission has agreed that national procedures can continue for the time being for bibliographic applications, including those for herbal products.

In 1997, upon the initiative of the European Parliament, the European Commission and the European Medicines Evaluation Agency (EMEA), an *ad hoc*

Working Group on Herbal Medicinal Products (HMPWG) was established at the EMEA. The main thrust of the HMPWG has been the protection of public health by preparing guidance to help facilitate mutual recognition of marketing authorisations in the field of herbal medicines, and to minimise CPMP (Committee on Proprietary Medicinal Products) arbitrations.

A major study undertaken by the AESGP (Association of the European Self-medication Industry) in 1998 at the request of the European Commission confirmed the different approaches taken by Member States in the regulation of herbal medicinal products.[15] Different traditions in the therapeutic use of herbal preparations, coupled with different national approaches to their assessment, have resulted in differences in the availability of some herbal medicines. For example, ginkgo (*Ginkgo biloba*) is available as a prescription-only medicine in some EU countries, but as a food supplement in others. Similarly, St. John's wort (*Hypericum perforatum*) is accepted as a treatment for depression in some Member States, but not in others.

The AESGP study revealed that, in general, herbal medicinal products were either fully licensed with efficacy proven by clinical trials or by bibliography (in accordance with Article 4.8a (ii) of Council Directive 65/65/EEC), or that herbal products had a more or less simplified proof of efficacy, according to their national use. Furthermore, the study found major discrepancies between Member States in the classification of individual herbal preparations and products into one of these categories, as well as in the requirements for obtaining a marketing authorisation (product licence). The report highlighted the need for clarification of the regulatory framework and harmonisation of the regulatory requirements to ensure that herbal products could have access to the single market for pharmaceuticals.

An important initiative in the harmonisation process has been the formation of the European Scientific Cooperative on Phytotherapy (ESCOP), an organisation representing national associations for phytotherapy. ESCOP was founded in 1989 by six EU national scientific associations with the objective of establishing a scientific umbrella organisation to provide harmonised criteria for the assessment of herbal medicinal products, to support scientific research and contribute to the acceptance of phytotherapy in Europe.[16]

ESCOP now comprises 13 national associations across Europe, and the American Botanical Council. The ESCOP Scientific Committee has published 60 monographs for individual herbal drugs; the monographs follow the European Summary of Product Characteristics (SPC) format.[17] To date, four ESCOP monographs (frangula bark, senna fruit: angustifoliae and acutifoliae, senna leaf) have been adopted by the CPMP as the basis of core SPCs for herbal medicinal products.[18] The EMEA Herbal Medicinal Products Working Party (HMPWP, formerly the *ad hoc* HMPW Group) is continuing the work with developing core SPCs from ESCOP monographs. Draft documents are available for valerian and ispaghula.[19]

Future regulation of herbal medicinal products in the EU

From the late 1980s, the need for a new regulatory framework for herbal products has been under discussion. In 1987, the European Parliament acknowledged in a resolution

'that there does exist a large number of well-known medicinal plants, traditionally used by the population and fully described in scientific literature whose very slight pharmacological effect allows their authorisation on the basis of a list to ensure correct identification of the species, variety, conservation, labelling and specified dosage and application; this group would not require the same kind of monitoring as proprietary medicinal products.'[20]

Furthermore, the European Parliament called on the European Commission

'to help to ensure that, profiting by the results of research work to date, a scientific approach to phytopharmaceuticals is developed, which will not only incorporate centuries of practical experience but will also respect the indispensable requirement of scientific precision.'

In September 1999, the European Pharmaceutical Committee set up a working group of Member States to investigate the possibility of a directive for traditionally used medicines. Work on the new directive commenced in April 2000. At the time of going to press, a formal draft of a Directive on Traditional Medicinal Products was under discussion in Member States. The draft directive provides a framework for the regulation of traditionally used herbal medicinal products.[21] The proposed definition of traditional use is 30 years continuous use within the EU (with possible flexibility to allow up to 15 years non-EU use provided the product was available in the Community for at least 15 years).

It is proposed that a licence application will include a bibliographic review of the safety data associated with the use of the herbal product in a particular indication. In addition, this review will need to be accompanied by an expert report on the safety data submitted. The criteria of quality, safety and efficacy may be addressed as follows.

Quality All the usual requirements apply, including good manufacturing practice (GMP) and European Pharmacopoeia standards.

Safety The use of bibliographic data and the possibility of a negative list for toxic products on a national or EU basis. The directive will not cover prescription only herbal medicinal products, i.e. those considered to require medical supervision.

Efficacy Evidence will not be required, but a 'traditionally used for...' statement and 'the effectiveness of this product has not been proven' (or similar wording) will be required in the product labelling.

In the future, it is possible that the directive will extend to traditional medicines which include non-herbal active ingredients.

Current regulatory position of herbal products in the UK

Herbal products are available in the UK through various retail outlets, such as pharmacies, health-food shops, mail order companies, supermarkets and department stores. Some herbal products consist solely of loose, dried plant material; others are presented as pre-packaged formulated products in a variety of pharmaceutical forms for both internal (tablets, capsules, liquids) and external use (creams, ointments) and may contain one or several herbal ingredients which may be dried herbs or their extracts. The current regulatory position is complicated by the fact that herbal products can fall into one of three categories: licensed herbal products, those exempt from licensing and those marketed as food supplements.

The majority of herbal products are marketed without medicinal claims either exempt from licensing (*see below*) or as food supplements. Those supplied as food supplements are controlled under food legislation whilst those exempt from licensing are controlled under medicines legislation. Difficulties in defining the status of products occupying the borderline between medicines and foods have resulted in similar products being marketed in both these categories. Provided the products were marketed without reference to medicinal claims, the Medicines Control Agency (MCA), the government body responsible for regulating medicinal products has, in the past, generally been satisfied that the products were not subject to medicines legislation.[22] However, implementation of the definition of a medicinal product in accordance with EC Directives has meant that greater emphasis is now being placed on the nature of the herbal ingredients being supplied as food supplements.

Licensed herbal medicinal products

Almost all of the licensed herbal medicines on the UK market have been available for some time and most originally held Product Licences of Right (PLR) (*see* Review of Herbal Medicines in the UK). The MCA regulates medicinal products for human use in accordance with the Medicines for Human Use (Marketing Authorisations Etc.) Regulations 1994 SI 3144 (The Regulations)[23] and the Medicines Act 1968.[24] The Regulations which took effect from January 1995 arose out of the need to implement EC legislation establishing the new EC marketing authorisation procedures (Future Systems). The Regulations effectively implement the full range of controls set out in Directive 65/65/ EEC which apply to 'relevant medicinal products' (as defined in the Regulations). The main controls include application requirements and procedures for the grant, variation and renewal of UK licences, requirements in relation to pharmacovigilance, labelling and package leaflets as well as provisions for suspension, compulsory variation or revocation and related enforcement measures.

The Medicines Act and secondary legislation made under it remain the legal basis for other aspects of medicines control including manufacturer and wholesale dealers' authorisations, controls on sale and supply and controls on promotion. Further explanation may be obtained by reference to a chapter on herbal remedies in Dale and Appelbe's *Pharmacy Law and Ethics*.[25]

Therefore, prior to marketing, all new licensed herbal products are assessed by the MCA for quality, safety and efficacy in accordance with EC and UK legislation. Specific EC guidelines exist on the quality, specifications and manufacture of herbal medicinal products.[26–28]

Herbal remedies exempt from licensing

Under the Medicines Act, herbal remedies manufactured and sold or supplied in accordance with specific exemptions set out in Sections 12(1) or (2) or Article 2 of the Medicines (Exemptions from Licences) (Special and Transitional Cases) Order 1971 (SI 1450)[29] are exempt from the requirement to hold product licences. The exempt products are those compounded and supplied by herbalists on their own recommendation, those comprised solely of dried, crushed or comminuted plants sold under their botanical name with no written recommendations as to their use, and those made by a holder of a Specials Manufacturing Licence on behalf of a herbalist.

The exemptions are intended, for example, to give herbal practitioners the flexibility they need to prepare their own remedies for individual patients without the burden of licensing, and to enable simple dried herbs to be readily available to the public. During consideration of the UK legislation to implement the EC Future Systems legislation, the question arose as to whether or not herbal medicines exempted under the Medicines Act were eligible for exemption under Directive 65/65/EEC as amended. The Directive requires herbal medicinal products to possess marketing authorisations if they are 'industrially produced' but this term is not defined in UK or EC law. The UK Government has, however, adopted the view that herbal medicines currently exempted under the Medicines Act are manufactured or supplied on a small scale or by traditional processes which take them outside the meaning of 'industrially produced'. As a result these products fall outside the scope of the new Regulations and retain their exempt status.[30]

More recently, it has been suggested that this situation is not ideal and that special licensing requirements should be made in order to control all herbal medicine-like products.[31] This view has been endorsed by two UK medical practitioners following hepatic failure and subsequent death of a 32-year-old man attributed to a herbal ingredient in a Chinese herbal remedy.[32] The MCA is also now of the view that the present regulatory arrangements for unlicensed herbal medicines have significant weaknesses.[3] The regime for unlicensed herbal products is considered not to provide sufficient protection or information for the public and there are no specific safeguards in place to ensure adequate product quality and safety.[33]

Control of herbal ingredients in the UK

Most of the herbal ingredients used in licensed herbal medicines have been used as traditional remedies for centuries without major safety problems, and the majority is included in the General Sales List (GSL).[34] Potentially hazardous plants such as digitalis, rauwolfia and nux vomica are specifically controlled under the Medicines Act as prescription-only medicines (POM),[35] and thus are not available other than via a registered medical practitioner. In addition, certain herbal ingredients are controlled under The Medicines (Retail Sale and Supply of Herbal Remedies) Order 1977 SI 2130.[36] This Order (Part I) specifies 25 plants which cannot be supplied except via a pharmacy, and includes well-known toxic species, such as *Areca*, *Crotalaria*, *Dryopteris* and *Strophanthus*. In Part II, the Order specifies plant species, such as *Aconitum*, *Atropa*, *Ephedra* and *Hyoscyamus*, which can be supplied by 'herbal practitioners', and in

Part III defines the dosages and routes of administration permitted.

Legislation has now been introduced to prohibit the use of *Aristolochia* species or species likely to be confused with *Aristolochia* in unlicensed medicines.[37] These measures were introduced in the wake of cases of serious toxicity and evidence showing widespread substitution of certain ingredients in traditional Chinese medicines with *Aristolochia* (*see below*). The MCA has also announced the need to update the list of herbal ingredients subject to restrictions or prohibitions in use in unlicensed medicines to take account of the herbal ingredients used in traditional Chinese and Ayurvedic medicines.[38]

Review of herbal medicines in the UK

The majority of licensed herbal remedies available in the UK have been marketed for a long time, in fact, for many from before the Medicines Act or any medicines licensing system. In September 1971, a registration exercise issued all medicinal products already on the market with a Product Licence of Right (PLR); no scientific assessment was undertaken. In order to be issued with PLRs for their products, pharmaceutical companies had simply to provide details of the products and evidence that the products had been marketed prior to 1971. This procedure applied to all medicinal products, including herbal medicines, and in total 39 000 PLRs were granted. It was obvious that at some future date all PLR products (including herbal medicines) would have to be assessed by the Licensing Authority for their quality, safety, and efficacy in the same manner as those products which had applied for a product licence after 1971. European Community (EC) legislation required that this review of all PLR products be completed by May 1990.

During the UK review of herbal medicinal products holding a PLR, the Licensing Authority agreed to accept bibliographic evidence of efficacy for herbal medicinal products which were indicated for minor, self-limiting conditions.[39] No evidence was required from new clinical trials provided the manufacturers agreed to label their products as 'a traditional herbal remedy for the symptomatic relief of. . .' and to include the statement 'if symptoms persist consult your doctor'. The Licensing Authority considered it inappropriate to relax the requirements for proof of efficacy for herbal medicinal products indicated for more serious conditions. Thus, evidence was required from controlled clinical trials for herbal medicinal products indicated for conditions considered inappropriate for self-diagnosis and treatment.

In its assessment of the safety of herbal medicinal products, the Licensing Authority agreed to rely as far as possible on the work of other agencies. Thus, supporting evidence of safety included, for example, acceptance of a herbal ingredient for food use, or inclusion of a herbal ingredient on Schedule 1 of the General Sales List (GSL).[34]

Regulatory control of herbal medicines world-wide

The World Health Organization (WHO) has reviewed the regulatory control of herbal medicines in 50 countries and summarised the wide differences in the approach to regulation between these countries.[40] Herbal products are well established as phytomedicines in some countries, whereas in others they are regarded as foods, and therapeutic claims are not allowed. In the context of this book, it should be noted that many of the herbs included in the monographs are of economic importance in some non-European countries, particularly Australia, Canada and the USA.

In Australia, therapeutic goods for human use which are imported or manufactured are subject to the Therapeutic Goods Act, 1989. For the purpose of labelling requirements, herbs are included in the List of Australian Approved Names for Pharmaceutical Substances, which is published by the Therapeutic Goods Administration.[40]

Herbal medicines are regulated as drugs in Canada and must conform to labelling and other requirements as set out in the Food and Drugs Act and Regulations.[40] Herbal remedies used for minor self-limiting conditions are allocated a Drug Identification Number (DIN) based on pharmacological rationale. In order to facilitate registration of products containing herbs, a series of Standardised Drug Monographs (SDM) has been prepared. The Drugs Directorate has provided guidelines for the manufacture and sale of botanical products which fall into three categories: food supplements (no DIN required, no therapeutic claims); phytopharmaceuticals with full drug status (approved therapeutic indications, approved dosage, efficacy supported by scientific evidence, DIN required); traditional herbal medicines (self-medication only, efficacy supported from the herbal literature, approved therapeutic indications and dosage).[41] In November 2001, the Natural Health Products Directorate published a series of further developments on the working draft of the proposed regulatory framework for Natural Health Products.[42] Product licences, compliance with good manufacturing practice (GMP), and a definition of natural products are currently being subject to a review procedure.

The majority of medicinal herbs and their products are regulated in the USA as foods or food additives, and most of the regulatory action has been concerned with safety.[40] In 1990, the Food and Drugs Administration (FDA) reported on over-the-counter drugs, including herbs.[43] Some herbs (e.g. cascara, senna) were pronounced safe and effective, but the majority were not. Overall, 250 herbs, primarily based on their use as food additives, i.e. flavours and fragrances, were designated GRAS (Generally Regarded As Safe) status; however, this does not mean that such herbs (e.g. ginger, liquorice) are FDA-approved for therapeutic purposes. In 1994, the Dietary Supplement Health and Education Act (DSHEA) became law. In theory, this Act allows publications, book chapters and scientific reports to support the sale of dietary supplements.[43] Although medicinal claims cannot be made for such products, labelling may describe effects on general well-being. DSHEA and its regulations seek to define herbs in the context of the modern market place, but they can only be regarded as an interim legislative step.[43]

It is apparent that not only is the regulation of medicinal herbs different from one country to another, but also that the regulatory processes are not necessarily ideal and are under current review.

Quality, Safety and Efficacy of Herbal Medicines

In order to ensure public health, medicinal products must be safe, efficacious and of suitable quality for use. To obtain a marketing authorisation (product licence) within the EU, manufacturers of herbal medicinal products are required to demonstrate that their products meet acceptable standards of quality, safety and efficacy.

Quality

Over the past decade the quality of herbal products has continued to be a major concern. The importance of quality in ensuring the safety and efficacy of herbal products has been reviewed extensively.[44–48]

Problems with unregulated herbal products The vast majority of quality-related problems are associated with unregulated herbal products. There is substantial evidence that many ethnic medicines, in particular, those used in traditional Chinese medicine (TCM) and traditional Asian medicines (Ayurvedic and Unani), lack effective quality controls and may give rise to serious public health concerns. The problems include deliberate or accidental inclusion of prohibited or restricted ingredients, substitution of ingredients, contamination with toxic substances and differences between the labelled and actual contents. These problems are further compounded by demand outstripping supply of good-quality ingredients, confusing nomenclature over plant species, cultural differences of view over toxicity and traditional practices such as substituting one ingredient for another having a reportedly similar action.

The MCA has established an ethnic medicines forum to encourage and assist the UK ethnic medicines sector to achieve improvements to safety and quality standards in relation to unlicensed ethnic medicines in advance of any improvements to the regulatory regime which might emerge from current policy initiatives within the EU on the traditional use directive.[49] Although individual herbs present in traditional Chinese medicines and traditional Asian medicines are not the subject of monographs in this book, they do illustrate the problems that may be associated with the quality and safety of herbal medicines.

Substitution and adulteration *Aristolochia* Inadvertent exposure to *Aristolochia* species in unlicensed herbal medicines has resulted in cases of nephrotoxicity and carcinogenicity in Europe, China, Japan and the USA. Concerns were first raised about the effects of products containing aristolochic acids in Belgium where, since 1993, over 100 cases of irreversible nephropathy have been reported in young women using a preparation claimed to aid weight loss. The nephrotoxicity was traced to the inadvertent use of the toxic *Aristolochia fangchi* root in the formulation as a substitute for *Stephania tetrandra*. Aristolochic acids, the toxic components of *Aristolochia* species, are known to be nephrotoxic, carcinogenic and mutagenic. A number of the Belgian patients have subsequently developed urothelial cancer as a result of exposure to the toxic aristolochic acids.[50–53]

Seven cases of nephropathy involving substitution of *Aristolochia fangchi* and *Stephania tetrandra* have been reported in France.[10] Toxicity has also resulted from the substitution of *Aristolochia manshuriensis* stem for the stem of *Clematis* and *Akebia* species.[10] In the UK, two such cases of end-stage renal failure were reported in 1999.[54] Other cases have been reported in China (17 cases with 12 fatalities) and Japan (ten cases of renal failure).[10] Also, the FDA has reported two cases of serious renal disease due to *Aristolochia* being substituted for *Clematis* species in a dietary supplement.[55]

Substitution of one plant species for another, often of a completely different genus, is an established practice in TCM. Furthermore, herbal ingredients are traded using their common Chinese Pin Yin names, and this can lead to confusion. For example, the name Fang ji can be used to describe the roots of *Aristolochia fangchi*, *Stephania tetrandra* or *Cocculus* species, and the name Mu Tong can be used to describe the stem of *Aristolochia manshuriensis*, *Clematis* or *Akebia* species.

The widespread substitution with *Aristolochia* species in TCM products available in the UK has been confirmed in a recent MCA study which reported the presence of aristolochic acids in at least 40% of TCM products containing Fang ji and Mu Tong.[56]

The problems associated with *Aristolochia* have prompted regulatory action world-wide and new legislation has been introduced in the UK to prohibit the use of *Aristolochia* species in unlicensed medicines in the UK (*see above*).

Digitalis Cases of serious cardiac arrhythmias were reported in the USA in 1997 following the accidental substitution of plantain with *Digitalis lanata*.[57] Subsequent investigation revealed that large quantities of the contaminated plantain had been shipped to more than 150 manufacturers, distributors and retailers over a two-year period.

Podophyllum Fourteen cases of podophyllum poisoning have been reported from Hong Kong following the inadvertent use of the roots *Podophyllum hexandrum* instead of *Gentiana* and *Clematis* species.[58] It is reported that this accidental substitution arose because of the apparent similarity in morphology of the roots.

Aconitum Cases of cardiotoxicity resulting from the ingestion of *Aconitum* species used in TCM have been reported from Hong Kong.[59] In TCM, *Aconitum* rootstocks are processed by soaking or boiling them in water in order to hydrolyse the aconite alkaloids into their less toxic aconine derivatives. Toxicity can, however, result when such processes are uncontrolled and unvalidated. In the UK, the internal use of aconite is restricted to prescription only.

Adulteration with heavy metals/toxic elements and synthetic drugs The adulteration of ethnic medicines with heavy metals/toxic elements and synthetic drugs continues to be a major international problem. A comprehensive review has summarised test results on products and case histories of patients who had experienced toxic effects.[44] Similar findings continue to be reported. In most cases involving synthetic drugs, the drugs are undeclared in the product and only come to light when the user experiences adverse effects which are sufficiently serious to warrant medical intervention. Exposure to the undeclared drug is revealed in the subsequent investigation of the clinical case.

The situation with the heavy metals/toxic elements differs in that whilst these ingredients may arise from the plant ingredients themselves or be introduced as trace contaminants during processing, they are also frequently added intentionally and declared as ingredients within some TCM and Asian medicine formulations. The Chinese Pharmacopoeia, for example, includes monographs for realgar (arsenic disulfide), calomel (mercurous chloride), cinnabaris (mercuric sulfide) and hydrargyri oxydum rubrum (red mercuric oxide), and includes formulations for nearly 50 products that include one or more of these substances.[60]

A US survey reported widespread inconsistencies and adulterations in imported Asian medicines.[61] Of 260 imported products tested, at least 83 (32%) contained undeclared pharmaceuticals (most commonly ephedrine, chlorpheniramine, methyltestosterone and phenacetin) or heavy metals (lead, arsenic or mercury). Another survey found evidence of a continuing problem, with 10% of 500 OTC products testing positive for undeclared drugs and/or toxic amounts of lead, mercury or arsenic.[62]

Elsewhere, health departments have reported similar conclusions based on their findings. A survey conducted in Singapore between 1990 and 1997 on TCM products reported that 42 different products were found to contain excessive amounts of heavy metals (mercury, lead, arsenic) and that 32 different TCM products were found to contain a total of 19 drugs.[63] In total, 93 cases of excessive content of toxic heavy metals and undeclared drugs were detected. The drugs detected included berberine, antihistamines (chlorpheniramine, promethazine, cyproheptadine), non-steroidal anti-inflammatory drugs (diclofenac, indomethacin, ibuprofen), analgesic antipyretics (paracetamol, dipyrone), corticosteroids (prednisolone, dexamethasone, fluocinonide), sympathomimetics agents (ephedrine), bronchodilators (theophylline), diuretics (hydrochlorthiazide) and the antidiabetic phenformin. A study in Taiwan found that more than 20% of 2609 products were found to be adulterated with synthetic drugs, most commonly caffeine, paracetamol, indomethacin and hydrochlorthiazide.[64]

Other examples of adultered products come from a report from the Singapore Ministry of Health which identified sildenafil in two Chinese proprietary medicines,[65] and a report from the USA FDA which described the recall of a herbal product after traces of chlordiazepoxide were found in the capsules.[66] In 2001, the UK MCA reported presence of mercury (due to the inclusion of cinnabaris) in samples of the product Shugan Wan on the UK market.[49]

Cases of toxicity associated with synthetic drugs present in ethnic medicines include a case of poisoning in Hong Kong resulting from the use of a TCM product containing anticonvulsant agents (phenytoin, carbamazepine and valproate).[67] In 2000, the USA FDA issued a public health warning on five herbal products following adverse effects in patients.[68] The products were found to contain the antihyperglycaemic prescription drugs glibenclamide and phenformin. In March 2001, the UK MCA reported a serious case of hypoglycaemic coma in a patient who had taken a TCM product, Xiaoke Wan, which contained glibenclamide.[69]

Cases of toxicity associated with heavy metals in ethnic medicines include a patient from Taiwan who developed a unique syndrome of multiple renal tubular dysfunction after taking a Chinese herbal medicine contaminated with cadmium.[70] In the USA, two cases of alopecia and sensory polyneuropathy resulting from thallium in a TCM product have been reported.[71] In the UK, cases have been reported of two patients with heavy metal intoxication following ingestion of an Indian remedy containing inorganic arsenic and mercury,[72] and of a patient with lead poisoning after exposure to an Indian medicine containing toxic amounts of lead, arsenic and mercury.[73] In a case reported from Macau, death of a 13-year-old girl from arsenic poisoning has been linked with a Chinese herbal product Niu Huang Chieh Tu Pien.[74]

Quality of regulated herbal products   Compared with conventional preparations, herbal medicinal products present a number of unique problems when quality aspects are considered. These arise because of the nature of the herbal ingredients, which are complex mixtures of constituents, and it is well documented that concentrations of plant constituents can vary considerably depending on environmental and genetic factors. Furthermore, the constituents responsible for the claimed therapeutic effects are frequently unknown or only partly explained and this precludes the level of control which can routinely be achieved with synthetic drug substances in conventional pharmaceuticals. The position is further complicated by the traditional practice of using combinations of herbal ingredients, and it is not uncommon to have as many as five herbal ingredients in one product.

In recognition of the special problems associated with herbal medicinal products, the CPMP has issued specific guidelines dealing with quality aspects and manufacture.[26,28] These guidelines have recently been updated by the CPMP Quality Working Party (QWP) and the EMEA HMPWP. In addition, a new guideline has been developed on specifications 'Note for guidance on specifications: test procedures and acceptance criteria for herbal drugs, herbal drug preparations and herbal medicinal products (CPMP/

QWP/2820/00)'.[27] The EMEA HMPWP has also developed the guidance document 'Points to consider on Good Agricultural and Collection Practice for starting materials of herbal origin'.[75]

The CPMP Guidelines highlight the need for good control of both the starting materials and the finished product, and emphasise the importance of good manufacturing practice in the manufacture of herbal medicinal products.

The WHO has also published guidelines dealing with the quality control of medicinal plant materials.[76]

European Pharmacopoeia Since its creation in 1964, the European Pharmacopoeia (Ph Eur) has devoted part of its work to the establishment of monographs on herbal drugs which are used either in their natural state after drying or extraction, or for the isolation of natural active ingredients. The Ph Eur includes over 120 monographs on herbal drugs, and a similar number of monographs are under development. Many general methods of analysis are also described in the Ph Eur, including tests for pesticides and for microbial contamination.[77]

Herbal ingredients Control of the starting materials is essential in order to ensure reproducible quality of herbal medicinal products.[78–81] The following points are to be considered in the control of starting materials.

Authentication and reproducibility of herbal ingredients The problems associated with unregulated herbal products, as illustrated above, highlight the major public health issues that can arise when their herbal ingredients have not been authenticated correctly. Herbal ingredients must be accurately identified by macroscopical and microscopical comparison with authentic material or accurate descriptions of authentic herbs.[79] It is essential that herbal ingredients are referred to by their binomial Latin names of genus and species; only permitted synonyms should be used. Even when correctly authenticated, it is important to realise that different batches of the same herbal ingredient may differ in quality due to a number of factors.

Inter- or intraspecies variation For many plants, there is considerable inter- and intraspecies variation in constituents, which is genetically controlled and may be related to the country of origin.

Environmental factors The quality of a herbal ingredient can be affected by environmental factors, such as climate, altitude and growing conditions.

Time of harvesting For some herbs the optimum time of harvesting should be specified as it is known that the concentrations of constituents in a plant can vary during the growing cycle or even during the course of a day.

Plant part used Active constituents usually vary between plant parts and it is not uncommon for a herbal ingredient to be adulterated with parts of the plant not normally utilised. In addition, plant material that has been previously subjected to extraction and is therefore 'exhausted' is sometimes used to increase the weight of a batch of herbal ingredient.

Post-harvesting factors Storage conditions and processing treatments can greatly affect the quality of a herbal ingredient. Inappropriate storage after harvesting can result in microbial contamination, and processes such as drying may result in a loss of thermolabile active constituents.

Adulteration/substitution Instances of herbal remedies adulterated with other plant material and conventional medicines, and the consequences of this, have been discussed above. In particular, the serious public health consequences that may arise from the substitution of herbal ingredients by toxic *Aristolochia* species have been highlighted. Reports of herbal products devoid of known active constituents have reinforced the need for adequate quality control of herbal remedies.

Identity tests In order to try to ensure the quality of licensed herbal medicines, it is essential therefore not only to establish the botanical identity of a herbal ingredient but also to ensure batch-to-batch reproducibility. Thus, in addition to macroscopical and microscopical evaluation, identity tests are necessary. Such tests include simple chemical tests, e.g. colour or precipitation and chromatographic tests. Thin-layer chromatography is commonly used for identification purposes but for herbal ingredients containing volatile oils a gas–liquid chromatographic test may be used. Although the aim of such tests is to confirm the presence of active principle(s), it is frequently the case that the nature of the active principle has not been established. In such instances chemical and chromatographic tests help to provide batch-to-batch comparability and the chromatogram may be used as a 'fingerprint' for the herbal ingredient by demonstrating the profile of some common plant constituents such as flavonoids.

Assay For those herbal ingredients with known active principles, an assay should be established in order to set the criterion for the minimum accepted percentage of active substance(s). Such assays should, wherever possible, be specific for individual chemical substances and high-pressure liquid chromatography or gas–liquid chromatography are the methods of choice. Where such assays have not been established then non-specific methods such as titration or colorimetric assays may be used to determine the total content of a group of closely related compounds.

Contaminants of herbal ingredients Herbal ingredients should be of high quality and free from insect, other animal matter and excreta. It is not possible to remove completely all contaminants and hence specifications should be set in order to limit them:

Ash values Incineration of a herbal ingredient produces ash which constitutes inorganic matter. Treatment of the ash with hydrochloric acid results in acid-insoluble ash which consists mainly of silica and may be used to act as a measure of soil present. Limits may be set for ash and acid-insoluble ash of herbal ingredients.

Foreign organic matter It is not possible to collect a herbal ingredient without small amounts of related parts of plant or other plants. Standards should be set in order to limit the percentage of such unwanted plant contaminants.

Microbial contamination Aerobic bacteria and fungi are normally present in plant material and may increase due to faulty growing, harvesting, storage or processing. Herbal ingredients, particularly those with high starch content, may be prone to increased microbial growth. It is not uncommon for herbal ingredients to have aerobic bacteria present at 10^2–10^8 colony forming units per gram. Pathogenic organisms including *Enterobacter*, *Enterococcus*, *Clostridium*, *Pseudomonas*, *Shigella* and *Streptococcus* have been shown to contaminate herbal ingredients. It is essential that limits be set for microbial contamination and the Ph Eur now gives non-mandatory guidance on acceptable limits.[77]

Pesticides Herbal ingredients, particularly those grown as cultivated crops, may be contaminated by DDT (dichlorodiphenyltrichloroethane) or other chlorinated hydrocarbons, organophosphates, carbamates or polychlorinated biphenyls. Limit tests are necessary for acceptable levels of pesticide contamination of herbal ingredients. The Ph Eur includes details of test methods together with mandatory limits for 34 potential pesticide residues.[77]

Fumigants Ethylene oxide, methyl bromide and phosphine have been used to control pests which contaminate herbal ingredients. The use of ethylene oxide as a fumigant with herbal drugs is no longer permitted in Europe.

Toxic metals Lead, cadmium, mercury, thallium and arsenic have been shown to be contaminants of some herbal ingredients. Limit tests for such toxic metals are essential for herbal ingredients.

Other contaminants As standards increase for the quality of herbal ingredients it is possible that tests to limit other contaminants such as endotoxins, mycotoxins and radionuclides will be utilised to ensure high quality for medicinal purposes.

Herbal products Quality assurance of herbal products may be ensured by control of the herbal ingredients and by adherence to good manufacturing practice standards. Some herbal products have many herbal ingredients with only small amounts of individual herbs being present. Chemical and chromatographic tests are useful for developing finished product specifications. Stability and shelf life of herbal products should be established by manufacturers. There should be no differences in standards set for the quality of dosage forms, such as tablets or capsules, of herbal medicines from those of other pharmaceutical preparations.

The quality of an unlicensed herbal remedy will not have been assessed by a Regulatory Authority and may thus potentially affect the safety and efficacy of the product. In view of this, it may be concluded that a pharmacist should only sell or recommend herbal medicinal products that hold a product licence. However, the majority of herbal medicinal products are only available as unlicensed products. When deciding upon the suitability of such products, a pharmacist should consider the intended use and the manufacturer. It is highly likely that unlicensed herbal remedies manufactured by an established pharmaceutical company will have been subjected to suitable in-house quality control procedures.

Safety

As with all forms of self-treatment, the use of herbal medicinal products presents a potential risk to human health.[80] There are concerns that the patient may be exposed to potentially toxic substances either from the herbal ingredients themselves or as a result of exposure to contaminants present in the herbal product. Furthermore, self-administration of any therapy in preference to orthodox treatment may delay a patient seeking qualified advice, or cause a patient to abandon conventional treatment without first seeking appropriate advice. Emerging evidence suggests that herbal medicinal products may in some cases compromise the efficacy of conventional medicines, for example through herb–drug interactions.

The safety of all medicinal products is of the utmost importance. All applications for marketing authorisations for new medicines undergo extensive evaluation of their risks and benefits and, once granted, licensed products are closely monitored for the occurrence of suspected adverse effects. The safety of herbal medicinal products is of particular importance as the majority of these products is self-prescribed and is used to treat minor and often chronic conditions.

The extensive traditional use of plants as medicines has enabled those medicines with acute and obvious signs of toxicity to be well recognised and their use avoided. However, the premise that traditional use of a plant for perhaps many hundreds of years establishes its safety does not necessarily hold true.[80,81] The more subtle and chronic forms of toxicity, such as carcinogenicity, mutagenicity and hepatotoxicity, may well have been overlooked by previous generations and it is these types of toxicities that are of most concern when assessing the safety of herbal remedies.

A UK Medical Toxicology Unit conducted a study of potentially serious adverse reactions associated with exposure to traditional medicines and food supplements during 1991 to 1995.[82] Of 1297 enquiries from healthcare professionals, a total of 785 cases were identified as possible ($n = 738$), probable ($n = 35$) or confirmed ($n = 12$) cases of poisoning caused by traditional medicines or food supplements. The report concluded that the overall risk to public health from these types of products was low. However, clusters of cases were identified that gave cause for concern. Twenty-one cases of liver toxicity, including two deaths were associated with the use of traditional Chinese medicines, although no causative agent was identified.

Intrinsically toxic constituents of herbal ingredients Limited toxicological data are available on medicinal plants. However, there exists a considerable overlap between those herbs used for medicinal purposes and those used for cosmetic or culinary purposes, for which a significant body of information exists. For many culinary herbs used in herbal remedies, there is no reason to doubt their safety providing the intended dose and route of administration is in line with their food use. When intended for use in larger therapeutic doses the safety of culinary herbs requires re-evaluation.

Culinary herbs Some culinary herbs contain potentially toxic constituents. The safe use of these herbs is ensured by limiting the amount of constituent permitted in a food product to a concentration not considered to represent a health hazard.

Apiole The irritant principle present in the volatile oil of parsley is held to be responsible for the abortifacient action.[83] Apiole is also hepatotoxic and liver damage has been documented as a result of excessive ingestion of parsley, far exceeding normal dietary consumption, over a prolonged period.[83] *See* Parsley.

β-Asarone Calamus rhizome oil contains β-asarone as the major component, which has been shown to be carcinogenic in animal studies.[83] Many other culinary herbs contain low levels of β-asarone in their volatile oils and therefore the level of β-asarone permitted in foods as a flavouring is restricted.

Estragole (Methylchavicol) Estragole is a constituent of many culinary herbs but is a major component of the oils of tarragon, fennel, sweet basil and chervil. Estragole has been reported to be carcinogenic in animals.[83] The level of estragole permitted in food products as a flavouring is restricted.

Safrole Animal studies involving safrole, the major component of sassafras oil, have shown it to be hepatotoxic and carcinogenic.[83] The permitted level of safrole as a flavouring in foods is 0.1 mg/kg.

Other intrinsically toxic constituents Aristolochic acids are reported to occur only in the Aristolochiaceae family. They have been reported in *Aristolochia* species, and appear to occur throughout the plant in the roots, stem, herb and fruit. The aristolochic acids are a series of substituted nitrophenanthrene carboxylic acids. The main constituents are 3,4-methylenedioxy-8-methoxy-10-nitrophenanthrene-1-carboxylic acid. Low concentrations of aristolochic acids have been reported in *Asarum* species, another member of the Aristolochiaceae family. Aristolochic acids have been shown to be nephrotoxic, carcinogenic and mutagenic.[84]

Pyrrolizidine alkaloids are present in a number of plant species, notably *Crotalaria*, *Heliotropium* and *Senecio*. Many of these plants have been used in African, Caribbean and South American countries as food sources and as medicinal 'bush teas'. Hepatotoxicity associated with their consumption is well documented and has been attributed to the pyrrolizidine alkaloid constituents.[85,86] Pyrrolizidine alkaloids can be divided into two categories based on their structure, namely those with an unsaturated nucleus (toxic) and those with a saturated nucleus (considered to be non-toxic).

Several herbs currently used in herbal remedies contain pyrrolizidines; they include liferoot (*Senecio aureus*), borage, comfrey, coltsfoot and echinacea (*see* individual monographs).

In addition to data from various animal studies, cases of human hepatotoxicity associated with the ingestion of comfrey have been documented (*see* Comfrey). The concentrations of pyrrolizidine alkaloids present in borage and coltsfoot are thought to be too low to be of clinical significance, although the dangers associated with low-dose exposure are unclear. The use of borage oil as a source of gamma-linolenic acid and as an alternative to evening primrose oil is currently very popular. Whether or not pyrrolizidine alkaloids are present in borage oil is unclear from published data. The pyrrolizidine alkaloids identified in echinacea to-date have been of the non-toxic saturated type.

Benzophenanthridine alkaloids are present in bloodroot and in prickly ash. Although some of these alkaloids have exhibited cytotoxic properties in animal studies, their toxicity to humans has been refuted (*see* Bloodroot).

Lectins are plant proteins that possess haem-agglutinating and potent mitogenic properties. Both mistletoe and pokeroot contain lectins. Systemic exposure to pokeroot has resulted in haematological aberrations. Mistletoe lectins may also inhibit protein synthesis.[87] (*see* Mistletoe and Pokeroot).

Viscotoxins, constituents of mistletoe, are low molecular weight proteins which possess cytotoxic and cardiotoxic properties.[87] For many years, mistletoe preparations have been used in Europe as cancer treatments. Clinical trials carried out with Iscador, a product produced from the naturally fermented plant juice of mistletoe, have concluded that Iscador may exhibit some weak antitumour effects but should only be used alongside conventional therapy in the long-term treatment of cancer.

Lignans. Hepatotoxic reactions reported for chaparral have been associated with the lignan constituents (*see* Chaparral).

Saponins. Pokeroot also contains irritant saponins which have produced severe gastrointestinal irritation involving intense abdominal cramping and haematemesis. Systemic exposure to these saponins has resulted in hypotension and tachycardia. In May 1979, the US Herb Trade Association requested that all its members should stop selling pokeroot as a herbal beverage or food because of its toxicity.[88]

Diterpenes. The irritant properties of many diterpenes are well documented and queen's delight contains diterpene esters which are extremely irritant to all mucosal surfaces (*see* Queen's Delight).

Cyanogenetic glycosides are present in the kernels of a number of fruits including apricot, bitter almond, cherry, pear and plum seeds. Gastric hydrolysis of these compounds following oral ingestion results in the release of hydrogen cyanide (HCN), which is rapidly absorbed from the upper gastrointestinal tract and which can lead to respiratory failure. It has been estimated that oral doses of 50 mg of HCN, equivalent to about 50–60 apricot kernels, can be fatal[89] (*see* Apricot). However, variation in cyanogenetic glycoside content of the kernels could reduce or increase the number required for a fatal reaction. In the early 1980s a substance called amygdalin was promoted as a 'natural' non-toxic cure for cancer. Amygdalin is a cyanogenetic glycoside that is also referred to as laetrile and 'vitamin B$_{17}$'. Two near-fatal episodes of HCN poisoning were recorded in which the patients had consumed apricot kernels as an alternative source of amygdalin, due to the poor availability of laetrile. Scientific research did not support the claims made for laetrile, although a small number of anecdotal reports suggested that laetrile may have some slight anticancer activity. As a result, legislation drawn up in 1984[90] restricted the availability of cyanogenetic substances so that amygdalin can only be administered under medical supervision.

Furanocoumarins are found predominantly in the families Umbelliferae (e.g. parsley, celery), Rutaceae (e.g. bergamot, *Citrus* species), Moraceae and Leguminosae. The furanocoumarins occur as linear and branched forms: the most commonly reported linear furanocoumarins are 8-methoxypsoralen, 5-methoxypsoralen (bergapten) and psoralen. The furanocoumarins are phototoxic. Severe phototoxic reactions have been reported in humans following the use of bergamot oil in topical preparations. Severe phototoxic burns have been reported in a Swedish patient following a visit to a suntan parlour after ingestion of a large quantity of celery soup.[91] In the UK, a patient developed severe phototoxicity during oral photochemotherapy with psoralen and ultraviolet A (PUVA) after eating a large quantity of soup made from celery, parsley and parsnip.[92] The authors highlighted the potential hazards of eating foods containing psoralens during PUVA therapy. In the UK, the MCA received two reports describing severe skin burns in patients who had been treated with TCM preparations derived from *Psoralea corylifolia* fruit.[93]

Volatile oils. See Precautions in specific patient groups, Pregnant breastfeeding mothers (pp. 18–20).

Herbal ingredients that may cause adverse effects Examples of adverse effects that have been documented in humans or animals for the herbal ingredients described in the monographs are summarised in Table 1. These adverse effects include allergic, cardiac, hepatic, hormonal, irritant and purgative effects, and a range of toxicities. Some of the potential adverse effects of the herbal ingredients which are the subject of the 148 monographs are listed in Table 2. For further detailed information, including literature references, the reader should consult individual monographs. The following few examples are illustrative of some of the adverse effects caused by herbal ingredients.

Comfrey, coltsfoot Hepatotoxic reactions have been documented for comfrey and coltsfoot. Both of these herbal ingredients contain pyrrolizidine alkaloids, compounds known to be hepatotoxic. However, it was later reported that the reaction documented for coltsfoot may have in fact involved a herbal tea containing a *Senecio* species rather than coltsfoot.[44] The *Senecio* genus is characterized by its pyrrolizidine alkaloid constituents.

Mistletoe, scullcap A case of hepatitis has been reported for a woman who was taking a multi-constituent herbal product (*see* Mistletoe). Based on the known toxic constituents of mistletoe and other herbal ingredients present in the product, it was concluded that mistletoe was the component responsible for the hepatitis. Lectins and viscotoxins, the toxic constituents in mistletoe, are not known to be hepatotoxic and no other reports of liver damage associated with mistletoe ingestion have been documented. The product also contained scullcap, which is recognised to be frequently adulterated with a *Teucrium* species. Recently, hepatotoxic reactions have been associated with germander (*Teucrium chamaedrys*) (*see* Scullcap).

Pokeroot Severe gastrointestinal irritation and haematological abnormalities documented for pokeroot can be directly related to the saponin and lectin constituents of pokeroot.[44]

Sassafras Hepatotoxicity has been associated with the consumption of a herbal tea containing sassafras. The principal component of sassafras volatile oil is safrole, which is known to be hepatotoxic and carcinogenic.[83]

Table 1 Examples of adverse effects that may occur with herbal ingredients

Potential adverse effect	Constituent/Herbal ingredient
Allergic (*see* Appendix 12) Hypersensitive	Sesquiterpene lactones: arnica, chamomile, feverfew, yarrow
Phototoxic Immune Cardiac (*see* Appendix 3) Endocrine	Furanocoumarins: angelica, celery, wild carrot Canavanine: alfalfa Cardiac glycosides: pleurisy root, squill
Hypoglycaemic (*see* Appendix 9) Hyperthyroid Hormonal (*see* Appendix 10) Mineralocorticoid Oestrogenic Anti-androgen	Alfalfa, fenugreek Iodine: fucus Triterpenoids: liquorice Isoflavonoids: alfalfa, red clover Saponins: ginseng, saw palmetto
Irritant (*see* Appendix 13) Gastrointestinal	Numerous compounds including anthraquinones (purgative), capsaicinoids, diterpenes, saponins, terpene-rich volatile oils
Renal Toxic Hepatotoxic/carcinogenic	Aescin: horse-chestnut; terpene-rich volatile oils Pyrrolizidine alkaloids: comfrey, liferoot; β-asarone: calamus; lignans: chaparral; safrole: sassafras
Mitogenic Cyanide poisoning Convulsant	Proteins: mistletoe, pokeroot Cyanogenetic glycosides: apricot Camphor/thujone-rich volatile oils

Table 2 Potential adverse effects of herbal ingredients listed in the monographs

Herb	Adverse effect	Reasons/Comments
Agnus Castus	Allergic reactions	–
Alfalfa	Systemic lupus erythematosus syndrome	Canavanine, toxic amino acid
Aloes	Purgative, irritant to GI tract	Anthraquinones
Angelica	Phototoxic dermatitis	Furanocoumarins
Aniseed	Contact dermatitis	Anethole in volatile oil
Apricot[1]	Cyanide poisoning, seed	Cyanogenetic glycosides
Arnica[1]	Dermatitis, irritant to GI tract	Sesquiterpene lactones
Artichoke	Allergenic, dermatitis	Sesquiterpene lactones
Asafoetida	Dermatitis, irritant	Gum, related species
Bayberry	Carcinogenic to rats	–
Blue Flag	Nausea, vomiting, irritant to GI tract and eyes	Fresh root, furfural (volatile oil)
Bogbean	Purgative, vomiting	In large doses
Boldo	Toxicity, irritant	Volatile oil
Boneset	Dermatitis, cytotoxic	Sesquiterpene lactones
Borage[1]	Genotoxic, carcinogenic, hepatotoxic	Pyrrolizidine alkaloids
Broom	Cardiac depressant	Sparteine (alkaloid)
Buchu	Irritant to GI tract, kidney	Volatile oil
Calamus[1]	Carcinogenic, nephrotoxic, convulsions	β-Asarone in oil
Capsicum	Irritant	Capsaicinoids
Cascara	Purgative, irritant to GI tract	Anthraquinones
Cassia	Allergenic, irritant	Cinnamaldehyde in volatile oil
Celery	Phototoxic, dermatitis	Furanocoumarins
Cereus	Irritant to GI tract	Fresh juice
Chamomile, German	Allergic reactions	Sesquiterpene lactones
Chamomile, Roman	Allergic reactions	Sesquiterpene lactones
Chaparral	Dermatitis, hepatotoxic	Lignans
Cinnamon	Allergenic, irritant	Cinnamaldehyde in volatile oil
Clove	Irritant	Eugenol in volatile oil
Cohosh, Black	Nausea, vomiting	High doses
Cohosh, Blue	Irritant to GI tract	Seeds poisonous
Cola	Sleeplessness, anxiety, tremor	Caffeine
Coltsfoot[1]	Genotoxic, carcinogenic, hepatotoxic	Pyrrolizidine alkaloids
Comfrey[1]	Genotoxic, carcinogenic, hepatotoxic	Pyrrolizidine alkaloids
Corn Silk	Allergenic, dermatitis	–
Cowslip	Allergenic	Quinones
Damiana	Convulsions	High dose (one report only), quinones, cyanogenetic glycosides
Dandelion	Allergenic, dermatitis	Sesquiterpene lactones
Echinacea	Allergenic, irritant	Polysaccharide
Elecampane	Allergenic, irritant	Sesquiterpene lactones
Eucalyptus	Nausea, vomiting	Oil
Evening Primrose Oil	Mild indigestion, increased risk of epilepsy	Schizophrenic patients on phenothiazines
Eyebright	Mental confusion, raised intraocular pressure	Tincture
Feverfew	Allergenic, dermatitis	Sesquiterpene lactones
Frangula	Purgative, irritant to GI tract	Anthraquinones
Fucus	Hyperthyroidism	Iodine content
Garlic	Irritant to GI tract, dermatitis	Sulfides
Ginkgo	Gastric upset, headache	–
Ginseng	Mastalgia, vaginal bleeding, insomnia	Various effects (see Ginseng)
Golden Seal	Gastric upset	Berberine, potentially poisonous

Herb	Adverse effect	Reasons/Comments
Gravel Root[1]	Genotoxic, carcinogenic, hepatotoxic	Pyrrolizidine alkaloids
Ground Ivy	Irritant to GI tract, kidneys	Pulegone in volatile oil
Guaiacum	Allergenic, dermatitis	Lignans
Hops	Allergenic, dermatitis	Oleo-resin
Horehound, White	Dermatitis, irritant	Plant juice
Horse-chestnut	Nephrotoxic	Aescin
Horseradish	Allergenic, irritant	Glucosinolates
Hydrangea	Dermatitis, irritant to GI tract	–
Hydrocotyle	Phototoxic, dermatitis	–
Ispaghula	Oesophageal obstruction, flatulence	If swallowed dry
Jamaica Dogwood	Irritant, numbness, tremors	High doses
Juniper	Irritant, abortifacient	Volatile oil, confusion with savin
Lady's Slipper	Allergenic, dermatitis, hallucinations	–
Liferoot[1]	Genotoxic, carcinogenic, hepatotoxic	Pyrrolizidine alkaloids
Liquorice	Hyperaldosteronism	Excessive ingestion
Lobelia	Nausea, vomiting, diarrhoea	Lobeline (alkaloid)
Maté	Sleeplessness, anxiety, tremor	Caffeine
Mistletoe	Hepatitis, hypotension, poisonous	Mixed herbal preparation
Motherwort	Phototoxic dermatitis	Volatile oil
Nettle	Irritant	Amines
Parsley	Irritant, hepatitis, phototoxic, abortifacient	Apiole in volatile oil, excessive ingestion
Pennyroyal	Irritant, nephrotoxic, hepatotoxic	Pulegone in volatile oil
Pilewort[1]	Irritant	Protoanemonin
Plantain	Allergenic, dermatitis, irritant	Mustard-type oil
Pleurisy Root	Dermatitis, irritant, cardiac activity	Cardenolides
Pokeroot	Mitogenic, toxic, nausea, vomiting, cramp	Lectins
Prickly Ash, Southern	Toxic to animals	–
Pulsatilla[1]	Allergenic, irritant	Protanemonin
Queen's Delight[1]	Irritant to GI tract	Diterpenes
Red Clover	Oestrogenic	Isoflavonoids
Rhubarb	Purgative, irritant to GI tract	Anthraquinones
Rosemary	Convulsions	Camphor in volatile oil
Sage	Toxic, convulsant	Thujone, camphor in volatile oil
Sassafras[1]	Carcinogenic, genotoxic	Safrole in volatile oil
Scullcap	Hepatotoxicity	Mixed product; adulteration with *Teucrium* spp.
Senega	Irritant to GI tract	Saponins
Senna	Purgative, irritant to GI tract	Anthraquinones
Shepherd's Purse	Irritant	Isothiocyanates
Skunk Cabbage	Itch, inflammation	–
Squill	Irritant, cardioactive	Saponins
St. John's Wort	Phototoxic	Hypericin
Tansy[1]	Severe gastritis, convulsions	Thujone in volatile oil
Thyme	Irritant to GI tract	Thymol in volatile oil
Wild Carrot	Phototoxic, dermatitis	Furanocoumarins
Yarrow	Allergenic, dermatitis	Sesquiterpene lactones
Yellow Dock	Purgative, irritant to GI tract	Anthraquinones

[1] Not recommended for internal use

Excessive ingestion

Ginseng Excessive doses of ginseng have been reported to cause agitation, insomnia, and raised blood pressure and have been referred to as abuse of the remedy. However, side-effects have also been reported for ginseng following the ingestion of recommended doses, and include mastalgia and vaginal bleeding.[94]

Liquorice Excessive ingestion of liquorice has resulted in typical corticosteroid-type side-effects of oedema and hypertension.[85]

Parsley Parsley volatile oil contains apiole which is structurally related to the recognised hepatocarcinogen, safrole. Ingestion of apiole has resulted in a number of cases of fatal poisoning.[83]

Hypersensitivity reactions

Chamomile Sesquiterpene lactones are known to possess allergenic properties. They occur predominantly in herbs of the Compositae (Asteraceae) family, of which chamomile is a member. Hypersensitivity reactions have been reported for chamomile and other plants from the same family. Cross-sensitivity to other members of the Compositae family is well recognised.

Feverfew The sesquiterpene lactones present in feverfew are considered to be the active principles in the herb. It is unknown whether documented side-effects for feverfew, such as mouth ulcers and swollen tongue, are also attributable to these constituents.[95]

Phototoxic reactions

Parsley Furanocoumarins, compounds known to cause phototoxic reactions, are constituents of parsley. Excessive ingestion of parsley has been associated with the development of photosensitive rash which resolved once parsley consumption ceased.[83]

Precautions in specific patient groups

Pregnant/breastfeeding mothers Few conventional medicines have been established as safe to take during pregnancy and it is generally recognised that no medicine should be taken unless the benefit to the mother outweighs any possible risk to the foetus. This rule should also be applied to herbal medicinal products. However, one of the major problems is that herbal products are often promoted to the public as being 'natural' and completely 'safe' alternatives to conventional medicines. Table 3 lists some herbal ingredients taken from the following 148 monographs that specifically should be avoided or used with caution during pregnancy. As with conventional medicines, no herbal products should be taken during pregnancy unless the benefit outweighs the potential risk.

Table 3 Herbal Ingredients Best Avoided or used with Caution during Pregnancy
Absence of a herbal ingredient from this list does not signify safety and as with all medicines, herbal remedies should only be used where the perceived benefit outweighs any possible risk. For a number of herbs the chemistry and pharmacology are poorly documented and their use in pregnancy should be avoided. Some of the herbs listed are reputed to be abortifacient or to affect the menstrual cycle although no recent clinical or experimental data exists. In view of the potential serious effects caution in their use is advised.

Herb	Effect
Agnus Castus	Hormonal action
Aloes	Cathartic, reputed abortifacient
Apricot	Cyanide toxicity
Asafoetida	Reputed abortifacient and to affect menstrual cycle
Avens	Reputed to affect menstrual cycle
Blue Flag	Irritant oil
Bogbean	Irritant, possible purgative
Boldo	Irritant oil
Boneset	Cytotoxic constituents (related species)
Borage	Pyrrolizidine alkaloids
Broom	Sparteine is oxytoxic
Buchu	Irritant oil

Herb	Effect
Burdock	Uterine stimulant, *in vivo*
Calendula	Reputed to affect menstrual cycle, uterine stimulant, *in vitro*
Cascara	Anthraquinones, non-standardised preparations to be avoided
Chamomile, German	Reputed to affect menstrual cycle, uterine stimulant with excessive use
Chamomile, Roman	Reputed abortifacient and to affect menstrual cycle with excessive use
Chaparral	Uterine activity, hepatotoxic
Cohosh, Black	Uterine oestrogen receptor binding *in vitro*
Cohosh, Blue	Reputed abortifacient and to affect menstrual cycle
Cola	Caffeine, consumption should be restricted
Coltsfoot	Pyrrolizidine alkaloids
Comfrey	Pyrrolizidine alkaloids
Cornsilk	Uterine stimulant, *in vivo*
Damiana	Cyanogenetic glycosides, risk of cyanide toxicity in high doses
Eucalyptus	Oil should not be taken internally during pregnancy
Euphorbia	Smooth muscle activity, *in vitro*
Fenugreek	Oxytoxic, uterine stimulant, *in vitro*
Feverfew	Reputed abortifacient and to affect menstrual cycle
Frangula	Anthraquinones, non-standardised preparations to be avoided
Fucus	Thyroid gland activity, possible heavy metal contamination
Gentian	Reputed to affect menstrual cycle
Ginseng, Eleutherococcus	Hormonal activity
Ginseng, Panax	Hormonal activity
Golden Seal	Alkaloids with uterine stimulant activity, *in vitro*
Ground Ivy	Irritant oil
Hawthorn	Uterine activity, *in vivo*, *in vitro*
Hops	Uterine activity, *in vitro*
Horehound, Black	Reputed to affect menstrual cycle
Horehound, White	Reputed abortifacient and to affect menstrual cycle
Horseradish	Irritant oil; avoid excessive ingestion
Hydrocotyle	Reputed abortifacient and to affect menstrual cycle
Jamaica Dogwood	Uterine activity, *in vitro*, *in vivo*; irritant
Juniper	Reputed abortifacient and to affect menstrual cycle. Confusion over whether oil is toxic
Liferoot	Pyrrolizidine alkaloids
Liquorice	Oestrogenic activity, reputed abortifacient
Lobelia	Lobeline, toxicity
Maté	Caffeine, consumption should be restricted
Meadowsweet	Uterine activity, *in vitro*
Mistletoe	Toxic constituents, uterine stimulant, animal
Motherwort	Uterine activity, *in vitro*, reputed to affect menstrual cycle
Myrrh	Reputed to affect menstrual cycle
Nettle	Reputed abortifacient and to affect menstrual cycle
Passionflower	Harman, harmaline uterine stimulants, animal
Pennyroyal	Abortifacient, irritant oil (pulegone)
Plantain	Uterine activity, *in vitro*; laxative
Pleurisy Root	Uterine activity, *in vivo*; cardioactive constituents
Pokeroot	Toxic constituents, uterine stimulant, reputed to affect menstrual cycle
Poplar	Conflicting reports over use of aspirin in pregnancy; salicylates excreted in breast milk may cause rashes in babies
Prickly Ash, Northern	Pharmacologically active alkaloids and coumarins
Prickly Ash, Southern	Pharmacologically active alkaloids
Pulsatilla	Reputed to affect menstrual cycle, uterine activity, *in vitro*, *in vivo*; irritant (fresh plant)
Queen's Delight	Irritant diterpenes

Herb	Effect
Raspberry	Uterine activity, *in vitro*, traditional use to ease parturition
Red Clover	Oestrogenic activity
Rhubarb	Anthraquinones, non-standardised preparations to be avoided
Sassafras	Abortifacient (oil), hepatotoxic (safrole)
Scullcap	Traditional use to eliminate afterbirth and promote menstruation; potential hepatotoxicity
Senna	Anthraquinones, non-standardised preparations to be avoided
Shepherd's Purse	Reputed abortifacient and to affect menstrual cycle
Skunk Cabbage	Reputed to affect menstrual cycle
Squill	Reputed abortifacient and to affect menstrual cycle
St. John's Wort	Slight uterine activity, *in vitro*
Tansy	Uterine activity, abortifacient (thujone in oil)
Uva-Ursi	Large doses, oxytocic
Vervain	Reputed abortifacient, oxytocic, utero-activity *in vivo*
Wild Carrot	Oestrogenic activity, irritant oil
Willow	Conflicting reports over use of aspirin in pregnancy; salicylates excreted in breast milk may cause rashes in babies
Yarrow	Reputed abortifacient and to affect menstrual cycle (thujone in oil)
Yellow Dock	Anthraquinones, non-standardised preparations to be avoided

Volatile oils Many herbs are traditionally reputed to be abortifacient and for some this reputation can be attributed to their volatile oil component.[83] A number of volatile oils are irritant to the genito-urinary tract if ingested and may induce uterine contractions. Herbs that contain irritant volatile oils include ground ivy, juniper, parsley, pennyroyal, sage, tansy and yarrow. Some of these oils contain the terpenoid constituent, thujone, which is known to be abortifacient. Pennyroyal oil also contains the hepatotoxic terpenoid constituent, pulegone. A case of liver failure in a woman who ingested pennyroyal oil as an abortifacient has been documented (*see* Pennyroyal).

Utero-activity A stimulant or spasmolytic action on uterine muscle has been documented for some herbal ingredients including blue cohosh, burdock, fenugreek, golden seal, hawthorn, jamaica dogwood, motherwort, nettle, raspberry and vervain. Raspberry is a popular remedy taken during pregnancy to help promote an easier labour by relaxing the uterine muscles. The pharmacological activity exhibited by raspberry may vary between different preparations and from one individual to another. Raspberry should not be used during pregnancy unless under medical supervision.

Herbal teas Increased awareness of the harmful effects associated with excessive tea and coffee consumption has prompted many individuals to switch to herbal teas. Whilst some herbal teas may offer pleasant alternatives to tea and coffee, some contain pharmacologically active herbal ingredients, which may have unpredictable effects depending on the quantity of tea consumed and strength of the brew. Some herbal teas contain laxative herbal ingredients such as senna, frangula and cascara. In general stimulant laxative preparations are not recommended during pregnancy and the use of unstandardised laxative preparations is particularly unsuitable. A case of hepatotoxicity in a newborn baby has been documented in which the mother consumed a herbal tea during pregnancy as an expectorant.[96] Following analysis the herbal tea was reported to contain pyrrolizidine alkaloids which are known to be hepatotoxic.

Breastfeeding mothers A drug substance taken by a breastfeeding mother presents a hazard if it is transferred to the breast milk in pharmacologically or toxicologically significant amounts. Limited information is available regarding the safety of conventional medicines taken during breastfeeding. Much less information exists for herbal ingredients, and generally the use of herbal remedies is not recommended during lactation.

Paediatric use Herbal medicines have traditionally been used to treat both adults and children. Herbal medicines may offer a milder alternative to some conventional medicines, although the suitability of a herbal remedy needs to be considered with respect to quality, safety and efficacy. Herbal medicines should be used with caution in children and medical advice should be sought if in doubt. Chamomile is a popular remedy used to treat teething pains in babies. However, chamomile is known to contain allergenic sesquiterpene lactones and should therefore be used with caution. The administration of herbal teas to children is generally unwise unless used according to professional advice.[97]

Older patients   A review has considered the available evidence on the use of several herbal medicinal products (St. John's wort, valerian, ginkgo, horse-chestnut, saw palmetto and yohimbe) by older patients.[98] Whilst the treatments may offer considerable benefits for a range of conditions, the review raised the need for caution, particularly with regard to potential drug–herb interactions and possible adverse effects, when herbal medicinal products are used by older patients.

Patients with cardiovascular disease   Concerns have been raised about the use of herbal medicinal products for cardiovascular disease, in particular, because of the lack of scientific assessment and the potential for toxic effects and major drug–herb interactions.[99]

Peri-operative use   The need for patients to discontinue herbal medicinal products prior to surgery has been proposed.[100] From the available evidence, it has been suggested that the potential exists for direct pharmacological effects, pharmacodynamic interactions and pharmacokinetic interactions with eight commonly used herbal medicinal products (echinacea, ephedra, garlic, ginkgo, ginseng, kava, St. John's wort, valerian). The need for physicians to have a clear understanding of the herbal medicinal products being used by patients and to take a detailed history was highlighted.

The American Society of Anaesthesiologists (ASA) has reported that a number of anaesthesiologists have noted significant changes in heart rate or blood pressure in some patients who have been taking herbal medicinal products, including St. John's Wort, ginkgo and ginseng, and has advised patients to tell their doctor if they are taking herbal products before surgery.[101]

Herb–drug interactions   Generally speaking, limited information is available regarding interactions between herbal products and conventional medicines. However, awareness of this issue is increasing, and the potential for drug–herb interactions has been discussed.[102–105] Concerns have been raised in the literature about herbal medicines interfering with breast cancer treatment,[106] and potential interactions between herbal products and cardiac drugs.[107]

Instances of drug interactions have been tentatively linked, retrospectively, to the concurrent use of herbal medicines. The rationale for such interactions is often difficult to explain if knowledge regarding the phytochemical constituents of the herbal product, their pharmacological activity and metabolism are poorly understood. The emergence of significant problems associated with the ingestion of grapefruit juice concurrently with certain medicines has emphasised the fact that clinically relevant interactions between drugs and natural products (both herbs and foods) may occur.[108]

As with conventional drug interactions, herb–drug interactions may be pharmacodynamic or pharmacokinetic. Pharmacodynamic interactions could result when a herbal drug and a conventional drug have similar or antagonistic pharmacological effects or adverse effects. These interactions are usually predictable from a knowledge of the pharmacology of the interacting herb and drug. Pharmacokinetic interactions could occur when a herb alters the absorption, distribution, metabolism or excretion of a drug (and vice versa). These interactions are not easy to predict.

As with all potential drug interactions there are particular concerns when patients are stabilised on conventional medicines, such as warfarin, digoxin, anticonvulsants (e.g. phenytoin) and ciclosporin that are known to have a narrow therapeutic window.

St. John's wort   Since 1998 evidence has emerged from spontaneous reports and published case reports of the interactions between St. John's wort and certain prescribed medicines leading to a loss of or reduction in therapeutic effect of these prescribed medicines (*see* St. John's Wort).[11] Drugs that may be affected include indinavir, warfarin, ciclosporin, digoxin, theophylline and oral contraceptives. There have also been reports of increased serotonergic effects in patients taking St. John's wort concurrently with selective serotonin reuptake inhibitors (e.g. sertraline, paroxetine). Results of drug interaction studies have provided some evidence that St. John's Wort may induce some cytochrome P450 (CYP) drug-metabolising enzymes in the liver as well as affecting P-glycoprotein (a transport protein). Regulatory Authorities throughout the EU and elsewhere have issued advice to patients and healthcare professionals.

The evidence for and understanding of most drug–herb interactions is limited. An attempt can be made, however, to identify herbal ingredients that have the potential to interfere with specific categories of conventional drugs, based on known phytochemical and pharmacological properties of the herb, and on any documented adverse effects.

For example, herbs containing substantial levels of coumarins may potentially increase blood coagulation time if taken in large doses. Prolonged or excessive use of a herbal diuretic may potentiate existing diuretic therapy, interfere with existing hypo/hypertensive therapy, or potentiate the effect of certain cardioactive drugs due to hypokalaemia. Herbs which have been documented to lower blood sugar concentrations may cause hypoglycaemia if taken in sufficient amounts and interfere with existing hypoglycaemic therapy. An individual receiving antihypertensive therapy may be more susceptible to the hypertensive adverse effects that have been documented with, for example, ginseng or which are associated with the excessive ingestion of plants such as liquorice.

This approach has been used in drawing up Appendices 1–13 (pp. 497–506), which provide information on potential drug–herb interactions. Appendix 1 groups together various therapeutic categories of medicines that may be affected by a particular herb or group of herbs. Appendices 2–13 list herbal ingredients that are claimed to have a specific activity alphabetically within each Appendix, including laxative, cardioactive, diuretic, hypo/hypertensive, anticoagulant/coagulant, hypo/hyperlipidaemic, sedative, hypo/hyperglycaemic, hormonal, immunostimulant, allergenic or irritant. Some commonly occurring groups of natural products found within these 148 herbal ingredients contribute towards their activities, toxicities or adverse effects. Appendices 14–22 list those herbal ingredients that contain amines, alkaloids or have sympathomimetic anti-inflammatory or antispasmodic activities, coumarins, flavonoids, iridoids, saponins, tannins or volatile oils.

Interactions of herbal products in therapeutic drug monitoring There are also examples of herbal medicinal products which appear to cross-react with diagnostic markers in therapeutic drug monitoring, e.g. where the constituents of a Chinese medicine and *Eleutherococcus* cross-reacted with digoxin assays.[104]

Reporting of adverse reactions to herbal medicinal products It is essential that information on the risks associated with the use of herbal products is systematically collected and analysed in order to protect public health. In 1996, the UK MCA extended its 'Yellow Card Scheme' for adverse drug reaction reporting to include reporting of suspected adverse reactions to unlicensed herbal products. This followed a report from a UK Medical Toxicology Unit on potentially serious adverse reactions associated with herbal remedies. Twenty-one cases of liver toxicity,

including two deaths, were associated with the use of TCM.[82]

The need to further improve pharmacovigilance on herbal products was highlighted in a study of patients' perceived behaviour towards reporting adverse reactions.[109] The study found that patients would be less likely to consult their doctor for suspected adverse drug reactions (minor or severe) to herbal remedies than for similar adverse reactions to a conventional over-the-counter medicine. This illustrates the need for greater public awareness that adverse reactions can occur and that such reactions should be reported. It also highlights the need for healthcare professionals to take a detailed medical history including use of herbal products and to be aware that patients may be reluctant to provide information.

The Uppsala Monitoring Centre of the World Health Organization plays an important role in the international monitoring of adverse health effects associated with herbal medicines.[110] The Centre has carried out an analysis of the suspected adverse reactions to herbal medicines reported over a period of 20 years. In 21 (0.8%) of the 2487 case reports reported to occur with single-ingredient herbal products, the suspected adverse reaction had a fatal outcome. Three of these reports concerned intestinal perforation after administration of a senna-containing laxative, presumed to be prior to X-ray examination because of intestinal pathology. Three reports concerned respiratory failure in association with the use of psyllium mucilloid-containing products and three other of respiratory failure in association with ispaghula husk. One patient had an anaphylactic shock after the injection of a horse-chestnut extract. In the remaining cases no pattern was recognizable. The Centre has highlighted the need for improved reporting in particular with regard to the precise identity and composition of the products.

Efficacy

Despite the growing popularity of herbal medicines world-wide there is a dearth of scientific evidence of efficacy. Indeed, many of the herbs used medicinally in Europe have a traditional reputation for their uses, but there is little scientific documentation of their active constituents, pharmacological actions or clinical efficacy. Examples of this group include avens, boneset, burdock, clivers, damiana, Jamaica dogwood, parsley piert, pulsatilla and wild lettuce. For other herbs, documented phytochemical data or pharmacological data from animal studies may provide a plausible basis for their traditional uses, but evidence of efficacy from clinical studies is limited.

The current emphasis on evidence-based medicine requires evidence of efficacy from rigorous randomised controlled trials. Where possible, the evidence is best evaluated by systematic reviews and meta-analyses of available clinical trial data, as such approaches minimise both selection bias and random error.

Such approaches are now being applied to herbal medicines. Reports of systematic reviews undertaken for a number of herbal ingredients, e.g. aloe vera, artichoke, echinacea, evening primrose, feverfew, garlic, ginger, ginkgo, ginseng, hawthorn, horse-chestnut, mistletoe, peppermint, saw palmetto, St. John's wort and valerian have been published.[111–113] Several systematic reviews have been prepared by the Cochrane Collaboration (the international association dedicated to preparing and maintaining systematic reviews of the effects of healthcare interventions).[114] Several reviews highlight that, in some cases, the evidence base is weak and studies are often flawed. In other cases, studies have been methodologically sound and evidence of efficacy has been compelling.

St. John's wort, a widely used herbal product, has been investigated in many clinical studies. Evidence from randomised controlled trials has confirmed the efficacy of St. John's wort products over placebo in the treatment of mild-to-moderate depression (*see* St. John's Wort).[11] There is, however, a need for further studies to evaluate efficacy compared with that of standard treatments, particularly newer antidepressant agents, in well-defined patient groups and conducted over longer time periods.

One of the fundamental problems characteristic of herbal medicinal products is that the individual herbal ingredients contain a vast array of chemical constituents. Further, herbal medicines traditionally involve mixtures of different herbal ingredients, although in developed countries, recent trends indicate that single-ingredient herbal products are becoming increasingly popular. Herbalists would argue that combinations of ingredients are designed to provide the best therapeutic outcome while reducing adverse effects and toxicity. Evidence is emerging that different constituents within a herbal preparation may contribute to the overall therapeutic effect of the product and that in some cases synergistic and additive effects play an important role.[115]

In most cases there is a lack of knowledge of the phytochemical constituents responsible for the claimed therapeutic effects. To further complicate matters, it is well known that herbal products derived from the same herbal drug can vary considerably in terms of their phytochemical constituents depending on the source of plant material, the manufacture of the extracts and formulation of the dosage forms. As a result, efforts to establish clinical efficacy are hampered by how far results for a specific product can be extrapolated to other products containing the same plant but different extracts. Where the active constituents of a herbal ingredient are known it is possible and, in most cases, desirable to standardise the extract/product. The aim of standardisation is to obtain an optimum and consistent quality of a herbal drug preparation by adjusting it to give a defined content of a constituent or a group of constituents with known therapeutic activity. Examples of herbal drugs with constituents with accepted, known therapeutic activity are few. Herbs with documented activities (and known active constituents) include: senna, frangula (hydroxyanthracenes); belladonna (alkaloids) and horse-chestnut (saponins).

In the case of St. John's wort, early studies concentrated on the hypericin constituents but more recent work suggests that hyperforin and possibly flavonoids also contribute to the antidepressant properties.[11] Studies analysing St. John's wort products have reported differing contents of hypericin and hyperforin.[116,117] Furthermore, some products showed consistent batch-to-batch concentrations of hypericin and hyperforin, whilst others exhibited significant interbatch variability.[116]

Despite the dearth of documented clinical evidence for the effects of the majority of herbal ingredients, there is no reason why herbal medicinal products should not be available for use in minor conditions, providing that these are consistent with traditional uses and that the herbal ingredients are of suitable quality and safety. It would seem to be more appropriate to use those herbal ingredients for which documented phytochemical and pharmacological data support the traditional use. Herbal medicines intended for use in more serious medical conditions require evidence of efficacy to support their use.

Herbal Medicinal Products of Current Interest

Echinacea Echinacea is widely used throughout Europe for the prevention and treatment of colds and other upper respiratory tract infections. A recent Cochrane review of 16 clinical trials has reported that the overall results suggest that some products may have an effect greater than placebo, but that overall the results were inconclusive (*see* Echinacea).[118]

Garlic Numerous studies and systematic reviews have investigated the effects of garlic preparations in lowering raised serum cholesterol concentrations (*see* Garlic). Generally, the studies report beneficial results for garlic. However the evidence at present is insufficient to recommend garlic as routine treatment for hypercholesterolaemia. One of the major problems in assessing the evidence available on garlic is the wide variation in the chemical composition of the products available, compared with fresh garlic. Further controlled studies are needed using standardised preparations to investigate efficacy in reducing serum lipids, blood pressure, platelet aggregation and antimicrobial activity (*see* Garlic).

Ginger   Some clinical studies have reported ginger to be an effective prophylactic against motion sickness, although subsequent studies have found ginger to be ineffective (*see* Ginger).

Ginkgo   Ginkgo is widely used in France and Germany in authorised herbal medicinal products for the treatment of circulatory insufficiencies (peripheral and cerebral). Currently, no licensed herbal medicinal products containing ginkgo are available in the UK.

Several systematic reviews have been carried out analysing the available evidence on the effects of ginkgo in cerebral insufficiency, dementia, tinnitus and intermittent claudication (*see* Ginkgo). Overall the results suggest some beneficial effects, but further studies are needed.

Ginseng   Ginseng is widely renowned for its adaptogenic properties in Eastern countries, where it is used to help the body cope with stress and fatigue, and to promote recovery from illness or imbalance such as hypertension or hypoglycaemia. Generally, it is only recommended to be used for certain individuals with specific illnesses. By comparison, in the UK, ginseng is mainly self-administered and taken in the form of tablets or capsules containing dried extracts of the root. Ginseng products available in the UK are sold as food supplements, often in combination with vitamins and minerals. A wealth of research describing a wide range of pharmacological activities, particularly on the hypothalamic and pituitary regions of the brain, has been documented for ginseng (*see* Ginseng).

Saw palmetto   Saw palmetto is widely used in Europe, particularly in Germany, for symptoms associated with benign prostatic hypertrophy (BPH). In the UK, saw palmetto is licensed in a number of products for the symptomatic relief of short-term, male urinary discomfort. Results of clinical trials indicate that saw palmetto is a potential agent for the symptomatic treatment of BPH (*see* Saw Palmetto).

Valerian   Valerian is widely used in Europe for nervous tension and for promoting sleep. The therapeutic indications proposed by the EMEA HMPWP include relief of temporary, mild nervous tension and temporary difficulty in falling asleep.[19] A systematic review of randomised, double-blind, placebo-controlled trials of valerian reported inconsistencies in methodology between studies, and that the evidence for efficacy was inconclusive (*see* Valerian). It is unclear whether the active principles in valerian are associated with the volatile oil, the iridoid components termed valepotriates or with some other, as yet unidentified, group of constituents.

Conclusion

The use of herbal medicinal products, including use in addition to or instead of conventional medicines, is continuing to increase. Healthcare professionals need to be aware that patients may be taking herbal medicinal products, and need to understand their effects and be aware of the potential problems associated with their use. This handbook provides the reader with factual information on almost 150 herbal ingredients present in herbal medicinal products in European and other developed countries. Herbal medicinal products can offer an alternative to conventional medicines in non-life-threatening conditions, providing they are of adequate quality and safety, and are used in an appropriate manner by suitable individuals.

References

1   Kessler RC *et al* Long-term trends in the use of complementary and alternative medical therapies in the United States. *Ann Intern Med* 2001; **135**: 262–268.

2   Barnes J. Herbal medicine. *Pharm J* 1998; **260**: 344–348.

3   House of Lords Select Committee on Science and Technology Session 1999–2000, 6th Report. Complementary and Alternative Medicine. 21st November 2000.

4   Ernst E, White AR. The BBC survey of complementary medicine use in the UK. *Complement Ther Med* 2000; **8**: 32–36.

5   Thomas KJ *et al.* Use and expenditure on complementary medicine in England: a population based survey. *Complement Ther Med* 2001; **9**: 2–11.

6   Brevoort P. The US botanical market – an overview. *Herbalgram* 1996; **36**: 49–57.

7   Brevoort P. The booming US botanical market. A new overview. *Herbalgram* 1998; **44**: 33–46.

8   Blumenthal M. Herbs and phytomedicines in the European Community. In: Blumenthal M, ed. *The Complete German Commission E Monographs. Therapeutic Guide to Herbal Medicines*. Austin, Texas: American Botanical Council, 1998.

9   Institute of Medical Statistics (IMS) Self-Medication International. *Herbals in Europe*. London: IMS Self-Medication International, 1998.

10 EMEA Herbal Medicinal Products Working Party. Position paper on the risks associated with the use of herbal products containing *Aristolochia* species. EMEA website: www.eudra.org/emea.html. October 2001.

11 Barnes J *et al*. St. John's Wort (*Hypericum perforatum* L.): a review of its chemistry, pharmacology and clinical properties. *J Pharm Pharmacol* 2001; **53**: 583–600.

12 Evans WC. *Trease and Evans' Pharmacognosy*, 14th edn. London: WB Saunders, 1998.

13 Council Directive 65/65/EEC. *Official Journal of the European Communities* 1965; **22**: 369.

14 Britt R. The New EC Systems in the UK, *Regulatory Affairs J* 1995; **6**: 380–384.

15 AESGP (Association of the European Self-medication Industry). Herbal Medicinal Products in the European Union, 15 March 1999. http://www.aesgp.be.

16 Steinhoff B. The contribution of the European Scientific Cooperative on Phytotherapy and World Health Organisation monographs. *Drug Inform J* 1999; **33**: 17–22.

17 *Monographs on the Medicinal Uses of Plant Drugs*, Fascicules 1 and 2 (1996), Fascicules 3, 4 and 5 (1997), Fascicule 6 (1999). Exeter: European Scientific Cooperative on Phytotherapy (ESCOP)

18 European Commission, CPMP Guidelines on Information on Medicinal Products: Core SPCs for Frangulae Cortez, Sennae Fructus Angustifoliae, Sennae Fructus Acutifoliae, Sennae Folium, February 1994.

19 European Medicines Evaluation Agency. Herbal Medicinal Products Working Party Draft Core Summary of Product Characteristics for Valerian and Ispaghula. http://www.eudra.org/emea.html. October, 2001.

20 *Official Journal of the European Communities* No. C 305 of 16 October 1987.

21 Draft of Provisions of a Directive on Traditional Herbal Medicinal Products. http://www.mca.gov.uk. February 2002.

22 Medicines Act Leaflet (MAL) 8. A Guide to the Status under the Medicines Act of Borderline Products for Human Use. London: Medicines Control Agency.

23 Statutory Instrument (SI) 1994:3144, The Medicines for Human Use (Marketing Authorisations Etc) Regulations.

24 The Medicines Act, l968. London: HM Stationery Office.

25 Appelbe GE, Wingfield J. *Dale and Appelbe's Pharmacy Law and Ethics*, 6th edn. London: The Pharmaceutical Press, 1997.

26 CPMP/QWP 2819/00 (EMEA/CVMP 814/00) Note for Guidance. Quality of Herbal Medicinal Products. EMEA website: www.eudra.org/emea.html. October 2001.

27 CPMP/QWP 2820/00 (EMEA/CVMP 814/00) Note for Guidance. Specifications: test procedures and acceptance criteria for herbal drugs, herbal drug preparations and herbal medicinal products. EMEA website: www.eudra.org/emea.html. October 2001.

28 CPMP/CVMP Note for Guidance on Manufacture of Herbal Medicinal. Products. The Rules Governing Medicinal Products in the European Union 1992, vol. IV: 127–129.

29 Statutory Instrument (SI) 1971: 1450, The Medicines (Exemptions from Licences) (Special and Transitional Cases) Order.

30 Anon. Herbal licensing position confirmed. *Pharm J* 1994; **253**: 746.

31 De Smet PAGM. Should herbal medicine-like products be licensed as medicines? *BMJ* 1995; **310**: 1023–1024.

32 Vautier G, Spliller RC. Safety of complementary medicines should be monitored. *BMJ* 1995; **311**: 633.

33 Holder S. Regulatory aspects of herbal medicines: a global view. *The Regulatory Review* 2001; **4**: 13–17.

34 Statutory Instrument (SI) 1984: 769, The Medicines (Products Other than Veterinary Drugs) (General Sales List) Order, 1984, as amended by SI 1985:1540, SI 1987: 910, SI 1989: 969 and SI 1990: 1129.

35 Statutory Instrument (SI) 1983: 1212, The Medicines (Products Other than Veterinary Drugs) (Prescription Only) Order 1983, as amended.

36 Statutory Instrument (SI) 1977: 2130, (The Medicines Retail Sale or Supply of Herbal Remedies) Order, 1977.

37 Statutory Instrument (SI) 2001:1841, The Medicines (Aristolochia and Mu Tong etc) (Prohibition) Order, 2001.

38 Medicines Control Agency. Review of herbal ingredients for use in unlicensed herbal medicinal products. September 2001. www.mca.gov.uk.

39 Medicines Act Leaflet (MAL 2). Guidelines on Safety and Efficacy Requirements for Herbal Medicinal Products. Guidance Notes on Applications for Product Licences; 1989, 53–54.

40 Anon. *Regulatory Situation of Herbal Medicines – a Worldwide Review*. Geneva: WHO, 1998: 1–45.

41 Boon H, Smith M. *The Botanical Pharmacy – the Pharmacology of 47 Common Herbs*, 2nd edn. Kingston, Ontario: Quarry Health and the College of Naturopathic Medicine, 2000.

42 Anon. Further developments to the NHPD working draft of the proposed regulatory framework for NHPs. Health Canada. www.hc-sc.gc.ca/hpb/onhp/nph_reg_frame_nov21_upd_e.html. October, 2001.

43 Foster S, Tyler VE. *Tyler's Honest Herbal*, 4th edn. New York: Haworth Press, 1999.

44 De Smet PAGM. Toxicological outlook on quality assurance of herbal remedies. In: *Adverse Effects of Herbal Drugs*, vol 1. Berlin: Springer Verlag, 1992.

45 De Smet PAGM. Overview of Herbal Quality Control. *Drug Inform J* 1999; **33**: 717–724.

46 Bauer R. Quality Criteria and Standardization of Phytopharmaceuticals: Can acceptable drug standards be achieved? *Drug Inform J* 1998, **32**: 101–110.

47 Busse W. The significance of quality for efficacy and safety of herbal medicinal products. *Drug Inform J* 2000, **34**: 15–23.

48 Corbin Winslow L. Herbs as Medicines. *Arch Intern Med* 1998: **158**: 2192–2199.

49 Medicines Control Agency. Traditional Medicines: Public Health and Compliance with Medicines Law. www.mca.gov.uk. November 2001.

50 Vanherweghem, J-L, *et al*. Rapidly progressive interstitial renal fibrosis in young women: association with slimming regimen including Chinese herbs. *Lancet* 1993; **341**: 135–139.

51 Cosyns, J-P *et al*. Chinese herbs nephropathy: A clue to Balkan endemic nephropathy. *Kidney Int* 1994; **45**: 1680–1688.

52 Van Ypersele C, Vanherweghem J-L. The tragic paradigm of Chinese herb nephropathy. *Nephrol Dial Transplant* 1995; **10**: 157–160

53 Cosyns J-P *et al*. Urothelial lesions in Chinese-herb nephropathy. *Am J Kidney Dis* 1999; **33**: 1011–1017.

54 Lord G *et al*. Nephropathy caused by Chinese herbs in the UK. *Lancet* 1999; **354**: 481–482.

55 FDA Press Release. Vital Nutrients Recalls Joint Ease & Verified Quality Brand Joint Comfort Complex because of adverse health risk associated with aristolochic acid. www.fda.gov-USA. June 2001.

56 Charvill A. Investigation of formulated Traditional Chinese Medicines (TCM) and raw herbs for the presence of *Aristolochia* species. British Pharmaceutical Conference Science Proceedings 2001. London: Pharmaceutical Press, 2001: 295.

57 Slifman NR. Contamination of botanical dietary supplements by *Digitalis lanata*. *N Engl J Med* 1998; **339**: 806–811.

58 But PPH *et al*. Adulterants of herbal products can cause poisoning. *BMJ* 1996; **313**: 117.

59 Tai Y-T *et al*. Cardiotoxicity after accidental herb-induced aconite poisoning. *Lancet* 1992; **340**: 1254–1256.

60 *Pharmacopoeia of the People's Republic of China* (English edition). Chemical Industry Press, 2000.

61 Ko R. Adulterants in Asian patent medicines. *N Engl J Med* 1998; **339**: 847.

62 Au AM *et al*. Screening methods for drugs and heavy metals in Chinese patent medicines. *Bull Environ Contam Toxicol* 2000; **65**: 112–119.

63 Koh H-L, Woo S-O. Chinese Proprietary Medicine in Singapore: Regulatory control of toxic heavy metals and undeclared drugs. *Drug Safety* 2000; **23**: 351–362.

64 Huang WF *et al*. Adulteration by synthetic substances of traditional Chinese medicines in Taiwan. *J Clin Pharmacol* 1997; **37**: 344–350.

65 Singapore Ministry of Health Press Statement. Chinese Proprietary Medicine Found Adulterated with Sildenafil. 3 March 2001.

66 FDA Press Release. Anso Comfort Capsules Recalled by Distributor. 13 February 2001. www.fda.gov-USA

67 Lau KK *et al*. Phenytoin poisoning after using Chinese proprietary medicines. *Hum Exp Toxicol* 2000; **19**: 385–386.

68 FDA Press Release. State Health Director Warns Consumers about Prescription Drugs in Herbal Products. 15 February 2000. www.fda.gov-USA.

69 Medicines Control Agency. Hypoglycaemia following the use of Chinese herbal medicine Xiaoke Wan. *Curr Probl Pharmacovigilance* 2001; **27**: 8.

70 Wu M-S. Multiple tubular dysfunction induced by mixed Chinese herbal medicines containing cadmium. *Nephrol Dialysis Transplant* 1996; **11**: 867–870.

71 Schaumburg HH *et al*. Alopecia and sensory polyneuropathy from thallium in a Chinese herbal medication. *JAMA.* 1992; **268**: 3430–3431.

72 Kew J *et al*. Arsenic and mercury intoxication due to Indian ethnic remedies. *BMJ* 1993; **306**: 506–507.

73 Sheerin NS *et al*. Simultaneous exposure to lead, arsenic and mercury from Indian ethnic medicines. *Br J Clin Pharmacol* 1994; **48**: 332–333.

74 Cuncha J *et al*. Arsenic and acute lethal intoxication. *Hong Kong Pharm J* 1998; 7: 50–53.

75 EMEA Herbal Medicinal Products Working Party. Points to Consider on Good Agricultural and Collection Practice for Starting Materials of Herbal Origin. EMEA website: www.eudra.org/emea.html. October 2001.

76 World Health Organization. *Quality Control of Medicinal Plant Materials*. Geneva: World Health Organization, 1998.

77 *European Pharmacopoeia*, 4th edn. 2002. Strasbourg: Council of Europe, 2002.

78 Phillipson JD. Quality assurance of medicinal plants. In: Franz C *et al*. First World Congress on medicinal and aromatic plants for human welfare, WOCMAP, quality, phytochemistry, industrial aspects, economic aspects. *Acta Horticult* 1993; **333**: 117–122.

79 Houghton P. Establishing identification criteria for botanicals. *Drug Inform J* 1998; **32**: 461–469.

80 De Smet PAGM. Health risks of herbal remedies. *Drug Safety* 1995; **13**: 81–93.

81 De Smet PAGM. Adverse effects of herbal remedies. *Adverse Drug React Bull* 1997; **183**: 695–698.

82   Shaw D *et al*. Traditional remedies and food supplements. A 5-year toxicological study (1991–1995). *Drug Safety* 1997; **17**: 342–356.

83   Tisserand R, Balacs T. *Essential Oil Safety*. Edinburgh: Churchill Livingstone, 1995.

84   De Smet PAGM. Aristolochia species. In: *Adverse Effects of Herbal Drugs*, vol 1. Berlin: Springer Verlag, 1992.

85   D'Arcy PF. Adverse reactions and interactions with herbal medicines. Part 1. Adverse reactions. *Adverse Drug React Toxicol Rev* 1991; **10**: 189–208.

86   Mattocks AR. *Chemistry and Toxicology of Pyrrolizidine Alkaloids*. New York: Academic Press, 1986.

87   Anderson LA, Phillipson JD. Mistletoe – the magic herb. *Pharm J* 1982; **229**: 437–439.

88   Tyler VE. *The Honest Herbal*, 3rd edn. New York: Howarth Press, 1993.

89   Chandler RF *et al*. Controversial laetrile. *Pharm J* 1984; **232**: 330–332.

90   Statutory Instrument (SI) 1984:87. The Medicines (Cyanogenetic Substances) Order 1984.

91   Ljunggren B. Severe phototoxic burn following celery ingestion. *Arch Dermatol* 1990; **126**: 1334–1336.

92   Boffa MJ *et al*. Celery soup causing severe phototoxicity during PUVA therapy. *Br J Dermatol* 1996; **135**: 330–345.

93   Medicines Control Agency. *Psoralea corylifolia* fruit in Traditional Chinese Medicines causing severe skin reaction. *Curr Probl Pharmacovigilance* 2001; **27**: 12.

94   Baldwin CA *et al*. What pharmacists should know about ginseng. *Pharm J* 1986; **237**: 583–586.

95   Baldwin CA *et al*. What pharmacists should know about feverfew. *Pharm J* 1987; **239**: 237–238.

96   Roulet M *et al*. Hepatic veno-occlusive disease in newborn infant of a woman drinking herbal tea. *J Pediatr* 1988; **112**: 433–436.

97   Allen JR *et al*. Are herbal teas safe for infants and children. *Aust Family Physician* 1989; **18**: 1017–1019.

98   Ernst E. Herbal Medications for common ailments in the elderly. *Drugs Ageing* 1999; **15**: 423–428.

99   Mashour NH. Herbal medicine for the treatment of cardiovascular disease. *Arch Intern Med* 1998; **158**: 2225–2234.

100   Ang-lee MK *et al*. Herbal medicines and perioperative care. *JAMA* 2001; **286**: 208–216.

101   American Society of Anesthesiologists (ASA). www.asahq.org/PublicEducation/herbal.html. September 2001.

102   Ernst E. Possible interactions between synthetic and herbal medicinal products. *Perfusion* 2000; **13**: 4–15.

103   Fugh-Berman A. Herb–drug interactions. *Lancet* 2000; **355**: 134–138.

104   Miller L. Selected clinical considerations focusing on known and potential drug–herb interactions. *Arch Intern Med* 1998; **158**: 2200–2211.

105   Brown R. Potential interactions of herbal medicines with antipsychotics, antidepressants and hypnotics. *Eur J Herb Med* 1997; **3**: 25–28.

106   Boyle F. Herbal medicines can interfere with breast cancer treatment. *Med J Aust* 1997; **167**: 286.

107   Cheng TO. Herbal interactions with cardiac drugs. *Arch Intern Med* 2000; **160**: 870–871.

108   Anon. Grapefruit and drug effects. *Drugs Q* 1999; **3**: 25–28.

109   Barnes J *et al*. Different standards for reporting ADRs to herbal remedies and conventional OTC medicines: face-to-face interviews with 515 users of herbal remedies. *Br J Clin Pharmacol* 1998; **45**: 496–500.

110   Farah MH *et al*. International reporting of adverse health effects associated with herbal medicines. *Pharmacoepidemiol Drug Safety* 2000; **9**: 105–112.

111   Ernst E, Pittler MH. The efficacy of herbal drugs. In: *Herbal Medicine: a Concise Overview for Professionals*. London: Butterworth-Heinemann, 2000: 69–81.

112   Ernst E. The clinical efficacy of herbal treatments: an overview of recent systematic reviews. *Pharm J* 1999; **262**: 85–87.

113   Ernst E. Herbal medicines: where is the evidence? *BMJ* 2000; **321**: 395–396.

114   The Cochrane Library. http://www.update-software.com/cochrane/

115   Williamson EM. Synergy – myth or reality? In: *Herbal Medicine: a Concise Overview for Professionals*. London: Butterworth-Heinemann, 2000: 43–58.

116   Wurglics M *et al*. Comparison of German St John's Wort Products according to hyperforin and total hypericin content. *J Am Pharm Assoc* 2001; **41**: 560–566.

117   Bergonzi MC *et al*. Variability in the content of the constituents *of Hypericum perforatum* L. and some commercial extracts. *Drug Dev Indust Pharm* 2001; **26**: 491–497.

118   Melchart D *et al*. Echinacea for the prevention and treatment of the common cold (Cochrane review). *The Cochrane Library*, Issue 1, 2002. Oxford: Update Software.

General References

G1 American Herbal Pharmacopoeia and Therapeutic Compendium. Analytical, quality control and therapeutic monographs. Santa Cruz, California: American Herbal Pharmacopoeia, 1997–2002.

G2 Bisset NG, ed. *Herbal Drugs and Phytopharmaceuticals* (Wichtl M, ed., German edition). Stuttgart: Medpharm, 1994.

G3 Blumenthal M *et al.*, eds. *The Complete German Commission E Monographs*. Austin, Texas: American Botanical Council, 1998.

G4 Blumenthal M *et al.*, eds. *Herbal Medicine*. Expanded Commission E Monographs. Austin, Texas: American Botanical Council, 2000.

G5 Boon H, Smith M. *The Botanical Pharmacy*. The Pharmacology of 47 Common Herbs. Kingston: Quarry Press, 1999.

G6 Bradley PR, ed. *British Herbal Compendium*, vol 1. Bournemouth: British Herbal Medicine Association, 1992.

G7 *British Herbal Pharmacopoeia*. Keighley: British Herbal Medicine Association, 1983.

G8 *British Herbal Pharmacopoeia, 1990*, vol 1. Bournemouth: British Herbal Medicine Association, 1990.

G9 *British Herbal Pharmacopoeia, 1996*. Exeter: British Herbal Medicine Association, 1996

G10 *British Pharmaceutical Codex 1934*. London: Pharmaceutical Press, 1934.

G11 *British Pharmaceutical Codex 1949*. London: Pharmaceutical Press, 1949.

G12 *British Pharmaceutical Codex 1973*. London: Pharmaceutical Press, 1973.

G13 *British Pharmacopoeia 1993*. London: HMSO, 1993.

G14 *British Pharmacopoeia 1999*. London: The Stationery Office, 1999

G15 *British Pharmacopoeia 2001*. London: The Stationery Office, 2001.

G16 Council of Europe. *Flavouring Substances and Natural Sources of Flavourings*, 3rd edn. Strasbourg: Maisonneuve, 1981.

G17 Council of Europe. *Natural Sources of Flavourings*. Report No. 1. Strasbourg: Council of Europe, 2000.

G18 Cupp MJ, ed. *Toxicology and Clinical Pharmacology of Herbal Products*. Totawa, New Jersey: Humana Press, 2000.

G19 De Smet PAGM *et al.*, eds. *Adverse Effects of Herbal Drugs*, vol 1. Berlin: Springer-Verlag, 1992.

G20 De Smet PAGM *et al.*, eds. *Adverse Effects of Herbal Drugs*, vol 2. Berlin: Springer-Verlag, 1993.

G21 De Smet PAGM *et al.*, eds. *Adverse Effects of Herbal Drugs*, vol 3. Berlin: Springer-Verlag, 1997.

G22 Duke JA. *Handbook of Medicinal Herbs*. Boca Raton: CRC, 1985.

G23 European Medicines Evaluation Agency. Herbal Medicinal Products Working Party Draft Core Summary of Product Characteristics for Valerian and Ispaghula. http://www.eudra.org/emea.html (accessed 20 February 2002).

G24 *European Pharmacopoeia*, 2nd edn. Strasbourg: Maisonneuve, 1980.

G25 *European Pharmacopoeia*, 3rd edn. Strasbourg: Council of Europe, 1997.

G26 *European Pharmacopoeia*, 3rd edn, 1998 Supplement. Strasbourg: Council of Europe, 1998.

G27 *European Pharmacopoeia*, 3rd edn, 1999 Supplement. Strasbourg: Council of Europe, 1999.

G28 *European Pharmacopoeia*, 4th edn, 2002. Strasbourg: Council of Europe, 2002.

G29 Evans WC. *Trease and Evans' Pharmacognosy*, 14th edn. London: WB Saunders Company, 1998.

G30 Farnsworth NR. Potential value of plants as sources of new antifertility agents I. *J Pharm Sci* 1975; **64**: 535–598.

G31 Fetrow CW, Avila JR. *Professional's Handbook of Complementary and Alternative Medicines*. Springhouse: Springhouse Corporation, 1999.

G32 Foster S, Tyler VE. *Tyler's Honest Herbal*, 4th edn. New York: The Haworth Herbal Press, 1999.

G33 Frohne D, Pfänder HJ. *A Colour Atlas of Poisonous Plants*. London: Wolfe, 1984.

G34 Grieve M. *A Modern Herbal*. Thetford, Norfolk: Lowe and Brydon, 1979.

G35 Gruenwald J *et al.*, eds. *PDR for Herbal Medicines*, 1st edn. Montvale: Medical Economics Company, 1998.

G36 Gruenwald J *et al.*, eds. *PDR for Herbal Medicines*, 2nd edn. Montvale: Medical Economics Company Inc, 2000.

G37 The Medicines (Products other than Veterinary Drugs) (General Sales List), SI No.769: 1984, as amended SI No.1540: 1985; SI No.1129: 1990; and SI No.2410: 1994.

G38 Guenther E. *The Essential Oils*, six volumes. New York: Van Nostrand, 1948–1952.

G39 Hamon NW, Blackburn JL. *Herbal Products – A Factual Appraisal for the Health Care Professional*. Winnipeg: Cantext, 1985.

G40 Hoppe HA. *Taschenbuch der Drogenkunde*. Berlin: de Gruyter, 1981.

G41 Leung AY. *Encyclopedia of Common Natural Ingredients Used in Food, Drugs and Cosmetics*. New York-Chichester: Wiley, 1980.

G42 Mabey R., ed. *The Complete New Herbal*. London: Elm Tree Books, 1988.

G43 *Martindale. The Complete Drug Reference*, 32nd edn. (Parfitt K, ed.). London: The Pharmaceutical Press, 1999.

G44 *Martindale: The Extra Pharmacopoeia*, 28th edn. (Reynolds JEF, ed.). London: The Pharmaceutical Press, 1982.

G45 *Martindale: The Extra Pharmacopoeia*, 29th edn. (Reynolds JEF, ed.). London: The Pharmaceutical Press, 1989.

G46 *Martindale, The Extra Pharmacopoeia*: 30th edn. (Reynolds JEF, ed.). London: The Pharmaceutical Press, 1993.

G47 *Martindale. The Extra Pharmacopoeia*, 31st edn. (Reynolds JEF, ed.). London: The Pharmaceutical Press, 1996.

G48 *The Merck Index. An Encyclopedia of Chemicals, Drugs and Biologicals*, 11th edn. Rahway, NJ: Merck, 1989.

G49 Mills SY. *The Dictionary of Modern Herbalism*. Wellingborough: Thorsons, 1985.

G50 Mills S, Bone K. *Principles and Practice of Phytotherapy*. Edinburgh: Churchill Livingstone, 2000.

G51 Mitchell J, Rook A. *Botanical Dermatology – Plants and Plant Products Injurious to the Skin*. Vancouver: Greengrass, 1979.

G52 *Monographs on the Medicinal Uses of Plant Drugs*, Fascicules 1 and 2 (1996), Fascicules 3, 4 and 5 (1997), Fascicule 6 (1999). Exeter: European Scientific Cooperative on Phytotherapy.

G53 Morelli I *et al. Selected Medicinal Plants*. Rome: FAO, 1983.

G54 Robbers JE, Tyler VE. *Tyler's Herbs of Choice*. New York: The Haworth Herbal Press, 1999.

G55 Schulz V, Hänsel R, Tyler V. *Rational Phytotherapy. A Physicians' Guide to Herbal Medicine*. Berlin: Springer-Verlag, 1998.

G56 Schulz V, Hänsel R, Tyler V. *Rational Phytotherapy. A Physicians' Guide to Herbal Medicine*, 4th edn. Berlin: Springer-Verlag, 2000.

G57 Simon JE *et al. Herbs – An Indexed Bibliography, 1971–80*. Oxford: Elsevier, 1984.

G58 Tisserand R, Balacs T. *Essential Oil Safety*. Edinburgh: Churchill Livingstone, 1995.

G59 Trease GE, Evans WC. *Pharmacognosy*, 13th edn. London: Baillière Tindall, 1989.

G60 Tyler VE. *The Honest Herbal*, 3rd edn. Philadelphia: Strickley, 1993.

G61 *United States Pharmacopeia 24 and National Formulary 19 and Supplements*. Rockville, Maryland, US: United States Pharmacopeial Convention, 2000

G62 Wagner H *et al. Plant Drug Analysis*. Berlin: Springer-Verlag, 1983.

G63 World Health Organization. *WHO Monographs on Selected Medicinal Plants*, vol 1. Geneva: World Health Organization, 1999.

G64 Wren RC. *Potter's New Cyclopedia of Botanical Drugs and Preparations* (revised, Williamson EW, Evans FJ). Saffron Walden: Daniel, 1988.

G65 www.cfsan.fda.gov/~dms/eafus.html (US Food and Drug Administration)

Agnus Castus

Species (Family)

Vitex agnus-castus L. (Verbenaceae)

Synonym(s)

Chasteberry, Chaste Tree, Monk's Pepper

Part(s) Used

Fruit

Pharmacopoeial and Other Monographs

American Herbal Pharmacopoeia[G1]
BHP 1996[G9]
Complete German Commission E[G3]
ESCOP 1997[G52]
Martindale 32nd edition[G43]
Mills and Bone [G50]
PDR for Herbal Medicines 2nd edition[G36]

Legal Category (Licensed Products)

GSL[G37]

Constituents[G40]

Alkaloids Viticin

Diterpenes Rotundifuran (labdane-type), vitexilacton and 6β,7β-diacetoxy-13-hydroxy-labda-8,14-diene.[1]

Flavonoids Flavonol (kaempferol, quercetagetin) derivatives, the major constituent being casticin. Other identified flavonoids include penduletin and chrysophanol D.[2–4]

Iridoids In the leaf: 0.3% aucubin, 0.6% its *p*-hydroxybenzoyl derivative agnuside and 0.07% unidentified glycosides.[3,5]

Other constituents Fatty acids, including stearic and palmitic, volatile oil 0.5% with cineol and pinene as main components; castine (a bitter principle).[6,7]

Food Use

Agnus castus is not used in foods.

Herbal Use

Traditionally, agnus castus has been used for menstrual problems resulting from corpus luteum deficiency, including premenstrual symptoms and spasmodic dysmenorrhoea, for certain menopausal conditions, and for insufficient lactation.[G4,G49] The German Commission E approved it for internal use for irregularities of the menstrual cycle, premenstrual complaints and mastodynia.[G3]

Dosage

Fruit 0.5–1.0 g three times daily;[G49] by contrast, 30–40 mg daily of crushed fruit.[G3]

Tincture 1 : 5 (g/mL), 50–70% ethanol (v/v) 0.15–0.2 mL.[G4]

Pharmacological Actions

In vitro and animal studies

Agnus castus does not contain any oestrogenic constituents but has been reported to diminish release of follicle-stimulating hormone from the anterior pituitary whilst increasing the release of luteinising hormone and prolactin.[8,9]

Extracts of agnus castus act at dopamine receptors and affect prolactin release. Dopamine D_2-receptor binding of extracts has been demonstrated for three different dopamine receptors (rat striatum, calf striatum and human recombinant receptors) and for two separate ligands (sulpiridine and spiroperidol).[1,10,11] The active compounds acted as dopamine agonists and were characterised as labdane diterpenes. The two most active diterpenes, rotundifuran and 6β,7β-diacetoxy-13-hydroxy-labda-8,14-diene, had IC_{50} values (calf striatum preparation, ^{3}H-spiroperidol ligand) of 45 µg/mL (124 nmol/mL) and 79 µg/mL (194 nmol/mL), respectively.[11] A lyophilised extract of agnus castus (5 mg/mL) was similar in activity to 10^{-4} mol/L dopamine in receptor–ligand binding assays, displacing ^{3}H-spiroperidol from calf brain striatal preparations.[10]

An extract of agnus castus inhibited release of acetylcholine from ^{3}H-choline loaded rat brain striatal cells on electrical stimulation, and had an IC_{50} value of 30 µg/mL.[11]

Hexane fractions of agnus castus bind to human opiate receptors with IC$_{50}$ values of 20 µg/mL (µ-receptors) and 10 µg/mL (κ-receptors).[12]

Agnus castus extracts and fractions dose-dependently stimulated galactosidase activity in yeast cells; this may be indicative of oestrogen-receptor binding. Radioligand–receptor binding assays have demonstrated that agnus castus only binds weakly to oestrogen receptors in comparison to dopamine receptor binding.[12]

Clinical studies

A proprietary preparation containing an alcoholic extract of agnus castus (0.2% w/w) has been available in Germany since the 1950s. It is used in the treatment of breast disease and pain, ovarian insufficiency, and dysfunctional uterine bleeding.[8,13–17] The clinical effects of agnus castus have been reviewed.[18,19] Details of clinical studies described in these reviews are summarised below.

Effects on prolactin secretion   Several open, uncontrolled studies involving small numbers of women with fertility disorders, hyperprolactinaemia and menstrual disorders have explored the effects of treatment with extracts of agnus castus (e.g. Mastodynon and Agnucaston; Bionorica), generally at doses equivalent to 30–40 mg drug for several months. These studies report decreased prolactin concentrations at the end of treatment, compared with baseline values.[18,19]

A double-blind, placebo-controlled study involving women with cyclic mastalgia compared the effects of Mastodynon tablets ($n = 32$) and Mastodynon solution ($n = 31$) with those of placebo ($n = 38$) over three menstrual cycles. Prolactin concentrations in the two treated groups were significantly reduced, compared with those in the placebo group.

Other studies have reported that women with normal basal prolactin concentrations do not experience significant reduction in the concentration following treatment with agnus castus.

In a double-blind, placebo-controlled trial, 37 women with deficiencies in corpus luteal phase and latent hyperprolactinaemia received an agnus castus preparation ($n = 17$) or placebo ($n = 20$) for three menstrual cycles. In the treated group, the luteal phase was extended to 10.5 days from an initial 3.4–5.5 days.

The effects of agnus castus have also been investigated in men. In an open, uncontrolled study, 20 healthy men were given a commercial preparation of agnus castus extract (BP 1095E1) at doses ranging from 120 to 480 mg extract (3–12 times higher than doses used in women) for 14 days.[20] The lowest

dose was reported to increase serum prolactin concentrations, whereas the higher dose decreased prolactin concentrations.

Effects on mastodynia   In an open, uncontrolled trial, 825 women with mastodynia received Mastodynon for three months. At the end of the study, 465 patients (56%) said they were symptom-free, and a further 198 patients (24%) reported that their symptoms had improved. A subsequent trial involving 121 women reported that 75% of participants experienced relief of symptoms.

In a randomised, double-blind, placebo-controlled study, 104 patients with breast pain were treated for three menstrual cycles with either Mastodynon solution ($n = 34$), tablets ($n = 32$) or placebo ($n = 38$). Patients in both treated groups claimed to have reduced breast pain; the findings were reported to be statistically significant for treatment, compared with placebo.

Another randomised, double-blind, placebo-controlled trial involving 97 patients with cyclic mastalgia compared Mastodynon solution ($n = 48$) with placebo ($n = 49$).[21] After two menstrual cycles, pain intensity, as assessed by visual analogue scale (VAS) scores was reduced in both groups; the reduction was significantly greater in the agnus castus group ($p = 0.006$). However, at the end of the study (after three cycles), the reduction in pain intensity between the two groups was no longer statistically significant ($p = 0.064$). It was reported that Mastodynon was well-tolerated.

Effects on premenstrual syndrome   Five postmarketing surveillance studies involving more than 5000 women have monitored the effects of agnus castus preparations in premenstrual syndrome (PMS).[19]

A randomised, double-blind, controlled trial involving 175 women with PMS compared Agnolyt (Madaus) one capsule daily (equivalent to 3.5–4.2 mg dry extract) ($n = 90$) and pyridoxine two capsules daily ($n = 85$) over three menstrual cycles.

Therapeutic response was measured using a premenstrual tension scale (self-assessment) and a clinical global impression (CGI) scale (physician assessment). Reductions in PMS scale scores (of around 48%) were reported for both groups.[22] It was concluded that the two treatments were equally effective in the treatment of symptoms of PMS.

In a randomised, double-blind, placebo-controlled, parallel-group trial, 170 women with PMS received agnus castus extract ZE 440 (60% ethanol, extract ratio 6 to 12 : 1; standardised for casticin) 20 mg daily ($n = 86$) or placebo ($n = 84$) for three menstrual cycles.[23] The main outcome measure was the participant's self-assessment of PMS symptoms (irritability, mood alteration, anger, headache, breast fullness and bloating). At the end of the third cycle, improvements in the PMS symptoms were significantly greater in the agnus castus group, compared with the placebo group ($p < 0.001$). Clinical global impression scores for severity of condition, global improvement and overall risk/benefit were also significantly better for agnus castus, compared with placebo ($p < 0.001$). Mild adverse events were reported by four agnus castus recipients and three placebo recipients. All resolved without treatment. It was concluded that agnus castus dry extract is an effective and well-tolerated treatment for symptoms of PMS.[23]

Agnus castus has also been reported to be effective in the treatment of endocrine disorders such as menstrual neuroses and dermatoses [24] and has been used for the treatment of acne.[25,26]

A lactogenic action has been documented for agnus castus;[27] chemical analysis of the breast milk revealed no changes in composition.

The precise mode of action of agnus castus and the active constituents has not been established. However, it is thought to act on the pituitary–hypothalamic axis rather than directly on the ovaries.

Side-effects, Toxicity

Agnus castus is generally well-tolerated, although allergic reactions (which resolved following discontinuation of agnus castus therapy), headaches and an increase in menstrual flow have been reported.[8,24]

Contra-indications, Warnings

Agnus castus has dopaminergic activity and should not be used with dopamine receptor antagonists or agonists.

Pregnancy and lactation In view of the documented pharmacological actions and lack of toxicity data, the use of agnus castus during pregnancy should be avoided. Agnus castus has been reported to stimulate milk secretion without altering the composition of the breast milk.[24,27] Nevertheless, agnus castus should be avoided during lactation until further information is available.

Pharmaceutical Comment

The chemistry and pharmacology of agnus castus are well-documented. There is clinical evidence indicating that raised prolactin concentrations are reduced following agnus castus treatment, and that there are beneficial effects in mastodynia and in symptoms of PMS.

References

See also General References G1, G3, G5, G9, G31, G36, G40, G43, G49 and G50.

1 Hoberg E *et al.* Diterpene aus agni-casti fructus und ihre analytik. *Z Phytother* 1999; **20**: 140–158.

2 Belic I *et al.* Constituents of *Vitex agnus castus* seeds. Part 1. Casticin. *J Chem Soc* 1961; 2523–2525.

3 Gomaa CS *et al.* Flavonoids and iridoids from *Vitex agnus castus*. *Planta Med* 1978; **33**: 277.

4 Wollenweber E, Mann K. Flavonols from fruits of *Vitex agnus castus*. *Planta Med* 1983; **48**: 126–127.

5 Rimpler H. Verbenaceae. Iridoids and ecdysones from *Vitex* species. *Phytochemistry* 1972; **11**: 2653–2654.

6 Kustrak D *et al.* The composition of the volatile oil of *Vitex agnus castus*. *Planta Med* 1992; **58**(Suppl.1): A681.

7 Zwaving JH, Bos R. Composition of the essential fruit oil of *Vitex agnus castus*. *Pharm World Sci* 1993; **15**(Suppl.H): H15.

8 Houghton PJ. Agnus castus. *Pharm J* 1994; **253**: 720–721.

9 Amann W. Umkehrung der pharmakologischen wirkung von *Agnus castus* bei niedriger dosierung. (Gleichzeitig ein beitrag zur endokrinologie der sexualhormone). *Z Forsch Praxis Fortbildung (Med)* 1966; **7**: 229–233.

10 Jarry H *et al.* Auf der suche nach dopaminergen substanzen in agni-casti-fructus-präparaten: warum eigentlich? *Z Phytother* 1999; **20**: 140–158.

11 Berger D *et al.* Rezeptorbindungsstudien mit extrakten und daraus isolierten substanzen. *Z Phytother* 1999; **20**: 140–158.

12 Brugisser R *et al.* Untersuchungen an opioid-rezeptoren mit *Vitex agnus-castus* L. *Z Phytother* 1999; **20**: 140–158.

13 Amann W. Prämenstruelle Wasserretention. Günstige wirkung von *Agnus castus* (Agnolyt[R]) auf prämenstruelle wasserretention. *Z Allg Med* 1979; **55**: 48–51.

14 Amann W. Das 'prämenstruelle syndrom' hat viele gesichter. Häufig bringt schon die gezielte anamnese aufschluss. *Arztl Praxis* 1979; **31**: 3091–3092.

15 Amann W. Amenorrhoe. Günstige wirkung von *Agnus castus* (Agnolyt[R]) auf amenorrhoea. *Z Allg Med* 1982; **58**: 228–231.

16 Turner S, Mills S. A double-blind clinical trial on a herbal remedy for premenstrual syndrome; a case study. *Complementary Ther Med* 1993; **1**: 73–77.

17 Milewicz A *et al. Vitex agnus castus* extract in the

treatment of luteal phase defects due to latent hyperprolactinaemia. Results of a randomized placebo-controlled double blind study. *ArzneimittelForsch* 1993; **43**: 752–756.

18 Gorkow C. Klinischer Kenntnisstand von agnicasti fructus-Klinisch-pharmakologische untersuchungen und wirksamkeitsbelege. *Z Phytother* 1999; **20**: 159–168.

19 Gorkow C *et al*. Evidence of efficacy of *Vitex agnus castus* preparations. In: Loew D, Blume H, Dingermann TH, eds. *Phytopharmaka V, Forschung und Klinische Anwendung*. Darmstadt: Steinkopf Verlag, 1999: 189–208.

20 Merz PG *et al*. The effects of a special *Agnus castus* (BP1095E1) on prolactin secretion in healthy male subjects. *Exp Clin Endrocrinol Diabetes* 1996; **104**: 447–453.

21 Halaška M *et al*. Treatment of cyclical mastalgia with a solution containing a *Vitex agnus castus* extract: results of a placebo-controlled double-blind study. *The Breast* 1999; **8**: 175.

22 Lauritzen CH *et al*. Treatment of premenstrual tension syndrome with *Vitex agnus castus* – Controlled, double-blind study versus pyridoxine. *Phytomedicine* 1997; **4**: 183–189.

23 Schellenberg R. Treatment for the premenstrual syndrome with agnus castus fruit extract: prospective, randomised, placebo controlled study. *BMJ* 2001; **322**: 134–137.

24 Kartnig T. *Vitex agnus-castus* – Mönchspfeffer oder Keuschlamm. Ein arzeipflanze mit indirektluteotroper wirkung. *Z Phytother* 1986; **7**: 119–122.

25 Amann W. Akne vulgaris und *Agnus castus* (Agnolyt[R]). *Z Allg Med* 1975; **51**: 1645–1648.

26 Amann W. Ist die acne vulgaris eine psychosomatische erkrankung? Versuch einer klärung: Der psychosomatische aspekt der acne vulgaris. *Artzliche Kosmetol* 1984; **14**: 162–170.

27 Bruckner C. In mitteleuropa genutzte heilpflanzen mit milchsekretionsfördernder wirkung (galactagoga). *Gleditschia* 1989; **17**: 189–201.

Agrimony

Species (Family)

Agrimonia eupatoria L. (Rosaceae)

Synonym(s)

Agrimonia

Part(s) Used

Herb

Pharmacopoeial and Other Monographs

BHP 1996 [G9]
Complete German Commission E[G3]
PDR for Herbal Medicines 2nd edition[G36]

Legal Category (Licensed Products)

GSL[G37]

Constituents[1,2,G2,G22,G31,G40,G64]

Acids Palmitic acid, salicylic acid, silicic acid and stearic acid.

Flavonoids Apigenin, luteolin, luteolin-7-glucoside, quercetin, quercitrin, kaempferol and glycosides.[3]

Tannins 3–21%. Condensed tannins in herb; hydrolysable tannins (e.g. ellagitannin).

Vitamins Ascorbic acid (vitamin C), nicotinamide complex (about 100–300 µg/g leaf), thiamine (about 2 µg/g leaf) and vitamin K.

Other constituents Bitter principle, triterpenes (e.g. α-amyrin, ursolic acid, euscapic acid), phytosterols and volatile oil 0.2%.

Food Use

Agrimony is listed by the Council of Europe as a natural source of food flavouring (category N2). This category indicates that agrimony can be added to foodstuffs in small quantities, with a possible limitation of an active principle (as yet unspecified) in the final product.[G16]

Herbal Use

Agrimony is stated to possess mild astringent and diuretic properties.[1] It has been used for diarrhoea in children, mucous colitis, grumbling appendicitis, urinary incontinence, cystitis, and as a gargle for acute sore throat and chronic nasopharyngeal catarrh.[G2,G7]

Dosage

Dried herb 2–4 g by infusion three times daily.[G7]

Liquid extract 1–3 mL (1 : 1 in 25% alcohol) three times daily.[G7]

Tincture 1–4 mL (1 : 5 in 45% alcohol) three times daily.[G7]

Pharmacological Actions

In vitro and animal studies

Significant uricolytic activity has been documented for agrimony infusions and decoctions (15% w/v), following their oral administration to male rats at a dose of 20 mL/kg body weight (equivalent to 3 g dry drug).[4] Diuretic activity was stated to be minimal and elimination of urea unchanged. A hypotensive effect in anaesthetised cats has been documented for an agrimony extract given by intravenous injection; blood pressure was lowered by more than 40%.[5]

Marked antibacterial activity against *Staphylococcus aureus* and α-haemolytic streptococci has been reported for agrimony.[6]

An aqueous ethanol extract of the herb was tested for immunomodulative activity in the peritoneal cavities of mice.[7] Immunostimulant activity resulted in an increase in phagocytic activity and increases in the activities of lysozyme and peroxidase. *Agrimonia eupatoria* given in the diet of mice for 12 days prior to intraperitoneal administration of streptozotocin resulted in a reduction in hyperglycaemia.[8] Further investigation revealed stimulation of 2-deoxyglucose transport, glucose oxidation and incorporation of glucose into glycogen in mouse abdominal muscle. An aqueous extract (0.25–1 mg/mL) stimulated insulin secretion from a BRIN-BD11 pancreatic B cell line.[9] These findings demonstrate that *A. eupatoria* aqueous extract given orally to mice has antihyperglycaemic, insulin-releasing and insulin-like activity.[9]

A related species, *A. pilosa*, has also been investigated. *In vivo* antitumour activity in mice has been attributed to the tannin agrimoniin[10] which has not been reported as a constituent of *A. eupatoria*. Agrimoniin was administered intraperitoneally into ascites-type and solid tumours in rodents.[11] At doses of greater than 10 mg/kg, given before or after intraperitoneal inoculation with MM2 cells, it completely rejected tumour growth in mice.[11] Solid tumours of MH134 and Meth-A were inhibited by agrimoniin, and the number of peripheral blood cells was increased, indicating that agrimoniin has antitumour activity and that it exerts its effect by enhancing the immune response. *In vitro* studies have reported that agrimoniin induces the cytotoxicity of murine peritoneal exudate cells,[12] and that it induces interleukin 1 in human peripheral blood mononuclear cells and in mouse adherent peritoneal exudate cells *in vivo*.[13] Several phloroglucinols isolated from *A. pilosa* have demonstrated activity against *Staphylococcus aureus*,[14] and a methanol extract of the herb inhibited HIV-1 protease activity.[15] An aqueous suspension of *A. pilosa* herb (1 mg/kg and 5 mg/kg) given orally or intraperitoneally significantly reduced blood glucose concentrations in streptozotocin-induced diabetic rats.[16]

Clinical studies
The successful treatment of cutaneous porphyria in a group of 20 patients receiving agrimony infusions has been described.[17] An improvement in skin eruptions together with a decrease in serum iron concentrations and in urinary porphyrins was noted.

A compound herb preparation containing agrimony has been used to treat 35 patients suffering from chronic gastroduodenitis.[18] After 25 days of therapy, 75% of patients claimed to be free from pain, 95% from dyspeptic symptoms and 76% from palpitation pains. Gastroscopy was said to indicate that previous erosion and haemorrhagic mucous changes had healed. No side-effects or signs of toxicity were documented.

Side-effects, Toxicity
None documented for *A. eupatoria*. A polar fraction containing flavonoids and triterpenes, but not tannins, produced a negative result in the Ames test.[1]

In mice, agrimoniin has been documented to cause stretching and writhing reactions when administered by intraperitoneal injection, and cyanosis and necrosis at the site of intravenous injection.[11] These reactions were considered to be inflammatory reactions. The LD_{50} of agrimoniin in mice has been estimated as 33 mg/kg (by intravenous injection), 101 mg/kg (by intraperitoneal injection), and greater than 1 g/kg (by mouth).[11] Cytotoxic activity has been reported for *A. pilosa*[10] (*see In vitro and animal studies*).

Contra-indications, Warnings

Excessive doses may interfere with existing drug treatment for high or low blood pressure, and anticoagulant therapy. In view of the tannin constituents, excessive use should be avoided.

Pregnancy and lactation Agrimony is reputed to affect the menstrual cycle.[G22] In view of the lack of toxicity data, excessive use of agrimony should be avoided during pregnancy and lactation.

Pharmaceutical Comment

Relatively limited information is available on the chemistry of agrimony, although more is known about the tannin constituents of the related species *A. pilosa*. Human studies have indicated that agrimony may be useful in the treatment of certain cutaneous and gastrointestinal disorders, although further studies are needed to confirm these reports. The tannin constituents may justify the astringent activity attributed to the herb. In view of the lack of toxicity data, excessive use of agrimony should be avoided.

References

See also General References G2, G3, G9, G16, G22, G31, G36, G37, G40, G42 and G64.

1 Bilia AR *et al*. Constituents and biological assay of *Agrimonia eupatoria*. *Fitoterapia* 1993; **64**: 549–550.
2 Carnat A *et al*. L'aigremoine: étude comparée d'*Agrimonia eupatoria* L. et *Agrimonia procera* Wallr. *Plantes médicinales et phytothérapie* 1991; **25**: 202–211.
3 Sendra J, Zieba J. Flavonoids from *Agrimonia eupatoria* L. *Diss Pharm Pharmacol* 1971; **24**: 79–83.
4 Giachetti D *et al*. Ricerche sull'attivita diuretica ed uricosurica di *Agrimonia eupatoria*. *Boll Soc Ital Biol Sper* 1986; **62**: 705–711.
5 Petkov V. Plants with hypotensive, antiatheromatous and coronarodilatating action. *Am J Chin Med* 1979; **7**: 197–236.
6 Petkov V. Bulgarian traditional medicine: A source of ideas for phytopharmacological investigations. *J Ethnopharmacol* 1986; **15**: 121–132.
7 Bukovsky M, Blanárik P. Immunomodulative

effects of ethanolic-aqueous extracts of herba Agrimoniae, flos Chamomillae and flos Calendulae cum calyce. *Farmaceutiky Obzor* 1994; **63**: 149–156.

8 Swanston-Flatt SK *et al*. Traditional plant treatments for diabetes in normal and streptozotocin diabetic rats. *Diabetologia* 1990; **33**: 462–464.

9 Gray AM, Flatt PR. Actions of the traditional antidiabetic plant, *Agrimonia eupatoria* (agrimony): effects on hyperglycaemia, cellular glucose metabolism and insulin secretion. *Br J Nutr* 1998; **80**: 109–114.

10 Miyamoto K *et al*. Isolation of agrimoniin, an antitumour constituent, from the roots of *Agrimonia pilosa* Ledeb. *Chem Pharm Bull (Tokyo)* 1985; **33**: 3977–3981.

11 Miyamoto K *et al*. Antitumour effect of agrimoniin, a tannin of *Agrimonia pilosa* Ledeb., on transplantable rodent tumors. *Jpn J Pharmacol* 1987; **43**: 187–195.

12 Miyamoto K *et al*. Induction of cytotoxicity of peritoneal exudate cells by agrimoniin, a novel immunomodulatory tannin of *Agrimonia pilosa* Ledeb. *Cancer Immunol Immunother* 1988; **27**: 59–62.

13 Murayama T *et al*. Agrimoniin, an antitumour tannin of *Agrimonia pilosa* Ledeb., induces interleukin-1. *Anticancer Res* 1992; **12**: 1471–1474.

14 Yamaki M *et al*. Antimicrobial activity of naturally occurring and synthetic phloroglucinols against *Staphylococcus aureus*. *Phytother Res* 1994; **8**: 112–114.

15 Min BS *et al*. Screening of Korean plants against human immunodeficiency virus type 1 protease. *Phytother Res* 1999; **13**: 680–682.

16 Hsu F-L, Cheng J-T. Investigation in rats of the antihyperglycaemic effect of plant extracts used in Taiwan for the treatment of diabetes mellitus. *Phytother Res* 1992; **6**: 108–111.

17 Patrascu V *et al*. Rezultate terapeutice favorabile in porfiria cutanata cu *Agrimonia eupatoria*. *Dermato-venerologia* 1984; **29**: 153–157.

18 Chakarski I *et al*. Clinical study of a herb combination consisting of *Agrimonia eupatoria*, *Hipericum perforatum*, *Plantago major*, *Mentha piperita*, *Matricaria chamomila* for the treatment of patients with chronic gastroduodenitis. *Probl Vatr Med* 1982; **10**: 78–84.

Alfalfa

Species (Family)

Medicago sativa L. (Fabaceae/Leguminosae)

Synonym(s)

Lucerne, Medicago, Purple Medick

Part(s) Used

Herb

Pharmacopoeial and Other Monographs

BHP 1996[G9]
Martindale 32nd edition [G43]
PDR for Herbal Medicines 2nd edition[G36]

Legal Category (Licensed Products)

GSL[G37]

Constituents[G19,G22,G41,G64]

Acids Lauric acid, maleic acid, malic acid, malonic acid, myristic acid, oxalic acid, palmitic acid and quinic acid.

Alkaloids Pyrrolidine-type (e.g. stachydrine, homostachydrine); pyridine-type (e.g. trigonelline) in the seeds only.

Amino acids Arginine, asparagine (high concentration in seeds), cystine, histidine, isoleucine, leucine, lysine, methionine, phenylalanine, threonine, tryptophan and valine. The non-protein toxic amino acid canavanine is present in leaves (0.9–1.2 mg/g), stems (0.6–0.9 mg/g) and seeds (5–14 mg/g).[G19]

Coumarins Medicagol.

Isoflavonoids Coumestrol, biochanin A, daidzein, formononetin and genistein.

Saponins 2–3%. Hydrolysis yields aglycones, medicagenic acid, soyasapogenols A–F and hederagenin.[1] Sugar chain components include arabinose, galactose, glucuronic acid, glucose, rhamnose and xylose.

Steroids Campesterol, cycloartenol, β-sitosterol (major component), α-spinasterol and stigmasterol.

Other constituents Carbohydrates (e.g. arabinose, fructose, sucrose, xylose), vitamins (A, B_1, B_6, B_{12}, C, E, K), pectin methylesterase, pigments (e.g. chlorophyll, xanthophyll, β-carotene, anthocyanins), proteins, minerals and trace elements.

See reference G22 for more detailed chemical information.

Food Use

Alfalfa is widely used in foods and is listed by the Council of Europe as a source of natural food flavouring (categories N2 and N3). These categories indicate that alfalfa can be added to foodstuffs in small quantities, with a possible limitation of an active principle (as yet unspecified) in the final product.[G16] In the USA, alfalfa is listed as GRAS (Generally Recognised As Safe).[G41]

Herbal Use

The herb was not valued by ancient civilisations and is not detailed in classical herbals. Herbal use probably developed in the USA where claims have been made for it in the treatment of arthritis, high cholesterol, diabetes and peptic ulcers.[2,G19,G32] Reputedly, the herb has bactericidal, cardiotonic, diuretic, emetic, emmenagogue and oestrogenic properties.[2] Commercial preparations including teas, tablets and capsules are available.[G19] Alfalfa is stated to be a source of vitamins A, C, E and K, and of the minerals calcium, potassium, phosphorus and iron. It has been used for avitaminosis A, C, E or K, hypoprothrombinaemic purpura, and debility of convalescence.[G7,G64]

Dosage

Dried herb 5–10 g as an infusion three times daily.[G7]

Liquid extract 5–10 mL (1:1 in 25% alcohol) three times daily.[G7]

Pharmacological Actions

In vitro and animal studies

Alfalfa top (stem and leaves) saponins have been reported to decrease plasma cholesterol concentrations without changing high-density lipoprotein (HDL) cholesterol concentrations, decrease intestinal absorption of cholesterol, increase excretion of neutral steroids and bile acids, prevent atherosclerosis and induce the regression of atherosclerosis.[3]

Hypocholesterolaemic activity has been reported for root saponins, when given to monkeys receiving a high-cholesterol diet.[4] Alfalfa herb fed to monkeys reduced hypercholesterolaemia and atherosclerosis; the effect may be partially due to the saponin constituents.[G19] In mice fed with alfalfa (6.25% of diet) for 12 days before administration of streptozotocin, hyperglycaemia was reduced compared with values for control animals.[5]

Oestrogenic activity in ruminants has been documented for coumestrol and the isoflavone constituents.[G22,G41]

An investigation into the effect of various herbs on hepatic drug metabolising enzymes in the rat, showed that alfalfa potentiated the activity of aminopyrine N-demethylase but had no effect on glutathione S-transferase or epoxide hydrolase activities.[6]

The seeds are reported to contain trypsin inhibitors.[G41] Saponins isolated from the aerial parts have been reported to stimulate the lipolytic activity of neopancreatinum (a mixture of porcine pancreatic enzymes including lipase, amylase and proteases).[7]

Alfalfa root saponins have been documented to exhibit selective toxicity towards fungi.[1,8,9] A medicagenic acid glycoside with low haemolytic activity, isolated from alfalfa root, was found to exhibit both strong inhibitory and fungitoxic activities towards several medically important yeasts including *Candida* species, *Torulopsis* species, *Geotrichum canadidum* and *Rhodotorula glutinis*.[8] It has been proposed that the antimycotic activity of alfalfa saponins is related to their ability to complex steroids and that fungi sensitive to the saponins may contain relatively more steroids in their membranes.[8] Antifungal properties have also been documented for medicago.[G41]

The saponin constituents are documented to be haemolytic and to interfere with vitamin E utilisation, and are believed to be one of the causes of ruminant bloat.[G41] Haemolytic activity is associated with the medicagenic acid glycosides and not the hederagenin and soyasapogenol glycosides.

The effects of polysaccharides from medicago on mice lymphocytes *in vitro* indicated immunopotentiating activity.[10]

Clinical studies

In a short-term study involving three normolipidaemic individuals given alfalfa seeds (80–60 g daily), serum cholesterol concentrations were reported to be reduced.[G19] In another small study in which heat-treated alfalfa seeds (40 g three times daily for eight weeks) were taken by eight type-IIA hyperlipoproteinaemic patients and three type IIB patients, a significant decrease was noted in total serum cholesterol concentrations, low-density lipoprotein (LDL) cholesterol and apolipoprotein B. The LDL cholesterol concentration fell by less than 5% in two of the 11 patients.[11]

The manganese content of alfalfa (45.5 mg/kg) is reported to be the active principle responsible for a hypoglycaemic effect documented for the herb.[12] A diabetic patient, treated with soluble insulin but poorly controlled, found that an alfalfa extract adequately controlled his diabetes. When administered separately, only small doses of manganese chloride (5–10 mg) were required to have a hypoglycaemic effect. However, no effect was seen on the blood sugar concentrations of non-diabetic controls or of other diabetic patients, who were also administered manganese. It was concluded that manganese lowered the blood sugar concentration in this particular diabetic patient because he was unable to utilise manganese stored in his body.[12]

Side-effects, Toxicity

Both alfalfa seed and herb have been reported to induce a systemic lupus erythematosus (SLE)-like syndrome in female monkeys.[3,13,G19,G32] This activity has been attributed to canavanine, a non-protein amino acid constituent which has been found to have effects on human immunoregulatory cells *in vitro*.[14] Reactivation of quiescent SLE in humans has been associated with the ingestion of alfalfa tablets which, following analysis, were found to contain canavanine.[15] It was not stated whether the tablets contained seed or herb material. Canavanine is known to be toxic to all animal species because it is a structural analogue of arginine and may interfere with the binding of this amino acid to enzymes and its incorporation into proteins.[16,G19] Alfalfa seeds are reported to contain substantial quantities of canavanine (8.33–13.6 mg/kg), whereas the herb is stated to contain amounts that are considerably less.[16,17]

Pancytopenia has been associated with human ingestion of ground alfalfa seeds (80–160 g/day), which were taken to lower plasma cholesterol concentrations.[18]

Dietary studies using alfalfa top saponins (ATS) in the diet of rats and monkeys showed no evidence of toxicity and serum lipid concentrations were lowered.[3,19,20] In addition, when ATS were given to cholesterol-fed animals, a reduction in serum lipid concentrations was observed.[3,19,20] ATS are reported to be free of the SLE-inducing substance that is present in the seeds.[3]

Negative results were documented for alfalfa when tested for mutagenicity using *Salmonella* strains TA98 and TA100.[21]

Contra-indications, Warnings

Individuals with a history of SLE should avoid ingesting alfalfa. Ingestion of large amounts of alfalfa (exceeding amounts normally consumed in the diet) should be avoided in view of the documented oestrogenic activity and potential anticoagulant activity. Excessive doses may interfere with anticoagulant therapy and with hormonal therapy, including the oral contraceptive pill and hormone replacement therapy. Alfalfa may affect blood sugar concentrations in diabetic patients because of the manganese content.

Pregnancy and lactation   Alfalfa seeds are reputed to affect the menstrual cycle and to be lactogenic.[G30] Although the safety of alfalfa herb has not been established, it is probably acceptable for use during pregnancy and lactation provided that doses do not exceed the amounts normally ingested as a food. Alfalfa seeds should not be ingested during pregnancy or lactation.

Pharmaceutical Comment

The chemistry of alfalfa is well documented and it does appear to be a good source of vitamins and minerals, thereby supporting the herbal uses. However, normal human dietary intake of alfalfa is low and excessive ingestion should be avoided in view of the many pharmacologically active constituents (e.g. canavanine, coumarins, isoflavones and saponins), which may give rise to unwanted effects if taken to excess. Oestrogenic effects are generally associated with the ingestion of large amounts of the herb, such as in fodder for poultry and cattle. Reports of a possible SLE-inducing capacity for alfalfa, particularly the seeds, also suggests that excessive ingestion is not advisable. In view of the reports of arthralgia, alfalfa should not be recommended for the treatment of arthritis.

References

See also General References G5, G9, G16, G19, G22, G24, G30, G31, G32, G36, G37, G41, G43 and G64.

1   Oleszek W, Jurzysta M. Isolation, chemical characterization and biological activity of alfalfa (*Medicago media* Pers.) root saponins. *Acta Soc Bot Pol* 1986; **55**: 23–33.

2   Berry M. Alfalfa. *Pharm J* 1995; **255**: 353–354.

3   Malinow MR *et al.* Lack of toxicity of alfalfa saponins in cynomolgus macaques. *J Med Primatol* 1982; **11**: 106–118.

4   Malinow MR *et al.* Prevention of elevated cholesterolemia in monkeys by alfalfa saponins. *Steroids* 1977; **29**: 105–110.

5   Swanston-Flatt SK *et al.* Traditional plant treatments for diabetes in normal and streptozotocin-diabetic mice. *Diabetologia* 1990; **33**: 462–464.

6   Garrett BJ *et al.* Consumption of poisonous plants (*Senecio jacobaea*, *Symphytum officinale*, *Pteridium aquilinum*, *Hypericum perforatum*) by rats: chronic toxicity, mineral metabolism, and hepatic drug-metabolizing enzymes. *Toxicol Lett* 1982; **10**: 183–188.

7   Sroka Z *et al.* Stimulation of pancreatic lipase activity by saponins isolated from *Medicago sativa* L. *Z Naturforschung, Section C, J Biosci* 1997; **52**: 235–239.

8   Polacheck I *et al.* Activity of compound G2 isolated from alfalfa roots against medically important yeasts. *Antimicrob Agents Chemother* 1986; **30**: 290–294.

9   Jurzysta M, Waller GR. Antifungal and haemolytic activity of aerial parts of alfalfa (*Medicago*) species in relation to saponin composition. *Adv Expl Med Biol* 1996; **404**: 565–574.

10 Zhao WS *et al.* Immunopotentiating effects of polysaccharides isolated from *Medicago sativa* L. *Acta Pharmacol Sinica* 1993; **14**: 273–276.

11 Mölgaard J *et al.* Alfalfa seeds lower low density lipoprotein cholesterol and apolipoprotein B concentrations in patients with type II hyperlipoproteinemia. *Atherosclerosis* 1987; **65**: 173–179.

12 Rubenstein AH *et al.* Manganese-induced hypoglycaemia. *Lancet* 1962; **ii**: 1348–1351.

13 Malinow MR *et al.* Systemic lupus erythematosus-like syndrome in monkeys fed alfalfa sprouts: role of a nonprotein amino acid. *Science* 1982; **216**: 415–417.

14 Alcocer-Varela J *et al.* Effects of L-canavanine on T cells may explain the induction of systemic lupus erythematosus by alfalfa. *Arthritis Rheum* 1985; **28**: 52–57.

15 Roberts JL, Hayashi JA. Exacerbation of SLE associated with alfalfa ingestion. *N Engl J Med* 1983; **308**: 1361.

16 Natelson S. Canavanine to arginine ratio in alfalfa (*Medicago sativa*), clover (*Trifolium*), and the jack bean (*Canavalia ensiformis*). *J Agric Food Chem* 1985; **33**: 413–419.

17 Natelson S. Canavanine in alfalfa (*Medicago sativa*). *Experientia* 1985; **41**: 257–259.

18 Malinow MR *et al*. Pancytopenia during ingestion of alfalfa seeds. *Lancet* 1981; i: 615.

19 Malinow MR *et al*. The toxicity of alfalfa saponins in rats. *Food Cosmet Toxicol* 1981; **19**: 443–445.

20 René M *et al*. Lack of toxicity of alfalfa saponins in rats. *Cholesterol Metab* 1981; **40**: 349.

21 White RD *et al*. An evaluation of acetone extracts from six plants in the Ames mutagenicity test. *Toxicol Lett* 1983; **15**: 25–31.

Aloe Vera

Species (Family)

Aloe barbadensis Mill., *Aloe ferox* Mill. and hybrids with *Aloe africana* Mill. and *Aloe spicata* Baker (Liliaceae)

Synonyms

Aloe Gel, *Aloe vera* Tourn. ex L., *Aloe vera* (L.) Webb

Parts Used

Leaf gel

Pharmacopoeial and Other Monographs

Martindale 32nd edition[G43]
PDR for Herbal Medicines 2nd edition[G36]
WHO volume 1 1999[G63]

Legal Category (Licensed Products)

Aloe vera is not included in the GSL.

Constituents[G2,G6,G22,G41]

Aloe vera is reported to contain mono- and polysaccharides, tannins, sterols, organic acids, enzymes (including cyclooxygenase),[1] saponins, vitamins and minerals.[2]

Carbohydrates Glucomannan and other polysaccharides containing arabinose, galactose and xylose.

Lipids Includes cholesterol, gamolenic acid and arachidonic acid.[1] The polar, non-polar and fatty acid composition has been investigated.[1]

Food Use

Aloe vera is not used in foods.

Herbal Use

Traditionally, aloe vera has been used in ointments and creams to assist the healing of wounds, burns, eczema and psoriasis.[G2,G6,G41,G64]

Dosage

None documented.

Pharmacological Actions

Aloe vera refers to the mucilaginous tissue located in the leaf parenchyma of *Aloe vera* or related *Aloe* species. However, many documented studies for *Aloe vera* have utilised homogenised leaf extracts which therefore combine aloe vera with aloes, the laxative preparation obtained from the bitter, yellow juice also found in the leaf (*see* Aloes). Unless otherwise specified, the following studies will refer to a total leaf extract.

In vitro and animal studies

Gel preparations have been reported to be effective against radiation burns, skin ulcers and peptic ulcers.[2] However, the gel was also found to be ineffective against drug- and stress-induced gastric and peptic ulcers in rats.[2]

Anti-inflammatory activity has been observed in various rat and mouse models that received subcutaneous injections of *Aloe vera* leaf extract.[3] A positive response was noted in wound-healing (10 mg/kg, rat; 100 mg/kg, mouse), mustard oedema (10 mg/kg, rat) and polymorphonuclear leukocyte infiltration (2 mg/kg, mouse) tests, although no activity was demonstrated in the antifibrosis test (cotton pellet granuloma) (400 mg/kg, rat).

Anti-arthritic and anti-inflammatory activity has been documented for a cream containing homogenised *Aloe africana* leaves, ribonucleic acid, and ascorbic acid, following topical application to rats which had been injected (day 0) with *Mycobacterium butyricum* to cause adjuvant arthritis.[4] This model is considered a good experimental tool for studying rheumatoid arthritis.[4] The cream was found to be active when applied both as a prevention (days 1–13) and as a regression (days 21–35) treatment.[4] Subsequent work suggested that anthraquinone compounds (anthraquinone, anthracene and anthranilic acid) may be the active components in the aloe leaf mixture.[5] These compounds are, however, constituents of aloes rather than aloe vera (*see* Aloes). Aloe vera juice (presumably containing the anthraquinones contained in aloe preparation) has been applied directly to open pressure sores to assist in their healing.[6] The aloe vera extract exhibited an anaesthetic reaction, antibacterial action and increased local microcirculation.[6]

Endogenous cyclooxygenase in *Aloe vera* has been found to convert endogenous arachidonate to various prostanoids, namely PGE_2 (major), TXB_2, PGD_2, $PGF_{2\alpha}$, and 6-keto-$PGF_{1b\alpha}$.[1] The production of these compounds, especially PGE_2, has been associated with the beneficial effect of an aloe extract on human bronchial asthma[8] (see below).

Hypoglycaemic actions have been documented for aloes extracts (*see* Aloes).

Clinical studies

Enhancement of phagocytosis in adult bronchial asthma has been attributed to a non-dialysable fraction of the extract, consisting of active components that are a mixture of polysaccharide and protein or glycoprotein.[7] Despite the nature of these proposed active components, it has been proposed that activity of the fraction may be related to the previous observation that aloe vera synthesises prostaglandins from endogenous arachidonic acid using endogenous cyclooxygenase.[1] In this current study,[7] activity of the aloe vera extract required dark storage at 4–30°C for a period of 3–10 days.[3] These conditions are reported to be favourable for the hydrolysis of phospholipids, thus releasing arachidonic acid for synthesis of prostanoids.[1] In addition, activity was dependent on patients not having received prior treatment with a corticosteroid.[8] The gel has been reported to be effective in the treatment of mouth ulcers.[8]

Side-effects, Toxicity

None documented.

Contra-indications, Warnings

Hypoglycaemic activity has been documented for an aloe vera extract, although it is unclear whether this is associated with the true aloe vera gel or aloes extract.[9]

Pregnancy and lactation The external application of aloe vera gel during pregnancy is not thought to be any cause for concern. However, products stated to contain aloes extracts or aloe vera may well contain gastrointestinal stimulant anthraquinone components that are well recognised as the active constituents in aloes (laxative). As such, ingestion of such preparations during pregnancy and lactation should be avoided.

Pharmaceutical Comment

Aloe vera is obtained from the mucilaginous tissue in the centre of the *Aloe vera* leaf and consists mainly of polysaccharides and lipids. It should not be confused with aloes, which is obtained by evaporation of water from the bitter yellow juice that is drained from the leaf. Unlike aloes, aloe vera does not contain any anthraquinone compounds and does not, therefore, exert any laxative action. Studies have reported an anti-inflammatory and anti-arthritic action for total leaf extracts but the activity seems to be associated with anthraquinone compounds. Hypoglycaemic activity has been reported for aloe vera extract. Aloe vera is a source of gamolenic acid. The literature on burn management with aloe vera gel preparations is confused and further studies are required.[10]

References

See also General References G5, G6, G18, G19, G22, G29, G31, G32, G36, G41, G43, G63 and G64.

1 Afzal M *et al*. Identification of some prostanoids in *Aloe vera* extracts. *Planta Med* 1991; **57**: 38–40.
2 Parmar NS *et al*. Evaluation of *Aloe vera* leaf exudate and gel for gastric and duodenal anti-ulcer activity. *Fitoterapia* 1986; **57**: 380–381.
3 Davis RH *et al*. Biological activity of *Aloe vera*. *Med Sci Res* 1987; **15**: 235.
4 Davis RH *et al*. Topical effect of aloe with ribonucleic and vitamin C on adjuvant arthritis. *J Am Pod Med Assoc* 1985; **75**: 229–237.
5 Davis RH *et al*. Antiarthritic activity of anthraquinones found in aloe for podiatric medicine. *J Am Pod Med Assoc* 1986; **76**: 61–66.
6 Cuzzell JZ. Readers' remedies for pressure sores. *Am J Nurs* 1986; **86**: 923–924.
7 Shida T *et al*. Effect of Aloe extract on peripheral phagocytosis in adult bronchial asthma. *Planta Med* 1985; **51**: 273–275.
8 Plemons JM *et al*. Evaluation of acemannan in the treatment of aphthous stomatitis. *Wounds* 1994; **6**: 40–45.
9 Ghanam N *et al*. The antidiabetic activity of aloes: preliminary clinical and experimental observations. *Hormone Res* 1986; **24**: 288–294.
10 Marshall JM. Aloe vera gel: What is the evidence? *Pharm J* 1990; **244**: 360–362.

Aloes

Species (Family)

(i) *Aloe barbadensis* Mill. (Liliaceae)
(ii) *Aloe ferox* Mill. and its hybrids with *Aloe africana* Mill. and *Aloe spicata* Baker

Synonym(s)

Aloe vera Tourn. ex L., *A. vera* (L.) Webb, *A. vera* (L.) Burm. f.

Part(s) Used

Dried leaf juice

Pharmacopoeial and Other Monographs

BHC 1992[G6]
BHP 1996[G9]
BP 2001[G15]
Complete German Commission E[G3]
ESCOP 1997 (Cape Aloes)[G52]
Martindale 32nd edition[G43]
PDR for Herbal Medicines 2nd edition[G36]
Ph Eur 2002[G28]
USP24/NF19[G61]
WHO volume 1 1999[G63]

Legal Category (Licensed Products)

GSL[G37]

Constituents[G2,G20,G22,G41,G52,G64]

Anthranoids[1–6,G20,G52]   Cape aloes anthranoids are qualitatively identical to leaf exudate of *A. ferox*.[4] Anthrones (up to 30%), mainly the C-glycosides aloins A and B (= barbaloin, isobarbaloin, stereo-isomers of 10-glucosyl-aloe-emodin anthrone); other glycosides include 8-O-methyl-7-hydroxy aloins A and B, aloinosides A and B (aloin-11-O-α-L-rhamno-sides). Small quantities of 1,8-dihydroxyanthra-quinoid aglycones, including aloe-emodin and chrysophanol are also present.

Chromones[1,2,7,G20,G52]   Major constituents are aloesin (2-acetonyl-5-methyl-8-glucosyl chromone) and aloeresin E. Lesser quantities of isoaloeresin D, 8-C-glucosyl-7-O-methyl-aloesol and related glyco-sides which may be esterified at the glucose moiety by either cinnamic, *p*-coumaric or ferulic acids, are also present. Non-glycosylated chromones include 7-hydroxy-2,5-dimethylchromone, furoaloesone, 2-acetonyl-7-hydroxy-8-(3-hydroxyacetonyl)-5-methyl chromone and 2-acetonyl-8-(2-furoylmethyl)-7-hydroxy-5-methylchromone.[8,9]

Phenyl pyrones[1,2]   Glycosides include aloenin and aloenin B.

Other constituents[G52]   Cinnamic acid and 1-methyl-tetralin.

Food Use

Aloes is listed by the Council of Europe as a natural source of food flavouring (category N3).[G16] This category indicates that aloes can be added to food-stuffs in the traditionally accepted manner, although there is insufficient information available for an adequate assessment of potential toxicity. The con-centration of aloin present in the final product is limited to 0.1 mg/kg; 50 mg/kg in alcoholic beverages.[G16] In the USA, aloes is listed as GRAS (Generally Recognised As Safe).[G41]

Herbal Use

Aloes is recommended for the treatment of atonic constipation and suppressed menstrua-tion.[G2,G49,G64]

Dosage

Dried juice   50–200 mg or equivalent three times daily.[G6,G49]

In view of potential adverse effects, the dose recommended for adults and children aged over 10 years is 10–30 mg of hydroxyanthracene derivatives (calculated as barbaloin) once daily at night.[G52] Use of aloes as a laxative in self-treatment of con-stipation for more than two weeks is not recom-mended.[G52]

Pharmacological Actions

The activity of aloes can be attributed to the anthra-noid glycoside content. The glycosides are metabo-lised by glycosidases in the intestinal flora to form active anthrones. The laxative action is due to an increase in motility of the large intestine by inhibition of the Na^+/K^+ pump and chloride ion channels; enhanced fluid secretion occurs due to stimulation of mucus and chloride ion secretion.[G52]

In vitro and animal studies

Nine hours after oral administration, aloes produced diarrhoea at doses of 5 g/kg (in 20% of rats) and 20 g/kg (in 100% of rats).[10] Pretreatment of rats with the nitric oxide (NO) synthase inhibitor N-nitro-L-arginine methyl ester given intraperitoneally reduced diarrhoea induced by aloes (20 g/kg) 9 hours after oral administration. The results suggest that endogenous NO modulates the diarrhoeal effects of Cape aloes.[10]

Inhibitory effects of aqueous extracts of five genera of *Aloe*, including *A. ferox* and *A. barbadensis*, and aloe powder (Japanese Pharmacopoeia) on histamine release from rat peritoneal mast cells induced by antigen were investigated *in vitro*.[11] All extracts tested inhibited histamine release in a concentration-dependent manner under the test conditions. *Aloe ferox* extract, Japanese Pharmacopoeia aloes and barbaloin strongly inhibited histamine release (IC_{50} 0.16, 0.07 and 0.02 µg/mL, respectively).[11]

Aqueous extracts of aloes are said to elevate the rate of ethanol oxidation *in vivo*.[12] Oral administration of aloin (300 mg/kg) to rats 12 hours prior to administration of alcohol (3 g/kg) resulted in a significant decrease (40%) in blood alcohol concentration.[12] Pretreatment with intraperitoneal aloe-emodin 2 hours prior to alcohol administration significantly reduced blood alcohol concentrations; it was hypothesised that aloin is metabolised to aloe-emodin which exerts its effect on alcohol metabolism.[12] Activity-guided fractionation of the leaves of *A. aborescens* resulted in the isolation and characterisation of elgonica-dimers A and B (dimeric C-glycosides of anthrone emodin-10′-C-β-D-glucopyranoside and aloe-emodin) as potent inhibitors of cytosolic alcohol dehydrogenase and aldehyde dehydrogenase activities *in vitro*.[13]

Aloe-emodin and an alcoholic extract of aloes have been reported to possess antitumour activity.[G41]

Hypoglycaemic activity has been shown in alloxan-diabetic mice for aloes[14] and in diabetic rats for an aloe gum extract.[15,16]

Barbaloin is active *in vitro* against *Mycobacterium tuberculosis* and *Bacillus subtilis* (minimum inhibitory concentration 0.125 mg/mL and 0.25 mg/mL, respectively).[G18]

Clinical studies

The purgative action of the anthraquinone glycosides is well recognised (*see* Senna), although aloes is reported to be more potent than both senna and cascara.[G41,G45] Orally ingested anthranoid glycosides are not metabolised until they reach the colon. In humans, the intestinal flora break down O-glycosides readily and C-glycosides to some extent. The main active metabolite is aloe-emodin-9-anthrone.[G52]

An aloes extract in doses too small to cause abdominal cramps or diarrhoea had a significant hypoglycaemic effect in five patients with non-insulin-dependent diabetes.[14]

Side-effects, Toxicity

Aloes is a potent purgative that may cause abdominal pains, gastrointestinal irritation leading to pelvic congestion and, in large doses, may result in nephritis, bloody diarrhoea and haemorrhagic gastritis.[G41,G44] Like all stimulant purgatives, prolonged use of aloes may produce watery diarrhoea with excessive loss of water and electrolytes (particularly potassium), muscular weakness and weight loss.[G44]

Tests of the possible carcinogenicity of hydroxyanthraquinones and their glycosides showed that exposure to certain aglycones and glycosides may represent a human cancer risk.[17] Most of the aglycones tested were found to be mutagenic and some, such as emodin and aloe-emodin, were genotoxic in mammalian cells.

Administration of dried aloes extract 50 mg/kg per day for 12 weeks to mice did not result in the development of severe pathological symptoms, although a raised sorbitol dehydrogenase concentration was suggested to be indicative of liver damage.[G20] No mutagenic effects in *Salmonella typhimurium* and Va7 cells, or DNA repair induction in rat hepatocytes, were observed. These negative results are due to the inability of the test systems to release mutagenic anthranoids from the C-glycosides.[G20] Retrospective and prospective studies have shown no causal relationship between anthranoid laxative use and colorectal cancer.[G20]

Contra-indications, Warnings

Aloes has been superseded by less toxic laxatives.[G45] The drastic purgative action of aloes contra-indicates its use in individuals with haemorrhoids and existing kidney disease. Hypokalaemia resulting from laxative abuse potentiates the action of cardiac glycosides, interacts with anti-arrhythmic drugs, and with drugs which induce reversion to sinus rhythm, e.g. quinidine. Concomitant use with thiazide diuretics, adrenocorticosteroids and liquorice may aggregate electrolyte imbalance. In common with all purgatives, aloes should not be given to patients with inflammatory disease of the colon (e.g. Crohn's disease, ulcerative colitis), appendicitis, intestinal obstruction, abdominal pain, nausea or vomiting. Aloes colours alkaline urine red. Long-term use should be avoided and a doctor should be consulted within two weeks of treatment initiation if symptoms persist.

Pregnancy and lactation   In view of the irritant and cathartic properties documented for aloes, its use is contra-indicated during pregnancy.[G44] Anthraquinones may be secreted into breast milk and, therefore, aloes should be avoided during lactation (*see* Senna).

Aloes is reputed to be an abortifacient and to affect the menstrual cycle.[G22]

Pharmaceutical Comment

Aloes and aloe gel are often confused with each other. Aloes is obtained by evaporation of water from the bitter yellow juice drained from the leaves of *A. vera*. Commercial 'aloin' is a concentrated form of aloes.[G41] Aloe gel is prepared by many methods, but is obtained from the mucilaginous tissue in the centre of the leaf and does not contain anthraquinones (*see* Aloe Vera). Aloes is a potent purgative which has been superseded by less toxic drugs such as senna and cascara. Generally, the use of unstandardised preparations containing anthraquinone glycosides should be avoided, since their pharmacological effect is unpredictable and they may cause abdominal cramp and diarrhoea. In particular, the use of products containing combinations of anthraquinone laxatives should be avoided.

References

See also General References G2, G3, G6, G9, G15, G16, G20, G22, G25, G29, G31, G32, G36, G37, G41, G43, G49, G52, G56, G61, G63 and G64.

1 Park MK *et al*. Analysis of 13 phenolic compounds in *Aloe* species by high performance liquid chromatography. *Phytochem Anal* 1998; **9**: 186–191.
2 Okamura N *et al*. High-performance liquid chromatographic determination of phenolic compounds in *Aloe* species. *J Chromatogr A* 1996; **746**: 225–231.
3 Van Wyk E-E *et al*. Geographical variation in the major compounds of *Aloe ferox* leaf exudate. *Planta Med* 1995; **61**: 250–253.
4 Reynolds T. Chromatographic examination of some old samples of drug aloes. *Pharmazie* 1994; **49**: 524–529.
5 Rauwald HW, Sigler A. Simultaneous determination of 18 polyketides typical of *Aloe* by high performance liquid chromatography and photodiode array detection. *Phytochem Anal* 1994; **5**: 266–270.
6 Rauwald HW, Beil A. High-performance liquid chromatographic separation and determination of diastereomeric anthrone-C-glucosyls in Cape aloes. *J Chromatogr* 1993; **639**: 359–362.
7 Rauwald HW *et al*. Three 8-C-glucosyl-5-methylchromones from *Aloe barbadensis* (Ph. Eur. 1997). *Pharmazie* 1997; **52**: 962–964.
8 Speranza G *et al*. Studies on aloe, 12. Furoaloesone, a new 5-methylchromone from Cape aloe. *J Nat Prod* 1993; **56**: 1089–1094.
9 Speranza G *et al*. Studies on aloe, 15. Two new 5-methylchromones from Cape aloe. *J Nat Prod* 1997; **60**: 692–694.
10 Izzo AA *et al*. The role of nitric oxide in aloe-induced diarrhoea in the rat. *Eur J Pharmacol* 1999; **368**: 43–48.
11 Yamamoto M *et al*. Inhibitory effects of aloe extracts on antigen- and compound 48/80-induced histamine release from rat peritoneal mast cells. *Jpn J Toxicol Environ Health* 1993; **39**: 395–400.
12 Chung J-H *et al*. Acceleration of the alcohol oxidation rate in rats with aloin, a quinone derivative of aloe. *Biochem Pharmacol* 1996; **52**: 1461–1468.
13 Shin KH *et al*. Elongica-dimers A and B, two potent alcohol metabolism inhibitory constituents of *Aloe arborescens*. *J Nat Prod* 1997; **60**: 1180–1182.
14 Ghannam N *et al*. The antidiabetic activity of aloes: preliminary and experimental observations. *Horm Res* 1986; **24**: 288–294.
15 Al-Awadi FM, Gumaa KA. Studies on the activity of individual plants of an antidiabetic plant mixture. *Acta Diabetol Lat* 1987; **24**: 37–41.
16 Al-Awadi FM *et al*. On the mechanism of the hypoglycaemic effect of a plant extract. *Diabetologia* 1985; **28**: 432–434.
17 Westendorf J *et al*. Possible carcinogenicity of anthraquinone-containing medical plants. *Planta Med* 1988; **54**: 562.

Angelica

Species (Family)

Angelica archangelica L. (Apiaceae/Umbelliferae)

Synonym(s)

Archangelica officinalis Moench and Hoffm.

Part(s) Used

Fruit, leaf, rhizome, root

Pharmacopoeial and Other Monographs

BHP 1996[G9]
Complete German Commission E[G3]
PDR for Herbal Medicines 2nd edition[G36]

Legal Category (Licensed Products)

GSL[G37]

Constituents[G2,G22,G32,G41,G48,G57,G58,G64]

The literature mainly refers to constituents of the root.

Coumarins Over 20 furanocoumarins, including angelicin, archangelicin, bergapten, isoimperatorin and xanthotoxin.[1,G2] Also the coumarins osthol (major constituent in rhizome/root, 0.2%) and umbelliferone.[G2] The root also contains the furanocoumarins 2′-angeloyl-3′-isovaleryl vaginate,[2] heraclenol-2′-O-senecioate and heraclenol-2′-O-isovalerate.[3]

Volatile oils 0.35–1.3% in root and fruit. 80–90% monoterpenes, including α- and β-phellandrene, α- and β-pinene, sabinene, α-thujene, limonene, linalool, borneol[1,4] and four macrocyclic lactones.

Other constituents Archangelenone (a flavonoid), palmitic acid, caffeic and chlorogenic acids, sugars (fructose, glucose, sucrose, umbelliferose).

Food Use[1,G32]

Angelica is widely used in foods. Angelica is listed by the Council of Europe as a natural source of food flavouring (stem: category 1; other parts and preparations: category 4, with limits on coumarin and furanocoumarin) (*see* Appendix 23).[G17] In the USA, angelica is listed as GRAS (Generally Recognised As Safe).[G41]

Herbal Use[1,G32]

Angelica is stated to possess antispasmodic, diaphoretic, expectorant, bitter aromatic, carminative, diuretic and local anti-inflammatory properties. It has been used for respiratory catarrh, psychogenic asthma, flatulent dyspepsia, anorexia nervosa, rheumatic diseases, peripheral vascular disease, and specifically for pleurisy and bronchitis, applied as a compress, and for bronchitis associated with vascular deficiency.[G2,G7,G49,G64] The German Commission E monograph states that angelica can be used for lack of appetite and dyspeptic complaints such as mild stomach cramps and flatulence.[G4] Many related species, including *A. sinensis* (dong quai) are traditionally used in Chinese medicine.[G57]

Dosage

Dried leaf 2–5 g by infusion three times daily.[G7]

Leaf liquid extract 2–5 mL (1:1 in 25% alcohol) three times daily.[G7]

Leaf tincture 2–5 mL (1:5 in 45% alcohol) three times daily.[G7]

Dried rhizome/root Daily dose 4.5 g[G2] or 1–2 g by infusion three times daily.[G4,G7]

Rhizome/root liquid extract 0.5–2.0 mL (1:1 in 25% alcohol) three times daily.[G7]

Rhizome/root tincture 0.5–2 mL (1:5 in 50% alcohol) three times daily.[G7]

Fruit 1–2 g.[G49]

Pharmacological Actions

In vitro and animal studies

Minimal anti-inflammatory activity (1% inhibition of carrageenan-induced rat paw oedema) has been documented for fruit extracts (100 mg/kg body weight by mouth) given 45 minutes before eliciting oedema.[5] This was compared with 45% inhibition by indometacin (5 mg/kg by mouth). Angelica is reported to possess antibacterial and antifungal properties.[G41,G46] Antibacterial activity against *Mycobacterium avium* has been documented, with no activity exhibited against *Escherichia coli*, *Bacillus subtilis*, *Streptococcus faecalis* or *Salmonella typhi*.[6] Antifungal activity was reported in 14 of 15 fungi tested.[6]

A methanolic extract of *A. archangelica* root showed antispasmodic activity against spontaneous contractions of circular smooth muscle (IC$_{50}$ 265 µg/mL) and inhibited acetylcholine- and barium chloride-induced contractions of longitudinal smooth muscle (IC$_{50}$ values 242 and 146 µg/mL, respectively).[7]

Extracts of *A. archangelica* root exhibit calcium channel-blocking activity.[8] A series of isolated coumarins showed activity, the most active being archangelicin with an IC$_{50}$ 1.2 µg/mL (verapamil 2.0 µg/mL) as a calcium channel antagonist as assessed by inhibition of depolarisation in GH$_4$C$_1$ rat pituitary cells.[9]

Sixteen coumarin compounds isolated from *A. archangelica* were tested for activity in cyclooxygenase 1 (COX-1) and 5-lipoxygenase (5-LO) inhibition assays *in vitro*.[10] None of the compounds demonstrated activity against COX-1, but osthol and oxypeucedanin isovalerate were active in the 5-LO assay.

In rabbits, a uterotonic action has been documented for Japanese angelica root following intraduodenal administration of a methanolic extract (3 g/kg).[11] *A. sinensis* is reported to have induced uterine contraction and relaxation.[G57]

Clinical studies

None documented for angelica (*A. archangelica*). The furanocoumarin constituent bergapten (5-methoxypsoralen) has been used in the PUVA (psoralen (P) and high-intensity long-wavelength ultraviolet irradiation) treatment of psoriasis.[G45]

Side-effects, Toxicity

Both angelica and the root oil have been reported to cause [G32] photodermatitis and phototoxicity, respectively, following external contact.[6,G22,G33,G58] Angelica contains furanocoumarin constituents which are known to cause photosensitisation. Concern has been expressed at the possible carcinogenic risk of the furanocoumarin bergapten. Seven species of plants known to cause dermatitis were analysed for psoralen, 8-methoxypsoralen (xanthotoxin) and 5-methoxypsoralen (bergapten). The highest total yield was obtained from *A. archangelica*.[12]

The root oil has been reported to be non-irritant and non-sensitising on animal and human skin.[6]

Root and fruit oils obtained by steam distillation are claimed to be devoid of furanocoumarins, although extracts may contain them.[G41]

Toxicity studies have been documented for the root oil.[6] Acute LD$_{50}$ values have been reported as 2.2 g/kg body weight (mouse, by mouth) and 11.16 g/kg (rat, by mouth). Death was attributed to liver and kidney damage, although animals surviving for three days completely recovered with a reversal of organ damage. An acute LD$_{50}$ (rabbit, dermal) value was reported to be greater than 5 g/kg. Subacute toxicity studies, lasting eight weeks, suggested that the tolerated dose in the rat was 1.5 g/kg, although at lower doses the animals weighed less than the controls.[6]

Furanocoumarins isolated from a related Chinese species, *Angelica koreana*, have been reported to affect the hepatic metabolism of hexobarbitone. The compounds were found to cause a marked inhibition of drug metabolism in the first phase and an acceleration in the second phase, and were thought to be drug-metabolising enzyme inhibitors rather than enzyme inducers. Furanocoumarins investigated included imperatorin and oxypeucedanin, which are also documented as constituents of *A. archangelica*. It has been reported that a related Chinese species, *Angelica sinensis*, may be hepatoprotective and prevent the reduction of hepatic glycogen.

Contra-indications, Warnings

Angelica may provoke a photosensitive allergic reaction because of the furanocoumarin constituents. In addition, excessive doses may interfere with anticoagulant therapy because of the coumarin constituents.

The use of bergapten in cosmetic and suntan preparations is stated to be ill-advised by some regulatory authorities,[G45] in view of the concerns regarding the risk of skin cancer. The International Fragrance Association recommends that angelica root oil be limited to a maximum of 0.78% in products applied to skin which is then exposed to sunshine.[G58]

Pregnancy and lactation   Angelica root is reputed to be an abortifacient and to affect the menstrual cycle. In view of this and the photosensitising constituents, the use of angelica during pregnancy and lactation in amounts exceeding those used in foods should be avoided.

Pharmaceutical Comment

The chemistry of angelica is well documented. Although the traditional use of Chinese angelica species, such as *A. sinensis* and *A. acutiloba*, is well established in oriental medicine, there is limited documented pharmacological information available for *A. archangelica*, the species most commonly used in Europe, to justify its herbal uses. In view of the presence of known pharmacologically active constituents, especially bergapten, consumption of amounts exceeding normal human dietary intake should be avoided. Angelica contains furanocoumarins which are known to possess photosensitising properties.

The related species *A. sinensis* (dong quai) is popular in traditional Chinese medicine (TCM) and occurs in about 70% of all TCM prescriptions to treat dysmenorrhoea, postnatal disturbances, anaemia, constipation and chronic pelvic infections.[13] Western naturopaths recommend the use of dong quai in hypertension, for modification of high blood sugar concentrations, regulation of the immune system, liver detoxification, anaemia and to relieve allergic conditions. Several unlicensed over-the-counter (OTC) products containing dong quai are readily available.

The chemistry of dong quai is similar to that of *A. archangelica*, with coumarins and volatile oil being major components.[13] In addition, a series of phthalides (e.g. ligustilide, butylphthalide, butylidenephthalide) have been isolated. Pharmacological investigations have shown that phthalides and coumarins have antispasmodic activity. The volatile constituents generally exert a hypotensive effect. A polysaccharide component is active against Ehrlich ascites tumours in mice and has immunostimulating activity,[14] and protects the gastric mucosa against ethanol- and indomethacin-induced damage.[15] Clinical investigation has failed to support the claims for relieving menopausal symptoms.[16] *A. sinensis* has been reported to be effective in improving abnormal protein metabolism in patients with chronic hepatitis or hepatic cirrhosis.[17]

The furanocoumarins are phototoxic and have photocarcinogenic potential, but need ultraviolet (UV) light for activation. An extract of dong quai administered subcutaneously to rabbits did not affect prothrombin time given alone, but did after concurrent administration of a single dose of warfarin.[18] Elevation of prothrombin time was noted in a patient stabilised on warfarin who began taking dong quai.[19] Coagulation values returned to normal one month after discontinuing use of dong quai.

References

See also General References G2, G3, G9, G10, G16, G22, G31, G33, G36, G37, G41, G44, G48, G49, G57, G58 and G64.

1 Czygan F-C. (Root of the holy ghost or Angelica root – *Angelica archangelica*). *Z Phytother* 1998; **19**: 342–348.

2 Harmala P *et al.* A furanocoumarin from *Angelica archangelica*. *Planta Med* 1992; **58**: 287–289.

3 Sun H, Jakupovic J. Further heraclenol derivatives from *Angelica archangelica*. *Pharmazie* 1986; **41**: 888–889.

4 Holm Y *et al.* Enantiomeric composition of monoterpene hydrocarbons in n-hexane extracts of *Angelica archangelica* L. roots and seeds. *Flavour Fragrance J* 1997; **12**: 397–400.

5 Zielinska-Jenczylik J *et al.* Effect of plant extracts on the *in vitro* interferon synthesis. *Arch Immunol Ther Exp* 1984; **32**: 577.

6 Opdyke DLJ. Angelica root oil. *Food Cosmet Toxicol* 1975; **13**(Suppl.): 713.

7 Izzo AA *et al.* Spasmolytic activity of medicinal plants used for the treatment of disorders involving smooth muscles. *Phytother Res* 1996; **10**: S107–S108.

8 Harmala P *et al.* Choice of solvent in the extraction of *Angelica archangelica* roots with reference to calcium blocking activity. *Planta Med* 1992; **58**: 176–183.

9 Harmala P *et al.* Isolation and testing of calcium blocking activity of furanocoumarins from *Angelica archangelica*. *Planta Med* 1991; **57**: A58–A59.

10 Roos G *et al.* Isolation, identification and screening for COX-1 and 5-LO inhibition of coumarins from *Angelica archangelica*. *Pharmaceut Pharmacol Lett* 1997; **7**: 157–160.

11 Harada M *et al.* Effect of Japanese angelica root and peony root on uterine contraction in the rabbit *in situ*. *J Pharm Dyn* 1984; **7**: 304–311.

12 Zobel AM, Brown SA. Dermatitis-inducing psoralens on the surface of seven medicinal plant species. *J Toxicol Cutan Ocul Toxicol* 1991; **10**: 223–231.

13 Awang DVC. Dong quai. *Can Pharm J* 1999; **132**: 38–41.

14 Choy YM *et al.* Immunological studies of low molecular weight polysaccharide from *Angelica sinensis*. *Am J Chin Med* 1994; **22**: 137–145.

15 Cho CH *et al.* Study of the gastrointestinal protective effects of polysaccharides from *Angelica sinensis* in rats. *Planta Med* 2000; **66**: 348–351.

16 Hirata JD *et al.* Does dong quai have oestrogenic effects in postmenopausal women? A double-blind, placebo-controlled trial. *Fertil Steril* 1997; **68**: 981–986.

17 Chang H-M, But PP-H. *Pharmacology and Appli-*

cations of Chinese Materia Medica, vol 1. Singapore: World Scientific, 1986: 499.

18   Lo ACT *et al*. Dong quai (*Angelica sinensis*) effects the pharmacodynamics but not the pharmaco-kinetics of warfarin in rabbits. *Eur J Drug Metab Pharmacokinet* 1995; **20**: 55–60.

19   Page RL, Lawrence JD. Potentiation of warfarin by dong quai. *Pharmacotherapy* 1999; **19**: 870–876.

Aniseed

Species (Family)

Pimpinella anisum L. (Apiaceae/Umbelliferae)

Synonym(s)

Anise, Anisi Fructus, Anisum, *Anisum officinarum* Moench., *Anisum vulgare* Gaertn.

Part(s) Used

Fruit

Pharmacopoeial and Other Monographs

BHP 1996[G9]
BP 2001[G15]
Complete German Commission E[G3]
ESCOP 1997[G52]
Martindale 32nd edition[G43]
PDR for Herbal Medicines 2nd edition[G36]
Ph Eur 2002[G28]

Legal Category (Licensed Products)

GSL[G37]

Constituents[G2,G22,G41,G52,G58,G64]

Coumarins Scopoletin, umbelliferone, umbelliprenine; bergapten (furanocoumarin).

Flavonoids Flavonol (quercetin) and flavone (apigenin, luteolin) glycosides, e.g. quercetin-3-glucuronide, rutin, luteolin-7-glucoside, apigenin-7-glucoside; isoorientin and isovitexin (C-glucosides).

Volatile oils 2–6%. Major components are *trans*-anethole (80–95%), with smaller amounts of estragole (methyl chavicol),[G52] anise ketone (*p*-methoxyphenylacetone) and β-caryophyllene. Minor components include anisaldehyde and anisic acid (oxidation products of anethole), linalool, limonene, α-pinene, pseudoisoeugenol-2-methyl butyrate, acetaldehyde, *p*-cresol, cresol, hydroquinone, β-farnesene, α-, β- and γ-himachalene, bisabolene, *d*-elemene, *ar*-curcumene and myristicin.[1]

Other constituents Carbohydrate (50%), lipids 16% (saturated and unsaturated), β-amyrin (triterpene), stigmasterol (phytosterol) and its palmitate and stearate salts.

Food Use

Aniseed is used extensively as a spice and is listed by the Council of Europe as a natural source of food flavouring (category N2). This category allows small quantities of aniseed to be added to foodstuffs, with a possible limitation of an active principle (as yet unspecified) in the final product.[G16] In the USA, aniseed is listed as GRAS (Generally Recognised As Safe).[2,G41]

Herbal Use

Aniseed is stated to possess expectorant, antispasmodic, carminative and parasiticide properties. Traditionally, it has been used for bronchial catarrh, pertussis, spasmodic cough, flatulent colic; topically for pediculosis and scabies; its most specific use is for bronchitis, tracheitis with persistent cough, and as an aromatic adjuvant to prevent colic following the use of cathartics.[G2,G7,G64]

Aniseed has been used as an oestrogenic agent.[3] It has been reputed to increase milk secretion, promote menstruation, facilitate birth, alleviate symptoms of the male climacteric and increase libido.[3]

Dosage

Dried fruit Adults: 1.0–5.0 g crushed fruits in 150 mL water as an infusion several times daily.[G52] Children: 0–1 year old, 1.0 g of crushed fruits as an infusion; 1–4 years of age, 2.0 g; over 4 years, use adult dose.[G52]

Oil 0.05–0.2 mL three times daily.[G7]

Spirit of anise (BPC 1949) 0.3–1.0 mL three times daily.

Distilled anise water (BPC 1934) 15–30 mL three times daily.

Pharmacological Actions

The pharmacological effects of aniseed are largely due to the presence of anethole, which is structurally related to the catecholamines adrenaline, noradrenaline and dopamine. Anethole dimers closely resemble the oestrogenic agents stilbene and stilboestrol.[3]

In vitro and animal studies

Antimicrobial, antifungal and insecticidal activities
The volatile oil has antibacterial, antifungal and insecticidal activities.[G41,G52] Anethole, anisaldehyde and myristicin have exhibited mild insecticidal properties.[(G41,)]

Antispasmodic activity
Anise oil (200 mg/L) was shown to antagonise carbachol-induced spasms in a guinea-pig tracheal muscle preparation.[G52]

Secretolytic and expectorant effect
Application of aniseed (6.4 g/140 mL) to isolated ciliated epithelium of frog trachea induces small increases in transport velocity.[G52] Dilutions of anise oil increased respiratory tract fluid in anaesthetised guinea-pigs, rats and cats. A similar action was observed in anaesthetised rabbits inhaling anise oil.[G52] The reputed lactogogic action of anise has been attributed to anethole, which exerts a competitive antagonism at dopamine receptor sites (dopamine inhibits prolactin secretion), and to the action of polymerised anethole, which is structurally related to the oestrogenic compounds stilbene and stilboestrol.[3]

CNS activities
Whole plant aqueous infusions have been reported to delay (but not prevent) the onset of picrotoxin-induced seizures and to reduce the mortality rate in mice following intraperitoneal injection.[4] Aniseed has also been found to slightly elevate γ-aminobutyric acid (GABA) concentrations in brain tissue.[4] The anticonvulsant effect is much weaker with aniseed than with conventional drug treatment and therefore its use as an anticonvulsant in Arabic folklore is not supported.[4] Anise oil diluted in sesame oil (0.25–1.0 mL/kg) given intraperitoneally to mice increased in a dose-dependent manner the dose of pentylenetetrazole needed to induce clonic and tonic seizures.[5] Activity was also observed against tonic seizures induced by maximal electric shock. Motor impairment was observed at higher doses of anise oil. Pentobarbital-induced sleeping time was prolonged by intraperitoneal administration of anise oil (50 mg/kg) to mice.[G52]

Other activities
Oral administration of anethole (250–1000 mg/kg) to Swiss albino mice with Ehrlich ascites tumour in the paws indicated antitumour activity.[6] The conclusions were based on biochemical changes (nucleic acids, proteins, malondialdehyde, glutathione), survival rate and tumour weight. Anise oil given to rats (100 mg/kg given subcutaneously) stimulated liver regeneration after partial hepatectomy.[G52]

Clinical studies
Aniseed is mainly used for the treatment of dyspeptic complaints and catarrh of the upper respiratory tract.[G2,G41,G52] There is a lack of documented clinical studies with aniseed.

Side-effects, Toxicity
Contact dermatitis reactions to aniseed and aniseed oil have been attributed to anethole.[7,G31,G51] Reactions have been reported with products, such as creams and toothpastes, flavoured with aniseed oil.[G51] The volatile oil and anethole have been stated to be both irritant and sensitising.[G31,G51] Two female workers in a cake factory developed severe dermatitis, and patch tests indicated sensitivity to anise oil and to anethole.[8] Soreness, dryness and cracking of lips and perioral skin occurred in an individual using a herbal (fennel) toothpaste; anethole was reported to be the sensitising agent.[9] Bergapten is known to cause photosensitivity reactions and concern has been expressed over the possible carcinogenic risk of bergapten.[G45]

Ingestion of as little as 1–5 mL of anise oil can result in nausea, vomiting, seizures, and pulmonary oedema.[7]

The LD_{50} values per kg body weight for anise oil and *trans*-anethole are 2.7 g and 2–3 g, respectively.[G52] Mild liver lesions were observed in rats fed repeated anethole doses (695 mg/kg) for an unspecified duration.[3] Hepatic changes have been described in rats fed anethole in their daily diet (1%) for 15 weeks,[G22] although at a level of 0.25% there were no changes after one year. Rats fed with 0.1% *trans*-anethole in their diet for 90 days showed no toxic effects, but higher concentrations (0.3%, 1.0% and 3.0%) resulted in liver oedema.[G52] In therapeutic doses, anethole is reported to cause minimal hepatotoxicity.[G22] *Trans*-anethole given orally to rats (50–80 mg/kg) resulted in dose-dependent anti-implantation activity.[10] Significant oestrogenic activity was observed, but no anti-oestrogenic, progestational, anti-progestational, androgenic or anti-androgenic activity.[10]

Oral administration (1% of diet) of *trans*-anethole to rats resulted in induction of parathion-degrading drug enzymes.[G52] Male Wistar rats were treated with *trans*-anethole (125 or 250 mg/kg) by gavage for 10 days and the activities of liver microsome and cytosol phase I and II biotransformation enzymes were determined.[11] There was no effect on cytochrome P450, but UDP-glucuronyltransferase activity in the cytosol towards the substrates 4-chlorophenol and 4-hydroxyphenol was significantly increased for both doses. It was concluded that *trans*-anethole preferentially induces phase II biotransformation in rat liver *in vivo*.[11]

The safety of *trans*-anethole (4-methoxy propenylbenzene) has been reviewed by the Expert Panel of the Flavour and Extract Manufacturer Association (FEMA).[2] The evaluation was based on whether the hepatotoxic metabolite anethole epoxide is produced. At low levels of exposure, *trans*-anethole is efficiently detoxicated in rodents and humans, primarily by O-demethylation and ω-oxidation, respectively, while epoxidation is only a minor pathway. At higher doses in rats, a metabolic shift occurs resulting in epoxidation and formation of anethole epoxide. The continuous intake of high doses of *trans*-anethole induces a continuum of cytotoxicity, cell necrosis and cell proliferation. In chronic dietary studies in rats, hepatotoxicity resulted when the daily production of anethole epoxide exceeded 30 mg anethole epoxide per kg body weight. Neither *trans*-anethole nor anethole epoxide showed any evidence of genotoxicity. The Expert Panel concluded that the hepatocarcinogenic effects in female rats occur via a non-genotoxic mechanism and are secondary to hepatotoxicity caused by continuous exposures to high hepatocellular concentrations of anethole epoxide. *Trans*-anethole was reaffirmed as GRAS, based on a thorough study of the scientific literature.[2] Because *trans*-anethole undergoes efficient metabolic detoxication in humans at low levels of exposure, the neoplastic effects in rats associated with dose-dependent hepatotoxicity are not indicators of any significant risk to human health from the use of *trans*-anethole as a flavouring substance.[2]

Contra-indications, Warnings

Aniseed may cause an allergic reaction. It is recommended that the use of aniseed oil should be avoided in dermatitis, and inflammatory or allergic skin conditions.[G31,G58] Aniseed should be avoided by persons with known sensitivity to anethole.[G52] Bergapten may cause photosensitivity in sensitive individuals. The documented oestrogenic activity of anethole and its dimers may affect existing hormone therapy, including the oral contraceptive pill and hormone replacement therapy, if excessive doses are ingested. In view of the structural similarity reported between anethole and myristicin, consumption of large amounts of aniseed may cause neurological effects similar to those documented for nutmeg.

Pregnancy and lactation Traditionally, aniseed is reputed to be an abortifacient[G22] and also to promote lactation. The safety of aniseed taken during pregnancy and lactation has not been established; however, there are no known problems provided that doses taken do not greatly exceed the amounts used in foods. It has been proposed that aniseed and preparations used at recommended dosages may be used during pregnancy and lactation.[G52]

Pharmaceutical Comment

The chemistry of aniseed is well studied and documented pharmacological activities support some of the herbal uses. Aniseed is used extensively as a spice and is widely used in conventional pharmaceuticals for its carminative, expectorant and flavouring properties. Aniseed contains anethole and estragole which are structurally related to safrole, a known hepatotoxin and carcinogen. Although both anethole and estragole have been shown to cause hepatotoxicity in rodents, aniseed is not thought to represent a risk to human health when it is consumed in amounts normally encountered in foods. Anethole was reaffirmed as GRAS in 1997 on the basis of the recognised metabolic detoxication of *trans*-anethole in humans at low levels of exposure (1 mg/kg body weight).[2] For medicinal use, it is recommended that treatment should not be continued for extended periods.

References

See also General References G2, G3, G9, G15, G16, G22, G25, G29, G31, G36, G37, G41, G43, G51, G52, G58 and G64.

1 Burkhardt G *et al*. Terpene hydrocarbons in *Pimpinella anisum* L. *Pharm Weekbl (Sci)* 1986; **8**: 190–193.

2 Newberne P *et al*. The FEMA GRAS assessment of trans-anethole used as a flavouring substance. *Food Chem Toxicol* 1999; **37**: 789–811.

3 Albert-Puleo M. Fennel and anise as estrogenic agents. *J Ethnopharmacol* 1980; **2**: 337–344.

4 Abdul-Ghani A-S *et al*. Anticonvulsant effects of some Arab medicinal plants. *Int J Crude Drug Res* 1987; **25**: 39–43.

5 Pourgholami MH *et al*. The fruit essential oil of *Pimpinella anisum* exerts anticonvulsant effects in mice. *J Ethnopharmacol* 1999; **66**: 211–215.

6 Al-Harbi MM *et al*. Influence of anethole treatment on the tumour induced by Ehrlich ascites carcinoma cells in paw of Swiss albino mice. *Eur J Cancer Prevent* 1995; **4**: 307–318.

7 Chandler RF, Hawkes D. Aniseed – a spice, a

flavor, a drug. *Can Pharm J* 1984; **117**: 28–29.

8 Garcia-Bravo B *et al*. Occupational contact dermatitis from anethole in food handlers. *Contact Dermatitis* 1997; **37**: 38.

9 Franks A. Contact allergy to anethole in toothpaste associated with loss of taste. *Contact Dermatitis* 1998; **38**: 354–355.

10 Dhar SK. Anti-fertility activity and hormonal profile of trans-anethole in rats. *Indian J Physiol Pharmacol* 1995; **39**: 63–67.

11 Rompelberg CJM *et al*. Effects of the naturally occurring alkenylbenzenes eugenol and trans-anethole on drug-metabolising enzymes in the rat liver. *Food Chem Toxicol* 1993; **31**: 637–645.

Apricot

Species (Family)

Prunus armeniaca L. (Rosaceae)

Synonym(s)

None

Part(s) Used

Kernel (seed), expressed oil

Pharmacopoeial and Other Monographs

Martindale 32nd edition[G43]

Legal Category (Licensed Products)

Apricot is not included in the GSL. Amygdalin (a cyanogenetic glycoside) is classified as a POM.[1]

Constituents

Acids Phenolic. Various quinic acid esters of caffeic, *p*-coumaric and ferulic acids.[2] Neochlorogenic acid major in kernel, chlorogenic in fruit.[3]

Glycosides Cyanogenetic. Amygdalin (mandeloni-Cyanide content of kernel varies from 2 to 200 mg/100 g.[3]

Tannins Catechins, proanthocyanidins (condensed).[4]

Other constituents Cholesterol, an oestrogenic fraction (0.09%) containing oestrone (both free and conjugated) and α-oestradiol.[5]

Other plant parts

Leaves and fruit contain various flavonol (kaempferol, quercetin) glycosides including rutin (major).[5]

Food Use

Apricot fruit is commonly eaten. Apricot is listed by the Council of Europe as a natural source of food flavouring (category N1 and N2). These categories limit the total amount of hydrocyanic acid permitted in the final product to 1 mg/kg. Exceptions to this are 25 mg/kg for confectionery, 50 mg/kg for marzipan and 5 mg/kg for fruit juices.[G16] In the USA, apricot kernel extract is listed as GRAS (Generally Recognised As Safe).[G65]

Herbal Use

Traditionally, the oil has been incorporated into cosmetic and perfumery products such as soaps and creams.[G34]

Dosage

None documented. Traditionally, apricot kernels have not been utilised as a herbal remedy.

Pharmacological Actions

During the late 1970s and early 1980s considerable interest was generated in apricot from claims that laetrile (a semi-synthetic derivative of amygdalin) was an effective treatment for cancer. Two review papers[6,7] discuss these claims for laetrile together with its chemistry, metabolism and potential toxicity.

The claims for laetrile were based on three different theories. The first claimed that cancerous cells contained abundant quantities of β-glucosidases, enzymes which release hydrogen cyanide from the laetrile molecule as a result of hydrolysis. Normal cells were said to be protected because they contained low concentrations of β-glucosidases and high concentrations of rhodanese, an enzyme which converts cyanide to the less toxic thiocyanate. However, this theory was disproved when it was shown that both cancerous and normal cells contain only trace amounts of β-glucosidases, and similar amounts of rhodanese. In addition, it was thought that amygdalin was not absorbed intact from the gastrointestinal tract.[6,7]

The second theory proposed that following ingestion, amygdalin was hydrolysed to mandelonitrile, transported intact to the liver and converted to a β-glucuronide complex. This complex was then carried to the cancerous cells, hydrolysed by β-glucuronidases to release mandelonitrile and subsequently hydrogen cyanide. This theory was considered to be untenable.[7]

A third theory proposed that laetrile is vitamin B_{17}, that cancer is a result of a deficiency of this vitamin, and that chronic administration of laetrile would prevent cancer. Again this was not substantiated by any scientific evidence.[7]

A retrospective analysis of the use of laetrile by cancer patients reported that it may have slight activity.[6,7] However, a subsequent clinical trial concluded that laetrile was ineffective in cancer treatment. Furthermore, it was claimed that patients taking laetrile reduced their life expectancy as a result of lack of proper medical care and chronic cyanide poisoning.[6,7]

In order to reduce potential risks to the general public, amygdalin was made a prescription-only medicine in 1984.[1]

Side-effects, Toxicity

Laetrile and apricot kernel ingestion are the most common sources of cyanide poisoning, with more than 20 deaths reported.[6,7] Apricot kernels are toxic because of their amygdalin content. Hydrolysis of the amygdalin molecule by β-glucosidases, heat, mineral acids or high doses of ascorbic acid (vitamin C) yields hydrogen cyanide (HCN), benzaldehyde, and glucose. β-Glucosidases are not generally abundant in the gastrointestinal tract, but they are present in the kernels themselves as well as certain foods including beansprouts, carrots, celery, green peppers, lettuce, mushrooms and sweet almonds. Hydrolysis of the amygdalin molecule is slow in an acid environment but much more rapid in an alkaline pH. There may therefore be a delay in the onset of symptoms of HCN poisoning as a result of the transit time from the acid pH of the stomach to the alkaline environment of the small intestine.

Acute poisoning

Cyanide is rapidly absorbed from the upper gastrointestinal tract, diffuses readily throughout the body and promptly causes respiratory failure if untreated. Symptoms of cyanide toxicity progress rapidly from dizziness, headache, nausea, vomiting and drowsiness to dyspnoea, palpitations, marked hypotension, convulsions, paralysis, coma and death, which may occur from 1 to 15 minutes after ingestion. Antidotes for cyanide poisoning include nitrite, thiosulfate, hydroxocobalamin, cobalt edetate and aminophenol.[6,7]

Chronic poisoning

Principal symptoms include increased blood thiocyanate, goitre, thyroid cancer, lesions of the optic nerve, blindness, ataxia, hypertonia, cretinism and mental retardation.[6] These symptoms may develop as a result of ingesting significant amounts of cyanide, cyanogenetic precursors in the diet, or cyanogenetic

drugs such as laetrile. Demyelinating lesions and other neuromyopathies reportedly occur secondary to chronic cyanide exposure, including long-term therapy with laetrile. Agranulocytosis has also been attributed to long-term laetrile therapy.[6,7]

Individual reports of adverse reactions and cyanide poisoning in patients using laetrile have been documented.[G45]

Normally, low concentrations of ingested cyanide are controlled naturally by exhalation or by rapid conversion to the less toxic thiocyanate by the enzyme rhodanese. Oral doses of 50 mg of hydrogen cyanide (HCN) can be fatal. This is equivalent to approximately 30 g kernels which represents about 50–60 kernels, and approximately 2 mg HCN/g kernel. Apricot seed has also been reported to contain 2.92 mg HCN/g.[8] A 500-mg laetrile tablet was found to contain between 5 and 51 mg HCN/g.

There may be considerable variation in the number of kernels required to be toxic, depending on the concentration of amygdalin and β-glucosidases present in the kernels, the timespan of ingestion, the degree of maceration of the kernels, individual variation in hydrolysing, and detoxifying abilities.

Systemic concentrations of β-glucosidases are low and therefore toxicity following parenteral absorption of amygdalin is low. However, cyanide poisoning has been reported in rats following intraperitoneal administration of laetrile, suggesting another mechanism of hydrolysis had occurred.[6,7]

It is thought that cyanogenetic glycosides may possess carcinogenic properties. Mandelonitrile (amygdalin = mandelonitrile diglucoside) is mutagenic and stimulates guanylate cyclase.[6,7]

Contra-indications, Warnings

Apricot kernels are toxic due to their amygdalin content. Following ingestion hydrogen cyanide is released and may result in cyanide poisoning. Fatalities have been reported following the ingestion of apricot kernels. Contact dermatitis has been reported for apricot kernels.[9]

Pregnancy and lactation Apricot kernels are toxic and should not be ingested. The ingestion of cyanogenetic substances may result in teratogenic effects.[6] However, one case has been reported where no acute toxicity was noted in the infant when laetrile was used during the third term of pregnancy. It was unknown whether chronic effects would be manifested at a later date.[6] Breeding rats fed ground apricot kernels had pups with normal birth weights, but with lower survival rates and lower weaning weights.[3]

Pharmaceutical Comment

Interest in apricot kernels was generated as a result of claims in the late 1970s that laetrile, a semi-synthetic derivative of the naturally occurring constituent amygdalin, was a natural, non-toxic cure for cancer. Apricot kernels were seen as an alternative source for this miracle cure. These claims have since been disproved and it has been established that laetrile (amygdalin) is far from non-toxic, particularly if administered orally. Fatal cases of cyanide poisoning have been reported following the ingestion of apricot kernels.

References

See also General References G10, G16, G32, G34, G43 and G57.

1 The Medicines (Cyanogenetic Substances) Order, SI 1984 No. 187, London: HMSO, 1984.

2 Möller B, Herrmann K. Quinic acid esters of hydroxycinnamic acids in stone and pome fruit. *Phytochemistry* 1983; **22**: 477–481.

3 Miller KW *et al.* Amygdalin metabolism and effect on reproduction of rats fed apricot kernels. *J Toxicol Environ Health* 1981; **7**: 457–467.

4 Awad O. Steroidal estrogens of *Prunus armeniaca* seeds. *Phytochemistry* 1973; **13**: 678–690.

5 Henning W, Herrmann K. Flavonol glycosides of apricots (*Prunus armeniaca* L.) and peaches (*Prunus persica* Batch). 13. Phenolics of fruits. *Z Lebensm Unters Forsch* 1980; **171**: 183–188.

6 Chandler RF *et al.* Laetrile in perspective. *Can Pharm J* 1984; **117**: 517–520.

7 Chandler RF *et al.* Controversial laetrile. *Pharm J* 1984; **232**: 330–332.

8 Holzbecher MD *et al.* The cyanide content of laetrile preparations, apricot, peach and apple seeds. *Clin Toxicol* 1984; **22**: 341–347.

9 Göransson K. Contact urticaria to apricot stone. *Contact Dermatitis* 1981; **7**: 282.

Arnica

Species (Family)

Arnica montana L. (Asteraceae/Compositae)
Arnica chamissonis Less. ssp.*foliosa* (Nutt.) Maguire
also allowed in German Pharmacopoeia.[G52]

Synonym(s)

Leopard's Bane, Mountain Tobacco, Wolf's Bane

Part(s) Used

Flower

Pharmacopoeial and Other Monographs

BHP 1996[G9]
BP 2001[G15]
ESCOP 1997[G52]
Martindale 32nd edition[G43]
Mills and Bone[G50]
PDR for Herbal Medicines 2nd edition[G36]
Ph Eur 2002[G28]

Legal Category (Licensed Products)

GSL, for external use only.[G37]

Constituents[1–3,G2,G22,G41,G52,G64]

Alkaloids Traces of non-toxic alkaloids tussilagine and isotussilagine[4] but these are reportedly artefacts produced during extraction.[5]

Amines Betaine, choline and trimethylamine.

Carbohydrates Mucilage, polysaccharides including inulin.

Coumarins Scopoletin and umbelliferone.

Flavonoids Betuletol, eupafolin, flavonol glucuronides,[1–3] hispidulin, isorhamnetin, kaempferol, laciniatin, luteolin, patuletin, quercetin, spinacetin, tricin and 3,5,7-trihydroxy-6,3′,4′-trimethoxyflavone.

Terpenoids Sesquiterpene lactones of the pseudo-guaianolide-type, 0.2–0.8%.[G52] Pharmacopoeial standard not less than 0.4%.[G15,G28] Helenalin,[6] 11α,13-dihydrohelenalin and their esters with acetic,

isobutyric, methacrylic, tiglic and other carboxylic acids.[G52] Diterpenes including z-labd-13-ene-8α,15-diol.[7]

Volatile oils Up to 1%, normally about 0.3%. Thymol and thymol derivatives.

Other constituents Amino acid (2-pyrrolidine acetic), bitter principle (arnicin), caffeic acid, carotenoids, fatty acids, phytosterols, polyacetylenes, resin, tannin (unspecified).

Food Use

Arnica is listed by the Council of Europe as a natural source of food flavouring (category N2). This category indicates that arnica can be added to foodstuffs in small quantities, with a possible limitation of an active principle (as yet unspecified) in the final product.[G16] In the USA, arnica is listed by the Food and Drugs Administration (FDA) as an 'unsafe herb',[G22] and is only approved for food use in alcoholic beverages.[G41]

Herbal Use[G2–G4,G32,G43,G50,G52,G54]

Arnica is stated to possess topical counter-irritant properties. It has been used for unbroken chilblains, alopecia neurotica, insect bites, gingivitis, aphthous ulcers, rheumatoid complaints and specifically for sprains and bruises.[G2,G7,G52,G64]

German Commission E approved external use for injuries and consequences of accidents, e.g. haematoma, dislocation, contusions, oedema due to fracture, rheumatoid muscle and joint pains, inflammation of oral and throat region, furuncolosis, inflammation caused by insect bites and superficial phlebitis.[G3,G4]

Arnica is mainly used in homeopathic preparations; it is used to a lesser extent in herbal products.

Dosage

Tincture of arnica flower (BPC 1949) 2–4 mL for external application only.

Preparations Ointments, creams, gels, compresses made with 5–25% v/v tinctures, 5–25% v/v fluid extracts, diluted tinctures or fluid extract (1:3–1:10), decoctions 2.0 g drug/100 mL water.[G3,G4]

Pharmacological Actions[G50,G52,G56]

In vitro and animal studies

Antimicrobial activity Arnica has been reported to exhibit bactericidal properties against *Listeria monocytogenes* and *Salmonella typhimurium*.[G41] Helenalin and related sesquiterpenes from arnica have antimicrobial activity against *Bacillus subtilis* and *Staphylococcus aureus*,[8] *Corynebacterium insidosum, Micrococcus roseus, Mycobacterium phlei, Sarcinia lutea* and *Proteus vulgaris*.[G52] Antifungal activity against *Trichophyton mentagrophytes, Epidermaphyton* spp. and *Botrytis cinerea* is reported for helenalin.[8,G52]

Antitumour activity The cytotoxicity of 21 flavonoids and five sesquiterpene lactones from *Arnica* spp. has been investigated *in vitro* in studies using GLC_4 (a human small cell lung carcinoma) and COLO 320 (a human colorectal cancer) cell lines.[9] The most potent compound, helenalin, had an IC_{50} value of 0.44 µmol/L against GLC_4 and 1.0 µmol/L against COLO 320 after 2 hours exposure.[9] Some of the individual flavonols and flavones of arnica at non-toxic concentrations significantly reduced helenalin-induced cytotoxicity *in vitro*.[10]

Anti-inflammatory activity Moderate (29%) anti-inflammatory effect in the carageenan rat paw model has been reported for arnica.[11] Helenalin is a potent inhibitor in this test and in chronic adjuvant arthritis tests in rats.[12] The α-methylene-γ-lactone moiety of sesquiterpenes is required for activity, and the potency of helenalin is enhanced by the presence of the 6-hydroxy group.[13] The mode of action of sesquiterpene lactones as anti-inflammatory agents is at multiple sites. At a concentration of 5×10^{-4} mol/L, the compounds uncoupled oxidative phosphorylation of human polymorphoneutrophils, elevated cyclic adenosine monophosphate (cAMP) levels of rat neutrophils, and rat and mouse liver cells, and inhibited free and total lysosomal enzyme activity.[12] Human polymorphonuclear neutrophil chemotaxis was inhibited at 5×10^{-4} mol/L, whereas prostaglandin synthetase activity was inhibited at concentrations of 10^{-3} mol/L. Helenalin and 11α-13-dihydrohelenalin inhibited collagen-induced platelet aggregation, thromboxane formation and 5-hydroxytryptamine secretion in a concentration-dependent manner.[14]

Other activities Helenalin has potent activity in the hotplate tail flick analgesic test in mice.[13]

Helenalin has also been reported to possess immunostimulant activity *in vitro*,[15] while high molecular weight polysaccharides have been found to exhibit immunostimulant activity *in vivo* in the carbon clearance test in mice.[15,16]

Arnica contains an adrenaline-like pressor substance and a cardiotonic substance.[G24]

Clinical studies

A gel preparation of arnica flowers applied externally to the limbs of 12 male volunteers was more effective than placebo in the treatment of muscle ache.[G50,G52] In a randomised, double-blind, placebo-controlled study, 89 patients with venous insufficiency received arnica gel (20% tincture) or placebo.[G50] It was reported that arnica treatment produced improvements in venous tone, oedema and in feeling of heaviness in the legs.

Side-effects, Toxicity

Arnica is poisonous if taken internally. It is irritant to mucous membranes and ingestion may result in fatal gastroenteritis, muscle paralysis (voluntary and cardiac), increase or decrease in pulse rate, palpitation of the heart, shortness of breath, and may even lead to death.[G33,G41] Helenalin is stated to be the toxic principle responsible for these effects.[G33] Thirty millilitres of a 20% arnica tincture, taken by mouth, was reported to produce serious, but not fatal, symptoms.[G41] The topical application of arnica has been documented to cause dermatitis.[17,G51] Arnica is a strong sensitiser, with the sesquiterpene lactone constituents implicated as the contact allergens: they possess an α-methylene group exocyclic to a γ-lactone ring, which is recognised as an immunological prerequisite for contact allergy.[17,18] Helenalin is also reported to possess cytotoxic activity and this has been attributed to its ability to alkylate with sulfhydryl groups.[G33] Helenalin was not mutagenic in the *Salmonella typhimurium* assay.[G52]

Contra-indications, Warnings

Arnica should not be taken internally except in suitable homeopathic dilutions.[G42]

Externally, arnica is poorly tolerated by some people, precipitating allergic reactions in sensitive individuals.[G42] It should only be applied to unbroken skin and withdrawn at the first sign of reaction.[G7] Toxic allergic skin reactions have occurred following application of the tincture.[G33]

Pharmaceutical Comment

The chemistry and pharmacology of arnica are well documented, but there is a paucity of clinical data. Anti-inflammatory properties associated with sesquiterpene lactones justify the herbal uses, although allergenic and cytotoxic properties are also associated with this class of constituents. Arnica is not suitable for internal use, although it is present in some homeopathic products. External use of arnica tincture, which is included as an ingredient in some cosmetics, hair shampoos and bath preparations, may cause an allergic reaction. The pyrrolizidine alkaloids tussilagine and isotussilagine, reportedly present in arnica, are non-toxic. Moreover, they are artefacts produced during the extraction process with methanol.

References

See also General References G2, G9, G11, G15, G16, G19, G22, G28, G29, G31, G32, G36, G37, G41, G42, G43, G48, G50, G51, G52, G54, G56 and G64.

1 Merfort I, Wendisch D. Flavonoidglycoside aus *Arnica montana* und *Arnica chamissonis*. *Planta Med* 1987; **53**: 434–437.
2 Merfort I. Flavonol glycosides of Arnicae flos DAB 9. *Planta Med* 1986; **52**: 427.
3 Merfort I, Wendisch D. Flavonolglucuronide aus den blüten von *Arnica montana*. *Planta Med* 1988; **54**: 247–250.
4 Passreiter CM *et al*. Tussilagine and isotussilagine: two pyrrolizidine alkaloids in the genus *Arnica*. *Planta Med* 1992; **58**: 556–557.
5 Passreiter CM. Co-occurrence of 2-pyrrolidine-acetic acid with the pyrrolizidines tussilaginic acid and isotussilaginic acid and their 1-epimers in *Arnica* species and *Tussilago farfara*. *Phytochem* 1992; **31**: 4135–4137.
6 Leven W, Willuhn G. Spectrophotometric determination of sesquiterpenlactone (S1) in 'Arnicae flos DAB 9' with m-dinitrobenzene. *Planta Med* 1986; **52**: 537–538.
7 Schmidt Th *et al*. First diterpenes from *Arnica*. *Planta Med* 1992; **58**: A713.
8 Lee K-H *et al*. Structure–antimicrobial activity relationships among the sesquiterpene lactones and related compounds. *Phytochemistry* 1977; **16**: 117–118.
9 Woerdenbag HJ *et al*. Cytotoxicity of flavonoids and sesquiterpene lactones from *Arnica* species against the GLC$_4$ and the COLO 320 cell lines. *Planta Med* 1994; **60**: 434–437.
10 Woerdenbag HJ *et al*. Decreased helenalin-induced cytotoxicity by flavonoids from *Arnica* as studied in a human lung carcinoma cell line. *Phytomedicine* 1995; **2**: 127–132.
11 Mascolo N *et al*. Biological screening of Italian medicinal plants for anti-inflammatory activity. *Phytother Res* 1987; **1**: 28–31.
12 Hall IH *et al*. Mode of action of sesquiterpene lactones as anti-inflammatory agents. *J Pharm Sci* 1980; **69**: 537–543.
13 Hall IH *et al*. Anti-inflammatory activity of sesquiterpene lactones and related compounds. *J Pharm Sci* 1979; **68**: 537–542.
14 Schröder H *et al*. Helenalin and 11α,13-dihydrohelenalin, two constituents from *Arnica montana* L., inhibit human platelet function via thiol-dependent pathways. *Thrombosis Res* 1990; **57**: 839–845.
15 Chang HM *et al*. *Advances in Chinese Medicinal Materials Research*. Philadelphia: World Scientific, 1985.
16 Puhlmann J, Wagner H. Immunologically active polysaccharides from *Arnica montana* herbs and tissue cultures. *Planta Med* 1989; **55**: 99.
17 Rudzki E, Grzywa Z. Dermatitis from *Arnica montana*. *Contact Dermatitis* 1977; **3**: 281–282.
18 Hausen BM. Identification of the allergens of *Arnica montana* L. *Contact Dermatitis* 1978; **4**: 308.

Artichoke

Species (Family)

Cynara scolymus L. (Asteraceae/Compositae)

Synonym(s)

Globe Artichoke.

Globe artichoke should not be confused with Jerusalem artichoke, which is the tuber of *Helianthus tuberosa* L.

Part(s) Used

Leaf

Pharmacopoeial and Other Monographs

BHP 1996[G9]
Complete German Commission E[G3]
Martindale 32nd edition[G43]
Mills and Bone[G50]
PDR for Herbal Medicines 2nd edition[G36]

Legal Category (Licensed Products)

GSL[G37]

Constituents[1,2,G41]

Acids Phenolic, up to 2%. Caffeic acid, mono- and dicaffeoylquinic acid derivatives, e.g. cynarin (1,5-di-O-caffeoylquinic acids) and chlorogenic acid (mono derivative).

Flavonoids 0.1–1%. Flavone glycosides e.g. luteolin-7β-rutinoside (scolymoside), luteolin-7β-D-glucoside and luteolin-4β-D-glucoside.

Volatile oils Sesquiterpenes β-selinene and caryophyllene (major); also eugenol, phenylacetaldehyde, decanal, oct-1-en-3-one, hex-1-en-3-one, and non-trans-2-enal.

Other constituents Phytosterols (taraxasterol and β-taraxasterol), tannins, glycolic and glyceric acids, sugars, inulin, enzymes including peroxidases,[3] cynaropicrin and other sesquiterpene lactones, e.g. grosheimin, cynarotriol.[4,5] The root and fully developed fruits and flowers are devoid of cynaropicrin; highest content reported in young leaves.[6]

Food Use

Artichoke is listed by the Council of Europe as a natural source of food flavouring (category N2). This category indicates that artichoke can be added to foodstuffs in small quantities, with a possible limitation of an active principle (as yet unspecified) in the final product.[G16] In the USA, artichoke leaves are approved for use in alcoholic beverages only, with an average maximum concentration of 0.0016% (16 ppm).[G41]

Herbal Use

Artichoke is stated to possess diuretic, choleretic, hypocholesterolaemic, hypolipidaemic, and hepatostimulating properties.[7–9] Modern use of artichoke is focused on its use in the treatment of hyperlipidaemia, hyperlipoproteinaemia, non-ulcer dyspepsia and conditions requiring an increase in choleresis. There is also interest in the potential hepatoprotective properties of globe artichoke, although this has not yet been tested in controlled clinical trials.[10,11]

Dosage

The German Commission E recommends an average daily dose of 6 g drug, or an equivalent dose of extract (based on the herb-to-extract ratio) or other preparations, for dyspeptic problems.[G3,G56] A recommended dosage regimen for liquid extract (1 : 2) is 3–8 mL daily.[G50]

Dosages used in clinical trials of globe artichoke leaf extract have assessed the effects of dosages of up to 1.92 g daily in divided doses for up to six months.[12]

Pharmacological Actions

Several pharmacological properties have been documented for artichoke leaf, including inhibition of cholesterol biosynthesis, hypolipidaemic, antioxidant and hepatoprotective activity. It remains unclear which of the constituents of artichoke are responsible for its pharmacological activities. The dicaffeoylquinic acids, which include cynarin, are likely to be an important group of constituents in this respect.[11,G50] The sesquiterpene lactones, such as cynaropicrin, and flavonoids, such as luteolin glycoside, may also exert biological effects.[11]

In vitro and animal studies

Hypolipidaemic, hypocholesterolaemic and choleretic activity Hypolipidaemic, hypocholesterolaemic and choleretic activities are well documented for globe artichoke leaf extract and particularly for the constituent cynarin; this literature has been reviewed.[10,11] Globe artichoke leaf extract not only increases choleresis and, therefore, cholesterol elimination, but also has been shown to inhibit cholesterol biosynthesis.[10] Preparations of globe artichoke leaf extract inhibit cholesterol biosynthesis in a concentration-dependent manner in studies in cultured rat hepatocytes.[13,14] Low concentrations ($<$0.1 mg/mL) of globe artichoke extract achieved around 20% inhibition, whereas 65% inhibition was noted with concentrations of 1 mg/mL. Luteolin was considered to be one of the most important constituents for this effect, and it was suggested that a possible mechanism of action might be indirect inhibition of hydroxymethylglutaryl-CoA reductase (HMG-CoA).[14] Other *in vitro* studies have documented a concentration-dependent inhibition of *de novo* cholesterol biosynthesis in cultured rat and human hepatocytes for globe artichoke leaf extract 0.03–0.1 mg/mL.[15]

Several other experimental studies have documented lipid-lowering effects for globe artichoke leaf extract and cynarin *in vivo*.[10,11] A study in rats explored the hypocholesterolaemic, hypolipidaemic and choleretic effects of purified (containing 46% caffeoylquinic acids, calculated as cholorogenic acid) and total extracts of globe artichoke leaf (containing 19% caffeoylquinic acids, calculated as cholorogenic acid).[7] The purified extract was found to be more potent than the total artichoke extract: purified extract 25 mg/kg intraperitoneally reduced plasma triglyceride and cholesterol concentrations by 33% and 45%, respectively, whereas reductions of only 18% and 14%, respectively, were observed with the total extract (100 mg/kg intraperitoneally).[7] Both purified (25 mg/kg intraperitoneally) and total extract (200 mg/kg intraperitoneally) significantly enhanced bile secretion following treatment, compared with baseline values; the increase in bile secretion seen with the purified extract was still statistically significant 3 hours after treatment. The more potent pharmacological activities observed with the purified extract were attributed to the higher concentration of monocaffeoylquinic acids

(e.g. chlorogenic, neochlorogenic) compared with dicaffeoylquinic acids (e.g. cynarin) present.

Another study investigated the effects of cynarin on total cholesterol concentrations in serum and liver of rats given ethanol (6 g/kg/day by gavage over three days).[16] In rats given ethanol alone, serum cholesterol concentrations rose significantly by 44%, compared with controls ($p < 0.01$). Rats given ethanol plus cynarin (30 mg/kg intraperitoneally 30 minutes before gavage) showed a significant reduction in serum cholesterol concentrations, compared with controls ($p < 0.05$).

Antioxidant and hepatoprotective activity In *vitro*, a luteolin-rich globe artichoke leaf aqueous extract (flavonoid content around 0.4% w/w) retarded low-density lipoprotein (LDL) oxidation in a concentration-dependent manner (determined by a prolongation of the lag phase to conjugated diene formation).[17] The same tests carried out with the pure aglycone luteolin at concentrations of 0.1–1 µmol/L showed that this constituent had a similar concentration-dependent effect on LDL oxidation in this model. Luteolin-7-O-glucoside also demonstrated a concentration-dependent reduction in LDL oxidation, but was less potent than luteolin.

Several *in vitro* and *in vivo* studies have investigated the antioxidative and hepatoprotective properties of globe artichoke leaf extracts, and their constituents, against liver cell damage induced by different hepatotoxins.

The hepatoprotective effect of polyphenolic compounds isolated from artichoke has been investigated *in vitro* using rat hepatocytes.[8] Cynarin was the only compound reported to exhibit significant cytoprotective activity, with a lesser action demonstrated by caffeic acid. A standardised extract of globe artichoke (Hepar-SL forte) significantly inhibited the formation of malondialdehyde induced by *tert*-butyl-hydroperoxide (*t*-BHP) in a concentration-dependent manner within 40 minutes of incubation, compared with control.[18] The protective antioxidant effect of globe artichoke was reported to be significant, compared with control, even at a concentration of 1 µg/mL. A reduction in *t*-BHP-induced cell death with globe artichoke extract was also observed. Further studies assessed the antioxidative and protective potential of the same extract (Hepar-SL forte) in cultures of primary rat hepatocytes exposed to *t*-BHP.[19] Incubation of cultured hepatocytes with globe artichoke extract and *t*-BHP inhibited *t*-BHP-induced malondialdehyde formation in a concentration-dependent manner. Globe artichoke extract was significantly effective, compared with control, at concentrations down to 0.001 mg/mL. Furthermore, concentrations of globe artichoke extract down to 0.005 mg/mL significantly enhanced hepatocyte survival. The antioxidative effect of the extract was not affected by various pretreatments (including tryptic digestion, boiling and acidification), although it was sensitive to alkalinisation. Incubation with the globe artichoke constituents chlorogenic acid and cynarin resulted in significant inhibition, and incubation with both compounds was reported to have a synergistic effect, although an additive effect may be a more accurate description of the findings. Chlorogenic acid and cynarin were not solely responsible for the antioxidant effect, as reduction of malondialdehyde formation by the extract was at least twofold that seen with the chlorogenic acid and cynarin.[19] The antioxidative and hepatoprotective potential of globe artichoke extract was confirmed in other studies which also indicated that several constituents of the extract may contribute to the effects.[20]

The effects of globe artichoke leaf extract and its constituents have also been investigated for activity against oxidative stress in studies using human leukocytes.[21] Globe artichoke leaf extract demonstrated a concentration-dependent inhibition of oxidative stress induced by several agents, such as hydrogen peroxide and phorbol-12-myristate-13-acetate, that generate reactive oxygen species. The constituents cynarin, caffeic acid, chlorogenic acid and luteolin also showed concentration-dependent inhibitory activity in these models.

In vivo hepatoprotectivity against tetrachloromethane-induced hepatitis has been documented for globe artichoke leaf extract (500 mg/kg) administered orally to rats 48 hours, 24 hours and 1 hour before intoxication.[9] Concentrations of liver transaminases were significantly lower in rats given globe artichoke leaf extract, compared with those in controls. A hepatoregenerating effect has also been described for an aqueous extract of globe artichoke leaf administered orally to rats for three weeks following partial hepatectomy.[22] Regeneration was determined by stimulation of mitosis and increased weight in the residual liver when animals were sacrificed in globe artichoke-treated rats, compared with controls. In a similar study, aqueous extract of globe artichoke leaf (0.5 mL daily for five days preceding hepatectomy) was found to be more potent than a root extract.[23]

Clinical studies

Several clinical trials have explored the choleretic and hypolipidaemic properties of globe artichoke leaf extract, and its effects in patients with symptoms of dyspepsia.

A randomised, double-blind, placebo-controlled, crossover trial involving 20 male volunteers assessed the choleretic effects of a single intraduodenal dose (1.92 g in 300 mL water) of the globe artichoke leaf extract Hepar-SL forte.[24] Intraduodenal bile secretion, the primary outcome variable, was measured using multichannel probes starting 30 minutes after drug administration and continuing for up to 4 hours afterwards. An increase in bile secretion was observed in both groups; maximal increases for globe artichoke leaf extract and placebo were 152% at 60 minutes after drug administration, and 40% at 30 minutes, respectively. Differences between globe artichoke leaf extract and placebo were statistically significant at 30, 60 and 90 minutes after drug administration ($p < 0.01$) and at 120 and 150 minutes after drug administration ($p < 0.05$). In another randomised controlled trial, 60 patients with dyspepsia received a combination preparation containing extracts of globe artichoke 50 mg, boldo (*Peumus boldus*) 30 mg and chelidonium (*Chelidonium majus*) 20 mg per tablet, or placebo, three times daily for 14 days.[25] The volume of bile secreted, measured using a duodenal probe, increased significantly in the treatment group, compared with the placebo group ($p < 0.01$). Also, an improvement in symptoms was reported for 50% of the treatment group, compared with 38% of the placebo group. There are also clinical studies in the older literature (some of which were placebo-controlled trials, whereas others were open, uncontrolled studies) which report choleretic effects with globe artichoke leaf extract. These trials have been summarised in several reviews.[10,24,G50]

The effects of globe artichoke leaf extract have also been monitored in several postmarketing surveillance (phase IV) studies in patients with non-specific gastrointestinal complaints, including dyspepsia,[12] functional biliary tract complaints, constipation and gastric irritation.[11] The studies monitored the effects of globe artichoke leaf extract (Hepar-SL forte; one capsule contains 320 mg standardised aqueous extract; drug–extract ratio: 3.5 to 5.5 : 1) up to six capsules daily for six weeks[11] or six months.[12] Both studies reported improvements in clinical symptoms and reductions in serum total cholesterol and triglyceride concentrations, compared with baseline values. A subgroup analysis of 279 patients with at least three of five symptoms of irritable bowel syndrome reported significant reductions in the severity of symptoms and favourable evaluations of overall effectiveness by both physicians and participants.[26] The findings from postmarketing surveillance studies provide supporting data for the effects of globe artichoke leaf extract, but these are open studies and do not include a control group and, therefore, are not designed to assess efficacy.

The efficacy of globe artichoke leaf extract in patients with hyperlipoproteinaemia has been assessed in a randomised, double-blind, placebo-controlled, multicentre trial involving 143 patients with initial total cholesterol concentrations of >7.3 mmol/L (>280 mg/dL).[27] Participants received globe artichoke leaf extract (CY450; drug–extract ratio: 25 to 35:1) 1800 mg daily in two divided doses, or placebo, for six weeks. At the end of the study, mean total cholesterol concentrations had decreased by 18.5% to 6.31 mmol/L and by 8.6% to 7.03 mmol/L in the CY450 and placebo groups, respectively ($p < 0.0001$). CY450 treatment also led to a significant reduction in LDL cholesterol, compared with placebo ($p = 0.0001$). There was no difference between CY450 recipients and placebo recipients in blood concentrations of the liver enzyme gamma-glutamyltransferase (GGT).

A published abstract reports the findings of a previous randomised, double-blind, placebo-controlled trial of a globe artichoke leaf extract (Hepar-SL forte; 640 mg three times daily for 12 weeks) involving 44 healthy volunteers.[15] Mean baseline total cholesterol concentrations for participants in this study were low (placebo group: 203.0 mg/dL; globe artichoke extract group: 204.2 mg/dL). Subgroup analysis suggested lipid-lowering effects with globe artichoke extract for participants with baseline total cholesterol concentrations of >200 mg/dL. However, numbers of participants included in this analysis were small. The study indicates only that trials in patients with hyperlipoproteinaemia are required.

A series of three open, uncontrolled studies involved the administration of pressed globe artichoke juice (obtained from fresh leaves and flower buds) 10 mL three times daily for up to 12 weeks to a total of 84 patients with secondary hyperlipidaemia (total cholesterol $\geqslant$260 mg/dL).[28] After six weeks' treatment, total cholesterol, LDL cholesterol and triglyceride concentrations decreased, whereas high-density lipoprotein cholesterol tended to increase. Another uncontrolled study involved the administration of cynarin to 17 patients with familial type IIa or type IIb hyperlipoproteinaemia for whom blood lipid concentrations were maintained with dietary treatment alone.[29] Cynarin was taken 15 minutes before meals at either 250 mg or 750 mg daily dose. Over a period of three months, cynarin was reported to have no effect on mean serum cholesterol and triglyceride concentrations.[29] The results were in agreement with the findings of some previous workers, but

also in contrast to other studies that have reported cynarin to be effective in lowering serum concentrations of cholesterol and triglycerides when taken in daily doses ranging from 60 mg to 1500 mg.[29]

Side-effects, Toxicity

A randomised, double-blind, placebo-controlled trial involving 143 patients with hyperlipoproteinaemia reported a similar frequency of adverse events for globe artichoke leaf extract (CY450) and placebo groups.[27] A total of 28 adverse events were reported during the study, 26 of which related to mild changes in laboratory values. The relationship to the globe artichoke was considered to be 'unlikely' in all cases.

Postmarketing surveillance (phase IV) studies have monitored patients with non-specific gastrointestinal complaints receiving treatment with globe artichoke leaf extract (Hepar-SL forte; up to 1.92 g daily for six weeks[11] or six months[12]). In one study involving 533 patients with non-specific gastrointestinal complaints, including dyspepsia, functional biliary tract complaints, constipation and gastric irritation, seven adverse events (weakness, hunger, flatulence) were reported (1.3% of participants).[11] No serious adverse events were reported. A second postmarketing surveillance study involved 203 patients with symptoms of dyspepsia who received globe artichoke leaf extract up to 1.92 g daily for up to six months.[12] It was reported that no adverse events were recorded during the study, and that the physician's overall judgement of tolerability was given as 'good' or 'excellent' in 98.5% of cases.

Allergic contact dermatitis, with cross-sensitivity to other Compositae plants, has been documented for globe artichoke.[30,G51] A case of occupational contact urticaria syndrome in a 20-year-old woman has been reported in association with globe artichoke. The woman developed acute generalised urticaria, angioedema of the hands, forearms and face, and respiratory symptoms after handling globe artichokes. The clinical history and results of skin-prick tests indicated that the woman had developed type I allergy to globe artichoke antigen(s).[31] An isolated case of allergy to ingested globe artichoke has also been described.[32]

Cynaropicrin and other sesquiterpene lactones with allergenic potential have been isolated from globe artichoke.[30,G53] Purified globe artichoke extract is more toxic than a total extract. LD_{50} values (rat, by intraperitoneal injection) have been documented as greater than 1000 mg/kg (total extract) and 265 mg/kg (purified extract).[7]

Contra-indications, Warnings

Globe artichoke yields cynaropicrin, a potentially allergenic sesquiterpene lactone.[G51] Individuals with an existing hypersensitivity to any member of the Compositae family may develop an allergic reaction to globe artichoke.

Pregnancy and lactation In view of the lack of toxicity data, excessive use of globe artichoke should be avoided during pregnancy and lactation.

Pharmaceutical Comment

Globe artichoke is characterised by the phenolic acid constituents, in particular cynarin. Experimental studies (*in vitro* and *in vivo*) support some of the reputed uses of artichoke. Traditionally, the choleretic and cholesterol-lowering activities of globe artichoke have been attributed to cynarin.[7] However, studies in animals and humans have suggested that these effects may in fact be due to the monocaffeoylquinic acids present in globe artichoke (e.g. chlorogenic and neochlorogenic acids). Clinical trials investigating the use of globe artichoke and cynarin in the treatment of hyperlipidaemia generally report positive results. However, further rigorous clinical trials are required to establish the benefit of globe artichoke leaf extract as a lipid- and cholesterol-lowering agent. Hepatoprotective and hepatoregenerating activities have been documented for cynarin *in vitro* and in animals (rats). However, these effects have not yet been documented in clinical studies.

References

See also General References G3, G9, G16, G19, G36, G41, G43, G49, G50 and G51.

1   Brand N. Cynara scolymus L. – Die Artischocke. *Z Phytother* 1990; **11**: 169–175.
2   Hammouda FM *et al*. Quantitative determination of the active constituents in Egyptian cultivated *Cynara scolymus*. *Int J Pharmacog* 1993; **31**: 299–304.
3   Kamel MY, Ghazy AM. Peroxidases of *Cyanara scolymus* (global artichoke) leaves: purification and properties. *Acta Biol Med Germ* 1973; **31**: 39–49.
4   Jouany JM *et al*. Dosage indirect de la cynaropicrine dans la *Cynara scolymus* (Compositae) par libération de sa chaîne latérale hydroxyméthylacrylique. *Plant Méd Phytothér* 1975; **9**: 72–78.
5   Barbetti P *et al*. Grosulfeimin and new related guaianolides from *Cynara scolymus* L. *Ars Pharmac* 1992; **33**: 433–439.
6   Schneider G, Thiele Kl. Die Verteilung des Bitterstoffes Cynaropicrin in der Artischocke. *Planta Med* 1974; **26**: 174–183.
7   Lietti A. Choleretic and cholesterol lowering properties of two artichoke extracts. *Fitoterapia* 1977; **48**: 153–158.
8   Adzet T *et al*. Hepatoprotective activity of polyphenolic compounds from *Cynara scolymus* against CCl4 toxicity in isolated rat hepatocytes. *J Nat Prod* 1987; **50**: 612–617.
9   Adzet T *et al*. Action of an artichoke extract against CCl4-induced heptotoxicity in rats. *Acta Pharm Jugosl* 1987; **37**: 183–187.
10 Kraft K. Artichoke leaf extract – recent findings reflecting effects on lipid metabolism, liver and gastrointestinal tracts. *Phytomedicine* 1997; **4**: 369–378.
11 Fintelmann V, Menssen HG. Artichoke leaf extract. Current knowledge concerning its efficacy as a lipid-reducer and antidyspeptic agent. *Dtsch Apoth Ztg* 1996; **136**: 1405–1414.
12 Fintelmann V, Petrowicz O. Long-term administration of an artichoke extract for dyspepsia symptoms. Results of an observational study. *Natura Med* 1998; **13**: 17–26.
13 Gebhardt R. Artischockenextrakt. In vitro Nachweis einer Hemmwirkung auf die Cholesterin-Biosynthese. *Med Welt* 1995; **46**: 348–350.
14 Gebhardt R. Inhibition of cholesterol biosynthesis in primary cultured rat hepatocytes by artichoke (*Cynara scolymus* L.) extracts. *J Pharmacol Exp Ther* 1998; **286**: 1122–1128.
15 Petrowicz O *et al*. Effects of artichoke leaf extract (ALE) on lipoprotein metabolism in vitro and in vivo. *Atherosclerosis* 1997; **129**: 147.
16 Wójcicki J. Effect of 1,5-dicaffeylquinic acid (Cynarine) on cholesterol levels in serum and liver of acute ethanol-treated rats. *Drug Alcohol Depend* 1978; **3**: 143–145.
17 Brown JE, Rice-Evans CA. Luteolin-rich artichoke extract protects low density lipoprotein from oxidation *in vitro*. *Free Radic Res* 1998; **29**: 247–255.
18 Gebhardt R. Protektive antioxidative Wirkungen von Artischocken-extrakt an der Leberzelle. *Med Welt* 1995; **46**: 393–395.
19 Gebhardt R. Antioxidative and protective properties of extracts from leaves of the artichoke (*Cynara scolymus* L.) against hydroperoxide-induced oxidative stress in cultured rat hepatocytes. *Toxicol Appl Pharmacol* 1997; **144**: 279–286.
20 Gebhardt R, Fausel M. Antioxidant and hepatoprotective effects of artichoke extracts and constituents in cultured rat hepatocytes. *Toxicology in Vitro* 1997; **11**: 669–672.
21 Perez-Garcia F *et al*. Activity of artichoke leaf extract on reactive oxygen species in human leukocytes. *Free Radic Res* 2000; **33**: 661–665.

22 Maros T *et al.* Wirkungen der *Cynara scolymus*-Extrakte auf die Regeneration der Rattenleber. *Arzneimittelforschung* 1966; **16**: 127–129.

23 Maros T *et al.* Wirkungen der *Cynara scolymus*-extrakte auf die Regeneration der Rattenleber. *Arzneimittelforschung* 1968; **18**: 884–886.

24 Kirchhoff R *et al.* Increase in choleresis by means of artichoke extract. *Phytomedicine* 1994; **1**: 107–115.

25 Kupke D *et al.* Prüfung der choleretischen Aktivität eines pflanzlichen Cholagogums. *Z Allg Med* 1991; **67**: 1046–1058.

26 Walker A *et al.* Artichoke leaf extract reduces symptoms of irritable bowel syndrome in a post-marketing surveillance study. *Phytother Res* 2001; **15**: 58–61.

27 Englisch W *et al.* Efficacy of artichoke dry extract in patients with hyperlipoproteinemia. *Arzneim-Forsch/Drug Res* 2000; **50**: 260–265.

28 Dorn M. Improvement in raised lipid levels with artichoke juice (*Cynara scolymus* L.). *Br J Phytother* 1995/96; **4**: 21–26.

29 Heckers H *et al.* Inefficiency of cynarin as therapeutic regimen in familial type II hyperlipoproteinaemia. *Atherosclerosis* 1977; **26**: 249–253.

30 Meding B. Allergic contact dermatitis from artichoke, *Cynara scolymus*. *Contact Dermatitis* 1983; **9**: 314.

31 Quirce S *et al.* Occupational contact urticaria syndrome caused by globe artichoke (*Cynara scolymus*). *J Allergy Clin Immunol* 1996; **97**: 710–711.

32 Romano C *et al.* A case of allergy to globe artichoke and other clinical cases of rare food allergy. *J Invest Allergol Clin Immunol* 2000; **10**: 102–104.

Asafoetida

Species (Family)

Ferula species including:
(i) *Ferula assafoetida* L. (*Ferula rubricaulis* Boiss)
(ii) *Ferula foetida* (Bunge) Regel (Apiaceae/Umbelliferae)

Synonym(s)

Asafetida, Asant, Devil's Dung, Gum Asafetida

Part(s) Used

Oleo gum resin obtained by incising the living rhizomes and roots.

Pharmacopoeial and Other Monographs

BHC 1992[G6]
BHP 1996[G9]
Martindale 32nd edition[G43]
PDR for Herbal Medicines 2nd edition[G36]

Legal Category (Licensed Products)

GSL[G37]

Constituents[G6,G41,G46,G48,G58,G59,G62,G64]

Gum fraction 25%. Glucose, galactose, L-arabinose, rhamnose and glucuronic acid.

Resins 40–64%. Ferulic acid esters (60%), free ferulic acid (1.3%), asaresinotannols and farnesiferols A, B and C, coumarin derivatives (e.g. umbelliferone), coumarin–sesquiterpene complexes (e.g. asacoumarin A and asacoumarin B).[1] Free ferulic acid is converted to coumarin during dry distillation.

Volatile oils 3–17%. Sulfur-containing compounds with disulfides as major components, various monoterpenes.[1]
   The oleo gum resins of different *Ferula* species are not identical and many papers have documented their phytochemistry,[2–11] reporting polysulfanes,[2–11] complex acetylenes,[3] phenylpropanoids[7] and many sesquiterpene derivatives.[2,4,5,6,8,9]
   C-3 prenylated 4-hydroxycoumarin derivatives (e.g. ferulenol) are thought to represent the toxic principles in the species *Ferula communis*.[12]

Food Use

Asafoetida is used widely in foods. Asafoetida (essential oil, fluid extract and gommo-oleoresin) is listed by the Council of Europe as a source of natural food flavouring (category 5) (see Appendix 23).[G17] Asafoetida is approved for food use in the USA.[G41]

Herbal Use

Asafoetida is stated to possess carminative, antispasmodic and expectorant properties. It has been used for chronic bronchitis, pertussis, laryngismus stridulus, hysteria and specifically for intestinal flatulent colic.[G6,G7]

Dosage

Powdered resin   0.3–1 g three times daily[G6,G7]

Tincture of asafoetida   (BPC 1949) 2–4 mL

Pharmacological Actions

In vitro and animal studies

Asafoetida has been reported to possess anticoagulant and hypotensive properties.[G41] Asafoetida is an ingredient of a plant mixture reported to have antidiabetic properties in rats.[13] However, when the individual components of the mixture were studied asafoetida was devoid of antidiabetic effect with myrrh and aloe gum extracts representing the active hypoglycaemic principles.[14]
   Oestrogenic activity in rats has been documented for carotane sesquiterpenes and ferujol (a coumarin) isolated from *Ferula jaeschkeana*.[15,16]

Clinical studies

A protective action against fat-induced hyperlipidaemia has been documented for asafoetida and attributed to the sulfur compounds in the volatile oil fraction of the resin.[17] Two double-blind studies have reported the efficacy of asafoetida in the treatment of irritable bowel syndrome to be just below the 5% significance level in one study[18] and at 1% in the other.[19]

Side-effects, Toxicity

Asafoetida is documented to be relatively non-toxic; ingestion of 15 g produced no untoward effects.[G45] A report of methaemoglobinaemia has been associated with the administration of asafoetida (in milk) to a five-week-old infant for the treatment of colic.[20] Asafoetida was found to exert an oxidising effect on fetal haemoglobin but not on adult haemoglobin.

Toxic coumarin constituents of a related species, *Ferula communis*, have been documented to reduce prothrombin concentrations and to cause haemorrhaging in livestock.[21,G51]

Two other species, *Ferula galbaniflua* and *Ferula rubicaulis*, are stated to contain a gum that is rubefacient and irritant, causing contact dermatitis in sensitive individuals.[G51,G58]

A weak sister chromatid exchange-inducing effect in mouse spermatogonia[22] and clastogenicity in mouse spermatocytes[23] has been documented for asafoetida. Chromosomal damage by asafoetida has been associated with the coumarin constituents.

Contra-indications, Warnings

Asafoetida should not be given to infants because of the oxidising effect on fetal haemoglobin resulting in methaemoglobinaemia.[20] The gum of some *Ferula* species is reported to be irritant and therefore may cause gastrointestinal irritation or induce contact dermatitis in some individuals. Excessive doses may interfere with anticoagulant therapy and with hypertensive and hypotensive therapy.

Pregnancy and lactation   Asafoetida has a folkloric reputation as an abortifacient and an emmenagogue.[G30] However the use of asafoetida during pregnancy is probably acceptable, provided doses do not exceed amounts normally ingested in foods. In view of the toxic effect to infants (e.g. methaemoglobinaemia), asafoetida should be avoided during breast feeding.

Pharmaceutical Comment

Asafoetida is a complex oleo gum resin consisting of many constituents that vary according to the different species used. Asafoetida is commonly used in foods but little scientific evidence is available to justify the herbal uses. In view of the known pharmacologically active constituents, asafoetida should not be taken in amounts exceeding those used in foods.

References

See also General References G6, G7, G9, G16, G19, G30, G36, G37, G41, G43, G46, G48, G51, G58, G59, G62 and G64.

1   Kajimoto T *et al*. Sesquiterpenoid and disulphide derivatives from *Ferula assa-foetida*. *Phytochemistry* 1989; **28**: 1761–1763.

2   Dawidar A-A *et al*. Marmaricin, a new sesquiterpenoid coumarin from *Ferula marmarica* L. *Chem Pharm Bull* 1979; **27**: 3153–3155.

3   de Pascual Teresa J *et al*. Complex acetylenes from the roots of *Ferula communis*. *Planta Med* 1986; **52**: 458–462.

4   Miski M. Fercoperol, an unusual cyclic-endoperoxynerolidol derivative from *Ferula communis* subsp. *communis*. *J Nat Prod* 1986; **49**: 916–918.

5   Garg SN *et al*. Feruginidin and ferugin, two new sesquiterpenoids based on the carotane skeleton from *Ferula jaeschkeana*. *J Nat Prod* 1987; **50**: 253–255.

6   Garg SN *et al*. New sesquiterpenes from *Ferula jaeschkeana*. *Planta Med* 1987; **53**: 341–342.

7   Gonzalez AG *et al*. Phenylpropanoid and stilbene compounds from *Ferula latipinna*. *Planta Med* 1988; **54**: 184–185.

8   Miski M. New daucane and germacrane esters from *Ferula orientalis* var. *orientalis*. *J Nat Prod* 1987; **50**: 829–834.

9   Miski M. New daucane esters from *Ferula tingitana*. *J Nat Prod* 1986; **49**: 657–660.

10   Samimi MN and Unger W. Die gummiharze afghanischer asa foetida-liefernder ferula-arten. Beobachtungen zur herkunft und qualität afghanischer asa foetida. *Planta Med* 1979; **36**: 128–133.

11   Zhi-da M *et al*. Polysulfanes in the volatile oils of *Ferula* species. *Planta Med* 1987; **53**: 300–302.

12   Valle MG *et al*. Prenylated coumarins and sesquiterpenoids from *Ferula communis*. *Phytochemistry* 1987; **26**: 253–256.

13   Al-Awadi FM *et al*. On the mechanism of the hypoglycaemic effect of a plant extract. *Diabetologia* 1985; **28**: 432–434.

14   Al-Awadi FM, Gumaa KA. Studies on the activity of individual plants of an antidiabetic plant mixture. *Acta Diabetol Lat* 1987; **24**: 37–41.

15   Singh MM *et al*. Contraceptive efficacy and hormonal profile of ferujol: a new coumarin from *Ferula jaeschkeana*. *Planta Med* 1985; **51**: 268–270.

16   Singh MM *et al*. Antifertility and hormonal properties of certain carotane sesquiterpenes of *Ferula jaeschkeana*. *Planta Med* 1988; **54**: 492–494.

17   Bordia A, Arora SK. The effect of essential oil (active principle) of asafoetida on alimentary

lipemia. *Indian J Med Res* 1975; **63**: 707–711.

18 Rahlfs VW, Mössinger P. Zur Behandlung des Colon irritabile. *Arzneimittelforschung* 1976; **26**: 2230–2234.

19 Rahlfs VW, Mössinger P. Asa foetida bei colon irritabile. *Dtsch med Wochenschr* 1978; **104**: 140–143.

20 Kelly KJ *et al*. Methemoglobinemia in an infant treated with the folk remedy glycerited asafoetida. *Pediatrics* 1984; **73**: 717–719.

21 Aragno M *et al*. Experimental studies on the toxicity of *Ferula communis* in the rat. *Res Commun Chem Pathol Pharmacol* 1973; **59**: 399–402.

22 Abraham SK, Kesavan PC. Genotoxicity of garlic, turmeric and asafoetida in mice. *Mutat Res* 1984; **136**: 85–88.

23 Walia K. Effect of asafoetida (7-hydroxycoumarin) on mouse spermatocytes. *Cytologia* 1973; **38**: 719–724.

Avens

Species (Family)

Geum urbanum L. (Rosaceae)

Synonym(s)

Benedict's Herb, Colewort, Geum, Herb Bennet

Part(s) Used

Herb

Pharmacopoeial and Other Monographs

BHP 1983[G7]
PDR for Herbal Medicines 2nd edition[G36]

Legal Category (Licensed Products)

Avens is not included in the GSL.[G37]

Constituents[G40,G49,G64]

Limited information is available on the herb. Constituents reported include bitter principles, resin, tannins and volatile oil.

Other plant parts

The root has been more extensively studied and is reported to contain a phenolic glycoside (gein), yielding eugenol as the aglycone and vicianose (disaccharide) as the sugar component;[1] 30% tannin, including gallic, caffeic and chlorogenic acids (pseudotannins generally associated with condensed tannins);[1] a bitter substance, a flavonoid, and volatile oil.

Food Use

Avens is listed by the Council of Europe as a natural source of food flavouring (category N2). This category indicates that avens can be added to foodstuffs in small quantities, with a possible limitation of an active principle (as yet unspecified) in the final product.[G16]

Herbal Use

Avens is stated to possess antidiarrhoeal, antihaemorrhagic, and febrifugal properties. It has been used for diarrhoea, catarrhal colitis, passive uterine haemorrhage, intermittent fevers, and specifically for ulcerative colitis.[G7,G64]

Dosage

Dried herb 1–4 g or by infusion three times daily.[G7]

Liquid extract 1–4 mL (1 : 1 in 25% alcohol) three times daily.[G7]

Pharmacological Actions

In vitro and animal studies

A 20% aqueous decoction of avens, administered by intravenous injection, has been reported to produce a reduction in blood pressure in cats.[2] Tannins are generally known to possess astringent properties.

Side-effects, Toxicity

None documented.

Contra-indications, Warnings

In view of the reported tannin constituents and the lack of toxicity data, it is advisable to avoid excessive use of avens.

Pregnancy and lactation Avens is reputed to affect the menstrual cycle.[G30] In view of the lack of phytochemical, pharmacological and toxicological data, the use of avens during pregnancy should be avoided.

Pharmaceutical Comment

Limited phytochemical or pharmacological data are available for avens, although reported tannin constituents would indicate an astringent action thus supporting the traditional use in diarrhoea and haemorrhage. In view of the lack of toxicity data, excessive use should be avoided.

References

See also General References G2, G7, G16, G30, G31, G36, G37, G40, G49 and G64.

1 Psenák M *et al.* Biochemical Study on *Geum urbanum*. *Planta Med* 1970; **19**: 154–159.
2 Petkov V. Plants and hypotensive, antiatheromatous and coronarodilating action. *Am J Chin Med* 1979; **7**: 197–236.

Bayberry

Species (Family)

Myrica cerifera L. (Myricaceae)

Synonym(s)

Candleberry Bark, Myrica, Wax Myrtle Bark

Part(s) Used

Root bark

Pharmacopoeial and Other Monographs

BHP 1996[G9]
PDR for Herbal Medicines 2nd edition[G36]

Legal Category (Licensed Products)

GSL[G37]

Constituents[G22,G41,G48,G64]

Flavonoids Myricitrin.

Tannins 3.9% (bark), 34.82% (total aqueous extract).

Terpenoids Myricadiol, taraxerol and taraxerone.[1]

Other constituents Albumen, red dye, gum, resin, starch, wax containing palmitic, myristic and lauric acid esters.

Food Use

Bayberry is not used in foods.

Herbal Use

Bayberry is stated to possess antipyretic, circulatory stimulant, emetic and mild diaphoretic properties. It has been used for diarrhoea, colds and specifically for mucous colitis. An infusion has been used as a gargle for a sore throat, and as a douche for leucorrhoea. Powdered root bark has been applied topically for the management of indolent ulcers.[G7,G41,G64]

Dosage

Powdered bark 0.6–2.0 g by infusion or decoction three times daily.[G7]

Liquid extract 0.6–2.0 mL (1:1 in 45% alcohol) three times daily.[G7]

Pharmacological Actions

In vitro and animal studies

Myricitrin has been reported to exhibit choleretic, bactericidal, paramecicidal, and spermatocidal activity; myricadiol has mineralocorticoid activity.[G41] Tannins are known to possess astringent properties.

Side-effects, Toxicity

A total aqueous extract, tannin fraction, and tannin-free fraction from bayberry were all reported to produce tumours in NIH black rats, following weekly subcutaneous injections for up to 75 weeks.[2,3] The number of tumours that developed were stated to be statistically significant for the tannin fraction and tannin-free fraction. Analysis of the tannin-free fraction revealed the presence of four phenolic compounds, one of which was identified as myricitrin. No tumours were reported in a later study, in which rats were given subcutaneous injections of total aqueous extract for 78 weeks.

Large doses may cause typical mineralocorticoid side-effects (e.g. sodium and water retention, hypertension).

Contra-indications, Warnings

Large doses may interfere with existing hypertensive, hypotensive or steroid therapy. Excessive use of tannin-containing herbs is not recommended.

Pregnancy and lactation The safety of bayberry has not been established. In view of the possible mineralocorticoid activity and the reported carcinogenic activity, the use of bayberry during pregnancy and lactation should be avoided.

Pharmaceutical Comment

Limited chemical information is available for bayberry. Documented tannin constituents justify some of the herbal uses. In addition, mineralocorticoid activity has been reported for one of the triterpene constituents. In view of this and the tannin constituents, excessive use of bayberry should be avoided.

References

See also General References G9, G11, G22, G31, G32, G36, G37, G41, G44, G48 and G64.

1 Paul BD *et al.* Isolation of myricadiol, myricitrin, taraxerol, and taraxerone from *Myrica cerifera* L. root bark. *J Pharm Sci* 1974; **63**: 958–959.

2 Kapadia GJ *et al.* Carcinogenicity of *Camellia sinensis* (tea) and some tannin-containing folk medicinal herbs administered subcutaneously in rats. *J Natl Cancer Inst* 1976; **57**: 207–209.

3 Kapadia GJ *et al.* Carcinogenicity of some folk medicinal herbs in rats. *J Natl Cancer Inst* 1978; **60**: 683–686.

Bilberry

Species (Family)

Vaccinium myrtillus L. (Ericaceae)

Synonym(s)

Blueberry, bogberry, huckleberry, *Myrtilus niger* Gilib., *Vaccinium angulosum* Dulac, *Vaccinium montanum* Salisb., whortleberry

Part(s) Used

Fruit (berries), leaves

Pharmacopoeial and Other Monographs

Complete German Commission E[G3]
Martindale 32nd edition (Myrtillus)[G43]
Mills and Bone[G50]
PDR for Herbal Medicines 2nd edition[G36]

Legal Category (Licensed Products)

Bilberry is not included in the GSL.

Constituents[G2,G55]

Berries

Flavonoid glycosides Anthocyanins (particularly glycosides of delphinidin, cyanidin, petunidin, peonidin, malvidin),[1,2] quercetin-3-glucuronide and hyperoside.[3]

Polyphenols Catechin, epicatechin and tannins.

Other constituents Pectins[1] and vitamin C.

Leaves

Flavonoids Quercetin and its glycosides (hyperoquercitrin).[1]

Phenolic acids Caffeic, *p*-coumaric, *p*-hydroxybenzoic, protocatechuic and melilotic.[4]

Other constituents Tannins and iridoids.[1]

Food Use

Bilberries are used in foods.[1] Bilberry is listed by the Council of Europe as a natural source of food flavouring (category N1). This category indicates that there are no restrictions on the use of bilberry in foods.[G16]

Herbal Use[G64]

Bilberry is stated to possess astringent, tonic and antiseptic properties and has traditionally been used in the treatment of diarrhoea, dysentry, haemorrhoids, gastrointestinal inflammations, mouth infections, scurvy and urinary complaints.[1] It has also been used in diabetes, gout and rheumatism and applied locally in eye inflammation, burns and skin infections.[1]

Dosage

Dried fruit 20–60 g daily as a decoction for the treatment of diarrhoea.[G2]

Pharmacological Actions

Several pharmacological activities have been documented for bilberry, including ophthalmic activity and anti-inflammatory, wound-healing, anti-ulcer, anti-atherosclerotic and vasoprotective properties. The biochemical, biological, pharmacological and clinical effects of bilberry have been reviewed.[1]

In vitro and animal studies

An anthocyanidin extract of *V. myrtillus* has been reported to act as a superoxide anion scavenger[1,5] and as an inhibitor of lipid peroxidation in rat liver microsomes[1,5,6] and in mouse liver tissue *in vivo*,[5] and to inhibit potassium ion loss induced by free radicals in human erythrocytes.[1] *V. myrtillus* extract is stated to have a potent protective antioxidant action on human low-density lipoproteins (LDLs) *in vitro* during copper-mediated oxidation.[7] Oxidative activity is recognised as a major process in tissue damage in a variety of pathological conditions, such as atherosclerosis and carcinogenesis. In addition, oxidative stress is thought to be involved in brain ageing and age-related neurodegenerative disease. A study in rats reported that, compared with rats fed a control diet, dietary supplementation of blueberry (bilberry) extract for eight weeks reversed age-related deficits in several neuronal and behavioural parameters, such as enhancement of dopamine release from striatal slices and a water maze performance test.[8]

V. myrtillus anthocyanins have been reported to inhibit aggregation of human platelets *in vitro* in a dose-dependent manner[9] and, in rats, *V. myrtillus* anthocyanins administered orally at doses ranging from 5 to 400 mg/kg have been shown to prolong bleeding time markedly.[10] Inhibition of platelet aggregation has also been reported in humans treated with *V. myrtillus* anthocyanins (see Clinical studies).[11]

In vitro inhibition of elastase, a proteolytic enzyme involved with elastic fibre and connective tissue degeneration and with some pathological vascular conditions, has been demonstrated in studies using anthocyanins extracted from *V. myrtillus*.[12]

The hypolipidaemic activity of oral administration of extracts of *V. myrtillus* leaves has been demonstrated in rats.[13,14] In genetically hyperlipidaemic rats, plasma triglyceride and cholesterol concentrations, but not free fatty acids, decreased significantly.[13] In streptozotocin-induced diabetic rats, plasma glucose concentrations as well as plasma triglyceride concentrations decreased significantly compared with values in control rats.[14] In further experiments using blueberry and clofibrate, both preparations reduced plasma triglyceride concentrations in a dose-dependent manner in rats fed a hyperlipidaemic diet and in ethanol-treated normolipidaemic rats.[14] Blueberry, however, did not prevent fructose-elicited increases in plasma triglyceride concentrations. Other studies in glucose-loaded mice failed to demonstrate hypoglycaemic activity following oral administration of blueberry leaf extract.[15]

Several *in vitro* studies have demonstrated the relaxing effects of *V. myrtillus* anthocyanins on isolated vascular smooth muscle preparations, including the thoracic vein and splenic and coronary arteries.[16–18] There is evidence that the mechanism for this smooth muscle relaxant effect is via stimulation of prostaglandin release within vessel walls.[19]

Effects of *V. myrtillus* anthocyanins on enhancing arterial vasomotion (rhythmic variation of arteriole diameter in the microvasular network which influences microvascular blood flow and the formation of interstitial fluid) have been shown in experimental models, including the cheek pouch microcirculation of hamsters.[20] This model has also been used to investigate the effects of *V. myrtillus* anthocyanins on ischaemia–reperfusion injury.[21] Oral administration for two and four weeks of Myrtocyan, a commercially available product comprising bilberry anthocyanin complex, reduced the increase in capillary permeability, decreased leukocyte adhesion and improved capillary perfusion compared with controls. In rats, oral administration of *V. myrtillus* anthocyanins for 12 days before the induction of hypertension (by ligature of the abdominal aorta) limited the increase in vascular permeability and maintained a normal blood–brain barrier permeability.[22]

Components of bilberry have been reported to exhibit potential anticarcinogenic activity *in vitro* as demonstrated by inhibition of the induction of ornithine decarboxylase (ODC) by the tumour promoter phorbol 12-myristate 13-acetate (TPA).[23]

Myrtocyan and one of its anthocyanin constituents have been shown to have anti-ulcer activity in various experimental models of acute gastric ulcer and in chronic ulcer induced by acetic acid.[24] The mechanism for this may be by potentiation of the defensive barriers of the gastrointestinal mucosa, such as the secretion of gastric mucus or stimulation of cellular regeneration.[24]

Extracts of *V. myrtillus* leaves have demonstrated antibacterial activity against several species, including *Staphylococcus aureus* and *Escherichia coli*, as determined by the hole-plate diffusion method and the microdilution broth method.[25] *V. myrtillus* fruit extracts were less active.

The pharmacokinetics of *V. myrtillus* anthocyanins have been studied in rats.[26] Following a single oral administration, plasma anthocyanin concentrations peaked after 15 minutes and declined rapidly within 2 hours. No hepatic first-pass effect was observed; elimination occurred mostly through the urine and bile.

Clinical studies

Clinical studies with extracts of *V. myrtillus* fruits (berries) have focused mainly on its therapeutic applications in certain ophthalmological conditions and in altered microcirculation and peripheral venous insufficiency. The clinical efficacy of *V. myrtillus* fruits has been reviewed.[1]

A study involving 30 healthy subjects with normal platelet aggregation investigated the effects of administration of *V. myrtillus* anthocyanins (Myrtocyan) (480 mg) daily, ascorbic acid 3 g daily and *V. myrtillus* anthocyanins plus ascorbic acid on collagen- and ADP-induced platelet aggregation.[11] Platelet aggregation in blood samples taken from participants after 30 and 60 days' treatment was clearly reduced in all subjects compared with baseline values. The reduction in platelet aggregation was greater in subjects who received *V. myrtillus* anthocyanins alone than in those who received ascorbic acid alone and was most marked in subjects who received both preparations. Platelet aggregation returned to baseline values when tested 120 days after discontinuation of treatment.[11]

Early studies involving healthy subjects and patients with visual disorders who received *V. myrtillus* extracts alone or in combination with β-carotene and vitamin E reported improvements in night vision and faster adjustment to darkness and restoration of visual acuity following exposure to a bright flash of light.[1] Other studies reported improvements in retinal sensitivity and the visual field in patients with myopia or glaucoma following short- or long-term (six months) treatment with *V. myrtillus* anthocyanins.[1] However, all these studies appear to have been uncontrolled. Other uncontrolled studies in small numbers of patients with retinal pathologies have reported improvements in retinal function, compared with pretreatment values (e.g. ref. 27).

In a randomised, double-blind, placebo-controlled trial, 40 patients with diabetic and/or hypertensive retinopathy received Myrtocyan (160 mg) twice daily or placebo for one month.[28] At the end of the study, the placebo group received Myrtocyan for one month. It was reported that 77–90% of treated patients experienced improvement compared with the pretreatment period, as determined by ophthalmoscopy and fluorescein fundus angiography.[28] However, there does not appear to have been a statistical comparison between the treatment and placebo groups. A similar placebo-controlled trial involving 40 patients with early-phase diabetic retinopathy who received Myrtocyan for 12 months also reported improvements in Myrtocyan-treated patients.[29]

In a randomised, double-blind trial involving 51 patients with mild senile cortical cataract who received *V. myrtillus* anthocyanins plus vitamin E twice daily for four months, treated patients showed significant improvements in lens opacity compared with placebo recipients.[30]

Studies involving patients with peripheral vascular disorders of various origins are stated to have demonstrated clinical benefits with *V. myrtillus* extracts.[1] Other studies in patients with ulcerative dermatitis secondary to post-thrombotic or venous varicose stasis, capillary fragility secondary to liver disorders and other conditions, or chronic venous insufficiency have been reported to have shown improvements in clinical signs and symptoms.[1] However, several of these studies appear to have been uncontrolled (e.g. refs 31–33) and/or included only small numbers of patients (e.g. refs 31 and 32). A double-blind, placebo-controlled study involving 47 patients with peripheral vascular disorders reported reductions in subjective symptoms, such as paraesthesia, pain and

heaviness and improved oedema in patients treated with Myrtocyan (480 mg/day) for 30 days.[1] A single-blind study involving 60 patients with venous insufficiency who received Myrtocyan (480 mg/day) or placebo for 30 days reported significant improvements in oedema, paraesthesia, cramp-like pain and pressure sensation in Myrtocyan-treated patients compared with pretreatment values in these patients.[1]

V. myrtillus anthocyanins have been investigated in a variety of other disorders.

A randomised, double-blind, placebo-controlled trial of *V. myrtillus* anthocyanins (320 mg/day) taken for three days before menstruation was conducted involving 30 patients with chronic primary dysmenorrhoea.[34] Significant differences between the active treatment and placebo groups were reported for several symptoms investigated, including nausea and vomiting and breast tenderness; there was no effect on headache.

A trial involving 60 patients who had undergone haemorrhoidectomy who were randomised to receive *V. myrtillus* anthocyanins (320–480 mg/day) postoperatively in addition to usual medical care or to no additional treatment reported reductions in itch and oedema, but no effect on other symptoms, in bilberry recipients.[35]

Other studies, all of which were uncontrolled, have reported beneficial effects following administration of *V. myrtillus* extracts in patients with fibrocystic mastopathy[36] and type II diabetes mellitus,[37] in infantile dyspepsia[38] and in pregnant women with lower limb venous insufficiency and acute-phase haemorrhoids.[39]

Side-effects, Toxicity

A review of clinical trials of *V. myrtillus* extracts stated that no adverse effects had been observed, even following prolonged treatment.[1] However, most trials involved relatively small numbers of patients and, therefore, would only be able to detect very common acute adverse effects.

The same review summarised the results of an unpublished postmarketing surveillance study which had involved 2295 subjects who had taken Myrtocyan, usually 160 mg twice daily for 1–2 months, for lower limb venous insufficiency, capillary fragility, functional changes in retinal microcirculation or haemorrhoids. Ninety-four subjects reported side-effects, mainly relating to the skin and gastrointestinal and nervous systems.[1]

Long-term consumption of bilberry leaves may lead to toxicity. Chronic administration of doses of

1.5 g/kg per day or more to animals has been reported to be fatal.[G2]

Unpublished animal toxicity data for Myrtocyan have also been summarised.[1] In mice and rats, the LD_{50} for Myrtocyan is over 2000 mg/kg and, in dogs, single doses of 3000 mg/kg produced no adverse effects other than marked darkening of urine and faeces (demonstrating absorption). Oral daily doses to rats and dogs of 125–500 and 80–320 mg/kg, respectively, for six months did not induce mortality or toxic effects.[1] Pharmacokinetic studies of *V. myrtillus* anthocyanins in rats demonstrated that anthocyanins are removed rapidly from the systemic circulation within 2 hours of oral administration.[26]

Contra-indications, Warnings

In view of the inhibitory effects of *V. myrtillus* anthocyanins on platelet aggregation, the use of bilberry concurrently with other antiplatelet agents and anticoagulants may enhance the risk of bleeding.

Pregnancy and lactation   In an uncontrolled study, *V. myrtillus* anthocyanin extract (Tegens) (80 or 160 mg) twice or three times daily for three months was administered to pregnant women with lower limb venous insufficiency and acute-phase haemorrhoids with no apparent adverse effects.[39] However, the safety of bilberry has not been established and, in view of the lack of toxicity data, the use of bilberry during pregnancy and lactation should be avoided.

Pharmaceutical Comment

The chemistry of bilberry is well documented and there is good evidence that the anthocyanin constituents are responsible for the pharmacological effects of bilberry.

Documented scientific evidence from *in vitro* and animal studies provides supportive evidence for some of the uses of bilberry. There have been several clinical studies investigating the effects of bilberry in a range of conditions. However, many studies have been uncontrolled, involved only small numbers of patients and had other methodological flaws. Further, well-designed clinical trials are required to establish the efficacy of bilberry.

There are some limited toxicity and safety data for bilberry which together with data on adverse effects reported in clinical trials provide some support for the safety of bilberry when used at recommended doses in the short term. However, further data on the long-term safety of bilberry use are required and, therefore, excessive use of bilberry should be avoided.

Patients wishing to use bilberry for medicinal purposes should be advised to consult a pharmacist, doctor or other suitably trained health care professional for advice.

References

See also General References G2, G3, G31, G36, G43, G50 and G55.

1   Morazzoni P, Bombardelli E. *Vaccinium myrtillus* L. *Fitoterapia* 1996; **66**: 3–29.
2   Di Pierro F, Morazzoni P. Reaping the benefits: the role of two edible plants (*Vaccinium myrtillus* and *Glycine max*). Proceedings of the Herbal Medicine in the New Millenium Conference, Lismore, NSW, Australia, 1999: 146–150.
3   Fraisse D *et al.* Composition polyphénolique de la feuille de myrtille. *Ann Pharm Fr* 1996; **54**: 280–283.
4   Dombrowicz E *et al.* Phenolic acids in leaves of *Arctostaphylos uva ursi* L., *Vaccinium vitis idaea* L. and *Vaccinium myrtillus* L. *Pharmazie* 1991; **46**: 680–681.
5   Martín-Aragon S *et al. In vitro* and *in vivo* antioxidant properties of *Vaccinium myrtillus*. *Pharm Biol* 1999; **37**: 109–113.
6   Martín-Aragon S *et al.* Antioxidant action of *Vaccinium myrtillus* L. *Phytother Res* 1998; **12**(Suppl.): S104–S106.
7   Laplaud PM *et al.* Antioxidant action of *Vaccinium myrtillus* extract on human low-density lipoproteins *in vitro*: initial observations. *Fund Clin Pharmacol* 1997; **11**: 35–40.
8   Joseph JA *et al.* Reversals of age-related declines in neuronal signal transduction, cognitive, and motor behavioral deficits with blueberry, spinach, or strawberry dietary supplementation. *J Neurosci* 1999; **19**: 8114–8121.
9   Bottecchia D *et al.* Preliminary report on the inhibitory effect of *Vaccinium myrtillus* anthocyanosides on platelet aggregation and clot retraction. *Fitoterapia* 1987; **58**: 3–8.
10   Morazzoni P, Magistretti MJ. Activity of Myrtocyan, an anthocyanin complex from *Vaccinium myrtillus* (VMA), on platelet aggregation and adhesiveness. *Fitoterapia* 1990; **61**: 13–21.
11   Pulliero G *et al. Ex vivo* study of the inhibitory effects of *Vaccinium myrtillus* anthocyanosides on human platelet aggregation. *Fitoterapia* 1989; **60**: 69–75.
12   Jonadet M *et al.* Anthocyanosides extraits de *Vitis vinifera*, de *Vaccinium myrtillus* et de *Pinus maritimus*. *J Pharm Belg* 1983; **38**: 41–46.
13   Cignarella A *et al.* Hypolipidaemic activity of *Vaccinium myrtillus* leaves on a new model of genetically hyperlipidaemic rat. *Planta Med* 1992; **58**(Suppl.1): A581–A582.
14   Cignarella A *et al.* Novel lipid-lowering properties of *Vaccinium myrtillus* L. leaves, a traditional

antidiabetic treatment, in several models of rat dyslipidaemia: a comparison with clofibrate. *Thromb Res* 1996; **84**: 311–322.

15 Neef H *et al.* Hypogylcaemic activity of selected European plants. *Phytother Res* 1995; **9**: 45–48.

16 Bettini V *et al.* Effects of *Vaccinium myrtillus* anthocyanosides on vascular smooth muscle. *Fitoterapia* 1984; **55**: 265–272.

17 Bettini V *et al.* Interactions between *Vaccinium myrtillus* anthocyanosides and serotonin on splenic artery smooth muscle. *Fitoterapia* 1984; **55**: 201–208.

18 Bettini V *et al.* Mechanical responses of isolated coronary arteries to barium in the presence of *Vaccinium myrtillus* anthocyanosides. *Fitoterapia* 1985; **56**: 3–10.

19 Morazzoni P, Magistretti MJ. Effects of *Vaccinium myrtillus* anthocyanosides on prostacyclin-like activity in rat arterial tissue. *Fitoterapia* 1986; **57**: 11–14.

20 Colantuoni A *et al.* Effects of *Vaccinium myrtillus* anthocyanosides on arterial vasomotion. *Arzneimittelforschung* 1991; **41**: 905–909.

21 Bertuglia S *et al.* Effect of *Vaccinium myrtillus* anthocyanosides on ischaemia reperfusion injury in hamster cheek pouch microcirculation. *Pharmacol Res* 1995; **31**: 183–187.

22 Detre Z *et al.* Studies on vascular permeability in hypertension: action of anthocyanosides. *Clin Physiol Biochem* 1986; **4**: 143–149.

23 Bomser J *et al.* In vitro anticancer activity of fruit extracts from *Vaccinium* species. *Planta Med* 1996; **62**: 212–216.

24 Magistretti MJ *et al.* Antiulcer activity of an anthocyanidin from *Vaccinium myrtillus*. *Arzneimittelforschung* 1988; **38**: 686–690.

25 Brantner A, Grein E. Antibacterial activity of plant extracts used externally in traditional medicine. *J Ethnopharmacol* 1994; **44**: 35–40.

26 Morazzoni P *et al. Vaccinium myrtillus* anthocyanosides pharmacokinetics in rats. *Arzneimmittelforschung* 1991; **41**: 128–131.

27 Forte R *et al.* Fitotherapy and ophthalmology: considerations on dynamized myrtillus retinal effects with low luminance visual acuity. *Ann Ottal Clin Ocul* 1996; **122**: 325–333.

28 Perossini M *et al.* Diabetic and hypertensive retinopathy therapy with *Vaccinium myrtillus* anthocianosides (Tegens) double-blind placebo-controlled clinical trial. *Ann Ottal Clin Ocul* 1988; **113**: 1173–1190.

29 Repossi P *et al.* The role of anthocyanosides on vascular permeability in diabetic retinopathy. *Ann Ottal Clin Ocul* 1987; **113**: 357–361.

30 Bravetti GO *et al.* Preventive medical treatment of senile cataract with vitamin E and *Vaccinium myrtillus* anthocianosides: clinical evaluation. *Ann Ottal Clin Ocul* 1989; **115**: 109–116.

31 Coget J, Merlen JF. Étude clinique d'un nouvel agent de protection vasculaire le difrarel 20, composé d'anthocyanosides extraits du *Vaccinum myrtillus*. *Phlebologie* 1968; **21**: 221–228.

32 Piovella F *et al.* Impiego di antocianosidi da *Vaccinium myrtillus* al 25% come antocianidine nel trattamento della diatesi emorragica da deficit dell'emostasi primaria. *Gaz Med It* 1981; **140**: 445–449.

33 Tori A, D'Errico F. Gli antocianosidi da *Vaccinium myrtillus* nella cura delle flebopatie da stasi degli arti inferiori. *Gaz Med It* 1980; **139**: 217–224.

34 Colombo D, Vescovini R. Studio clinico controllato sull'efficacia degli antocianosidi del mirtillo cel trattamento della dismenorrea essenziale. *Giorn It Ost Gin* 1985; **7**: 1033–1038.

35 Pezzangora V *et al.* La terapia medica con antocianosidi del mirtillo nei pazienti operati di emorroidectomia. *Gaz Med It* 1984; **143**: 405–409.

36 Leonardi M. Il trattamento della mastopatia fibrosa con antocianosidi di mirtillo. *Minerva Ginecol* 1993; **45**: 617–621.

37 Ionescu-Tirgoviste C *et al.* Efectul unui amestec pe plante asupra echilibrului metabolic la bolnavii cu diabet zaharat de tip 2. *Med Intern* 1989; **41**: 185–192.

38 Tolan L *et al.* Utilizarea prafului de afine in dispepsiile sugarului. *Pediatria* 1969; **18**: 375–379.

39 Teglio L *et al. Vaccinium myrtillus* anthocyanosides in the treatment of venous insufficiency of inferior limbs and acute piles in pregnancy. *Quaderni Clin Osterica Ginecol* 1987; **42**: 221–231.

Bloodroot

Species (Family)

Sanguinaria canadensis L. (Papaveraceae)

Synonym(s)

Red Indian Paint, Red Root, Sanguinaria, Tetterwort

Part(s) Used

Rhizome

Pharmacopoeial and Other Monographs

BHP 1983[G7]
Martindale 32nd edition[G43]
PDR for Herbal Medicines 2nd edition[G36]

Legal Category (Licensed Products)

Bloodroot is not included in the GSL.[G37]

Constituents[G22,G41]

Alkaloids Isoquinoline type. 3.0–7.0%.[1] Sanguinarine (approx. 1%), sanguidimerine, chelerythrine, protopine; others include oxysanguinarine, α- and β-allocryptopine, sanguilutine, dihydrosanguilutine, berberine, coptisine and homochelidonine.

Other constituents Resin, starch, organic acids (citric, malic).
Alkaloid content of other plant parts recorded as 0.08% (leaf), 1.8% (root).

Food Use

Bloodroot is listed by the Council of Europe as a natural source of food flavouring (category N3). This category indicates that bloodroot can be added to foodstuffs in the traditionally accepted manner, although there is insufficient information available for an adequate assessment of potential toxicity.[G16]

Herbal Use

Bloodroot is stated to act as an expectorant, spasmolytic, emetic, cathartic, antiseptic, cardioactive, topical irritant and escharotic (scab-producing). Traditionally it is indicated for bronchitis (subacute or chronic), asthma, croup, laryngitis, pharyngitis, deficient capillary circulation, nasal polyps (as a snuff), and specifically for asthma and bronchitis with feeble peripheral circulation.[G7]

Dosage

Rhizome 0.06–0.5 g (1–2 g for emetic dose) three times daily.[G7]

Liquid extract 0.06–0.3 mL (1 : 1 in 60% alcohol) (1–2 mL for emetic dose) three times daily.[G7]

Tincture 0.3–2 mL (1 : 5 in 60% alcohol) (2–8 mL for emetic dose) three times daily.[G7]

Pharmacological Actions

Activities documented for bloodroot are principally attributable to the isoquinoline alkaloid constituents, in particular sanguinarine. In the last 10 years, interest has focused on the use of sanguinarine in dental hygiene products. Unless otherwise stated, the following actions refer to sanguinarine.

In vitro and animal studies

Considerable antimicrobial activity has been documented against both Gram-positive and Gram-negative bacteria, *Candida* and dermatophytes (fungi), and *Trichomonas* (protozoa).[2] In addition, anti-inflammatory activity has been described against carrageenan-induced rat paw oedema.[3]

Prolongation of the ventricular refractory period has been attributed to an inhibition of Na$^+$K$^+$ ATPase.[4,5] However, a single intravenous injection of sanguinarine to anaesthetised dogs reportedly exerted no effect on cardiovascular parameters monitored.[4]

In vitro inhibition of bone resorption and collagenase has been documented.[2]

Clinical studies

Many studies have investigated the efficacy of bloodroot extracts in oral hygiene.[2] Preparations containing bloodroot extracts, such as oral rinses and toothpastes, have been reported to significantly lower plaque, gingival and bleeding indices.[2] Alteration of the oral microbial flora, or development of resistant microbial strains has not been observed with the use of bloodroot extracts.[2]

Side-Effects, Toxicity

None documented for bloodroot. Much has been documented concerning the potential toxicity of the alkaloid constituents in bloodroot, in particular of sanguinarine.

In the 1920s contamination of cooking oil with *Argemone mexicana* seed oil was proposed as the causative factor for epidemic dropsy and associated glaucoma, with sanguinarine considered the toxic component of the seed oil.[1,6,7] However, subsequent workers disputed this theory and the toxicity of *A. mexicana* oil has been attributed to a fatty acid constituent.[1,7]

Conclusions reached in the 1960s over the carcinogenic potential of sanguinarine have more recently been disproved.[8] In addition, negative mutagenic activity has been observed in the Ames test (microbial, with and without activation).[8]

Sanguinarine is poorly absorbed from the gastrointestinal tract. This is reflected in stated acute oral LD_{50} values (rat) of 1.7 g/kg (sanguinarine) and 1.4 g/kg (sanguinaria extract), compared with an acute intravenous LD_{50} (rat) value of 28.7 mg/kg (sanguinarine).[1] Symptoms of diarrhoea, ataxia and reduced activity were observed in animals receiving high oral doses of sanguinarine.[5] The acute dermal toxicity (LD_{50}) of sanguinarine is stated to be greater than 200 mg/kg in rabbits.[1] The first experimental study of sanguinarine toxicity (1876) reported prostration and severe respiratory distress as the most marked signs of oral toxicity.[1] However, in more recent short-term toxicity studies no toxic signs were observed in the fetuses of rats following maternal administration of 5–30 mg/kg/day of sanguinarine.[1]

The reproductive and developmental toxicity potential of an *S. canadensis* extract has been evaluated in rats and rabbits.[8] Developmental toxicity (increase in postimplantation loss, slight decrease in fetal and pup body weights) was only evident at maternally toxic doses. No effect was reported on reproductive capabilities, on parturition or on lactation. It was concluded that oral ingestion of sanguinaria extract has no selective effect on fertility, reproduction, or on fetal or neonatal development.[8]

Hepatotoxicity has been documented in rats following a single intraperitoneal administration (10 mg/kg) of sanguinarine.[5] Toxicity was indicated by an increase in serum alanine aminotransferase and serum asparate aminotransferase activity, and by a significant reduction in microsomal cytochrome P450 and benzphetamine *N*-demethylase activities.[5] Macroscopic lesions were also observed but the authors stated that the two events could not be conclusively directly related.[5] No hepatotoxicity has been observed in short-term toxicity studies involving oral administration of sanguinarine.[1]

Animal studies have indicated sanguinarine to be non-irritant and to exhibit no allergenic or anaphylactic potential.[4] Human patch tests have shown sanguinarine to be non-irritant and non-sensitising.[4]

Contra-indications, Warnings

None documented.

Pregnancy and lactation Animal studies have indicated bloodroot to be non-toxic during pregnancy (see above). However, in view of its pharmacologically active constituents, use of bloodroot during pregnancy and lactation is best avoided.

Pharmaceutical Comment

Bloodroot is characterised by isoquinoline alkaloid constituents (benzophenanthridine-type), predominantly sanguinarine. A wide range of pharmacological activities has been documented for this class of compounds including antimicrobial, anti-inflammatory, antihistaminic, cardiotonic and antiplaque.[1,8] Other benzophenanthridine alkaloids have been associated with cytotoxic activities. However, recent interest over the potential use of bloodroot in oral hygiene has stimulated considerable research into both sanguinarine and bloodroot extracts. Results have indicated that products such as oral rinses and toothpastes containing either sanguinaria extracts or sanguinarine may be of value in dental hygiene, and are of low toxicity.

References

See also General References G7, G16, G22, G31, G36, G37, G41 and G43.

1 Becci PJ *et al.* Short-term toxicity studies of sanguinarine and of two alkaloid extracts of *Sanguinaria canadensis*. *J Toxicol Environ Health* 1987; **20**: 199–208.

2 Godowski KC. Antimicrobial action of sanguinarine. *J Clin Dent* 1989; **1**: 96–101.

3 Lenfield J *et al.* Antiinflammatory activity of quaternary benzophenanthridine alkaloids from *Chelidonium majus*. *Planta Med* 1981; **43**: 161–165

4 Schwartz HG. Safety profile of sanguinarine and Sanguinaria extract. *Compend Cont Educ Dent Suppl* 1986; **7**: S212–S217.

5 Dalvi RR. Sanguinarine: its potential as a liver toxic alkaloid present in the seeds of *Argemone mexicana*. *Experientia* 1985; **41**: 77–78.

6 Sood NN *et al.* Epidemic dropsy following transcutaneous absorption of *Argemone mexicana* oil. *Trans R Soc Trop Med Hyg* 1985; **79**: 510–512.

7 Lord G *et al*. Sanguinarine and the controversy concerning its relationship to glaucoma in epidemic dropsy. *J Clin Dent* 1989; **1**: 110–115.

8 Keller KA. Reproductive and developmental toxicological evaluation of Sanguinaria extract. *J Clin Dent* 1989; **1**: 59–66.

Blue Flag

Species (Family)

Iris versicolor L. or *Iris caroliniana* Watson (Irida-

Part(s) Used

Rhizome

Pharmacopoeial and Other Monographs

BHC 1992[G6]
BHP 1996[G9]
Martindale 32nd edition[G43]
PDR for Herbal Medicines 2nd edition[G36]

Legal Category (Licensed Products)

GSL[G37]

Constituents[G22,G40,G48,G64]

Acids Isophthalic acid 0.002%, salicylic acid, lauric acid, stearic acid, palmitic acid and 1-triacontanol.

Volatile oils 0.025%. Furfural.

Other constituents Iridin, β-sitosterol, iriversical[1] and tannin.

Food Use

Blue flag is not used in foods.

Herbal Use

Blue flag is stated to possess cholagogue, laxative, diuretic, dermatological, anti-inflammatory and anti-emetic properties. It has been used for skin diseases, biliousness with constipation and liver dysfunction, and specifically for cutaneous eruptions.[G7,G64]

Dosage

Dried rhizome 0.6–2.0 g or by decoction three times daily.[G6,G7,G10]

Liquid extract 1–2 mL (1:1 in 45% alcohol) three times daily.[G6,G7,G10]

Pharmacological Actions

None documented.

Side-effects, Toxicity

It has been stated that the fresh root of blue flag can cause nausea and vomiting.[G42]

Furfural, a volatile oil constituent, is known to be irritant to mucous membranes causing lachrymation, inflammation of the eyes, irritation of the throat, and headache.[G48] Whether these irritant properties are attributable to the volatile oil of blue flag has not been established. Acute oral toxicity (rat, LD_{50}) for furfural has been documented as 127 mg/kg body weight.[G48] Iridin has been reported to be poisonous in both humans and livestock.[G22] However, it is unclear whether this substance is the same iridin documented as a constituent of blue flag.

Contra-indications, Warnings

Only small doses of the dried root are advisable, because of the risk of nausea and vomiting.[G42] In view of the possible irritant nature of the volatile oil, blue flag may not be suitable for internal use, especially in sensitive individuals.

Pregnancy and lactation The safety of blue flag has not been established. In view of this, together with the documented irritant properties of some of the constituents, blue flag should not be taken during pregnancy.

Pharmaceutical Comment

Little is known about the phytochemical, pharmacological or toxicological properties of blue flag and its constituents, although related species are known to be toxic. In view of these factors, the use of blue flag is best avoided.

References

See also General References G6, G9, G10, G22, G31, G36, G37, G40, G42, G43, G48 and G64.

1 Krick W *et al.* Isolation and structural determination of a new methylated triterpenoid from rhizomes of *Iris versicolor* L. *Z Naturforsch* 1983; 38: 689–692.

Bogbean

Species (Family)

Menyanthes trifoliata L. (Menyanthaceae)

Synonym(s)

Buckbean, Marsh Trefoil, Menyanthes

Part(s) Used

Leaf

Pharmacopoeial and Other Monographs

BHP 1996[G9]
Complete German Commission E[G3]
Martindale 32nd edition[G43]
PDR for Herbal Medicines 2nd edition[G36]

Legal Category (Licensed Products)

GSL[G37]

Constituents[G2,G62,G64]

Acid Caffeic acid, chlorogenic acid, ferulic acid, *p*-hydroxybenzoic acid, protocatechuic acid, salicylic acid, vanillic acid;[1,2] folic acid and palmitic acid.[2]

Alkaloids Gentianin and gentianidine (pyridine-type); choline.[2]

Coumarins Scopoletin.[2]

Flavonoids Hyperin, kaempferol, quercetin, rutin and trifolioside.[1,2]

Iridoids 7′,8′-Dihydrofoliamenthin, foliamenthin, loganin, menthiafolin and sweroside.[2–4]

Other constituents Carotene, ceryl alcohol, enzymes (e.g. emulsin, invertin), α-spinasterol, an unidentified substance with haemolytic properties.[2] α-Spinasterol has been reported to be a mixture of five sterols with α-spinasterol and stigmast-7-enol as major components.[5]

Food Use

Bogbean is listed by the Council of Europe as a natural source of food flavouring (category N2). This category indicates that bogbean can be added to foodstuffs in small quantities, with a possible limitation of an active principle (as yet unspecified) in the final product.[G16]

Herbal Use

Bogbean is stated to possess bitter and diuretic properties. It has been used for rheumatism, rheumatoid arthritis, and specifically for muscular rheumatism associated with general asthenia.[G2,G7,G8,G64]

Dosage

Dried leaf 1–2 g or by infusion three times daily.[G7]

Liquid extract 1–2 mL (1 : 1 in 25% alcohol) three times daily.[G7]

Tincture 1–3 mL (1 : 5 in 45% alcohol) three times daily.[G7]

Pharmacological Actions

In vitro and animal studies

A choleretic action has been described for caffeic acid and ferulic acid; a stomachic secretive action has been reported for protocatechuic acid and *p*-hydroxybenzoic acid. The iridoids possess bitter properties.[1] The bitter index (BI) of bogbean is stated to be 4000–10 000 (compared to gentian BI 10 000–30 000).[G62] Bogbean extracts have antibacterial activities.[6,7]

Side-effects, Toxicity

Large doses of bogbean are stated to be purgative and may cause vomiting.[8] An unidentified substance with haemolytic activity has been isolated from bogbean.[2]

Contra-indications, Warnings

Excessive doses may be irritant to the gastrointestinal tract, causing diarrhoea, griping pains, nausea and vomiting.[8]

Pregnancy and lactation The safety of bogbean has not been established. In view of the lack of toxicity data and possible purgative action, the use of bogbean during pregnancy and lactation should be avoided.

Pharmaceutical Comment

The chemistry of bogbean is well studied, but no pharmacological information is available to justify the herbal uses. In view of the lack of toxicity data, excessive doses should be avoided.

References

See also General References G2, G3, G8, G9, G16, G31, G36, G37, G43, G56, G62 and G64.

1 Swiatek L *et al*. Content of phenolic acids in leaves of *Menyanthes trifoliata*. *Planta Med* 1986; **52**: 530.

2 Giaceri G. Chromatographic identification of coumarin derivatives in *Menyanthes trifoliata* L. *Fitoterapia* 1972; **43**: 134–138.

3 Battersby AR *et al*. Seco-cyclopentane glucosides from *Menyanthes trifoliata*: foliamenthin, dihydrofoliamenthin, and menthiafolin. *Chem Commun* 1968; 1277–1280.

4 Loew P *et al*. The structure and biosynthesis of foliamenthin. *Chem Commun* 1968; 1276–1277.

5 Popov S. Sterols of the Gentianaceae family. *Dokl Bolg Akad Nauk* 1969; **22**: 293–296.

6 Moskalenko SA. Preliminary screening of Far-Eastern ethnomedicinal plants for antibacterial activity. *J Ethnopharmacol* 1986; **15**: 231–259.

7 Bishop CJ, MacDonald RE. A survey of higher plants for antibacterial substances. *Can J Bot* 1951; **29**: 260–269.

8 Todd RG, ed. *Martindale: The Extra Pharmacopoeia*, 25th edn. London: Pharmaceutical Press, 1967.

Boldo

Species (Family)

Peumus boldus Molina (Monimiaceae)

Synonym(s)

Boldus, *Boldus boldus* (Mol.) Lyons

Part(s) Used

Leaf

Pharmacopoeial and Other Monographs

BHP 1996[G9]
BP 2001[G15]
Complete German Commission E[G3]
ESCOP 1996[G52]
Martindale 32nd edition[G43]
PDR for Herbal Medicines 2nd edition[G36]
Ph Eur 2002[G28]
WHO volume 1 1999[G63]

Legal Category (Licensed Products)

GSL[G37]

Constituents[G2,G22,G41,G52,G58,G62,G64]

Alkaloids Isoquinoline-type. 0.25–0.7%. Pharmacopoeial standard not less than 0.1% alkaloid calculated as boldine.[G15,G28] Boldine 0.06% (major, disputed), isoboldine, 6a,7-dehydroboldine, isocorydine, isocorydine-N-oxide, norisocorydine, laurolitsine, laurotetanine, N-methyllaurotetanine, reticuline (aporphines); (−)-pronuciferine (proaporphine) and sinoacutine (morphinandienone).[1–4]

Flavonoids Flavonols (e.g. isorhamnetin) and their glycosides.[5,6]

Volatile oils 2.5%. Some 38 components have been identified, including *p*-cymene 28.6%, ascaridole 16.1%, 1,8-cineole 16.0%, linalool 9.1%, terpinen-4-ol 2.6%, α-terpineol 0.9%, fenchone 0.8% and terpinolene 0.4%.

Other constituents Coumarin 0.5%, resin and tannin.

Food Use

Boldo is listed by the Council of Europe as a natural source of food flavouring (category N3). This category indicates that boldo can be added to foodstuffs in the traditionally accepted manner, although insufficient information is available for an adequate assessment of potential toxicity.[G16] In the USA, boldo is approved for food use in alcoholic beverages only.[G64]

Herbal Use[G2,G4,G32,G43,G52]

Boldo is stated to possess cholagogue, liver stimulant, sedative, diuretic, mild urinary demulcent, and antiseptic properties. It has been used for mild digestive disturbances, constipation, gallstones, pain in the liver or gall bladder, cystitis, rheumatism, and specifically for cholelithiasis with pain.[G2,G7,G64] The German Commission E approved use for treatment of dyspepsia and mild spastic gastrointestinal complaints.[G3]

Dosage

Dried leaf 60–200 mg or by infusion three times daily;[G7] 2–5 g as a tea.[G52]

Liquid extract 0.1–0.3 mL (1:1 in 45% alcohol) three times daily.[G7]

Tincture 0.5–2.0 mL (1:10 in 60% alcohol) three times daily.[G7]

Pharmacological Actions

In vitro and animal studies

Boldo has exhibited choleretic (highest activity in rats), diuretic, stomachic and cholagogic properties.[G41,G52] The choleretic activity may be due to synergy between flavonoids and alkaloids.[G52] Experiments in rats have failed to demonstrate choleretic activity after oral administration of 400 or 800 mg/kg aqueous ethanolic extract, intraduodenal administration of 200 mg or 800 mg/kg, and intravenous administration of 32.5–130 mg/kg of a dry ethanolic extract.[7]

An aqueous ethanolic extract (equivalent to 0.5–1.0 mg/mL dried ethanolic extract) and also boldine (33 µg/mL) gave significant hepatoprotection against *t*-butyl hydroperoxide-induced hepatotoxicity in rat hepatocytes *in vitro*.[7] Boldine at a concentration of 0.015 mol/L inhibited microsomal lipid peroxidation in a rat liver preparation by 50%.[8] A dried aqueous ethanolic extract (0.06–0.115%) of boldine at a dose of 500 mg/kg gave 70% protection against carbon tetrachloride-induced hepatotoxicity in mice, and boldine alone (10 mg/kg) gave 49% protection.[7] An aqueous ethanolic extract of boldo at doses of 50 and 100 mg/kg administered intraperitoneally showed anti-inflammatory activity in the rat paw carrageenan-induced oedema test, whereas boldine alone appeared to be inactive.[7]

Boldine showed concentration-dependent relaxant activity on isolated rat ileum (EC_{50} 1.7×10^{-4} mol/L), and acted as a competitive antagonist of acetylcholine and as a non-competitive antagonist of barium.[9] Boldine at low micromolar concentrations prevented oxidation in rat brain homogenate and lipid peroxidation of red cell plasma membranes, led to inactivation of lysozymes, indicating high reactivity of free radicals.[10]

Boldo essential oil contains terpinen-4-ol, the irritant and diuretic principle in juniper oil.

Clinical studies

Boldo, in combination with cascara, rhubarb and gentian, has been reported to exhibit a beneficial effect on a variety of symptoms such as loss of appetite, digestion difficulties, constipation, flatulence and itching.[11,12] Rhubarb and gentian were found to be more effective with respect to appetite-loss related symptoms, and boldo and cascara more effective in constipation-related symptoms.

Two preparations containing extracts of boldo and cascara have been documented to increase biliary flow without altering the lithogenic index or bile composition.[13] Boldine may provide relief to patients with gallstones for whom surgery is not an option or drugs have not been effective.[G56] The choleretic action of boldine releases bile and its diuretic action increases fluid secretion, possibly cleansing sediment or bacteria from the biliary tract.[G56] Treatment of 12 human volunteers with boldo dry extract resulted in prolongation of intestinal transit time.[G4]

Ascaridole, a component of the volatile oil, previously found a clinical use as an anthelmintic agent.[14] However, this use has declined with the development of synthetic compounds with lower toxicity and a wider range of activity.

Side-effects, Toxicity

Boldo volatile oil is stated to be one of the most toxic oils.[G58] Application of the undiluted oil to the hairless backs of mice has an irritant effect.[15] The oil contains irritant terpenes, including terpinen-4-ol, the irritant principle in juniper oil.

An acute oral LD_{50} value for boldo oil has been given as 0.13 g/kg body weight in rats, with doses of 0.07 g/kg causing convulsions.[15] The acute dermal LD_{50} in rabbits has been reported as 0.625–1.25 g/kg.[15] No acute toxicity was observed in rats given oral doses of 3 g/kg of dry aqueous ethanolic extract.[G52] In mice, an aqueous ethanolic extract (1:1) had an LD_{50} of 6 g/kg (intraperitoneal administration).[G52] The LD_{50} values of total alkaloids and of boldine in mice were 420 and 250 mg/kg (intraperitoneal administration), respectively.[G52] Total alkaloids (intraperitoneal administration) given to dogs produced vomiting, diarrhoea and epileptic symptoms with a recovery after 50 minutes.[G52]

Boldine was not genotoxic as indicated by the SOS chromotest with *Escherichia coli*, or in the Ames test, and did not induce mutations in *Saccharomyces cerevisiae*.[16] Boldine did not induce an increase in the frequency of chromosome aberrations in human lymphocytes *in vitro*, or in mouse bone marrow cells *in vivo*. There were no signs of genotoxicity in mouse bone marrow, as assessed by the micro nucleus test.[16]

Contra-indications, Warnings

Excessive doses of boldo may cause renal irritation, because of the volatile oil, and should be avoided by individuals with an existing kidney disorder. Boldo is contraindicated in individuals with obstruction of bile duct or severe liver disease. For gallstone patients, it should only be used after consultation with a physician.[G3] Ascaridole is toxic and use of the oil is not recommended.[G58]

Pregnancy and lactation The safety of boldo taken during pregnancy has not been established. In view of the potential irritant nature of the volatile oil, the use of boldo during pregnancy should be avoided.

Pharmaceutical Comment

The chemistry of boldo is well documented, and some pharmacological data are available. Clinical studies have described choleretic activity, although further well-designed studies are required to establish this. The reputed diuretic and mild urinary antiseptic properties of boldo are probably attributable to the irritant volatile oil. In view of the toxicity data and the irritant nature of the volatile oil, excessive use of boldo should be avoided. Boldo is not recommended for long-term use.[G56]

References

See also General References G2, G3, G9, G10, G15, G16, G22, G28, G31, G36, G37, G41, G43, G52, G54, G56, G57, G58, G62 and G64.

1 Urzúa A, Acuña P. Alkaloids from the bark of *Peumus boldus*. *Fitoterapia* 1983; **4**: 175–177.
2 Urzúa A, Torres R. 6a,7-Dehydroboldine from the bark of *Peumus boldus*. *J Nat Prod* 1984; **47**: 525–526.
3 Hughes DW *et al*. Alkaloids of *Peumus boldus*. Isolation of laurotetatine and laurolitsine. *J Pharm Sci* 1968; **57**: 1619–1620.
4 Hughes DW *et al*. Alkaloids of *Peumus boldus*. Isolation of (+)-reticuline and isoboldine. *J Pharm Sci* 1968; **57**: 1023–1025.
5 Bombardelli E *et al*. A new flavonol glycoside from *Peumus boldus*. *Fitoterapia* 1976; **46**: 3–5.
6 Krug H, Borkowski B. Neue Flavonol-Glykoside aus den Blättern von Peumus boldus Molina. *Pharmazie* 1965; **20**: 692–698.
7 Lanhers MC *et al*. Hepatoprotective and anti-inflammatory effects of a traditional medicinal plant of Chile, *Pneumus boldo*. *Planta Med* 1991; 57:110–115

8 Cederbaum AI *et al*. Inhibition of rat liver microsomal lipid peroxidation by boldine. *Biochem Pharmacol* 1992; **44**: 1765–1772.
9 Speisky H *et al*. Activity of boldine on rat ileum. *Planta Med* 1991; **57**: 519–522.
10 Speisky H *et al*. Antioxidant properties of the alkaloid boldine in systems undergoing lipid peroxidation and enzyme inactivation. *Biochem Pharmacol* 1991; **41**: 1575–1581.
11 Borgia M *et al*. Pharmacological activity of a herbs extract: A controlled clinical study. *Curr Ther Res* 1981; **29**: 525–536.
12 Borgia M *et al*. Studio policentrico doppio-cieco doppio-controllato sull'attività terapeutica di una nota associazione di erbe medicamentose. *Clin Ter* 1985; **114**: 401–409.
13 Salati R *et al*. Valutazione delle proprietà coleretiche di due preparati contenenti estratti di boldo e cascara. *Minerva Dietol Gastroenterol* 1984; **30**: 269–272.
14 Wagner H, Wolff P, eds. *New Natural Products and Plant Drugs with Pharmacological, Biological or Therapeutical Activity*. Berlin: Springer-Verlag, 1977.
15 Boldo leaf oil. *Food Chem Toxicol* 1982; 20(Suppl.B): 643.
16 Moreno PRH *et al*. Genotoxicity of the boldine aporphine alkaloid in prokaryotic and eukaryotic organisms. *Mutat Res* 1991; **260**: 145–152.

Boneset

Species (Family)

Eupatorium perfoliatum L. (Asteraceae/Compositae)

Synonym(s)

Feverwort, Thoroughwort. Snakeroot has been used to describe poisonous *Eupatorium* species.

Part(s) Used

Herb

Pharmacopoeial and Other Monographs

BHP 1983[G7]
PDR® for Herbal Medicines 2nd edition[G36]

Legal Category (Licensed Products)

GSL – as Boneset and *Eupatorium*.[G37]

Constituents[G22,G41,G48,G64]

Flavonoids Flavonol (kaempferol, quercetin) glycosides including astragalin, hyperoside and rutin; eupatorin (flavone) and dihydroflavonols.[1]

Terpenoids Sesquiterpene lactones including euperfolin and euperfolitin (germacranolides), eufoliatin (guianolide), eufoliatorin (dilactone guaiane) and euperfolide.[2] Sesquiterpenes, diterpenes (dendroidinic acid, hebeclinolide), triterpenes (α-amyrin, dotriacontane) and sterols (sitosterol, stigmasterol).

Other constituents Volatile oil, resin, wax, tannic and gallic acids, bitter glucoside, inulin, polysaccharides and sugars.

Food Use

Boneset is not used in foods.

Herbal Use

Boneset is stated to possess diaphoretic and aperient properties. Traditionally, it has been used for influenza, acute bronchitis, nasopharyngeal catarrh, and specifically for influenza with deep aching, and congestion of the respiratory mucosa.[G7,G64]

Dosage

Herb 1–2 g or by infusion three times daily.[G7]

Liquid extract 1–2 mL (1 : 1 in 25% alcohol) three times daily.[G7]

Tincture 1–4 mL (1 : 5 in 45% alcohol) three times daily.[G7]

Pharmacological Actions

In vitro and animal studies

Immunostimulant activity (*in vitro* stimulation of granulocyte phagocytic activity) has been demonstrated by high dilutions (10^{-5}–10^{-7} g/100 mL) of various sesquiterpene lactones isolated from *E. perfoliatum*.[3] In addition, immunostimulating actions (granulocyte, macrophage and carbon clearance tests) have been documented for polysaccharide fractions from *E. perfoliatum*.[3,4]

An ethanol extract of the whole plant has exhibited weak anti-inflammatory activity in rats.[G41] Many activities have been documented for flavonoid compounds including anti-inflammatory activity.

Side-effects, Toxicity

Contact dermatitis has been reported for *Eupatorium* species but not specifically for boneset (*E. perfoliatum*).[G51] Cytotoxic properties have been documented for a related species, *E. cannabinum*, and are attributed to the sesquiterpene lactone eupatoriopicrin. This compound has not been documented as a constituent of boneset. Hepatotoxic pyrrolizidine alkaloids (PAs) have been isolated from various *Eupatorium* species although none have been documented as constituents of boneset (*E. perfoliatum*).[5]

Instances of allergic and anaphylactic reactions have been associated with the sesquiterpene lactone constituents in German chamomile, although no reactions specifically involving boneset have been documented.

The US Food and Drugs Administration (FDA) has classified boneset as a herb of undefined safety.[G22]

Contra-indications, Warnings

The allergenic potential of sesquiterpene lactones is well recognised. Individuals with a known hypersensitivity to other members of the Asteraceae family (e.g. chamomile, feverfew, ragwort, tansy) should avoid using boneset. Individuals with existing hypersensitivities/allergies should use boneset with caution.

Pregnancy and lactation   The safety of boneset taken during pregnancy has not been established. In view of the lack of toxicity data and the possibility of constituents with allergenic activity, the use of boneset during pregnancy and lactation should be avoided.

Pharmaceutical Comment

The constituents of boneset are fairly well documented and include many pharmacologically active classes such as flavonoids, sesquiterpene lactones (typical for the Asteraceae family) and triterpenes. Immunostimulant activity (*in vitro*) has been reported for sesquiterpene lactone and polysaccharide components, possibly supporting the traditional use of boneset in influenza. Many pharmacological studies have focused on the cytotoxic/antitumour actions of sesquiterpene lactone components of various *Eupatorium* species, although these actions have not been reported for sesquiterpene lactones isolated from boneset. Little is known regarding the toxicity of boneset. Hepatotoxic pyrrolizidine alkaloids, which have been documented for other *Eupatorium* species, have not been reported for boneset.

References

See also General References G7, G20, G22, G31, G32, G36, G37, G41, G48, G51 and G64.

1 Herz W *et al*. Dihydroflavonols and other flavonoids of *Eupatorium* species. *Phytochemistry* 1972; **11**: 2859–2863.
2 Herz W *et al*. Sesquiterpene lactones of *Eupatorium perfoliatum*. *J Org Chem* 1977; **42**: 2264–2271.
3 Wagner H. Immunostimulants from medicinal plants. In: Chang HM *et al*., eds. *Advances in Chinese Medicinal Materials Research*. Singapore: World Scientific, 1985: 159–170.
4 Wagner H *et al*. Immunostimulating polysaccharides (heteroglycans) of higher plants. *Arzneimittelforschung* 1985; **35**: 1069.
5 Pyrrolizidine Alkaloids. Environmental Health Criteria 80. Geneva: World Health Organization, 1988.

Borage

Species (Family)

Borago officinalis L. (Boraginaceae)

Synonym(s)

Beebread, Bee Plant, Burrage, Starflower (oil)

Part(s) Used

Herb

Pharmacopoeial and Other Monographs

Martindale 32nd edition[G43]
PDR for Herbal Medicines 2nd edition[G36]

Legal Category (Licensed Product)

Borage is not included in the GSL.[G37]

Constituents[G22,G64]

Alkaloids Pyrrolizidine-type. Lycopsamine, intermedine, acetyllycopsamine, acetylintermedine, amabiline, supinine and thesinine (unsaturated).[1,2] Concentrations reported as 0.01% and 2–10 ppm for commercial dried samples. Alkaloid concentrations reportedly the same for fresh and dried samples; fresh samples revealed alkaloids as the free base in the roots and mainly as *N*-oxides in the leaves.

Mucilages 11.1%. Yielding glucose, galactose and arabinose.

Oil Rich in fatty acids, in particular gamolenic acid.

Other constituents Acids (acetic, lactic, malic, silicic), cyanogenetic compounds and tannins (up to 3%).

Food Use

Borage is occasionally used in salads and soups.

Herbal Use[G64]

Borage is stated to possess diaphoretic, expectorant, tonic, anti-inflammatory and galactogogue properties.[3] Traditionally, borage has been used to treat many ailments including fevers, coughs and depression.[3,G42] Borage is also reputed to act as a restorative agent on the adrenal cortex.[3] Borage oil (starflower oil) is used as an alternative source to evening primrose oil for gamolenic acid.

Dosage

Infusion Two 5-mL spoonfuls of dried herb to one cup boiling water three times daily.[3]

Tincture 1–4 mL three times daily.[3]

Pharmacological Actions

In vitro and animal studies

Borage oil has been reported to attenuate cardiovascular reactivity to stress in rats.[4]

Clinical studies

The effect of borage seed oil on the cardiovascular reactivity of humans to acute stress has been studied in 10 individuals, who each received a total daily dose of 1.3 g for 28 days.[4] The individuals were required to undertake an acute psychological task requiring sensory intake and vigilance (Stroop colour test). Borage oil was found to attenuate cardiovascular reactivity to stress, indicated by a reduction in systolic blood pressure and heart rate and by increased task performance. The specific mechanisms by which borage exerts this effect were unknown but a central mechanism of action of the fatty acids was suggested in view of the simultaneous reduction in heart rate and blood pressure.[4]

Side-effects, Toxicity

No side-effects of borage have been identified. Borage contains low concentrations of unsaturated pyrrolizidine alkaloids, which are known to be hepatotoxic in both animals and humans (*see* Comfrey).[5]

Contra-indications, Warnings

Evening primrose oil is recommended to be used with caution in epileptic patients, especially in those with schizophrenia and/or those taking phenothiazines (*see* Evening Primrose); as borage oil is used similarly it should also be used with caution. In view of the known toxic pyrrolizidine alkaloid constituents, excessive or prolonged ingestion of borage should be avoided. In particular, infusions (e.g. herbal teas) containing borage should be avoided.

Pregnancy and lactation In view of the documented pyrrolizidine constituents and lack of toxicity data, borage should not be used during pregnancy or lactation.

Pharmaceutical Comment

Limited information is available on the constituents of borage. No documented pharmacological data were located to support the traditional uses, although the mucilage content supports the use of borage as a demulcent. Interest has focused on the volatile oil as a source of gamolenic acid. Borage contains known toxic pyrrolizidine alkaloids, although at concentrations considerably lower than comfrey for which human toxicity has been documented. However, it would seem wise to avoid excessive or prolonged ingestion of borage. It is unclear whether borage oil, currently available in food supplements, contains any pyrrolizidine alkaloids.

References

See also General References G18, G20, G22, G31, G32, G36, G42 and G43.

1 Luthry J *et al.* Pyrrolizidin-Alkaloide in Arzneipflanzen der Boraginaceen: *Borago officinalis* and *Pulmonaria officinalis*. *Pharm Acta Helv* 1984; **59**: 242–246.
2 Larsen KM *et al.* Unsaturated pyrrolizidines from Borage (*Borage officinalis*) a common garden herb. *J Nat Prod* 1984; **47**: 747–748.
3 Hoffman D. *The Herb Users Guide, the Basic Skills of Medical Herbalism.* Wellingborough: Thorsons, 1987.
4 Mills DE. Dietary fatty acid supplementation alters stress reactivity and performance in man. *J Hum Hypertens* 1989; **3**: 111–116.
5 Mattock AR. *Chemistry and Toxicology of Pyrrolizidine Alkaloids.* London: Academic Press, 1986.

Broom

Species (Family)

Sarothamnus scoparius (L.) Koch. (Leguminosae/
Papilionaceae)

Synonym(s)

Cytisus scoparius (L.) Link, Hogweed, Scoparius,
Spartium scoparium L.

Part(s) Used

Flowerhead

Pharmacopoeial and Other Monographs

BHC 1992[G6]
BHP 1996[G9]
Martindale 32nd edition[G43]
PDR for Herbal Medicines 2nd edition[G36]

Legal Category (Licensed Products)

Broom is not included in the GSL.[G37]

Constituents[G2,G40,G41,G48,G62,G64]

Alkaloids Quinolizidine-type. 0.8–1.5%. Sparteine
0.3–0.8% (major component); minor alkaloids
include cytisine (presence disputed), genisteine (*d*-α-
isosparteine), lupanine, oxysparteine and sarotha-
mine.

Amines Epinine, hydroxytyramine and tyramine.

Flavonoids Scoparin and vitexin.

Other constituents Amino acids, bitter principles,
carotenoids, fat, resin, sugars, tannin, wax and
volatile oil.

Food Use

Broom is listed by the Council of Europe as a natural
source of food flavouring (category N3). This category indicates that broom can be added to foodstuffs
in the traditionally accepted manner, although there
is insufficient information available for an adequate
assessment of potential toxicity.[G16]

Herbal Use

Broom is stated to possess cardioactive, diuretic,
peripheral vasoconstrictor and antihaemorrhagic
properties. It has been used for cardiac dropsy,
myocardial weakness, tachycardia, profuse menstruation and specifically for functional palpitation
with lowered blood pressure.[G2,G7,G64] Broom is also
reported to possess emetic and cathartic properties.[G41]

Dosage

Dried tops 1–2 g as a decoction.[G7]

Liquid extract 1–2 mL (1:1 in 25% alcohol).[G7]

Tincture 0.5–2.0 mL (1:5 in 45% alcohol).[G7]

Pharmacological Actions

The pharmacological actions of broom are primarily
due to the alkaloid constituents.

In vitro and animal studies

Sparteine is reported to exhibit pharmacological
actions similar to those of quinidine. Low doses
administered to animals result in tachycardia,
whereas high doses cause bradycardia and may lead
to ventricular arrest. Sparteine has little effect on the
central nervous system (CNS), but peripherally,
paralyses motor nerve terminals and sympathetic
ganglia as a result of a curare-like action.[G44]

The flowers, seeds, root and whole herb have been
used to treat tumours.[G41]

Clinical studies

None documented for broom. However, sparteine is
known to decrease the irritability and conductivity of
cardiac muscle and has been used to treat cardiac
arrhythmias,[G44] restoring normal rhythm in previously arrhythmic patients.[G2] Sparteine is reported
to have a quinidine-like action rather than a digitalis-
like action.[G2] Sparteine is also stated to be a powerful oxytocic drug, which was once used to stimulate
uterine contractions.

Side-effects, Toxicity

The alkaloid constituents in broom are toxic. Sparteine sulfate has been reported to be a cardiac depressant and can also produce respiratory arrest.[G44] Symptoms of poisoning are characterised by tachycardia with circulatory collapse, nausea, diarrhoea, vertigo and stupor.

Contra-indications, Warnings

Broom is stated to be inappropriate for non-professional use.[G49] Its use is contra-indicated in individuals with high blood pressure[G49] or a cardiac disorder, because of the alkaloid constituents.

Pregnancy and lactation The use of sparteine is contra-indicated during pregnancy.[G42] Sparteine is stated to be a powerful oxytocic drug and is cardiotoxic. Broom should not be taken during lactation.

Pharmaceutical Comment

The chemistry of broom is well documented. The pharmacological actions are primarily due to the alkaloid constituents. Sparteine, the major alkaloid component, is a cardiac depressant with actions similar to those of quinidine. Although these actions support the documented traditional herbal uses, broom is not suitable for self-medication.

References

See General References G2, G9, G11, G16, G31, G32, G36, G37, G40, G41, G42, G43, G48, G49, G62 and G64.

Buchu

Species (Family)

Agathosma betulina (Berg.) Pillans (Rutaceae)

Synonym(s)

Barosma betulina Bart. & Wendl., Round Buchu, Short Buchu

Note that Oval Buchu refers to *Agathosma crenulata* (L.) Pillans (synonym *Barosma crenulata* (L.) Hook.) and Long Buchu refers to *Agathosma serratifolia* (Curt.) Spreeth (synonym *Barosma serratifolia* (Curt.) Willd.).[G12]

Part(s) Used

Leaf

Pharmacopoeial and Other Monographs

BHC 1992[G6]
BHP 1996[G9]
Martindale 32nd edition[G43]
Mills and Bone[G50]
PDR for Herbal Medicines 2nd edition[G36]

Legal Category (Licensed Products)

GSL[G37]

Constituents[G2,G22,G41,G48,G64]

Flavonoids Diosmetin, quercetin, diosmin, quercetin-3,7-diglucoside, rutin.

Volatile oils 1.0–3.5%. Over 100 identified compounds, including diosphenol, limonene, menthone and pulegone as the major components.

Other constituents Mucilage, resin. Coumarins have been reported for many other *Agathosma* species.[1]

Food Use

Buchu is listed by the Council of Europe as a natural source of food flavouring (category N3). This cate-gory allows buchu to be added to foodstuffs in the traditionally accepted manner, although there is insufficient information available for an adequate assessment of potential toxicity.[G16] In the USA, buchu volatile oil is approved for food use with concentrations usually up to about 0.002% (15.4 ppm).[G16,G41]

Herbal Use

Buchu is stated to possess urinary antiseptic and diuretic properties. It has been used for cystitis, urethritis, prostatitis, and specifically for acute catarrhal cystitis.[G2,G7,G8,G64]

Dosage

Dried leaf 1–2 g by infusion three times daily.[G6,G7]

Liquid extract 0.3–1.2 mL (1:1 in 90% alcohol).[G6,G7]

Tincture 2–4 mL (1:5 in 60% alcohol).[G6,G7]

Pharmacological Actions

In vitro and animal studies

None documented for buchu. Diosmin has documented anti-inflammatory activity against carrageenan-induced rat paw oedema, at a dose of 600 mg/kg body weight.[2]

Side-effects, Toxicity

None documented for buchu. The volatile oil contains pulegone, a known hepatotoxin (*see* Pennyroyal).[G20] The oil may cause gastrointestinal and renal irritation.

Contra-indications, Warnings

Excessive doses of buchu should not be taken in view of the potential toxicity of the volatile oil. Buchu should be avoided in kidney infections.[G42]

93

Pregnancy and lactation   The safety of buchu has not been established. In view of this, together with the potential toxicity and irritant action of the volatile oil, the use of buchu during pregnancy and lactation should be avoided.

Pharmaceutical Comment

Limited chemical data are available for buchu. No scientific evidence was found to justify the herbal uses, although reputed diuretic and anti-inflammatory activities are probably attributable to the irritant nature of the volatile oil and the flavonoid components, respectively. In view of the lack of documented toxicity data, together with the presence of pulegone in the volatile oil, excessive use of buchu should be avoided.

References

See also General References G2, G6, G8, G9, G16, G22, G31, G32, G36, G37, G41, G42, G43, G48, G50, G58 and G64.

1   Campbell WE *et al*. Coumarins of the Rutoideae: tribe Diosmeae. *Phytochemistry* 1986; **25**: 655–657.
2   Farnsworth NR, Cordell GA. A review of some biologically active compounds isolated from plants as reported in the 1974–1975 literature. *Lloydia* 1976, **39**: 420–455.

Burdock

Species (Family)

Arctium majus Bernh. (Asteraceae/Compositae)

Synonym(s)

Arctium lappa L. and other *Arctium* species, Lappa

Part(s) Used

Root

Pharmacopoeial and Other Monographs

BHC 1992[G6]
BHP 1996[G9]
Martindale 32nd edition[G43]
Mills and Bone[G50]
PDR for Herbal Medicines 2nd edition[G36]

Legal Category (Licensed Products)

GSL[G37]

Constituents[G2,G6,G22,G41,G48,G64]

Acids Acetic acid, butyric acid, caffeic acid, chlorogenic acid, gamma-guanidino-*n*-butyric acid, α-guanidino-*n*-isovaleric acid, *trans*-2-hexenoic acid, isovaleric acid, lauric acid, linoleic acid, linolenic acid, myristic acid, oleic acid, palmitic acid, propionic acid, stearic acid and tiglic acid.[1–3]

Aldehydes Acetaldehyde, benzaldehyde, butyraldehyde, caproicaldehyde, isovaleraldehyde, propionaldehyde and valeraldehyde.[1]

Carbohydrates Inulin (up to 45–50%), mucilage, pectin and sugars.

Polyacetylenes 0.001–0.002% dry weight. Fourteen identified compounds include 1,11-tridecadiene-3,5,7,9-tetrayne (50%), 1,3,11-tridecatriene-5,7,9-triyne (30%) and 1-tridecen-3,5,7,9,11-pentayne as the major components;[4] arctinone-a, arctinone-b, arctinol-a, arctinol-b, arctinal, arctic acid-b, arctic acid-c, methyl arctate-b and arctinone-a acetate (sulfur-containing acetylenic compounds).[5,6]

Other constituents Fats (0.4–0.8%), fixed and volatile oils (0.07–0.18%), sesquiterpene lactones (arc-[7] bitters (lappatin), resin, phytosterols (sitosterol and stigmasterol), tannin[8] and lignan-type compound.[9–11]

Other species Flavonol (kaempferol, quercetin) glycosides are present in *Arctium minus* (Hill) Bernh.[3]

Food Use

Burdock is listed by the Council of Europe as a natural source of food flavouring (category N2). This category indicates that burdock can be added to foodstuffs in small quantities, with a possible limitation of an active principle (as yet unspecified) in the final product.[G16]

Herbal Use

Burdock is stated to possess diuretic and orexigenic properties. It has been used for cutaneous eruptions, rheumatism, cystitis, gout, anorexia nervosa, and specifically for eczema and psoriasis.[G2,G6,G7,G8,G60]

Dosage

Dried root 2–6 g or by infusion three times daily.[G7]

Liquid extract 2–8 mL (1:1 in 25% alcohol) three times daily.[G7]

Tincture 8–12 mL (1:10 in 45% alcohol) three times daily.[G7]

Decoction 500 mL (1:20) per day.[G7]

Pharmacological Actions

In vitro and animal studies

The roots and leaves of burdock plants not yet flowering are stated to possess diuretic, hypoglycaemic and antifurunculous properties.[7] A burdock extract (plant part not stated) was reported to cause a sharp, long-lasting reduction in the blood sugar concentration in rats, together with an increase in carbohydrate tolerance and a reduction in toxicity.[12] The antimicrobial activity documented for burdock has been attributed to the polyacetylene constituents,[4] although only traces of these compounds are found in the dried commercial herb.[G62]

Furthermore, arctiopicrin is stated to be a bitter with antibiotic activity against Gram-positive bacteria.[7,13] Antibacterial activity against Gram-positive (e.g. *Staphylococcus aureus*, *Bacillus subtilis*, *Mycobacterium smegmatis*) and Gram-negative (*Escherichia coli*, *Shigella flexneri*, *Shigella sonnei*) bacteria has been documented for burdock leaf and flower, whereas the root was only found to be active towards Gram-negative strains.[14]

In vivo uterine stimulant activity has been reported.[G30]

Protection against mutagenic activity has also been documented for burdock.[9,15,16]

Burdock reduced the mutagenicity to *Salmonella typhimurium* (TA98, TA100) of mutagens both requiring and not requiring S9 metabolic activation.[10] A lignan-like structure was proposed for the desmutagenic factor.[9] *In vivo* studies have shown that fresh or boiled plant juice from burdock may cause a significant reduction in DMBA-induced chromosome aberrations.[16]

Burdock has been reported to exhibit antitumour activity.[17]

The addition of dietary fibre (5%) from burdock roots to the diet of rats has been documented to provide protection against the toxicity of various artificial food colours.[18]

Side-effects, Toxicity

A single report of human poisoning with burdock has been documented.[19] The patient exhibited symptoms of atropine-like poisoning following the ingestion of a commercially packaged burdock root tea. Atropine is not a constituent of burdock, and subsequent analysis indicated that the tea was contaminated with a herbal source of solanaceous alkaloids, possibly belladonna leaf. This report served to highlight the problems which may arise with inadequate quality control of herbal preparations.

The carcinogenicity of burdock was investigated in 12 rats fed dried roots (33% of diet) for 120 days, followed by a normal diet until 480 days.[20] Ten of the 12 rats survived 480 days and no tumours were detected. A urinary bladder papilloma and an oligodendroglioma were observed in one rat but these were considered to have been induced spontaneously.

Burdock has been reported to exhibit antitumour properties (*see In vitro* and animal studies).

Contra-indications, Warnings

Excessive doses may interfere with existing hypoglycaemic therapy (*see In vitro* and animal studies).

Pregnancy and lactation *In vivo* uterine stimulant action has been reported.[G30] In view of this, and the lack of toxicity data, the use of burdock during pregnancy and lactation should be avoided.

Pharmaceutical Comment

The chemistry of burdock and related *Arctium* species has been well studied. Various pharmacological activities have been reported in animals although none support the reputed herbal uses. Documented bitter constituents, however, may explain the traditional use of burdock as an orexigenic. In view of the lack of toxicity data, excessive use of burdock should be avoided.

References

See also General References G2, G5, G6, G9, G10, G16, G20, G22, G30, G31, G32, G36, G37, G41, G43, G48, G56, G60, G62 and G64.

1 Obata S *et al.* Studies on the components of the roots of *Arctium lappa* L. *Agric Biol Chem* 1970; **34**: A31.
2 Yamada Y *et al.* γ-Guanidino-*n*-butyric acid from *Arctium lappa*. *Phytochemistry* 1975; **14**: 582.
3 Saleh NAM, Bohm BA. Flavonoids of *Arctium minus* (Compositae). *Experientia* 1971; **27**: 1494.
4 Schulte KE *et al.* Polyacetylenes in burdock root. *Arzneimittelforschung* 1967; **17**: 829–833.
5 Washino T *et al.* New sulfur-containing acetylenic compounds from *Arctium lappa*. *Agric Biol Chem* 1986; **50**: 263–269.
6 Washino T *et al.* Structures of lappaphen-a and lappaphen-b, new guaianolides linked with a sulfur-containing acetylenic compound, from *Arctium lappa* L. *Agric Biol Chem* 1987; **51**: 1475–1480.
7 Bever BO, Zahnd GR. Plants with oral hypoglycaemic action. *Q J Crude Drug Res* 1979; **17**: 139–196.
8 Nakabayashi T. Tannin of fruits and vegetables. III. Polyphenolic compounds and phenol-oxidising enzymes of edible burdock. *Nippon Shokuhin Kogyo Gakkaishi* 1968; **15**: 199–206.
9 Morita K *et al.* Chemical nature of a desmutagenic factor from burdock (*A. lappa* L.). *Agric Biol Chem* 1985; **49**: 925–932.
10 Ichihara A *et al.* Lappaol A and B, novel lignans from *Arctium lappa* L. *Tetrahedron Lett* 1976; **44**: 3961–3964.
11 Ichihara A *et al.* New sesquilignans from *Arctium lappa* L. The structure of lappaol C, D and E. *Agric Biol Chem* 1977; **41**: 1813–1814.
12 Lapinina LO, Sisoeva TF. Investigation of some plants to determine their sugar lowering action.

Farmatsevt Zh 1964; **19**: 52–58.

13 Cappelletti EM *et al*. External antirheumatic and antineuralgic herbal remedies in the traditional medicine of North-eastern Italy. *J Ethnopharmacol* 1982; **6**: 161–190.

14 Moskalenko SA. Preliminary screening of far-eastern ethnomedicinal plants for antibacterial activity. *J Ethnopharmacol* 1986; **15**: 231–259.

15 Morita K *et al*. Desmutagenic factor isolated from burdock (*Arctium lappa* L.). *Mutat Res* 1984; **129**: 25–31.

16 Ito Y *et al*. Suppression of 7,12-dimethylbenz(a)-anthracene-induced chromosome aberrations in rat bone marrow cells by vegetable juices. *Mutat Res* 1986; **172**: 55–60.

17 Dombradi CA, Foldeak S. Anti-tumor activity of *A. lappa* ext. *Tumori* 1966; **52**: 173–175.

18 Tsujita J *et al*. Comparison of protective activity of dietary fiber against the toxicities of various food colors in rats. *Nutr Rep Int* 1979; **20**: 635–642.

19 Bryson PD *et al*. Burdock root tea poisoning. Case report involving a commercial preparation. *JAMA* 1978; **239**: 2157–2158.

20 Hirono I *et al*. Safety examination of some edible plants, Part 2. *J Environ Pathol Toxicol* 1977; **1**: 72–74.

Burnet

Species (Family)

Sanguisorba officinalis L. (Rosaceae)

Synonym(s)

Garden Burnet, Greater Burnet, Sanguisorba

Part(s) Used

Herb

Pharmacopoeial and Other Monographs

BHP 1983[G7]
PDR for Herbal Medicines 2nd edition[G36]

Legal Category (Licensed Products)

GSL (Sanguisorba)[G37]

Constituents[G40,G64]

All phytochemical data located refer to the underground plant parts and not to the herb.

Flavonoids Flavones, unstable flavonol derivatives.

Saponins Ziyu glycosides I and II (major glycosides),[1] pomolic acid as aglycone (not tomentosolic acid as documented in earlier work), sanguisorbin 2.5–4.0%.

Tannins Numerous compounds (condensed and hydrolysable) have been isolated, including 3,3,4-tri-O-methylellagic acid.[2–6]

Other constituents Volatile oil, ascorbic acid (vitamin C) in the fresh plant.

Food Use

Burnet is not used in foods.

Herbal Use

Burnet is stated to possess astringent, antihaemorrhagic, styptic and antihaemorrhoidal properties. It has been used for ulcerative colitis, metrorrhagia, and specifically for acute diarrhoea.[G7,G64]

Dosage

Dried herb 2–6 g or by infusion three times daily.[G7]

Liquid extract 2–6 mL (1 : 1 in 25% alcohol) three times daily.[G7]

Tincture 2–8 mL (1 : 5 in 45% alcohol) three times daily.[G7]

Pharmacological Actions

In vitro and animal studies

None documented for burnet. The roots have been reported to contain an antihaemorrhagic principle, 3,3,4-tri-O-methylellagic acid.[2]

Side-effects, Toxicity

None documented.

Contra-indications, Warnings

None documented.

Pregnancy and lactation In view of the lack of phytochemical, pharmacological and toxicity data, the use of burnet during pregnancy and lactation should be avoided.

Pharmaceutical Comment

The chemistry of burnet herb does not appear to have been studied, although data are available for the underground plant parts. If present in the herb as well as the root, the tannin constituents would support the reputed astringent and antihaemorrhagic actions of burnet. In view of the lack of toxicity data and the possible high tannin content of the herb, excessive use of burnet should be avoided.

References

See also General References G7, G36, G37, G40 and G64.

1   Yosioka I *et al*. Soil bacterial hydrolysis leading to genuine aglycone. III. The structures of glycosides and genuine aglycone of *Sanguisorbae radix*. *Chem Pharm Bull* 1971; **19**: 1700–1707.

2 Kosuge T *et al*. Studies on antihemorrhagic substances in herbs classified as hemostatics in Chinese medicine. III. On the antihemorrhagic principle in *Sanguisorba officinalis* L. *Chem Pharm Bull* 1984; **32**: 4478–4481.

3 Nonaka G-I *et al*. Tannins and related compounds. XVII. Galloylhamameloses from *Castanea crenata* L. and *Sanguisorba officinalis* L. *Chem Pharm Bull* 1984; **32**: 483–489.

4 Nonaka G-I *et al*. A dimeric hydrolyzable tannin, sanguiin H-6 from *Sanguisorba officinalis* L. *Chem Pharm Bull* 1982; **30**: 2255–2257.

5 Tanaka T *et al*. Tannins and related compounds. XVI. Isolation and characterization of six methyl glucoside gallates and a gallic acid glucoside gallate from *Sanguisorba officinalis* L. *Chem Pharm Bull* 1984; **32**: 117–121.

6 Tanaka T *et al*. 7-O-galloyl-(+)-catechin and 3-O-galloylprocyanidin B-3 from *Sanguisorba officinalis*. *Phytochemistry* 1983; **22**: 2575–2578.

Calamus

Species (Family)

Acorus calamus L. (Araceae)

Various genetic species (*n* = 12): diploid North American, triploid European, tetraploid Asian, Eastern, Indian.

Synonym(s)

Sweet Flag

Part(s) Used

Rhizome

Pharmacopoeial and Other Monographs

BHP 1996[G9]
Martindale 32nd edition[G43]
PDR for Herbal Medicines 2nd edition[G36]

Legal Category (Licensed Products)

GSL[G37]

Constituents[G19,G22,G41,G58]

Amines Dimethylamine, methylamine, trimethylamine and choline.

Volatile oil 1.5–3.5%. β-Asarone content varies between genetic species: 96% in tetraploid (Indian), 5% in triploid (European) and 0% in the diploid (North American) species.[1–4] Other identified components include calamenol (5%), calamene (4%), calamone (1%), methyl eugenol (1%), eugenol (0.3%) and the sesquiterpenes acolamone, acoragermacrone and isoacolamone. Considerable qualitative and quantitative differences have been reported between the volatile oil from different genetic species, and between the volatile fraction of an alcoholic extract and the essential oil from the same variety (European).[3,4]

Tannin 1.5%.

Other constituents Bitter principles (e.g. acorin), acoric and palmitic acids, resin (2.5%), mucilage, starch (25–40%), sugars.

Food Use

The level of β-asarone permitted in foods is restricted to 0.1 mg/kg in foods and beverages, 1 mg/kg in alcoholic beverages and in foods containing *Acorus calamus* or *Asarum europaeum*.[G16] Calamus is listed by the Council of Europe as a source of natural food flavouring (category N3). This category indicates that calamus can be added to foodstuffs in the traditionally accepted manner, although there is insufficient information available for an adequate assessment of potential toxicity.[G16] Calamus is classified as an 'unsafe herb' by the US Food and Drugs Administration (FDA),[G22] and the use of the rhizome and its derivatives (oil, extracts) are prohibited from use in human food.[G41]

Herbal Use

Calamus is stated to act as a carminative, spasmolytic and diaphoretic. Traditionally it has been indicated for acute and chronic dyspepsia, gastritis and gastric ulcer, intestinal colic and anorexia.[G7]

Dosage

Rhizome 1–3 g or by infusion three times daily.[G7]

Liquid extract 1–3 mL (1 : 1 in 60% alcohol) three times daily.[G7]

Tincture 2–4 mL (1 : 5 in 60% alcohol) three times daily.[G7]

Pharmacological Actions

In vitro and animal studies

Numerous documented studies have concentrated on activities associated with the oil. The pharmacology and toxicology of calamus oil have been reviewed.[5] Unless specified, all of the following actions refer to those exhibited by the oil.

Spasmolytic action *in vitro* versus various spasmogens in different smooth muscle preparations including tracheal, intestinal, uterine, bronchial and vascular has been reported for European and Indian varieties.[5–8] In one study activity was associated with a lack of β-asarone,[6] whereas oils with either low or high levels of β-asarone have also exhibited activity.[5,7] The pattern of spasmolytic activity has been compared to that of papaverine, and a direct musculotropic action has been proposed.[8] Unlike papaverine an acetylcholine-like action has also been observed with low dilutions of the oil and asarone.[8]

Inhibition of monoamine oxidase activity and a stimulation of D- and L-amino oxidase has been reported.[5] The mechanism for this activity, involving serotonin and adrenaline, has been disputed, and an alternative mechanism involving depression of hypothalamic function has been proposed.[9]

In vitro oil rich in β-asarone has been reported to reduce phenylbutazone-induced ulcers in the rat by 5–60%, although no effect was observed on stress- or ethanol-induced ulcers.[7] No spasmolytic activity was reported for oil free from or with low levels of β-asarone.

A sedative action and a potentiation of barbiturate effect (increased sleeping time, reduction in body temperature) have been described in a number of small animals (mice, rats, rabbits and cats) following intravenous or intraperitoneal administration of European (alcoholic and aqueous extracts) and Indian varieties.[5] Dexamphetamine has been found to block the potentiating action of the Indian variety on barbiturate sleeping time.[5] Potentiation of morphine activity has been reported for the European variety.

The Indian oil has been reported to deplete levels of serotonin and noradrenaline in the rat brain following intraperitoneal administration.[5] The mechanism of action was suggested as similar to that of reserpine, and a potentiation of the amphetamine-detoxifying effect of reserpine has also been described.[5] In contrast, the central action of the European variety has been stated to not resemble that of reserpine.[5] Anti-adrenergic activity demonstrated by antagonism of dexamphetamine-induced agitational symptoms has been reported for the Indian variety in various small animals.[5]

Anticonvulsant, anti-arrhythmic (like quinidine) and hypotensive (apparently not due to a nervous mechanism) activities in small animals have also been reported for the Indian variety.[5]

α-Asarone, isolated from *Asarum europaeum* (Aristolochiaceae), has a local anaesthetic activity similar to that of benzocaine.[10]

Antifungal activity has been documented for β-asarone[11] and for the oil (weak).[5] Insecticidal and leech repellant properties have been reported for the oil and may be synergised by synthetic pine oil.[5] Antibacterial activity primarily versus organisms responsible for gut and throat infections has been documented,[12] although a lack of antibacterial activity has also been reported.[5]

Side-Effects, Toxicity[G19,G58]

Concerns over the toxicity of calamus centre around the volatile oil and in particular on the β-asarone content. The level of β-asarone in the oil varies considerably between the different genetic species of calamus (*see* Constituents).

Feeding studies (rat) using the Indian oil (high β-asarone) have shown death, growth depression, hepatic and heart abnormalities, and serous effusion in abdominal and/or peritoneal cavities.[13,14] A two-year study involving diet supplemented with calamus oil at 0, 500, 1000, 2500 and 5000 ppm, reported growth depression, and malignant duodenal tumours after 59 weeks at all levels of dietary supplementation.[13,14] Tumours of the same type were not noted in the controls.

Genotoxic activity (strong induction of chromosomal aberrations, slight increase in the rate of sister chromatid exchanges) has been exhibited by β-asarone in human lymphocyte cultures in the presence of microsomal activation.[15] Mutagenic activity (Ames) has been documented for root extracts, a tincture and β-asarone in one (TA100) of the various *Salmonella typhimurium* strains (TA98, 100, 1535, 1537, 1538) tested, but only in the presence of a microsomal activation mix.[16] Lack of mutagenicity has also been reported for an organic extract, when tested in the above *Salmonella typhimurium* strains (except TA1538) with and without activation.[17]

Acute toxicities (LD_{50}) quoted for the volatile oil from the Indian variety (high β-asarone content) include 777 mg/kg (rat, oral), >5 g/kg (guinea-pig, dermal), 221 mg/kg (rat, intraperitoneal).[5] The oleoresin is stated to be toxic at 400 and 800 mg/kg (mouse, intraperitoneal).[5] The LD_{50} of asarone in mice is stated to be 417 mg/kg (oral) and 310 mg/kg (intraperitoneal).[9]

Generally the oil is considered to be non-irritant, non-sensitising and non-phototoxic.[5,G58] However, bath preparations containing the oil have reportedly caused erythema, and dermatitis has been reported in hypersensitive individuals.[5]

Contra-indications, Warnings

The toxicity of calamus oil has been associated with the β-asarone content.[16] It has therefore been advised that only roots free from, or with a low content of β-asarone should be used in human phytotherapy.[16] In foods and beverages, the level of β-asarone permitted in the final product is restricted (*see* Food use).

Use of the isolated oil is not recommended.[G49,G58] External contact with the oil may cause an irritant reaction in sensitive individuals.

Calamus may potentiate monoamine oxidase inhibitor (MAOI) therapy (*in vitro* MAOI activity, amine constituents), although the clinical significance of the *in vitro* action has not been established.

Pregnancy and lactation In view of the toxic properties associated with calamus, it should not be used during pregnancy or lactation. It is not known whether β-asarone is excreted into the breast milk. In general, the topical application of any undiluted oil is not recommended. Application of preparations containing calamus oil may provoke an irritant reaction and is therefore best avoided.

Pharmaceutical Comment

The phytochemistry of calamus, especially the oil, has been extensively investigated. Three genotypes (diploid, triploid and tetraploid) have been identified which are chemically distinct with respect to the β-asarone content. Spasmolytic and anti-ulcer effects documented for the oil support the traditional herbal uses of calamus. In addition, bitter principles documented as constituents may account for the use of the root in anorexia. However, in view of the toxic properties documented for the oil and associated with β-asarone, it has been recommended that only β-asarone-free calamus root should be used in phytotherapy. Use of the oil is not recommended due to its carcinogenic activity and its ability to cause kidney damage, tremors and convulsions.[G58] Studies carried out to investigate the mutagenic potential of calamus have produced conflicting results.

References

See also General References G2, G9, G10, G16, G18, G19, G22, G29, G31, G32, G36, G37, G41, G43 and G58.

1 Stahl E, Keller K. Zur Klassifizierung handelsüblicher Kalmusdrogen. *Planta Med* 1981; **43**: 128–140.
2 Keller K, Stahl E. Zusammensetzung des ätherischen Öles von β-asaronfreiem Kalmus. *Planta Med* 1983; **47**: 71–74.
3 Mazza G. Gas chromatographic and mass spectrometric studies of the constituents of the rhizome of calamus. I. The volatile constituents of the essential oil. *J Chromatogr* 1985; **328**: 179–194.
4 Mazza G. Gas chromatographic and mass spectrometric studies of the constituents of the rhizome of calamus. II. The volatile constituents of alcoholic extracts. *J Chromatogr* 1985; **328**: 195–206.
5 Opdyke DJL. Calamus oil. *Food Cosmet Toxicol* 1977; **15**: 623–626.
6 Keller K *et al.* Spasmolytische wirkung des isoasaronfreien kalmus. *Planta Med* 1985; 6–9.
7 Keller K *et al.* Pharmacological activity of calamus oil with different amount of cis-isoasaron. *Naunyn Schmiedeberg's Arch Pharmacol* 1983; **324**(Suppl.): R55.
8 Das PK *et al.* Spasmolytic activity of asarone and essential oil of *Acorus calamus*, Linn. *Arch Int Pharmacodyn* 1962; **135**: 167–177.
9 Calamus. *Lawrence Review of Natural Products*. St Louis, MO: JB Lippincott, 1989.
10 Gracza L. The active substances of *Asarum europaeum*. 16. The local anaesthetic activity of the phenylpropanoids. *Planta Med* 1983; **48**: 153–157.
11 Ohmoto T, Sung Y-I. Antimycotic substances in the crude drugs II. *Shoyakugaku Zasshi* 1982; **36**: 307–314.
12 Jain SR *et al.* Antibacterial evaluation of some indigenous volatile oils. *Planta Med* 1974; **26**: 196–199.
13 Taylor JM *et al.* Toxicity of oil of calamus (Jammu Variety). *Toxicol Appl Pharmacol* 1967; **10**: 405.
14 Gross MA *et al.* Carcinogenicity of oil of calamus. *Proc Am Assoc Cancer Res* 1967; **8**: 24.
15 Abel G. Chromosome damaging effect on human lymphocytes by β-asarone. *Planta Med* 1987; 251–253.
16 Göggelmann W, Schimmer O. Mutagenicity testing of β-asarone and commercial calamus drugs with Salmonella typhimurium. *Mutat Res* 1983; **121**: 191–194.
17 Riazuddin S *et al.* Mutagenicity testing of some medicinal herbs. *Environ Mol Mutagen* 1987; **10**: 141–148.

Calendula

Species (Family)

Calendula officinalis L. (Compositae)

Synonym(s)

Gold-bloom, Marigold, Marybud, Pot Marigold

Part(s) Used

Flower

Pharmacopoeial and Other Monographs

BHP 1996[G9]
BP 2001[G15]
Complete German Commission E[G3]
ESCOP 1996[G52]
Martindale 32nd edition[G43]
Mills and Bone[G50]
PDR for Herbal Medicines 2nd edition[G36]
Ph Eur 2002[G28]
WHO volume 1 1999[G63]

Legal Category (Licensed Products)

GSL (external use only)[G37]

Constituents[G2,G48,G52,G53,G62,G64]

Flavonoids Pharmacopoeial standard not less than 0.4% flavonoids.[G15,G28] Flavonol (isorhamnetin, quercetin) glycosides including isoquercitrin, narcissin, neohesperidoside, and rutin.[1]

Polysaccharides Three polysaccharides PS-I, -II and –III have a $(1\rightarrow3)$-β-D-galactan backbone with short side chains at C-6, comprising α-araban-$(1\rightarrow3)$-araban, α-L-rhamnan-$(1\rightarrow3)$-araban or simple α-L-rhamnan moieties.[2]

Terpenoids Many components, including α- and β-amyrin, lupeol, longispinogenin, oleanolic acid, arnidiol, brein, calenduladiol, erythrodiol, faradiol, faradiol-3-myristic acid ester, faradiol-3-palmitic acid ester,[3] helantriols A1, B0, B1 and B2, lupeol, maniladiol, urs-12-en-3,16,21-triol, ursadiol; oleanolic acid saponins including calendulosides C–H;[4] campesterol, cholesterol, sitosterol, stigmasterol and taraxasterol (sterols).[5]

Volatile oils Terpenoid components include menthone, isomenthone, caryophyllene and an epoxide and ketone derivative, pedunculatine, α- and β-ionone, a β-ionone epoxide derivative, dihydroactinidiolide.[6]

Other constituents Bitter (loliolide),[7] arvoside A (sesquiterpene glycoside),[8] carotenoid pigments[9] and calendulin (gum).[9]

Food Use

Calendula is not used in foods. In the USA, calendula is listed as GRAS (Generally Recognised As Safe).[G65]

Herbal Use[G2,G4,G7,G32,G43,G52,G54,G56,G64]

Calendula is stated to possess antispasmodic, mild diaphoretic, anti-inflammatory, anti-haemorrhagic, emmenagogue, vulnerary, styptic and antiseptic properties. Traditionally, it has been used to treat gastric and duodenal ulcers, amenorrhoea, dysmenorrhoea and epistaxis; crural ulcers, varicose veins, haemorrhoids, anal eczema, proctitis, lymphadenoma, inflamed cutaneous lesions (topically) and conjunctivitis (as an eye lotion). The German Commission E approved internal and external use for inflammation of oral and pharyngeal mucosa and external use in treatment of poorly healing sores.[G3]

Dosage

Dried florets 1–4 g or by infusion three times daily.[G7]

Liquid extract 0.5–1.0 mL (1:1 in 40% alcohol) three times daily.[G7]

Calendula Tincture (BPC 1934) 0.3–1.2 mL (1:5 in 90% alcohol) three times daily.[G7]

External use Tincture–liquid extract (1:1) in 40% alcohol or tincture 1:5 in 90% alcohol. Apply to wounds as such and dilute 1:3 with water for compresses. Ointment 2.5%.[G52]

Pharmacological Actions

In vitro and animal studies

Anti-inflammatory, antibacterial and antiviral activities have been reported for calendula.[10] Weak anti-inflammatory activity in rats (carrageenan-induced oedema) has been reported.[11,12] An aqueous ethanolic extract had mild dose-dependent action in the mouse croton oil test with 20% inhibition being reached at a dose of 1200 µg/ear, whereas a carbon dioxide extract exhibited 70% inhibition at the same concentration.[5,13] The activity was shown to be due to the triterpenoids, the most active being a monoester of faradiol. Further separation of the triterpenoids has shown that the three most active compounds in the croton oil mouse test are faradiol-3-myristic acid ester, faradiol-3-palmitic acid ester and 4-taraxosterol.[3]

A polysaccharide enriched extract showed strong concentration-dependent adhesive properties on porcine buccal membranes ex vivo.[14] Fluorescent labelled rhamnogalacturan indicated the presence of polysaccharide layers on buccal membranes, leading to the suggestion that irritated buccal membranes may be smoothed by mucilage.

The formation of new blood vessels is an essential part of the wound-healing process. Angiogenic activity has been shown for a freeze-dried aqueous extract of calendula utilising the chick chorioallantoic membrane (CAM) assay.[15] The number of microvessels in calendula-treated CAMs was significantly higher than in the control ($p < 0.0001$). Furthermore, calendula-treated CAMs were positive for the glycosaminoglycan hyaluronan (HA) associated with neovascularisation. The presence of HA was not demonstrated in control CAMs.

A combination of allantoin and calendula extract applied to surgically induced skin wounds in rats has been reported to stimulate physiological regeneration and epithelisation.[16] This effect was attributed to a more intensive metabolism of glycoproteins, nucleoproteins and collagen proteins during the regenerative period in the tissues.[16] Allantoin applied on its own was found to exert a much weaker action.[16]

A proprietary cream containing a combination of plant extracts, including calendula, has been reported to be effective in dextran and burn oedemas and in acute lymphoedema in rats. Activity against lymphoedema was primarily attributed to an enhancement of macrophage proteolytic activity.[17] Slight increases in foot oedema were attributed to a vasodilatory action.

The trichomonacidal activity of calendula has been associated with the essential oil terpenoid fraction.[6]

An in vitro uterotonic effect has been described for calendula extract on rabbit and guinea-pig preparations.[18]

Immunostimulant activity, assayed using granulocyte and carbon clearance tests, of calendula extracts has been attributed to polysaccharide fractions of high molecular weight.[19] Polysaccharides PS-I, -II and -III have immunostimulant activity at concentrations of 10^{-5} to 10^{-6} mg/mL, stimulating phagocytosis of human granulocytes in vitro.[2] A dry 70% ethanolic extract was not directly mitogenic, and was inhibitory in the mitogen-induced lymphocyte assay, causing stimulation at concentrations of 0.1–10 µg/mL, and inhibition at higher concentrations.[20]

A 70% methanolic extract of calendula was successively extracted with ether, chloroform, ethyl acetate and n-butanol, leaving a residual aqueous extract. Each of the five extracts were concentrated and dissolved in 50% ethanol to produce 6% (w/v) solutions which were assessed for activity on liposomal lipid peroxidation induced by Fe^{2+} and ascorbic acid. The ether, butanol and water extracts showed antioxidant activity.[21]

The triterpenoid constituents of calendula are reported to be effective as spermicides and as antiblastocyst and abortion agents.[G53]

In vitro cytotoxic activity and in vivo antitumour activity (against mouse Ehrlich carcinoma) have been documented for calendula extracts.[7] The most active fraction in vivo (saponin-rich) was not the most active in vitro.[10]

A 70% aqueous ethanolic extract had marked antiviral activity against influenza virus and herpes simplex virus.[G52] A dichloromethane–methanol (1 : 1) extract exhibited potent anti-HIV activity in an in vitro MTT/tetrazolium-based assay.[22] Uninfected Molt-4 cells were completely protected for up to 24 hours from fusion and subsequent death caused by co-cultivation with persistently infected U-937/HIV-1 cells. The organic extract caused a significant concentration- and time-dependent reduction of HIV-1 reverse transcriptase.[22]

In a study in mice fed for three weeks with a diet containing either 0.1% or 0.4% of a calendula extract (containing 37% of esters of the carotenoid lutein), mammary tumour cells were infused into the mammary glands. Tumour latency increased, and tumour growth was inhibited in a dose-dependent manner by dietary lutein. In addition, dietary lutein was reported to enhance lymphocyte proliferation.[23]

Clinical studies

A proprietary cream preparation containing several plant extracts, including calendula, has been reported to reduce pain associated with postmastectomy lymphoedema, although there was no significant clinical difference in the reduction of oedema between controls and experimental groups.[17] Calendula tincture 20% has been reported to be useful in the treatment of chronic suppurative otitis.[24] Calendula extracts are used to accelerate healing and to reduce inflammation.[9] Thirty patients with burns or scalds were treated three times daily with a hydrogel containing 10% aqueous ethanolic extract of calendula for 14 days in an open, uncontrolled, pilot study.[25] Improvement was noted for reddening, swelling, blistering, pain, soreness and heat sensitivity.

Side-effects, Toxicity

An aqueous extract of calendula had an LD_{50} of 375 mg/kg (intravenous administration) and an LD_{100} of 580 mg/kg (intraperitoneal administration) in mice.[G52] Aqueous ethanolic extracts (drug/extract ratio 1:1 and 0.5:1, 30% ethanol) had LD_{50} values of 45 mg/mouse (subcutaneous administration) and 526 mg/100 g in rat (intravenous administration). An aqueous extract was not toxic following chronic administration to mice. Six saponins at doses of 400 µg were non-mutagenic in the Ames test using *Salmonella typhimurium* TA98 with and without S9 activation mixture.[G52] *In vitro* cytotoxicity has been reported for calendula extracts.[10] Extracts have been reported to be non-carcinogenic in rats and hamsters.[G52]

Contra-indications, Warnings

Calendula may cause an allergic reaction in sensitive individuals, especially those with an existing hypersensitivity to other members of the Asteraceae/Compositae.

Pregnancy and lactation Calendula is traditionally reputed to affect the menstrual cycle. An uterotonic effect (*in vitro*) has been reported, and the triterpenoid constituents are reported to be effective as spermatocides and as antiblastocyst and abortion agents. In view of the lack of toxicity data, the use of calendula is best avoided during pregnancy and lactation.

Pharmaceutical Comment

Phytochemical studies have reported four main groups of constituents, for calendula, namely flavonoids, polysaccharides, volatile oil and triterpenes. The latter seems to represent the principal group, with many compounds isolated including pentacyclic alcohols, glycosides (saponins) and

sterols. Animal studies have reported wound-healing and anti-inflammatory effects, supporting the traditional uses of calendula in various dermatological conditions. The anti-inflammatory effect is due to the triterpenoid constituents although flavonoids may contribute to the activity. The reputed antispasmodic effect may be attributable to the volatile oil fraction. In addition, immunostimulant activity has been reported for high molecular weight polysaccharide components. Despite the popularity of calendula in herbal preparations there is little substantial clinical evidence to support its use.

References

See also General References G2, G3, G5, G9, G10, G15, G28, G31, G32, G36, G37, G43, G48, G52, G53, G54, G56, G62 and G64.

1 Vidal-Ollivier E *et al.* Flavonol glycosides from *Calendula officinalis* flowers. *Planta Med* 1989; **55**: 73.

2 Varljen J *et al.* Structural analysis of a rhamnoarabinogalactan and arabinogalactans with immunostimulating activity from *Calendula officinalis*. *Phytochemistry* 1989; **28**: 2379–2383.

3 Zitterl-Eglseer K *et al.* Anti-oedematous activities of the main triterpendiol esters of marigold (*Calendula officinalis* L.). *J Ethnopharmacol* 1997; **57**: 139–144.

4 Pizza C *et al.* Plant metabolites. Triterpenoid saponins from *Calendula arvensis*. *J Nat Prod* 1987; **50**: 927–931.

5 Della Loggia R *et al.* The role of triterpenoids in the topical anti-inflammatory activity of *Calendula officinalis* flowers. *Planta Med* 1994; **60**: 516–520.

6 Gracza L. Oxygen-containing terpene derivatives from *Calendula officinalis*. *Planta Med* 1987; **53**: 227.

7 Willuhn G, Westhaus R-G. Loliolide (Calendin) from *Calendula officinalis*. *Planta Med* 1987; **53**: 304.

8 Pizza C, de Tommasi N. Plants metabolites. A new sesquiterpene glycoside from *Calendula arvensis*. *J Nat Prod* 1987; **50**: 784–789.

9 Fleischner AM. Plant extracts: To accelerate healing and reduce inflammation. *Cosmet Toilet* 1985; **100**: 45.

10 Boucard-Maitre Y *et al.* Cytotoxic and antitumoral activity of *Calendula officinalis* extracts. *Pharmazie* 1988; **43**: 220.

11 Peyroux J *et al.* Propriétés anti-oedémateuses et anti-hyperhémiantes du *Calendula officinalis* L. *Plant Méd Phytothér* 1981; **15**: 210–216.

12 Mascolo N *et al.* Biological screening of Italian

medicinal plants for anti-inflammatory activity. *Phytother Res* 1987; **1**: 28–31.

13 Della Loggia R *et al*. Topical anti-inflammatory activity of *Calendula officinalis* extracts. *Planta Med* 1990; **56**: 658.

14 Schmidgall J *et al*. Evidence for bioadhesive effects of polysaccharides and polysaccharide-containing herbs in a *ex vivo* bioadhesion assay on buccal membranes. *Planta Med* 2000; **66**: 48–53.

15 Patrick KFM *et al*. Induction of vascularisation by an aqueous extract of the flowers of *Calendula officinalis* L. the European marigold. *Phytomedicine* 1996; **3**: 11–18.

16 Kioucek-Popova E *et al*. Influence of the physiological regeneration and epithelization using fractions isolated from *Calendula officinalis*. *Acta Physiol Pharmacol Bulg* 1982; **8**: 63–67.

17 Casley-Smith JR, Casley-Smith JR. The effect of 'Unguentum lymphaticum' on acute experimental lymphedema and other high-protein edemas. *Lymphology* 1983; **16**: 150–156.

18 Shipochliev T. Extracts from a group of medicinal plants enhancing the uterine tonus. *Vet Med Nauki* 1981; **4**: 94–98.

19 Wagner H *et al*. Immunostimulating polysaccharides (heteroglycans) of higher plants. *Arzneimittelforschung* 1985; **35**: 1069.

20 Amirghofran Z *et al*. Evaluation of the immunomodulatory effects of five herbal plants. *J Ethnopharmacol* 2000; **72**: 167–712.

21 Popović M *et al*. Combined effects of plant extracts and xenobiotics on liposomal lipid peroxidation. Part 1. Marigold extract-ciprofloxacin/pyralene. *Oxidation Commun* 1999; **22**: 487–494.

22 Kalvatchev Z *et al*. Anti-HIV activity of extracts from *Calendula officinalis* flowers. *Biomed Pharmacother* 1997; **51**: 176–180.

23 Chew BP *et al*. Effects of lutein from marigold extract on immunity and growth of mammary tumors in mice. *Anticancer Res* 1996; **16**: 3689–3694.

24 Shaparenko BA. On use of medicinal plants for treatment of patients with chronic suppurative otitis. *Zh Ushn Gorl Bolezn* 1979; **39**: 48–51.

25 Baranov von AP. Calendula – wie ist die wirksamkeit bei verbrennungen und verbrühungen?. *Dtsch Apotheker Zeitung* 1999; **139**: 2135–2138.

Capsicum

Species (Family)

Capsicum species (Solanaceae) including *C. annum* L., *C. baccatum* L., *C. chinense* Jacq., *C. frutescens* L., *C. pubescens* Ruiz & Pavon, *C. minimum* Roxb.

Synonym(s)

Cayenne, Chilli Pepper, Hot Pepper, Paprika, Red Pepper, Tabasco Pepper

Part(s) Used

Fruit

Pharmacopoeial and Other Monographs

BHP 1996[G9]
Complete German Commission E (Paprika)[G3]
Martindale 32nd edition[G43]
PDR for Herbal Medicines 2nd edition[G36]
USP24/NF19[G61]

Legal Category (Licensed Products)

GSL[G37]

Constituents[G22,G41,G64]

Capsaicinoids Up to 1.5%, usually 0.11%. Major components capsaicin (48.6%), 6,7-dihydrocapsaicin (36%), nordihydrocapsaicin (7.4%), homodihydrocapsaicin (2%) and homocapsaicin (2%).

Volatile oils Trace. Over 125 components have been isolated with at least 24 characterised.

Other constituents Carotenoid pigments (capsanthin, capsorubin, carotene, lutein), proteins (12–15%), fats (9–17%), vitamins including A and C.

Other plant parts The plant material contains solanidine, solanine and solasodine (steroidal alkaloidal glycosides) and scopoletin (coumarin).

Food Use

Capsicum (chilli) peppers are widely used as a spice. Capsicum is listed by the Council of Europe as a natural source of food flavouring (category N2). This category indicates that capsicum can be added to foodstuffs in small quantities, with a possible limitation of an active principle (as yet unspecified) in the final product.[G16] In the USA, capsicum is stated to be GRAS (Generally Recognised As Safe).[G41]

Herbal Use[G4,G7,G64]

Capsicum is stated to possess stimulant, antispasmodic, carminative, diaphoretic, counterirritant, antiseptic and rubefacient properties. Traditionally, it has been used for colic, flatulent dyspepsia without inflammation, chronic laryngitis (as a gargle), insufficiency of peripheral circulation and externally for neuralgia including rheumatic pains and unbroken chilblains (as a lotion/ointment). The German Commission E approved external use for treatment of painful muscle spasms in shoulder, arm and spine; arthritis, rheumatism, lumbago and chilblains.[G3]

Dosage

Fruit 30–120 mg three times daily.[G7]

Capsicum Tincture (BPC 1968) 0.3–1.0 mL; capsaicin content 0.005–0.01%.[G4]

Stronger Tincture of Capsicum (BPC 1934) 0.06–2.0 mL.

Oleoresin 0.6–2.0 mg.[G44]

Oleoresin, internal 1.2 mg (maximum dose), 1.8 mg (maximum daily dose).[G37]

Oleoresin, external 2.5% maximum strength.[G37]

Creams, ointments 0.02–0.05%.[G4]

Pharmacological Actions

The action of capsaicin on nervous, cardiovascular, respiratory, thermoregulatory and gastrointestinal systems has been reviewed.[1] Capsaicin has been used as a neurochemical tool for studying sensory neurotransmission.[1]

In vitro and animal studies

Infusion of capsaicin (200 µg/kg, by intravenous injection) has been reported to evoke dose-dependent catecholamine secretion (adrenaline, noradrenaline) from the adrenal medulla of pentobarbitone-anaesthetised rats.[2]

The addition of capsaicin (0.014%) to a high-fat (30%) diet fed to rats was found to reduce serum-triglyceride concentrations but to have no effect on serum cholesterol or pre-β-lipoprotein concentrations.[3] Capsaicin was thought to stimulate lipid mobilisation from adipose tissue. Lipid absorption was unaffected by capsaicin supplementation.[3]

Activities of two hepatic enzymes, glucose-6-phosphate dehydrogenase and adipose lipoprotein lipase, were elevated in rats when capsaicin was added to the diet.[3] Capsicum extracts fed orally to hamsters have been reported to significantly decrease hepatic vitamin A concentrations.[4] Serum vitamin A concentrations were not affected.[4]

Both the gastric and duodenal mucosae are thought to contain 'capsaicin-sensitive' areas which afford protection against acid- and drug-induced ulcers when stimulated by hydrochloric acid or by capsaicin itself. Stimulation causes an increase in mucosal blood flow and/or vascular permeability, inhibits gastric motility, and activates duodenal motility.[5] Desensitisation of these areas, using a regimen involving subcutaneous or oral administration of capsaicin, is thought to remove the protection.[5] However, capsaicin desensitisation was found to have little effect on peripheral responses to stress (i.e. ulcer formation) but did enhance central responses (increase in plasma corticosterone concentration) in rats.[6] The increase in plasma corticosterone concentration observed in capsaicin-desensitised rats was similar in stressed and non-stressed animals.[6]

Capsaicin was found to influence adrenal cortical activity independently of the presence of a stress factor and may represent a stressor in itself.[6] Capsaicin desensitisation was not found to influence basal gastric acid secretion in non-stressed rats, but did lower pentagastrin-stimulated gastric output.[6] However, other results have reported that capsaicin desensitisation does increase acid secretion.[6]

Capsicum (leaf and stem) has been reported to exhibit uterine stimulant activity in animal studies.[G30]

Pharmacokinetic studies in rats have reported that capsaicin is readily transported via the gastrointestinal tract and absorbed through non-active transport into the portal vein.[2] Capsaicin is partly hydrolysed during absorption and the majority is excreted in the urine within 48 hours.[2,7] Dihydrocapsaicin-hydro-

lysing enzyme is present in various organs of the rat but principally in the gastrointestinal tract and the liver. The biotransformation pathway of dihydrocapsaicin in the rat has been studied.[7] Metabolites are mainly excreted as glucuronide conjugates in the urine.[7]

Clinical studies

Ingestion of red chillies (10 g in wheatmeal) by controls and duodenal ulcer sufferers has been reported to have no significant effect on acid or pepsin secretion, or on sodium, potassium and chloride concentrations in the gastric aspirate.[8] There was reported to be no apparent change (qualitative or quantitative) in mucous and no gastric mucosal erosion was evident.[8] However, in contrast, capsicum has been shown to increase acid concentration and DNA content (indicating exfoliation of epithelial cells) of gastric aspirates in both control subjects and patients with duodenal ulcers.[1] A study involving 18 healthy volunteers suggested that chilli (20 g in 200 mL water) protected against aspirin-induced gastroduodenal mucosal injury, compared with control (water).[9]

Capsicum is applied externally as a counter-irritant in many preparations used for rheumatism, arthritis, neuralgia and lumbago. Clinical studies of topical preparations containing capsaicin have investigated its effectiveness in the treatment of chronic post-herpetic neuralgia, shingles, diabetic neuropathy, rhinopathy and neuropathic pain in cancer patients.[G4,]

A systematic review of randomised, double-blind, placebo-controlled trials of topical capsaicin included 13 trials involving patients with diabetic neuropathy, osteoarthritis, post-herpetic neuralgia, postmastectomy pain and psoriasis.[10] All the included trials reported that capsaicin was superior to placebo. However, the review drew cautious conclusions because blinding may have been compromised by the irritant effects of capsaicin.

Side-effects, Toxicity

Capsicum contains pungent principles (capsaicinoids) that are strongly irritant to mucosal membranes. Inhalation of paprika can produce a form of allergic alveolitis.[G51]

Chronic administration of capsicum extract (0.5 µg capsaicin/kg body weight) to hamsters has been reported to be toxic.[4] Treated animals did not survive beyond 17 months whereas all untreated controls survived beyond this period. In addition, eye abnormalities were observed in the treated animals. This effect was attributed to the depletion of substance P in primary afferent neurons by capsaicin, causing a loss of corneal pain sensation and subsequently the loss of protective corneal reflexes.[4]

It is thought that metabolism of capsaicin and related analogues may reduce their acute toxicity.[7] LD_{50} values stated for capsaicin in mice include 0.56 mg/kg (intravenous), 7.56 mg/kg (intraperitoneal), 9.00 mg/kg (subcutaneous) and 190 mg/kg (oral). In rats, an intraperitoneal LD_{50} of 10 mg/kg has been reported for capsaicin.[7] The toxicity of capsaicinoids has reportedly not been ascribed to any one specific action but may be due to their causing respiratory failure, bradycardia and hypotension.[7]

Contra-indications, Warnings

Capsicum may cause gastrointestinal irritation, although it has been stated that capsicum does not influence the healing of duodenal ulcers and does not need to be avoided by patients with this condition.[1] Excessive ingestion may cause gastroenteritis, hepatic or renal damage.[G42] Capsicum may interfere with monoamine oxidase inhibitors (MAOIs) and antihypertensive therapy (increased catecholamine secretion), and may increase the hepatic metabolism of drugs (glucose-6-phosphate dehydrogenase and adipose lipoprotein lipase activity elevated).

Pregnancy and lactation There are no known problems with the use of capsicum during pregnancy, although it may cause gastrointestinal irritation and should therefore be used with caution. Doses should not greatly exceed amounts normally ingested in foods. It is not known whether the pungent components in capsicum are secreted into the breast milk.

Pharmaceutical Comment

Capsicum is commonly used in both foods and in medicinal products. The capsaicinoids are principally responsible for the biological activity of capsicum. These pungent principles are thought to stimulate and aid digestion and to act as a counter-irritant when applied externally. Capsaicin has also been used as a neurochemical tool for studying sensory neurotransmission. Topical creams containing capsaicin 0.025% and 0.075% are licensed in the UK for the treatment of pain in osteoarthritis, and painful diabetic neuropathy and post-herpetic neuralgia, respectively.[11] Capsicum oleoresin and capsaicin are ingredients of a number of over-the-counter (OTC) topical preparations for relief of pain in muscle, tendon and joints.[11]

Conflicting reports have been documented concerning the effect of capsicum on acid secretion and on ulcer healing. Capsaicin-sensitive areas of the gastric and duodenal mucosa are thought to provide protection against mucosal damage. It has been suggested that this protection is lost if the sensory fibres are desensitised. Whether oral consumption of capsicum by humans can cause desensitisation is unclear. The toxicity of capsicum extracts observed in animals is considered to be due to the capsaicinoid components. However, ingestion of capsicum in the diet is not thought to represent a health risk. Capsicum should not be ingested in doses greatly exceeding amounts normally used in foods.

References

See also General References G3, G5, G9, G12, G16, G22, G30, G31, G32, G33, G36, G37, G41, G43, G48, G51, G56, G61 and G64.

1 Locock RA. Capsicum. *Can Pharm J* 1985; **118**: 517–519.
2 Watanabe T *et al*. Capsaicin, a pungent principle of hot red pepper, evokes catecholamine secretion from the adrenal medulla of anesthetized rats. *Biochem Biophys Res Commun* 1987; **142**: 259–264.
3 Kawada T *et al*. Effects of capsaicin on lipid metabolism in rats fed a high fat diet. *J Nutr* 1986; **116**: 1272–1278.
4 Agrawal RC *et al*. Chilli extract treatment and induction of eye lesions in hamsters. *Toxicol Lett* 1985; **28**: 1–7.
5 Maggi CA *et al*. Capsaicin-sensitive mechanisms and experimentally induced duodenal ulcers in rats. *J Pharm Pharmacol* 1987; **39**: 559–561.
6 Dugani A, Glavin GB. Capsaicin effects on stress pathology and gastric acid secretion in rats. *Life Sci* 1986; **39**: 1531–1538.
7 Kawada T, Iwai K. *In vivo* and *in vitro* metabolism of dihydrocapsaicin, a pungent principle of hot pepper in rats. *Agric Biol Chem* 1985; **49**: 441–448.
8 Pimparkar BND *et al*. Effects of commonly used spices on human gastric secretion. *J Assoc Physicians India* 1972: **20**: 901–910.
9 Yeoh KG *et al*. Chili protects against aspirin-induced gastroduodenal mucosal injury in humans. *Dig Dis Sci* 1995; **40**: 580–583.
10 Zhang WY *et al*. The effectiveness of topically applied capsaicin. *Eur J Clin Pharmacol* 1994; **46**: 517–522.
11 British Medical Association and Royal Pharmaceutical Society of Great Britain. *British National Formulary, number 41*, 2001. London: British Medical Association and Royal Pharmaceutical Society of Great Britain, 2001.

Cascara

Species (Family)

Rhamnus purshiana DC. (*Frangula purshiana* (DC). A. Gray ex J.C. Cooper) (Rhamnaceae)

Synonym(s)

Cascara Sagrada, Rhamni Purshianae Cortex, Rhamnus

Part(s) Used

Bark

Pharmacopoeial and Other Monographs

BHP 1996[G9]
BP 2001[G15]
Complete German Commission E[G3]
ESCOP 1997[G52]
Martindale 32nd edition[G43]
PDR for Herbal Medicines 2nd edition[G36]
Ph Eur 2002[G28]
USP24/NF19[G61]

Legal Category (Licensed Products)

GSL[G37]

Constituents[G2,G6,G41,G48,G52,G59,G62,G64]

Anthracene glycosides Pharmacopoeial standard, not less than 8% hydroxyanthracene glycosides.[G15,G28] Cascarosides A and B are anthrone C- and O-glycosides being 8-O-β-D-glucosides of 10-*S*-deoxyglucosyl aloe-emodin anthrone (aloin A) and of 10-*R*-deoxyglucosyl aloe-emodin anthrone (aloin B), respectively. Cascarosides C and D are the 8-O-β-D-glucosides of 10-(*R*)-(*S*)-deoxyglucosyl chrysophanol anthrone (chrysaloin A and B, respectively). Cascarosides E and F are the 8-O-β-D-glucosides of 10-deoxyglucosyl emodin-9-anthrone. The cascarosides comprise 60–70% of the total hydroxyanthracene complex. Aloins A and B, chrysaloins A and B account for 10–30% of the total hydroxyanthracene complex. The remaining 10–20% is a mixture of hydroxyanthracene O-glycosides including monoglucosides of aloe-emodin, chrysophanol, emodin and physcion.

Other constituents Linoleic acid, myristic acid, syringic acid, lipids, resin and tannin.

Food Use

Cascara is listed by the Council of Europe as a natural source of food flavouring (category N4). This category indicates that while the use of cascara for flavouring purposes is recognised, it cannot be classified into the categories N1, N2 or N3 because of insufficient information.[G16] In the USA, cascara has been approved for food use.[G41]

Herbal Use[G2,G4,G6,G8,G43,G52,G54,G64]

Cascara is stated to possess mild purgative properties and has been used for constipation. The German Commission E approved for use for treatment of constipation.[G3]

Dosage

Dried bark 0.3–1 g single daily dose.[G3]

Infusion 1.5–2 g in 150 mL water.[G3]

Cascara Liquid Extract (BP 1980) 2–5 mL.

Preparations Equivalent to 20–30 mg hydroxyanthracene derivatives calculated as cascaroside A, daily.[G3]

Pharmacological Actions

The laxative action of anthraquinone glycosides is well recognised (*see* Senna). Cascara has a laxative action.[G45]

Clinical studies
Studies involving elderly patients suggest that cascara treatment, compared with placebo, leads to relief of constipation and increased bowel movements.[1]

Side-effects, Toxicity

The side-effects and toxicity documented for anthraquinone glycosides are applicable (*see* Senna).[G22]

Contra-indications, Warnings

Cascara is contra-indicated for patients with intestinal obstruction, acute intestinal inflammation, e.g. Crohn's disease, colitis, appendicitis, abdominal pain of unknown origin, and in children under 12.[G3] Cascara should not be used over an extended period of time.[G3]

Pregnancy and lactation   Cascara should not be used during pregnancy and lactation.

Pharmaceutical Comment

The chemistry of cascara is characterised by the anthraquinone derivatives, especially the cascarosides. The laxative action of these compounds is well recognised. Cascara has been used extensively in conventional pharmaceutical preparations. Stimulant laxatives have largely been superseded by bulk-forming laxatives. However, the use of non-standardised anthraquinone-containing preparations should be avoided since their pharmacological effects will be variable and unpredictable. In particular, the use of products containing combinations of anthraquinone laxatives is not advisable.

References

See also General References G2, G3, G6, G9, G12, G15, G16, G18, G20, G22, G28, G29, G31, G36, G37, G41, G43, G48, G54, G61, G62 and G64.

1   Petticrew M *et al*. Epidemiology of constipation in the general adult population. *Health Technol Assess* 1997; 1: 1–52.

Cassia

Species (Family)

Cinnamomum cassia Bl. (Lauraceae)

Synonym(s)

Cassia Bark, Cassia Lignea, Chinese Cinnamon, *Cinnamomum aromaticum* Nees, False Cinnamon

Part(s) Used

Bark

Pharmacopoeial and Other Monographs

BHP 1996[G9]
Martindale 32nd edition[G43]
PDR for Herbal Medicines 2nd edition[G36]

Legal Category (Licensed Products)

GSL (oil)[G37]

Constituents[G41,G58,G59,G62,G64]

Volatile oils 1–2%. Mainly composed of cinnamaldehyde (75–90%). Other major components include salicylaldehyde, methylsalicylaldehyde, and methyleugenol. Eugenol is reported to be absent. Cassia oil contains no monoterpenoids or sesquiterpenoids.[1]

Other constituents Calcium oxalate, coumarin, mucilage (higher content compared to cinnamon), resins, sugars and tannins (condensed). Complex diterpenoids have been isolated from cinnamomi cortex, for which *C. cassia* is used as a source.[1]

Food Use

Cassia bark and oil are extensively used as food flavourings. A temporary estimated acceptable daily intake of cinnamaldehyde is 700 µg/kg body weight. In the USA, cassia is listed as GRAS (Generally Recognised As Safe).[G41]

Herbal Use

Cassia is stated to possess carminative, antispasmodic, anti-emetic, antidiarrhoeal and antimicrobial properties. It has been used for flatulent dyspepsia, flatulent colic, diarrhoea, the common cold, and specifically for colic or dyspepsia with flatulent distension and nausea.[G7] Cassia bark is also documented to possess astringent properties.[G41,G64] Carminative and antiseptic properties are documented for the oil.[G41]

Dosage

Dried bark 0.5–1 g or by infusion three times daily.[G7]

Oil of cassia (BPC 1949) 0.05–0.2 mL three times daily.[G7]

Pharmacological Actions

In vitro and animal studies

Anti-ulcerogenic properties have been described for two propionic derivatives isolated from cassia.[2] An *in vivo* study using rats reported activity against a variety of ulcerogens including serotonin, phenylbutazone, ethanol, water immersion and stress. The compounds were thought to act by improving gastric blood flow rather than by inhibiting gastric secretion.

Many pharmacological investigations have been carried out on cinnamomi cortex, for which sources include *C. cassia* (cassia) and *Cinnamomum zeylanicum* (cinnamon). These studies have either looked at the volatile oil, in particular the major constituent cinnamaldehyde, or at parts excluding the oil.[1]

Activities documented for cinnamaldehyde include CNS stimulation (low dose), sedation (high dose), hypothermic and antipyretic actions;[1,G41] antibacterial and antifungal activity, acceleration of catecholamine (mainly adrenaline) release from the adrenal glands, weak papaverine-like action, increase in peripheral blood flow, hypotension, bradycardia and hyperglycaemia have also been reported.[1] However, these actions are of low potency and, in addition, much of the cinnamaldehyde content of cassia is thought to be lost by evaporation and auto-oxidation during decoction of the crude drug. The contribution of cinnamaldehyde to the overall therapeutic efficacy of cassia has therefore been doubted.[1]

Actions observed for essential oil-free aqueous extracts have been reported to be weak, and the only appreciable effects are prolongation of barbiturate-induced sedation and a slight reduction of acetic acid-induced writhing.[1]

In vivo inhibitory activity against complement formation has been documented and attributed to the diterpenoid and condensed tannin constituents.[1] Anti-inflammatory activity exhibited by the Japanese plant *Cinnamomum sieboldii* Meisn (also used as a source for cassia bark), has been attributed to a series of condensed tannin constituents.[1] Antiplatelet aggregation and antithrombotic actions have also been reported. These actions, together with the documented anti-inflammatory activity, are thought to contribute to the suppression of thrombus formation in certain diseases.[1]

Antitumour activity has been described and the activity depends on the plant source used.[1]

Side-effects, Toxicity

Allergic reactions, mainly contact sensitivity, to cassia oil and bark have been reported.[G51,G58] Cinnamaldehyde in toothpastes and perfumes has also been reported to cause contact sensitivity.[G51] Cassia oil is stated to cause dermal and mucous membrane irritation.[G58] The irritant and sensitising properties of cassia oil have been attributed to cinnamaldehyde.[G58] The dermal LD_{50} value for cassia oil is stated as 320 mg/kg body weight.[G58]

Contra-indications, Warnings

Contact with cassia bark or oil may cause an allergic reaction. Cassia oil is stated to be one of the most hazardous oils and should not be used on the skin in concentrations of more than 0.2%.[G58]

Pregnancy and lactation There are no known problems with the use of cassia during pregnancy, provided that amounts taken do not exceed those generally used in foods.

Pharmaceutical Comment

Cassia is similar in composition to cinnamon and both are widely used as flavouring agents in foods, and in pharmaceutical and cosmetic preparations. Cassia oil is stated to be inferior in flavour to cinnamon oil. The reputed herbal uses of cassia have been attributed to the oil. Cassia contains an irritant and sensitising principle in the oil, cinnamaldehyde, and should not be used in amounts generally exceeding those used in foods. It has been recommended that the oil should never be applied topically.

References

See also General References G9, G11, G19, G20, G31, G36, G37, G41, G43, G51, G58, G59, G62 and G64.

1 Hikino H. Oriental medicinal plants. In: Wagner H *et al.*, eds. *Economic and Medicinal Plants*, vol 1. London: Academic Press, 1985: 69–70.
2 Tanaka S *et al.* Antiulcerogenic compounds isolated from Chinese Cinnamon. *Planta Med* 1989; 55: 245–248.

Cat's Claw

Species (Family)

Uncaria tomentosa (Willd.) DC., *Uncaria guianensis* (Aubl.) Gmel. (Rubiaceae)

Synonym(s)

Life-giving Vine of Peru, Savéntaro, Uña de gato

Part(s) Used

Roots, root bark, stem bark and leaves

Pharmacopoeial and Other Monographs

None

Legal Category (Licensed Products)

Cat's claw is not included in the GSL.[G37]

Constituents

Alkaloids Both *U. tomentosa* and *U. guianensis* yield oxindole alkaloids, including isorhynchophylline and rhynchophylline and their *N*-oxides, mitraphylline and the indole alkaloids dihydrocorynantheine, hirsutine and hirsuteine.[1] *U. tomentosa* also contains isomitraphylline, its *N*-oxide, dihydrocorynantheine *N*-oxide and hirsutine *N*-oxide.[1]

There are two chemotypes of *U. tomentosa* which differ markedly in their patterns of alkaloids present in the root bark; in addition, the alkaloidal pattern of individual plants changes with time.[2,3] One chemotype primarily contains the pentacyclic oxindole alkaloids pteropodine, isopteropodine, mitraphylline, isomitraphylline, uncarine F and speciophylline,[4] whereas the other chemotype primarily contains the tetracyclic oxindole alkaloids rhynchophylline and isorhynchophylline.[1] Although a particular plant may contain either tetracyclic or pentacyclic oxindole alkaloids predominantly, both types of alkaloids can co-occur in the same plant.[3,5]

Other constituents Quinovic acid glycosides have been isolated from both species.[6–9] Polyhydroxylated triterpenes[10] and steroids (β-sitosterol, stigmasterol, campesterol)[11] occur in *U. tomentosa*. An unidentified South American species of *Uncaria* (presumably either *U. guianensis* or *U. tomentosa*) contains polyphenols ((−)-epicatechin and procyanidins).[4]

Food Use

Cat's claw is not used in foods.

Herbal Use[G32]

Cat's claw is stated to possess anti-inflammatory, antiviral, antioxidant, immunostimulating, antirheumatic and anticancer properties. It is native to the Amazon and has been used traditionally to treat gonorrhoea, dysentry, arthritis, rheumatism, gastric ulcers and various tumours.[12] It is also reputed to be a contraceptive.

Dosage

Commercial products (tablets, capsules) contain varying amounts of material, ranging from 25 to 300 mg standardised extract and from 400 mg to 5 g of plant material.[G31]

Pharmacological Actions

Several pharmacological activities have been documented for cat's claw, including anti-inflammatory, antimutagenic, antitumour, antioxidant and immunostimulating properties. The pharmacological activities of cat's claw have been reviewed.[12,13]

In vitro and animal studies

Certain oxindole alkaloids isolated from *U. tomentosa* (isopteropodine, pteropodine, isomitraphylline, isorhynchophylline) have been shown to enhance phagocytosis markedly *in vitro*.[14] Pentacyclic oxindole alkaloids from *U. tomentosa* have been reported to induce the release of a lymphocyte proliferation-regulating factor from human endothelial cells; tetracyclic oxindole alkaloids were found to reduce the activity of pentacyclic oxindole alkaloids on these cells in a dose-dependent manner.[12,15] Stem bark extracts of *U. tomentosa* have also been shown to stimulate interleukin 1 (IL-1) and interleukin 6 (IL-6) production *in vitro* in rat alveolar macrophages in a dose-dependent manner (range 0.025–0.1 mg/mL) and to potentiate the production of IL-1 and IL-6 in lipopolysaccharide-stimulated macrophages.[16]

Extracts and fractions of *U. tomentosa* bark have shown no mutagenic effect but demonstrated a protective antimutagenic effect *in vitro* against 8-methoxypsoralen- and UVA-induced photomutagenesis in *Salmonella typhimurium* TA102.[17] It was suggested that this antimutagenic activity may be due to an antioxidant effect of *U. tomentosa*.[17]

In vitro antioxidant activity of stem bark and root extracts of *U. tomentosa* has been demonstrated in an assay using *tert*-butylhydroperoxide-initiated chemoluminescence in rat liver homogenates.[18] Extracts also prevented free radical-mediated DNA sugar damage.[18]

In vitro antitumour activity of water extracts of *U. tomentosa* (C-Med-100) has been shown in a human leukaemic cell line (HL-60) and a human Epstein–Barr virus (EBV)-transformed B lymphoma cell line (Raji).[19] The suppressive effect of *U. tomentosa* extracts on tumour cell growth appear to be mediated through induction of apoptosis.[19] The pentacyclic oxindole alkaloids uncarine C and uncarine E from *U. guianensis* have been identified as cytotoxic and DNA-damaging agents in a yeast-based assay.[20] These alkaloids also showed moderate cytotoxicity to several mammalian cell lines, including human lung carcinoma.[20] *In vitro*, aqueous extracts of *U. tomentosa* bark appear to interact with oestrogen receptor-binding sites.[21]

Rhynchophylline has been reported to inhibit rat[22] and rabbit platelet aggregation *ex vivo*.[23] Studies in cats and dogs have reported that rhynchophylline has a negative inotropic effect which can contribute to a hypotensive effect.[24] Rhynchophylline and isorhynchophylline have been reported to have negative chronotropic and inotropic effects in isolated guinea-pig atria.[25] Isorhynchophylline has been reported to have hypotensive effects in rats and dogs.[26]

Trichloromethane/methanol and aqueous extracts of cat's claw (*U. tomentosa*) bark have demonstrated anti-inflammatory activity in the rat paw carrageenan-induced oedema test; a quinovic acid glycoside was identified as one of the active principles.[8] An aqueous extract of cat's claw (*U. tomentosa*) bark was reported to protect against oxidant-induced stress *in vitro* and to attenuate indomethacin-induced chronic intestinal inflammation in rats.[27] Cat's claw extract was found to prevent the activation of the transcription factor NF-κB, which suggests a mechanism for the anti-inflammatory activity of cat's claw.[27]

Quinovic acid glycosides have demonstrated antiviral activity in *in vitro* tests against the RNA virus vesicular stomatitis virus.[7] Two quinovic acid glycosides also demonstrated *in vitro* activity against rhinovirus type 1B.[7]

Receptor-binding assays using dihydrocorynantheine isolated from the branchlet and hook of *Uncaria sinensis* (and also found in *U. tomentosa*) have shown that this alkaloid is a partial agonist for serotonin receptors.[28]

Clinical studies

There is a lack of clinical evidence to support the activities of cat's claw.

A decoction of *U. tomentosa* bark ingested daily for 15 days by a smoker decreased the mutagenicity induced in *S. typhimurium* TA98 and TA100 by the subject's urine; urine from a non-smoker who ingested the same regimen of *U. tomentosa* did not show any mutagenic activity before, during or after treatment.[17]

In an uncontrolled study, 13 HIV-positive individuals who refused to receive other therapies ingested 20 mg daily of an extract of *U. tomentosa* root (containing 12 mg total pentacyclic oxindole alkaloids per gram) for 2.2–5 months.[12] The total leukocyte number in the group was unchanged, compared with pretreatment values, whereas the relative and absolute lymphocyte count increased significantly. No significant changes in T4/T8 cell ratios were observed.[12]

Side-effects, Toxicity

There has been a report of acute renal failure in a Peruvian woman with systemic lupus erythematosus who had added a product containing cat's claw (one capsule four times daily, obtained from a local herbal shop) to her regimen of prednisone, atenolol, metolazone, frusemide and nifedipine.[29] The patient had a serum creatinine concentration of 3.6 mg/dL and was diagnosed with acute allergic interstitial nephritis. She was advised to discontinue cat's claw and, one month later, her renal function had improved (serum creatinine 2.7 mg/dL).

Data on the acute oral toxicity of *U. tomentosa* aqueous root extract (containing 35 mg total pentacyclic oxindole alkaloids per gram) in mice and four-week oral toxicity of an aqueous extract of *U. tomentosa* root (containing 7.5 mg total oxindole alkaloids per gram) in rats administered 1000 mg/kg/day have been summarised.[12] The acute median LD$_{50}$ to mice was found to be greater than 16 g/kg body weight. In the study in rats, a slight but statistically significant increase in the percentage of lymphocytes and a decrease in the percentage of neutrophil granulocytes were seen. In addition, an increase in the relative weight of the kidneys in rats of both sexes was noted, although kidney histology was normal.

In vitro, extracts of *U. tomentosa* have been shown to possess antitumour activity and to stimulate production of the cytokines IL-1 and IL-6, both of which are known to initiate a cascade of defence activities of the immune system. Oxindole alkaloids from *U. tomentosa* have been reported to enhance phagocytosis *in vitro* (see *In vitro* and animal studies).

The *in vitro* toxicity of aqueous extracts of *U. tomentosa* has been evaluated in bioassays using Chinese hamster ovary (CHO) cells and bacterial cells (*Photobacterium phosphoreum*).[30] At the concentrations used (10–100 mg/mL), the extracts did not show a significant cytotoxic effect in CHO cells and demonstrated a non-toxic effect in the bacterial cells used.

Contra-indications, Warnings

In view of its immunostimulant properties, cat's claw may interfere with immunosuppressive therapy. Extracts of the pentacyclic chemotype of *U. tomentosa* should be avoided where there is a risk of organ rejection in patients undergoing transplants; this includes bone marrow transplants.[13]

In view of the inhibitory effects of rhynchophylline on platelet aggregation,[22,23] it has been stated that cat's claw is contra-indicated in patients receiving anticoagulants and in those with coagulation disorders.[G31]

Animal studies have reported hypotensive effects with rhynchophylline[24] and isorhynchophylline;[26] thus, cat's claw should be used with caution in patients receiving antihypertensive agents.[G31]

Pregnancy and lactation   The safety of cat's claw has not been established. In view of the lack of toxicity data, use of cat's claw during pregnancy and lactation should be avoided. In addition, use in children (< 3 years) is not advised.

Pharmaceutical Comment

The chemistry of cat's claw is well documented. Reported pharmacological activities are mainly associated with the oxindole alkaloids and the quinovic acid glycosides.

The two species *U. tomentosa* and *U. guianensis* may be confused.[12] In addition, there are two chemotypes of *U. tomentosa*, one predominantly producing pentacyclic oxindole alkaloids, and the other tetracyclic oxindole alkaloids.[3,12] Since the tetracyclic oxindole alkaloids have been reported to

antagonise the immunostimulant effect of the pentacyclic oxindole alkaloids on human cells *in vitro*,[12,15] it has been stated that mixtures of the two chemotypes of cat's claw are unsuitable for therapeutic use unless certified to contain less than 0.02% tetracyclic oxindole alkaloids.[31]

Documented scientific evidence from *in vitro* and, to a lesser extent, animal studies provides some supportive evidence for some of the uses of cat's claw. However, there is a lack of clinical data, and well-designed clinical trials involving adequate numbers of patients and using standardised preparations manufactured from the appropriate chemotype are necessary.

In view of the lack of toxicity and safety data, excessive use of cat's claw should be avoided. Individuals wishing to use cat's claw concurrently with conventional medicines should first seek advice from an appropriate healthcare professional.

References

1   Hemingway SR, Phillipson JD. Alkaloids from South American species of *Uncaria* (Rubiaceae). *J Pharm Pharmacol* 1974; 26(Suppl.): P113.

2   Laus G, Keplinger D. Separation of stereoisomeric oxindole alkaloids from *Uncaria tomentosa* by high performance liquid chromatography. *J Chromatogr* 1994; 662: 243–249.

3   Laus G *et al*. Alkaloids of Peruvian *Uncaria tomentosa*. *Phytochemistry* 1997; 45: 855–860.

4   Montenegro de Matta S *et al*. Alkaloids and procyanidins of an *Uncaria* sp. from Peru. *Il Farmaco-Ed Sci* 1976; 31: 5227–5235.

5   Phillipson JD *et al*. Alkaloids of *Uncaria*. Part V. Their occurrence and chemotaxonomy. *Lloydia* 1978; 41: 503–570.

6   Cerri R *et al*. New quinovic acid glycosides from *Uncaria tomentosa*. *J Nat Prod* 1988; 51: 257–261.

7   Aquino R *et al*. Plant metabolites. Structure and *in vitro* antiviral activity of quinovic acid glycosides from *Uncaria tomentosa* and *Guettarda platypoda*. *J Nat Prod* 1989; 52: 679–685.

8   Aquino R *et al*. Plant metabolites. New compounds and anti-inflammatory activity of *Uncaria tomentosa*. *J Nat Prod* 1991; 54: 453–459.

9   Yepez AM *et al*. Quinovic acid glycosides from *Uncaria guaianensis*. *Phytochemistry* 1991; 30: 1635–1637.

10 Aquino R *et al*. New polyhydroxylated triterpenes from *Uncaria tomentosa*. *J Nat Prod* 1990; 53: 559–564.

11 Senatore A *et al*. Richerche fitochimiche e biologiche sull'*Uncaria tomentosa*. *Boll Soc It Biol Sper* 1989; 65: ¯17–520.

12 Keplinger K *et al*. *Uncaria tomentosa* (Willd.) DC. – ethnomedicinal use and new pharmacological, toxicological and botanical results. *J Ethnopharmacol* 1999; **64**: 23–34.

13 Reinhard K-H. *Uncaria tomentosa* (Willd.) D.C.: cat's claw, Uña de gato, Savéntaro. *J Alt Complement Med* 1999; **5**: 143–151.

14 Wagner H *et al*. Die alkaloide von *Uncaria tomentosa* und ihre Phagozytose-steigernde Wirkung. *Planta Med* 1985; **51**: 419–423.

15 Wurm M *et al*. Pentacyclic oxindole alkaloids from *Uncaria tomentosa* induce human endothelial cells to release a lymphocyte-proliferation-regulating factor. *Planta Med* 1998; **64**: 701–704.

16 Lemaire I *et al*. Stimulation of interleukin-1 and -6 production in alveolar macrophages by the Neotropical liana, *Uncaria tomentosa* (Uña de gato). *J Ethnopharmacol* 1999; **64**: 109–115.

17 Rizzi R *et al*. Mutagenic and antimutagenic activities of *Uncaria tomentosa* and its extracts. *J Ethnopharmacol* 1993; **38**: 63–77.

18 Desmarchelier C *et al*. Evaluation of the *in vitro* antioxidant activity in extracts of *Uncaria tomentosa* (Willd.) DC. *Phytother Res* 1997; **11**: 254–256.

19 Sheng Y *et al*. Induction of apoptosis and inhibition of proliferation in human tumor cells treated with extracts of *Uncaria tomentosa*. *Anticancer Res* 1998; **18**: 3363–3368.

20 Lee KK *et al*. Bioactive indole alkaloids from the bark of *Uncaria guianensis*. *Planta Med* 1999; **65**: 759–760.

21 Salazar E, Jayme V. Depletion of specific binding sites for estrogen receptor by *Uncaria tomentosa*. *Proc Western Pharmacol Soc* 1998; **41**: 123–124.

22 Jin RM *et al*. Effect of rhynchophylline on platelet aggregation and experimental thrombosis. *Acta Pharm Sin* 1991; **26**: 246–249.

23 Chen C-X *et al*. Inhibitory effect of rhynchophylline on platelet aggregation and thrombosis. *Acta Pharmacol Sin* 1992; **13**: 126–130.

24 Zhang W, Liu G-X. Effects of rhynchophylline on myocardial contractility in anesthetized dogs and cats. *Acta Pharmacol Sin* 1986; **7**: 426–428.

25 Zhu Y *et al*. Negatively chronotropic and inotropic effects of rhynchophylline and isorhynchophylline on isolated guinea pig atria. *Chin J Pharmacol Toxicol* 1993; **7**: 117–121.

26 Shi JS *et al*. Hypotensive and hemodynamic effects of isorhynchophylline in conscious rats and anesthetised dogs. *Chin J Pharmacol Toxicol* 1989; **3**: 205–210.

27 Sandoval-Chacón M *et al*. Antiinflammatory actions of cat's claw: the role of NF-κB. *Aliment Pharmacol Ther* 1998; **12**: 1279–1289.

28 Kanatani H *et al*. The active principles of the branchlet and hook of *Uncaria sinensis* Oliv. examined with a 5-hydroxytryptamine receptor binding assay. *J Pharm Pharmacol* 1985; **37**: 401–404.

29 Hilepo JN *et al*. Acute renal failure caused by 'cat's claw' herbal remedy in a patient with systemic lupus erythematosus. *Nephron* 1997; **77**: 361.

30 Santa Maria A *et al*. Evaluation of the toxicity of *Uncaria tomentosa* by bioassays *in vitro*. *J Ethnopharmacol* 1997; **57**: 183–187.

31 Laus G, Keplinger K. Radix *Uncariae tomentosae* (Willd.) DC. *Z Phytother* 1997; **18**: 122–126.

Celery

Species (Family)

Apium graveolens L. (Apiaceae/Umbelliferae)

Synonym(s)

Apii Fructus, Celery Fruit, Celery Seed, Smallage

Part(s) Used

Fruit

Pharmacopoeial and Other Monographs

BHC 1992[G6]
BHP 1996[G9]
Martindale 32nd edition[G43]
PDR for Herbal Medicines 2nd edition[G36]

Legal Category (Licensed Products)

GSL[G37]

Constituents[G2,G6,G22,G38,G41,G48,G57,G58,G64]

Flavonoids Apigenin, apiin, isoquercitrin and others.[1]

Furanocoumarins Apigravin, apiumetin, apiumoside, bergapten, celerin, celereoside, isoimperatorin, isopimpinellin, osthenol, rutaretin, seselin, umbelliferone and 8-hydroxy-5-methoxypsoralen.[1-9]

Low concentrations (not exceeding 1.3 ppm) of furanocoumarins have been identified in commercial celery,[10] although concentrations are reported to rise considerably in diseased stems.[11]

Volatile oils 2–3%. Many components including limonene (60%) and selenine (10–15%), and various sesquiterpene alcohols (1–3%), e.g. α-eudesmol and β-eudesmol, santalol.[12,13] Phthalide compounds, 3-*n*-butyl phthalide and sedanenolide, provide the characteristic odour of the oil (presence of sedanolide and sedanonic anhydride disputed).[14,15]

Other constituents Choline ascorbate,[16] fatty acids (e.g. linoleic, myristic, myristicic, myristoleic, oleic, palmitic, palmitoleic, petroselinic and stearic acids).

Food Use

Celery is listed by the Council of Europe as a natural source of food flavouring (category N2). This category indicates that celery can be added to foodstuffs in small quantities, with a possible limitation of an active principle (as yet unspecified) in the final product.[G16] Celery stem (not the fruit) is commonly used in foods. In the USA, celery seed is listed as GRAS (Generally Recognised As Safe).[G41]

Herbal Use

Celery is stated to possess antirheumatic, sedative, mild diuretic and urinary antiseptic properties. It has been used for arthritis, rheumatism, gout, urinary tract inflammation, and specifically for rheumatoid arthritis with mental depression.[G2,G6,G7,G8,G64]

Dosage

Dried fruits 0.5–2.0 g or by decoction 1:5 three times daily.[G7]

Liquid extract 0.3–1.2 mL (1:1 in 60% alcohol) three times daily.[G7]

Liquid Extract of Celery (BPC 1934) 0.3–1.2 mL.

Pharmacological Actions

In vitro and animal studies

In mice, sedative and antispasmodic activities have been documented for the phthalide constituents.[17,G22] Celery seed oil has been reported to exhibit bacteriostatic activity against *Bacillus subtilis*, *Vibrio cholerae*, *Staphylococcus aureus*, *Staphylococcus albus*, *Shigella dysenteriae*, *Corynebacterium diphtheriae*, *Salmonella typhi*, *Streptococcus faecalis*, *Bacillus pumilus*, *Streptococcus pyogenes* and *Pseudomonas solanacearum*.[9] No activity was observed against *Escherichia coli*, *Sarcina lutea* or *Pseudomonas aeruginosa*.

Apigenin has exhibited potent antiplatelet activity *in vitro*, inhibiting the aggregation of rabbit platelets induced by collagen, ADP, arachidonic acid and platelet-activating factor (PAF), but not that induced by thrombin or ionophore A23187.[18]

Studies with celery plant extracts have demonstrated anti-inflammatory activity in the mouse ear test and against carrageenan-induced rat paw oedema,[19] and a hypotensive effect in rabbits and dogs after intravenous administration.[G41] In addition, hypoglycaemic activity has been documented.[G22]

Celery juice has been reported to exhibit choleretic activity and the phthalide constituents are stated to possess diuretic activity.[13]

Clinical studies

None documented for celery fruit. Hypotensive activity was reported in 14 of the 16 hypertensive patients given a celery plant extract.[G41]

Side-effects, Toxicity

None documented for celery fruit. Photosensitivity reactions have been reported as a result of external contact with celery stems.[20,21,G51] These reactions have been attributed to the furanocoumarin constituents which are known to possess photosensitising properties.[11,22] The concentrations of these compounds are reported to increase considerably in diseased celery stems.[11,22] It is thought that psoralen, the most potent phototoxic furanocoumarin, acts as a transient precursor for other furanocoumarins and does not accumulate in celery.[5,11]

Instances of allergic and anaphylactic reactions to celery have also been documented[23] following oral ingestion of the stems.[24] Celery allergy is reported to be mediated by IgE antibodies and an association between pollen and celery allergy has been postulated, although the common antigen had not been determined.[25]

Cross-sensitivities to celery have been documented in patients with existing allergies to dandelion and wild carrot.[G51]

Acute LD_{50} values (rats, by mouth; rabbits, dermal) have been reported as greater than 5 g/kg body weight.[26] Celery seed oil is stated to be non-irritant, non-phototoxic and non-sensitising in humans.[26,G58]

Contra-indications, Warnings

Celery fruit contains phototoxic compounds, furanocoumarins, which may cause photosensitive reactions. Celery fruit may precipitate allergic reactions, particularly in individuals with existing plant, pollen or food allergies. Diseased celery stems (indicated by a browning of the stem) should not be ingested.

Pregnancy and lactation Celery fruit is reputed to affect the menstrual cycle and to be abortifa-

cient.[G30] Uterine stimulant activity has been documented for the oil,[G22,G30] and the use of celery fruits is contra-indicated during pregnancy.[G49] This does not refer to celery stems that are commonly ingested as a food, although excessive consumption should be avoided.

Pharmaceutical Comment

Celery fruit should not be confused with the commercial celery stem, which is commonly eaten as a food. The chemistry of celery fruit is well studied and the phototoxic furanocoumarin constituents are well documented. Phototoxicity appears to be associated with the handling of the celery stems, especially diseased plant material. Limited scientific evidence is available to justify the herbal uses of celery, although bacteriostatic activity has been documented for the oil. Celery fruit should be used cautiously in view of the documented allergic reactions.

References

See also General References G2, G6, G9, G11, G16, G22, G30, G31, G32, G36, G37, G38, G41, G43, G48, G49, G51, G57, G58 and G64.

1 Garg SK *et al.* Glucosides of *Apium graveolens*. *Planta Med* 1980; **38**: 363–365.
2 Garg SK *et al.* Apiumetin – a new furanocoumarin from the seeds of *Apium graveolens*. *Phytochemistry* 1978; **17**: 2135–2136.
3 Garg SK *et al.* Celerin, a new coumarin from *Apium graveolens*. *Planta Med* 1980; **38**: 186–188.
4 Garg SK *et al.* Minor phenolics of *Apium graveolens* seeds. *Phytochemistry* 1979; **18**: 352.
5 Dall'Acqua *et al.* Biosynthesis of O-alkylfurocoumarins. *Planta Med* 1975; **27**: 343–348.
6 Garg SK *et al.* Apiumoside, a new furanocoumarin glucoside from the seeds of *Apium graveolens*. *Phytochemistry* 1979; **18**: 1764–1765.
7 Garg SK *et al.* Coumarins from *Apium graveolens* seeds. *Phytochemistry* 1979; **18**: 1580–1581.
8 Innocenti G *et al.* Investigations of the content of furocoumarins in *Apium graveolens* and in *Petroselinum sativum*. *Planta Med* 1976; **29**: 165–170.
9 Kar A, Jain SR. Investigations on the antibacterial activity of some Indian indigenous aromatic plants. *Flavour Industry* 1971; February.
10 Beier RC *et al.* Hplc analysis of linear furocoumarins (psoralens) in healthy celery (*Apium graveolens*). *Food Chem Toxicol* 1983; **21**: 163–165.
11 Chaudhary SK *et al.* Increased furocoumarin content of celery during storage. *J Agric Food Chem* 1985; **33**: 1153–1157.
12 Fehr D. Untersuchung über aromastoffe von sellerie (*Apium graveolens* L.). *Pharmazie* 1979; **34**: 658–662.

13   Stahl E. *Drug Analysis by Chromatography and Microscopy*. Ann Arbor, Michigan: Ann Arbor Science, 1973.

14   Bjeldanes LF, Kim I-S. Phthalide components of celery essential oil. *J Org Chem* 1977; **42**: 2333–2335.

15   Bos R *et al*. Composition of the volatile oils from the roots, leaves and fruits of different taxa of *Apium graveolens*. *Planta Med* 1986; **52**: 531.

16   Kavalali G, Akcasu A. Isolation of choline ascorbate from *Apium graveolens*. *J Nat Prod* 1985; **48**: 495.

17   Gijbels MJM *et al*. Phthalides in roots of *Apium graveolens*, *A. graveolens* var. *rapaceum*. Bifora testiculata and *Petroselinum crispum* var. *tuberosum*. *Fitoterapia* 1985; **56**: 17–23.

18   Teng CM *et al*. Inhibition of platelet aggregation by apigenin from *Apium graveolens*. *Asia Pac J Pharmacol* 1988; **1**: 85–89.

19   Lewis DA *et al*. The anti-inflammatory activity of celery *Apium graveolens* L. (Fam. Umbelliferae). *Int J Crude Drug Res* 1985; **23**: 27–32.

20   Berkley SF *et al*. Dermatitis in grocery workers associated with high natural concentrations of furanocoumarins in celery. *Ann Intern Med* 1986; **105**; 351–355.

21   Austad J, Kavli G. Phototoxic dermatitis caused by celery infected by *Sclerotinia sclerotiorum*. *Contact Dermatitis* 1983; **9**: 448–451.

22   Ashwood-Smith MJ *et al*. Mechanisms of photosensitivity reactions to diseased celery. *BMJ* 1985; **290**: 1249.

23   Déchamp C *et al*. Choc anaphylactique au céleri et sensibilisation à l'ambroisie et à l'armoise. Allergie croisée ou allergie concomitante? *Presse Med* 1984; **13**: 871–874.

24   Forsbeck M, Ros A-M. Anaphylactoid reaction to celery. *Contact Dermatitis* 1979; **5**: 191.

25   Pauli G *et al*. Celery sensitivity: clinical and immunological correlations with pollen allergy. *Clin Allergy* 1985; **15**: 273–279.

26   Opdyke DLJ. Celery seed oil. *Food Cosmet Toxicol* 1974; **12**: 849–850.

Centaury

Species (Family)

Centaurium erythraea Rafin. (Gentianaceae)

Synonym(s)

Centaurium minus Moench,[G45] *C. umbellatum* Gilib., *Erythraea centaurium* Pers., Minor Centaury

Part(s) Used

Herb

Pharmacopoeial and Other Monographs

BHP 1996[G9]
BP 2001[G15]
Complete German Commission E[G3]
ESCOP 1999[G52]
Martindale 32nd edition[G43]
PDR for Herbal Medicines 2nd edition[G36]
Ph Eur 2002[G28]

Legal Category (Licensed Products)

GSL[G37]

Constituents[G2,G41,G64]

Acids Phenolic. Protocatechuic, *m*- and *p*-hydroxy-benzoic, vanillic, syringic, *p*-coumaric, ferulic, sinapic and caffeic, hydroxyterephthalic and 2,5-dihydroxyterephthalic acids among others.

Alkaloids Pyridine-type. Traces of gentianine, gentianidine, gentioflavine and others.

Monoterpenoids Iridoids (bitters).[1,2] Gentiopicroside (about 2%) as major, others include centapicrin, gentioflavoside, sweroside and swertiamarin; intensely bitter *m*-hydroxybenzoylesters of sweroside and catapicrin.

Triterpenoids Includes α- and β-amyrin, erythrodiol, crataegolic acid, oleanolic acid and sitosterol.

Xanthones Highly methylated xanthones, including eustomin and 8-demethyleustomin.

Other constituents Flavonoids, fatty acids, in, alkanes and waxes.

Food Use

Centaury is listed by the Council of Europe as a natural source of food flavouring (category N2). This category indicates that centaury can be added to foodstuffs in small quantities, with a possible limitation of an active principle (as yet unspecified) in the final product.[G16] In the USA, the bitter properties of centaury are utilised in alcoholic and non-alcoholic beverages with maximum permitted doses between 0.0002% and 0.0008%.[G41]

Herbal Use[G2,G7,G52]

Centaury is reputed to act as a bitter, aromatic and stomachic. Traditionally, it has been used for anorexia and dyspepsia.

Dosage

Herb 2–4 g or by infusion three times daily.[G7]

Liquid extract 2–4 mL (1 : 1 in 25% alcohol) three times daily.[G7]

Pharmacological Actions

Centaury is stated to have bitter tonic, sedative and antipyretic properties.[G41] The antipyretic activity is stated to be due to the phenolic acids.[G45] Gentiopicrin is stated to have antimalarial properties.[G48]

In vitro and animal studies

Anti-inflammatory activity has been documented in two rat models; subchronic inflammation (air pouch granuloma and polyarthritis) test,[3] and the carra-geenan rat paw oedema test (19% compared to 45% with indomethacin).[4] Antipyretic activity has also been exhibited by a centaury extract against experimentally induced hyperthermia in rats, although pretreatment with the extract did not prevent hyperthermia.[3] In the same study, no analgesic activity could be demonstrated in mice (writhing syndrome and hotplate models).[3] Gentiopicroside (30 mg/kg/day intraperitoneally) inhibited tumour necrosis factor (TNF) production in carbon tetrachloride-induced and bacillus Calmette–Guérin/lipopolysaccharide-induced models of hepatic injury in mice.[G52]

In rats, anticholinesterase activity has been demonstrated for swertiamarin in a dose-dependent manner following oral administration, demonstrated by inhibition of carbachol-induced contraction of proximal colon.[G52] In mice, gentianine has central nervous system (CNS)-depressant activity at oral doses of 30 mg/kg, demonstrated by inhibition of spontaneous movement and prolonged hexobarbital-induced sleeping time.[G52] Anti-ulcerogenic and inhibitory gastric secretion in rats (100 mg/kg) have been shown for gentianine.[G52]

Side-effects, Toxicity

An alcoholic extract of centaury (200 mL/plate) was antimutagenic in *Salmonella typhimurium* strains TA8 and TA100.[G52]

Contra-indications, Warnings

Centaury is contra-indicated for individuals with peptic ulcers.[G52]

Pregnancy and lactation The safety of centaury taken during pregnancy has not been established. In view of the lack of toxicity data, use of centaury during pregnancy and lactation is best avoided.

Pharmaceutical Comment

There is little published information specifically concerning *C. erythraea*. Bitter components support the traditional use of centaury as an appetite stimulant, although it is said to be less active than comparable bitter herbs, such as gentian.[G2] In view of the lack of pharmacological and toxicological data, excessive use should be avoided.

References

See also General References G2, G3, G9, G15, G16, G28, G31, G36, G37, G43, G48, G52, G56 and G64.

1　Van der Sluis WG, Labadie RP. Onderzok naar en van secoiridoid glucosiden en zanthonen in het gescglacht *Centaurium*. *Pharm Weekbl* 1978; **113**: 21–32.

2　Van der Sluis WG, Labadie RP. Secoiridoids and xanthones in the genus *Centaurium*. Part 3. Decentapicrins A, B and C, new *m*-hydroxybenzoyl esters of sweroside from *Centaurium littorale*. *Planta Med* 1981; **41**: 150–160.

3　Berkan T *et al*. Antiinflammatory, analgesic, and antipyretic effects of an aqueous extract of *Erythraea centaurium*. *Planta Med* 1991; **57**: 34–37.

4　Mascolo N *et al*. Biological screening of Italian medicinal plants for anti-inflammatory activity. *Phytother Res* 1987; **1**: 28–31.

Cereus

Species (Family)

Selenicereus grandiflorus (L.) Britt. & Rose (Cacta-

Synonym(s)

Cactus grandiflorus, *Cereus grandiflorus* Mill., Night Blooming Cereus

Part(s) Used

Stem

Pharmacopoeial and Other Monographs

PDR for Herbal Medicines 2nd edition[G36]

Legal Category (Licensed Products)

Cereus is not included in the GSL.[G37]

Constituents[G22,G40,G64]

Alkaloids Isoquinoline-type. Unidentified alkaloids.[1]

Amines Tyramine[2], hordenine,[3] previously referred to as cactine.

Flavonoids Rutin, kaempferitrin, hyperoside, isorhamnetin-3-β-(galactosyl)-rutinoside.

Other constituents Resin

Food Use

Cereus is not used in foods.

Herbal Use

Cereus is reputed to act as a cardiac stimulant and as a partial substitute for digitalis, although there is no proof of its therapeutic value. Cereus has been used in cases of dropsy and various cardiac affections.[G10,G64]

Dosage

Liquid extract of cereus (BPC 1934) 0.06–0.6 mL.

Tincture of cereus (BPC 1934) 0.12–2.0 mL.

Pharmacological Actions

In vitro and animal studies

None documented for cereus. Cereus is reported to contain a cardiotonic amine, tyramine, which has positive inotropic activity.

Side-effects, Toxicity

The fresh juice of cereus is irritant to the oral mucosa, causing a burning sensation, nausea and vomiting. Diarrhoea has also been reported following cereus consumption.[G22]

Contra-indications, Warnings

In view of the documented tyramine content, excessive doses of cereus may interact with concurrent monoamine oxidase inhibitor (MAOI) treatment and may affect patients with an existing cardiac disorder.

Pregnancy and lactation The safety of cereus has not been established. In view of the limited information available on cereus, its use during pregnancy and lactation should be avoided.

Pharmaceutical Comment

Little phytochemical or pharmacological information has been documented for cereus, although the presence of tyramine, a cardiotonic amine, may support the traditional use of cereus as a cardiac stimulant. Cardiac complaints are not considered to be suitable for self-medication.

References

See also General References G10, G22, G31, G36, G37, G40, G48 and G64.

1 Brown SD *et al.* Cactus alkaloids. *Phytochemistry* 1968; 7: 2031–2036.

2 Wagner H, Grevel J. Neue herzwirksame drogen II, nachweis und isolierung herzwirksamer amine durch ionenpaar-HPLC. *Planta Med* 1982; 44: 36–40.

3 Petershofer-Halbmayer H *et al.* Isolierung von

Hordenin (Cactin) aus *Selenicereus grandiflorus* (L.) Britt. & Rose und *Selenicereus pteranthus* (Link & Otto) Britt. & Rose. *Sci Pharm* 1982; 50: 29–34.

Chamomile, German

Species (Family)

Matricaria recutita L. (Asteraceae/Compositae)

Synonym(s)

Chamomilla recutita (L.) Rauschert, Hungarian Chamomile, *Matricaria chamomilla* L., Matricaria Flowers, Sweet False Chamomile, Wild Chamomile

Part(s) Used

Flowerhead

Pharmacopoeial and Other Monographs

BHC 1992[G6]
BHP 1996[G9]
BP 2001[G15]
Complete German Commission E[G3]
ESCOP 1999[G52]
Martindale 32nd edition[G43]
Mills and Bone[G50]
PDR for Herbal Medicines 2nd edition[G36]
Ph Eur 2002[G28]
USP24/NF19[G61]
WHO volume 1 1999[G63]

Legal Category (Licensed Products)

GSL[G37]

Constituents[G2,G6,G22,G38,G41,G48,G52,G64]

Coumarins Umbelliferone and its methyl ether, heniarin.

Flavonoids Apigenin, apigetrin, apiin, luteolin, quercetin, quercimeritrin and rutin.

Volatile oils 0.24–1.9%. Pharmacopoeial standard not less than 4 mg/kg blue oil.[G15,G28] Main components are $(-)$-α-bisabolol (up to 50%)[1] and chamazulene (1–15%).[2] Others include $(-)$-α-bisabolol oxide A and B, $(-)$-α-bisabolone oxide A, spiroethers (e.g. *cis*- and *trans*-en-yn-dicycloether), sesquiterpenes (e.g. anthecotulid), cadinene, farnesene, furfural, spanthulenol and proazulenes (e.g. matricarin and matricin).

Chamazulene is formed from matricin during steam distillation of the oil. It varies in yield depending on the origin and age of the flowers.[2]

Other constituents Amino acids, anthemic acid (bitter), choline, polysaccharide, plant and fatty acids, tannin and triterpene hydrocarbons (e.g. triacontane).

Food Use

German chamomile is listed by the Council of Europe as a natural source of food flavouring (category N2). This category indicates that chamomile can be added to foodstuffs in small quantities, with a possible limitation of an active principle (as yet unspecified) in the final product.[G16] German chamomile is commonly used in herbal teas. In the USA, German chamomile is listed as GRAS (Generally Recognised As Safe).[G41]

Herbal Use[G2,G4,G6,G7,G8,G43,G52,G64]

German chamomile is stated to possess carminative, antispasmodic, mild sedative, anti-inflammatory, antiseptic and anticatarrhal properties. It has been used for flatulent nervous dyspepsia, travel sickness, nasal catarrh, nervous diarrhoea, restlessness and specifically for gastrointestinal disturbance with associated nervous irritability in children. It has been used topically for haemorrhoids, mastitis and leg ulcers. German Commission E approved use for gastrointestinal spasms and inflammatory diseases of the gastrointestinal tract and externally for skin and mucous membrane inflammation and bacterial skin diseases including oral cavity and gums. It is also approved for inflammations and irritations of the respiratory tract (by inhalation) and ano-genital inflammation (baths and irrigation).[G3]

Dosage

Dried flowerheads 2–8 g or by infusion three times daily.[G7]

Liquid extract 1–4 mL (1:1 in 45% alcohol) three times daily.[G7]

Pharmacological Actions

In vitro and animal studies

A wide range of pharmacological activities have been documented for German chamomile, including antibacterial, anti-inflammatory, antispasmodic, anti-ulcer, antiviral and hypouraemic activities.

Anti-inflammatory and anti-allergic activity Anti-allergic and anti-inflammatory activities[2,3] are well documented for German chamomile. The azulene components of the volatile oil are thought to contribute by inhibiting histamine release and they have been reported to prevent allergic seizures in guinea-pigs.[2] Aqueous alcoholic extracts inhibited 5-lipoxygenase and cyclooxygenase activity, and oxidation of arachidonic acid, and a supercritical carbon dioxide extract had IC_{50} values of 6–25 µg/mL for these three activities.[G52] The active compounds identified included apigenin, chamazulene, *cis*-en-yn spiroether and (−)-α-bisabolol.[G52] Matricin, the precursor to chamazulene, is reported to be a more effective anti-inflammatory agent than chamazulene.[2,4] Anti-inflammatory activity has also been documented for the sesquiterpene bisabolol compounds, with greatest activity reported for (−)-α-bisabolol,[2,5] and for *cis*-spiroether.[2] Anti-inflammatory activity (rat paw carrageenan test) has also been documented for a *cis*-spiroether against dextran induced oedema; no activity was observed against oedema induced by serotonin, histamine or bradykinin.[6] In addition, flavonoids are known to possess anti-inflammatory activity.

Sedative activity Apigenin competitively inhibited binding of flunitrazepam to the central benzodiazepine receptor, but lacked activity at other receptors, including muscarinic, α1-adrenoreceptor and GABA_A.[G52] High-performance liquid chromatography (HPLC) fractions of a methanol extract displaced flunitrazepam from its receptors in rat cerebellum membranes and muscimol from GABA receptors in rat cortical membranes, due to the presence of GABA in the fractions. Prolongation of hexobarbital-induced sleeping time and reduction in activity of mice have been documented.[G52]

Anti-ulcerogenic activity Anti-ulcerogenic activity in rats has been reported for (−)-α-bisabolol; the development of ulcers induced by indomethacin, stress or ethanol was inhibited.[2,7]

Antimicrobial and antiviral activities German chamomile oil has been reported to have antifungal activity and antibacterial activity against Gram-positive bacteria.[G52] The coumarin herniarin has antibacterial and antifungal activities in the presence of UV light. Antibacterial activity has been documented for the coumarin constituents.[2] An ethanolic extract of the entire plant has been reported to inhibit the growth of poliovirus and herpesvirus.[8]

Antispasmodic activity Antispasmodic activity on the isolated guinea-pig ileum has been documented for the flavonoid and bisabolol constituents.[2,9] Greatest activity was exhibited by the flavonoids, especially apigenin which was found to be more than three times as potent as papaverine.[2] (−)-α-Bisabolol activity was found to be comparable to that of papaverine, while the total volatile oil was considerably less active.[2] Smooth muscle relaxant properties have also been documented for a *cis*-spiroether.[2,6,10]

Enhancement of uterine tone in the guinea-pig and rabbit has been reported for an aqueous extract at a concentration of 1–2 mg extract/cm^3.[11]

Other activities High molecular weight polysaccharides with immunostimulating activity have been isolated from German chamomile.[12] The oil has been reported to increase bile secretion and concentration of cholesterol in the bile, following the administration of 0.1 mL/kg by mouth to cats and dogs.[13] A dose of 0.2 mL/kg was stated to exhibit hypotensive, and cardiac and respiratory depressant properties.[13]

The ability of the volatile oil to regenerate liver tissue in partially hepatectomised rats has been attributed to the azulene constituents.[2]

The volatile oil has been documented to reduce the serum concentration of urea in rabbits with experimentally induced uraemic conditions.[14]

Clinical studies

German chamomile extracts have been reported to exhibit anti-inflammatory, antipeptic and antispasmodic activities on the human stomach and duodenum.[2]

Anti-inflammatory and wound-healing effects Clinical studies investigating the anti-inflammatory effects and wound-healing properties of German chamomile preparations have been reviewed.[G52] A summary of this information is given below.

A cream containing German chamomile extract was reported to have effects equivalent to 0.25% hydrocortisone, and superior effects to 0.1% diflucortolone and 5% bufexamax in inflammatory dermatoses, as assessed in 161 patients. Studies involving healthy volunteers who received German chamomile preparations have reported that German chamomile ointment was superior to 0.1% hydrocortisone acetate in dermatitis, and German chamomile cream (20 mg/g) reduced visual sores and redness of skin in an adhesive-tape stripping test. A randomised, double-blind trial involving 25 participants indicated that a cream containing an aqueous alcoholic extract of German chamomile was more effective than hydrocortisone against UVB-induced erythema.

In an open study involving 98 patients with cancer, an extract preparation (containing 50 mg α-bisabolol and 150–300 mg apigenin-7-glucoside/100 g) used three times daily was reported to reduce oral mucositis caused either by irradiation or chemotherapy. However, a double-blind, placebo-controlled trial involving 164 patients showed that a mouthwash containing German chamomile did not decrease 5-fluorouracil-induced stomatitis.

German chamomile has been reported to be an effective treatment for mucosal infections. Diluted extracts administered as a mouthwash 5 or 6 times daily provided cooling and astringent effects.[2]

A cream containing German chamomile has produced additional anti-inflammatory, slight anaesthetic, cooling and deodorant effects in patients with cutaneous leg infections, when used in conjunction with existing treatment.[2]

The healing effects of German chamomile ointment and dexapanthenol 5% cream administered for six days were reported to have comparable effects in a study involving 147 female patients who underwent episiotomy during childbirth. A standardised extract (50 mg α-bisabolol and 3 mg chamazulene/100 g) significantly decreased weeping wound area and drying of wound in 14 patients following removal of tattoos. An ointment preparation improved haemorrhage, itching, burning and oozing due to haemorrhoids in a study involving 120 patients.

Sedative effects Sedative effects have been documented for German chamomile. Oral administration of a German chamomile extract was reported to induce a deep sleep in 10 of 12 patients undergoing cardiac catheterisation.[2]

Side-effects, Toxicity

Reports of allergic reactions to chamomile are common, although in the majority of cases the plant species is not specified.[15] Two reports of anaphylactic reactions to chamomile (species unspecified) have been documented[16,17] and in both cases the individuals concerned had an existing hypersensitivity to ragweed (member of Asteraceae/Compositae).

The symptoms they experienced included abdominal cramps, thickness of the tongue and a tight sensation in the throat,[17] angioedema of the lips and eyes, diffuse pruritus, a full sensation of the ears, generalised urticaria, upper airway obstruction, and pharyngeal oedema.[16] Both patients made a full recovery following medical treatment. Patients with an existing hypersensitivity to German chamomile have demonstrated cross-sensitivities to other members of the family Asteraceae/Compositae[18,G51], and also to celery (family Umbelliferae).[G51]

Allergic skin reactions have been documented following external contact with German chamomile.[2,19,G51] Consumption of chamomile tea may exacerbate existing allergic conditions and the use of a chamomile enema has been documented to cause asthma and urticaria.[G51]

The allergenic properties documented for chamomile have been attributed to anthecotulid, a sesquiterpene lactone present in low concentrations,[15] and to matricarin, a proazulene which has produced positive patch tests in patients with an existing sesquiterpene lactone hypersensitivity.[G51]

Sesquiterpene lactones have been implicated in the allergenic activity of many plants, especially those belonging to the Asteraceae/Compositae family (*see* Feverfew). The prerequisite for allergenic activity is thought to be an exocyclic α-methylene group.[20]

The flowerheads contain anthemic acid, which is reported to act as an emetic in large doses.[G22]

The acute toxicity of chamomile oil (German and Roman) is reported to be low.[21] Oral and dermal LD_{50} values in rabbits have been documented as greater than 5 g/kg,[21] and the application of undiluted oil to the hairless backs of mice, to rabbit skin, and to human skin was not found to produce any observable irritation.[21] An LD_{50} value (mouse, by mouth) for German chamomile oil has been documented as 2.5 mL/kg.[13] The acute oral toxicity of (−)-α-bisabolol in mice and rats is reported to be low at approximately 15 mL/kg.[22] The subacute oral toxicity of (−)-α-bisabolol has been estimated to be between 1.0 and 2.0 mL/kg in rats and dogs.[22] An LD_{50} value (mouse, intraperitoneal injection) for *cis*-spiroether has been stated as 670 mg/kg.[6]

Contra-indications, Warnings

In view of the documented allergic reactions and cross-sensitivities, German chamomile should be avoided by individuals with a known hypersensitivity to any members of the Asteraceae/Compositae family. In addition, German chamomile may precipitate an allergic reaction or exacerbate existing symptoms in susceptible individuals (e.g. asthmatics).

Excessive doses may interfere with existing anti-coagulant therapy, because of the coumarin constituents.

The use of chamomile preparations for teething babies is not recommended.

Pregnancy and lactation German chamomile is reputed to affect the menstrual cycle[G30] and extracts are reported to be uterotonic.[2,11] Teratogenicity studies in rats, rabbits and dogs have been documented for (−)-α-bisabolol, with the oral toxic dose stated as 1–3 mL/kg.[22] A dose of 3 mL/kg was found to increase the number of fetuses reabsorbed and reduce the body weight of live offspring.[22] (−)-α-Bisabolol administered orally (250 and 500 mg/kg) to pregnant rats has been reported to have no effect on the fetus.[1] In view of the documented information, the excessive use of chamomile during pregnancy and lactation should be avoided.

Pharmaceutical Comment

The chemistry of German chamomile, especially of the volatile oil component, is well documented and is similar to that of Roman chamomile.[24] Pharmacological activity is associated with the flavonoid and volatile oil fractions. A wide range of pharmacological actions have been documented (e.g. anti-inflammatory and antispasmodic activities) and many of these support the reputed herbal uses[23,24]. A small number of studies in patients and healthy volunteers have reported anti-inflammatory, wound healing and sedative effects. Toxicity studies to date have indicated chamomile to be of low toxicity, although allergic reactions are documented.

References

See also General References G2, G3, G5, G6, G9, G11, G15, G16, G18, G19, G22, G28, G30, G31, G32, G36, G37, G38, G41, G43, G48, G50, G51, G52, G56, G63 and G64.

1 Isaac O. Pharmacological investigations with compounds of chamomile I. On the pharmacology of (−)-α-bisabolol and bisabolol oxides (review). *Planta Med* 1979; 35: 118–124.

2 Mann C, Staba EJ. The chemistry, pharmacology, and commercial formulations of chamomile. In: Craker LE, Simon JE, eds. *Herbs, Spices, and Medicinal Plants: Recent Advances in Botany, Horticulture, and Pharmacology*, vol 1. Arizona: Oryx Press, 1986: 235–280.

3 Tubaro A *et al.* Evaluation of antiinflammatory activity of a chamomile extract after topical application. *Planta Med* 1984; 50: 359.

4 Jakovlev V *et al.* Pharmacological investigations with compounds of chamomile VI. Investigations on the antiphlogistic effects of chamazulene and matricine. *Planta Med* 1983; 49: 67–73.

5 Jacovlev V *et al.* Pharmacological investigations with compounds of chamomile II. New investigations on the antiphlogistic effects of (−)-α-bisabolol and bisabolol oxides. *Planta Med* 1979; 35: 125–140.

6 Breinlich VJ, Scharnagel K. Pharmakologische Eigenschaften des EN-IN-dicycloäthers aus *Matricaria chamomilla*. *Arzneimittelforschung* 1968; 18: 429–431.

7 Szelenyi I *et al.* Pharmacological experiments with compounds of chamomile III. Experimental studies of the ulcerprotective effect of chamomile. *Planta Med* 1979; 35: 218–227.

8 Suganda AG *et al.* Effets inhibiteurs de quelques extraits bruts et semi purifiés de plantes indigènes françaises sur la multiplication de l'herpesvirus humain 1 et du poliovirus humain 2 en culture cellulaire. *J Nat Prod* 1983; 46: 626–632.

9 Achterrath-Tuckermann U *et al.* Pharmacological investigations with compounds of chamomile. V. Investigations on the spasmolytic effect of compounds of chamomile and Kamillosan on the isolated guinea pig ileum. *Planta Med* 1980; 39: 38–50.

10 Hölzl J *et al.* Preparation of ¹⁴C-spiro ethers by chamomile and their use by an investigation of absorption. *Planta Med* 1986; 52: 533.

11 Shipochliev T. Extracts from a group of medicinal plants enhancing the uterine tonus. *Vet Med Nauki* 1981; 18: 94–98.

12 Wagner VH *et al.* Immunstimulierend wirkende polysaccharide (heteroglykane) aus höheren pflanzen. *Arzneimittelforschung* 1985; 35: 1069.

13 Ikram M. Medicinal plants as hypocholesterolemic agents. *JPMA* 1980; 30: 278–282.

14 Grochulski VA, Borkowski B. Influence of chamomile oil on experimental glomerulonephritis in rabbits. *Planta Med* 1972; 21: 289–292.

15 Hausen BM *et al.* The sensitizing capacity of Compositae plants. *Planta Med* 1984; 50: 229–234.

16 Casterline CL. Allergy to chamomile tea. *JAMA* 1980; 4: 330–331.

17 Benner MH, Lee HJ. Anaphylactic reaction to chamomile tea. *J Allergy Clin Immunol* 1973; 52: 307–308.

18 Hausen BM. The sensitising capacity of Compositae plants. III. Test results and cross-reactions in Compositae-sensitive patients. *Dermatologica* 1979; 159: 1–11.

19 Kettel WG. Allergy to *Matricaria chamomilla*.

Contact Dermatitis 1987; **16**: 50–51.

20 Mitchell JC, Dupuis G. Allergic contact dermatitis from sesquiterpenoids of the Compositae family of plants. *Br J Derm* 1971; **84**: 139–150.

21 Opdyke DLJ. Chamomile oil German. *Food Cosmet Toxicol* 1974; **12**: 851–852.

22 Habersang S *et al.* Pharmacological studies with compounds of chamomile IV. Studies on toxicity of (−)-α-bisabolol. *Planta Med* 1979; **37**: 115–123.

23 Harris B, Lewis R. Chamomile – Part 1. *Int J Alt Complement Med* 1994; September.

24 Berry M. The chamomiles. *Pharm J* 1995; **254**: 191–193.

Chamomile, Roman

Species (Family)

Chamaemelum nobile (L.) All. (Asteraceae/Compositae)

Synonym(s)

Anthemis nobilis L.

Part(s) Used

Flowerhead

Pharmacopoeial and Other Monographs

BHC 1992[G6]
BHP 1996[G9]
BP 2001[G15]
Martindale 32nd edition[G43]
PDR for Herbal Medicines 2nd edition (English Chamomile)[G36]
Ph Eur 2002[G28]
USP24/NF19[G61]

Legal Category (Licensed Products)

GSL[G37]

Constituents[G2,G6,G22,G41,G48,G64]

Coumarins Scopoletin-7-glucoside.

Flavonoids Apigenin, luteolin, constituents in, quercetin and their glycosides (e.g. apiin, luteolin-7-glucoside, and rutin).

Volatile oils 0.4–1.75%. Angelic and tiglic acid esters (85%);[1] others include 1,8-cineole, *l-trans*-pinocarveol, *l-trans*-pinocarvone, chamazulene, farnesol, nerolidol; germacranolide-type sesquiterpene lactones (0.6%),[2] including nobilin, 3-epinobilin, 1,10-epoxynobilin, 3-dehydronobilin; various alcohols including amyl and isobutyl alcohols, anthemol.[1–4] Chamazulene is formed from a natural precursor during steam distillation of the oil, and varies in yield depending on the origin and the age of flowers.[1]

Other constituents Anthemic acid (bitter), phenolic and fatty acids, phytosterol, choline and inositol.

Food Use

Roman chamomile is listed by the Council of Europe as a natural source of food flavouring (category N2). This category indicates that Roman chamomile can be added to foodstuffs in small quantities, with a possible limitation of an active principle (as yet unspecified) in the final product.[G16] Chamomile is commonly used as an ingredient of herbal teas. In the USA, Roman chamomile is listed as GRAS (Generally Recognised As Safe).[G41]

Herbal Use

Roman chamomile is stated to possess carminative, anti-emetic, antispasmodic, and sedative properties. It has been used for dyspepsia, nausea and vomiting, anorexia, vomiting of pregnancy, dysmenorrhoea, and specifically for flatulent dyspepsia associated with mental stress.[G2,G6,G7,G8,G64]

Dosage

Dried flowerheads 1–4 g or by infusion three times daily.[G7]

Liquid extract 1–4 mL (1:1 in 70% alcohol) three times daily.[G7]

Pharmacological Actions

German and Roman chamomile possess similar pharmacological activities (*see* Chamomile, German for a fuller description of documented pharmacological actions).

In vitro and animal studies

Few studies have been documented specifically for Roman chamomile. The azulene compounds are reported to possess anti-allergic and anti-inflammatory properties; their mechanism of action is thought to involve inhibition of histamine release (*see* Chamomile, German). The volatile oil has been documented as having anti-inflammatory activity (carrageenan rat paw oedema test), and antidiuretic and sedative effects following intraperitoneal administration of doses up to 350 mg/kg body weight to rats.[5]

The azulenes have been reported to stimulate liver regeneration following oral, but not subcutaneous, administration.

The sesquiterpenoids nobilin, 1,10-epoxynobilin and 3-dehydronobilin have demonstrated *in vitro* antitumour activity against human cells.[1] The concentration of hydroxyisonobilin required for cytotoxic activity is reported to be low enough to warrant further investigations (ED$_{50}$ 0.56 µg/mL versus HeLa; ED$_{50}$ 1.23 µg/mL versus KB; arbitrary acceptable test level 4 µg/mL).

Side-effects, Toxicity

Instances of allergic and anaphylactic reactions to chamomile have been documented (*see* Chamomile, German) The allergenic principles in chamomile are thought to be the sesquiterpene lactones.[1] Roman chamomile yields nobilin, a sesquiterpene lactone that is reported to be potentially allergenic.[1] However, Roman chamomile oil has also been reported to be non-irritant and non-sensitising to human skin.[2] Animal studies have indicated the oil to be either mildly or non-irritant, and to lack any phototoxic effects.[2]

Large doses of Roman chamomile are stated to act as an emetic[G44] and this has been attributed to the anthemic acid content.[6]

The acute toxicity of Roman chamomile in animals is reported to be relatively low.[1] Acute LD$_{50}$ values in rabbits (dermal) and rats (by mouth) have been stated to exceed 5 g/kg.[2]

Contra-indications, Warnings

In view of the documented allergic reactions and cross-sensitivities (*see* Chamomile, German), Roman chamomile should be avoided by individuals with a known hypersensitivity to any members of the Asteraceae/Compositae family. In addition, Roman chamomile may precipitate an allergic reaction or exacerbate existing symptoms in susceptible individuals (e.g. asthmatics). Excessive doses may interfere with anticoagulant therapy because of the coumarin constituents.

The use of chamomile preparations in teething babies is not recommended.

Pregnancy and lactation Roman chamomile is reputed to be an abortifacient and to affect the menstrual cycle.[G30] In view of this and the potential for allergic reactions, the excessive use of chamomile during pregnancy and lactation should be avoided.

Pharmaceutical Comment

The chemistry of Roman chamomile, particularly of the volatile oil, is well documented and is similar to that of German chamomile.[7] Limited pharmacological data are available for Roman chamomile, although many actions have been reported for German chamomile. In view of the similar chemical compositions, many of the activities described for German chamomile are thought to be applicable to Roman chamomile and thus support the traditional herbal uses[8]. Roman chamomile is stated to be of low toxicity, although allergic reactions (mainly contact dermatitis) have been reported.[G51]

References

See also General References G2, G6, G9, G15, G16, G18, G22, G25, G29, G30, G31, G32, G36, G37, G41, G43, G48, G51, G56, G61 and G64.

1 Mann C, Staba EJ. The chemistry, pharmacology, and commercial formulations of chamomile. In: Craker LE, Simon JE, eds. *Herbs, Spices, and Medicinal Plants: Recent Advances in Botany, Horticulture, and Pharmacology*, vol 1. Arizona: Oryx Press, 1986: 235–280.

2 Opdyke DLJ. Chamomile oil roman. *Food Cosmet Toxicol* 1974: **12**: 853.

3 Casterline CL. Allergy to chamomile tea. *JAMA* 1980; **4**: 330–331.

4 Hausen BM *et al.* The sensitizing capacity of Compositae plants. *Planta Med* 1984; **50**: 229–234.

5 Melegari M *et al.* Chemical characteristics and pharmacological properties of the essential oils of *Anthemis nobilis*. *Fitoterapia* 1988; **59**: 449–455.

6 Achterrath-Tuckermann U *et al.* Pharmacologisch Untersuchungen von Kamillen-Inhaltestoffen. *Planta Med* 1980; **39**: 38–50.

7 Berry M. The chamomiles. *Pharm J* 1995; **254**: 191–193.

8 Harris B, Lewis R. Chamomile – Part 1. *Int J Alt Complement Med* 1994; September.

Chaparral

Species (Family)

Larrea tridentata (DC.) Coville (Zygophyllaceae)

Synonym(s)

Creosote Bush. *L. tridentata* (south-western USA and northern Mexico) is now regarded as a separate species to *Larrea divaricata* Gav. (north-western Argentina).[1]

Part(s) Used

Herb

Pharmacopoeial and Other Monographs

Martindale 32nd edition[G43]

Legal Category (Licensed Products)

Chaparral is not included in the GSL.[G37]

Constituents[G22]

Amino acids Arginine, aspartine, cystine, glutamic acid, glycine, isoleucine, leucine, phenylalanine, tryptophan, tyrosine and valine.

Flavonoids More than 20 different compounds reported, including isorhamnetin, kaempferol and quercetin and their glycosidic and ether derivatives; gossypetin, herbacetin, and their acetate derivatives;[1–7] two C-glucosyl flavones.

Lignans Major constituent nordihydroguaiaretic acid (NDGA) (up to 1.84%), norisoguaiacin, dihydroguaiaretic acid, partially demethylated dihydroguaiaretic acid, 3'- demethoxyisoguaiacin.[8–10]

Resins 20%. Phenolic constituents on external leaf surfaces of *L. divaricata* and *L. tridentata* are reported to be identical, containing a number of flavone and flavonol glycosides, and two lignans (including NDGA).[5]

Volatile oils Many identified terpene components include calamene, eudesmol, limonene, α- and β-pinene, and 2-rossalene.[11]

Other constituents Two pentacyclic triterpenes,[12] saponins.

Other plant parts A cytotoxic naphthoquinone derivative, larreantin, has been isolated from the roots.[13]

Food Use

Chaparral is not used in foods, although a related species, *Larrea mexicana* Moric., also termed creosote bush, is listed by the Council of Europe as a natural source of food flavouring (category N2). This category indicates that creosote bush can be added to foodstuffs in small quantities, with a possible limitation of an active principle (as yet unspecified) in the final product.[G16] In the USA, NDGA is no longer permitted to be used as an antioxidant in foods following the results of toxicity studies in animals (*see* Side-effects, Toxicity).

Herbal Use

Chaparral has been used for the treatment of arthritis, cancer, venereal disease, tuberculosis, bowel cramps, rheumatism and colds.[G60]

Dosage

None documented.

Pharmacological Actions

In vitro and animal studies

Amoebicidal action against *Entamoeba histolytica* has been reported for a chaparral extract (0.01%).[14] This action may be attributable to the lignan constituents, which are documented as both amoebicidal and fungicidal.[9] NDGA has been reported to have antimicrobial activity against a number of organisms including *Penicillium* spp., *Salmonella* spp., *Streptococcus* spp., *Staphylococcus aureus*, *Bacillus subtilis*, *Pseudomonas aeruginosa* and various other pathogens and moulds.[8,15]

NDGA is an antioxidant, and has been documented to cause inhibition of hepatic microsomal enzyme function.[15–17]

Clinical studies

Medical interest in chaparral increased following claims that an aqueous infusion of the herb had caused the regression of a malignant melanoma in the cheek of an 85-year-old man.[18] However, results of a subsequent study that investigated the antitumour action of chaparral, as a tea, were inconclusive.[G60]

Side-effects, Toxicity

Acute hepatitis has been associated with chaparral ingestion.[19–21] Contact dermatitis to chaparral has been reported.[22,23] Chaparral-induced toxic hepatitis has been reported for two patients in different parts of the USA. The adverse effects were attributed to ingestion of a herbal nutritional supplement derived from the leaves of chaparral. Five cases of serious poisoning in the USA and another three in Canada have been linked to chaparral-containing products.[20,24] Some patients have developed irreversible reno-hepatic failure. Early investigations into the toxicity of NDGA concluded it to be low.[15] NDGA has been administered to humans, by intramuscular injection, in doses of up to 400 mg/kg body weight for 5–6 months, with little or no toxicity reported.[15] Documented oral LD_{50} values for NDGA include 4 g/kg (mouse), 5.5 g/kg (rat) and 830 mg/kg (guinea-pig).[15] Results of chronic feeding studies (two years, 0.25–1.0% of diet) in rats and mice reported no abnormalities in histological tests of the liver, spleen and kidney. Inflammatory caecal lesions and slight cystic enlargement of lymph nodes near the caecum were observed in rats at the 0.5% feeding level. At this point NDGA was considered to be safe for food use. However, two later studies in rats (using NDGA at up to 3% of the diet) reported the development of cortical and medullary cysts in the kidney.[15] On the basis of these findings, NDGA was removed from GRAS (Generally Recognised As Safe) status in the USA and is no longer permitted to be used as an antioxidant in foods.[15]

Contra-indications, Warnings

In view of the reports of acute hepatitis associated with chaparral ingestion, and the uncertainty regarding NDGA toxicity, consumption should be avoided. Excessive doses may interfere with monoamine oxidase inhibitor (MAOI) therapy, because of the documented amino acid constituents.

Pregnancy and lactation In vitro utero activity has been documented for chaparral.[G30] In view of the concerns regarding toxicity, chaparral should not be ingested during pregnancy or lactation.

Pharmaceutical Comment

The chemistry of chaparral is well studied and extensive literature has been published on the principal lignan component, NDGA. However, little documented evidence is available to justify the herbal uses of chaparral. In view of the concerns over the hepatic toxicity, the use of chaparral as a herbal remedy cannot be recommended.

References

See also General References G16, G18, G20, G22, G30, G31, G32, G36, G37, G43 and G60.

1 Bernhard HO, Thiele K. Additional flavonoids from the leaves of *Larrea tridentata*. *Planta Med* 1981; **41**: 100–103.
2 Sakakibara M *et al*. 6,8-Di-C-glucosylflavones from *Larrea tridentata* (Zygophyllaceae). *Phytochemistry* 1977; **16**: 1113–1114.
3 Sakakibara M *et al*. A new 8-hydroxyflavonol from *Larrea tridentata*. *Phytochemistry* 1975; **14**: 2097–2098.
4 Sakakibara M *et al*. New 8-hydroxyflavonols from *Larrea tridenta*. *Phytochemistry* 1975; **14**: 849–851.
5 Sakakibara M *et al*. Flavonoid methyl ethers on the external leaf surface of *Larrea tridentata* and *L. divaricata*. *Phytochemistry* 1976; **15**: 727–731.
6 Chirikdjian JJ. Isolation of kumatakenin and 4′,5-dihydroxy-3,3′,7-trimethoxyflavone from *Larrea tridentata*. *Pharmazie* 1974; **29**: 292–293.
7 Chirikdjian JJ. Flavonoids of *Larrea tridentata*. *Z Naturforsch* 1973; **28**: 32–35.
8 Gisvold O, Thaker E. Lignans from *Larrea divaricata*. *J Pharm Sci* 1974; **63**: 1905–1907.
9 Fronczek FR *et al*. The molecular structure of 3′-demethoxynorisoguaiacin triacetate from creosote bush (*Larrea tridentata*). *J Nat Prod* 1987; **50**: 497–499.
10 Page JO. Determination of nordihydroguaiaretic acid in creosote bush. *Anal Chem* 1955; **27**: 1266–1268.
11 Bohnstedt CF, Mabry TJ. The volatile constituents of the genus *Larrea* (Zygophyllaceae). *Rev Latinoam Quim* 1979; **10**: 128–131.
12 Xue H-Z *et al*. 3-β-(3,4-Dihydroxycinnamoyl)-erythrodiol and 3β-(4-hydroxycinnamoyl)-erythrodiol from *Larrea tridentata*. *Phytochemistry* 1988; **27**: 233–235.
13 Luo Z *et al*. Larreatin, a novel, cytotoxic naphthoquinone from *Larrea tridentata*. *J Org Chem* 1988; **53**: 2183–2185.
14 Segura JJ *et al*. In-vitro amebicidal activity of *Larrea tridentata*. *Bol Estud Med Biol* 1979; **30**: 267–268.

15 Oliveto EP. Nordihydroguaiaretic acid. A naturally occurring antioxidant. *Chem Ind* 1972: 677–679.

16 Burk D, Woods M. Hydrogen peroxide, catalase, glutathione peroxidasequinones, nordihydro-guaiaretic acid, and phosphopyridine in relation to X-ray action on cancer cells. *Radiation Res Suppl* 1963; **3**: 212–246.

17 Pardini RS *et al.* Inhibition of mitochondrial electron transport by nor-dihydroguaiaretic acid (NDGA). *Biochem Pharmacol* 1970; **19**: 2695–2699.

18 Smart CR *et al.* An interesting observation on nordihydroguaiaretic acid (NSC-4291; NDGA) and a patient with malignant melanoma—a preliminary report. *Cancer Chemother Rep Part 1* 1969; **53**: 147.

19 Katz M, Saibil F. Herbal hepatitis: subacute hepatic necrosis secondary to chaparral leaf. *J Clin Gastroenterol* 1990; **12**: 203–206.

20 Clark F, Reed R. Chaparral-induced toxic hepatitis – California and Texas, 1992. *Morb Mortal Wkly Rep* 1992; **41**: 812–814.

21 Gordon DW *et al.* Chaparral ingestion – the broadening spectrum of liver injury caused by herbal medicines. *JAMA* 1995; **273**: 489–490.

22 Leonforte JF. Contact dermatitis from *Larrea* (creosote bush). *J Am Acad Dermatol* 1986; **14**: 202–207.

23 Shasky DR. Contact dermatitis from *Larrea tridentata* (creosote bush). *J Am Acad Dermatol* 1986; **15**: 302.

24 Anon. Toxic tea. *Pharm J* 1993; **250**: 366.

Cinnamon

Species (Family)

(i) *Cinnamomum zeylanicum* Bl. (Lauraceae)
(ii) *Cinnamomum loureirii* Nees
(iii) *Cinnamomum burmanii* (Nees) Bl.

Synonym(s)

(i) Ceylon Cinnamon, *Cinnamomum verum* J.S. Presl., True Cinnamon
(ii) *Cinnamomum obtusifolium* Nees var.*loureirii* Perr. & Eb., Saigon Cassia, Saigon Cinnamon
(iii) Batavia Cassia, Batavia Cinnamon, Padang-Cassia, Panang Cinnamon

Part(s) Used

Inner bark

Pharmacopoeial and Other Monographs

BHP 1996[G9]
BP 2001[G15]
Complete German Commission E[G3]
Martindale 32nd edition[G43]
Ph Eur 2002[G28]
WHO volume 1 1999[G63]

Legal Category (Licensed Products)

GSL[G37]

Constituents[G2,G41,G48,G58,G59,G62,G64]

Tannins Condensed.

Volatile oils Up to 4%. Cinnamaldehyde (60–75%), benzaldehyde and cuminaldehyde; phenols (4–10%) including eugenol, methyl eugenol and safrole, pinene, phellandrene, cymeme and caryophyllene (hydrocarbons), eugenol acetate, cinnamyl acetate and benzyl benzoate (esters), linalool (an alcohol). Of the various types of cinnamon bark the oil of *C. zeylanicum* is stated to contain the highest amount of eugenol. Cinnamon oil differs from the closely related cassia oil in that the latter is reported to be devoid of eugenol, monoterpenoids and sesquiterpenoids (*see* Cassia).

Other constituents Calcium oxalate, cinnzeylanin, cinnzeylanol, coumarin, gum, mucilage, resins and sugars.

Other plant parts Cinnamon leaf oil contains much higher concentrations of eugenol, from 80 to 96% depending on the species. A cinnamon leaf oil of Chinese origin, *Cinnamomum japonicum* Sieb., contains a high concentration of safrole (60%) and only about 3% eugenol.

Food Use

Cinnamon is listed by the Council of Europe as a natural source of food flavouring (category N2). This category indicates that cinnamon can be added to foodstuffs in small quantities, with a possible limitation of an active principle (as yet unspecified) in the final product.[G16] It is commonly used as a spice in cooking, although at levels much less than the stated therapeutic doses. The acceptable daily intake of cinnamaldehyde has been temporarily estimated as $700\,\mu g/kg$ body weight.[G45] In the USA, cinnamon is listed as GRAS (Generally Recognised As Safe).[G41]

Herbal Use

Cinnamon is stated to possess antispasmodic, carminative, orexigenic, antidiarrhoeal, antimicrobial, refrigerant and anthelmintic properties. It has been used for anorexia, intestinal colic, infantile diarrhoea, common cold, influenza, and specifically for flatulent colic, and dyspepsia with nausea.[G7] Cinnamon bark is also stated to be astringent, and cinnamon oil is reported to possess carminative and antiseptic properties.[G2,G41,G64]

Dosage

Dried bark 0.5–1.0 g as infusion three times daily.[G7]

Liquid extract 0.5–1.0 mL (1 : 1 in 70% alcohol) three times daily.[G7]

Tincture of Cinnamon (BPC 1949) 2–4 mL.

Pharmacological Actions

In vitro and animal studies

Cinnamon oil has antifungal, antiviral, bactericidal and larvicidal properties.[G41] A carbon dioxide extract of cinnamon bark (0.1%) has been documented to suppress completely the growth of numerous microorganisms including *Escherichia coli*, *Staphylococcus aureus* and *Candida albicans*.[G41] (*See* Cassia for details of the many pharmacological actions documented for cinnamaldehyde and cinnamomi cortex (cinnamon bark).)

Antiseptic and anaesthetic properties have been documented for eugenol[1] and two insecticidal compounds, cinnzeylanin and cinnzeylanol, have been isolated.[G41] Tannins are known to possess astringent properties.

Weak tumour-promoting activity on the mouse skin and weak cytotoxic activity against HeLa cells has been documented for eugenol.[G41]

Side-effects, Toxicity

None documented for cinnamon bark. Cinnamon oil contains cinnamaldehyde, an irritant and sensitising principle.[G58] The dermal LD_{50} of the oil is reported to be 690 mg/kg body weight (*see* Cassia). The accepted daily intake of eugenol is up to 2.5 mg/kg.[G45]

Contra-indications, Warnings

Contact with cinnamon bark or oil may cause an allergic reaction.[G51] Cinnamon oil is stated to be a dermal and mucous membrane irritant, and a dermal sensitiser.[G58] It is a hazardous oil and should not be used on the skin.[G58] The oil should not be taken internally.

Pregnancy and lactation There are no known problems with the use of cinnamon during pregnancy and lactation, provided that doses do not greatly exceed the amounts used in foods.

Pharmaceutical Comment

The reputed antimicrobial, antiseptic, anthelmintic, carminative and antispasmodic properties of cinnamon are probably attributable to the volatile oil. The astringent properties of tannins may account for the claimed antidiarrhoeal action. Cinnamon should not be used in amounts greatly exceeding those used in foods.

References

See also General References G2, G3, G9, G12, G15, G16, G19, G25, G29, G31, G36, G37, G41, G43, G48, G51, G58, G59, G62, G63 and G64.

1 Wagner H, Wolff P (eds). *New Natural Products and Plant Drugs with Pharmacological, Biological or Therapeutical Activity*. Berlin: Springer Verlag, 1977.

Clivers

Species (Family)

Galium aparine L. (Rubiaceae)

Synonym(s)

Cleavers, Galium, Goosegrass

Part(s) Used

Herb

Pharmacopoeial and Other Monographs

BHC 1992[G6]
BHP 1996[G9]
Martindale 32nd edition[G43]
PDR for Herbal Medicines 2nd edition[G36]

Legal Category (Licensed Products)

GSL[G37]

Constituents[G6,G34,G40,G44,G48,G64]

Acids Caffeic acid, *p*-coumaric acid, gallic acid, *p*-hydroxybenzoic acid, salicylic acid and citric acid.[1]

Coumarins Unspecified. Scopoletin and umbelliferone reported for related species *Galium cruciata* and *Galium tauricum*.[2]

Iridoids Asperuloside (rubichloric acid), monotropein.[3,4]

Tannins Unspecified;[5] gallic acid is usually associated with hydrolysable tannins.

Other constituents Alkanes (C_{19}–C_{31}),[4] flavonoids.

Other plant parts Anthraquinones have been documented for the roots, but not for the aerial parts.[1]

Food Use

Clivers is not used in foods.

Herbal Use

Clivers is stated to possess diuretic and mild astringent properties. It has been used for dysuria, lymphadenitis, psoriasis, and specifically for enlarged lymph nodes.[G6,G7,G8,G64]

Dosage

Dried herb 2–4 g or by infusion three times daily.[G6,G7]

Liquid extract 2–4 mL (1 : 1 in 25% alcohol) three times daily.[G6,G7]

Expressed juice 3–15 mL three times daily.[G6,G7]

Pharmacological Actions

In vitro and animal studies

None documented for clivers. Asperuloside and monotropein have been reported to elicit a mild laxative action in mice.[6] The action was stated to be approximately 15 times less potent than that of senna, and of shorter duration.

Clinical studies

None documented. Tannins are known to possess astringent activities.

Side-effects, Toxicity

None documented.

Contra-indications, Warnings

It has been stated that diabetics should only use the expressed juice with caution[G34] although no pharmacological data were located to support this statement.

Pregnancy and lactation In view of the lack of pharmacological and toxicological information, the use of clivers during pregnancy should be avoided.

Pharmaceutical Comment

Limited chemical information is available for clivers. No scientific evidence was found to support the herbal uses, although documented tannin constituents may account for the reputed mild astringent action. In view of the paucity of toxicity data, excessive use of clivers should be avoided.

References

See also General References G6, G9, G34, G36, G37, G40, G43, G48, G49 and G64.

1   Hegnauer R. *Chemotaxonomie der Pflanzen*, vol 6. Basel and Stuttgart: Birhauser Verlag, 1973: 158–159.

2   Borisov MI. Coumarins of the genus Asperula and Galium. *Khim Prir Soedin* 1974; **10**: 82.

3   Grimshaw J. Structure of asperuloside. *Chem Ind* 1961: 403–404.

4   Corrigan D *et al*. Iridoids and alkanes in twelve species of *Galium* and *Asperula*. *Phytochemistry* 1978; **17**: 1131–1133.

5   Buckova A *et al*. Contents of tannins in some species of the Asperula and Galium genera. *Acta Fac Pharm Univ Comeniana* 1970; **19**: 7–28.

6   Inouye H *et al*. Purgative activities of iridoid glucosides. *Planta Med* 1974; **25**: 285–288.

Clove

Species (Family)

Syzygium aromaticum (L.) Merr. & Perry (Myrta-

Synonym(s)

Caryophyllus aromaticus L., *Eugenia aromatica* (L.) Baill., *Eugenia caryophyllata* Thunb., *Eugenia caryophyllus* (Spreng.) Bull. & Harr.

Part(s) Used

Clove (dried flowerbud), leaf, stem

Pharmacopoeial and Other Monographs

BHP 1996[G9]
BP 2001[G15]
Complete German Commission E[G3]
Martindale 32nd edition[G43]
PDR for Herbal Medicines 2nd edition[G36]
Ph Eur 2002[G28]

Legal Category (Licensed Products)

GSL[G37]

Constituents[G2,G22,G41,G48,G58,G64]

Volatile oils Clove bud oil (15–18%) containing eugenol (80–90%), eugenyl acetate (2–27%), β-caryophyllene (5–12%). Others include methyl salicylate, methyl eugenol, benzaldehyde, methyl amyl ketone and α-ylangene.

Leaf oil (2%) containing eugenol 82–88%.

Stem oil (4–6%) with eugenol 90–95%. A more comprehensive listing is provided elsewhere. [G22]

Other constituents Campesterol, carbohydrates, kaempferol, lipids, oleanolic acid, rhamnetin, sitosterol, stigmasterol and vitamins.

Food Use

Clove is listed by the Council of Europe as a natural source of food flavouring (category N2). This category indicates that clove can be added to foodstuffs in small quantities, with a possible limitation of an active principle (as yet unspecified) in the final product.[G16] Clove is commonly used in cooking, and as a flavouring agent in food products. In the USA, clove is listed as GRAS (Generally Recognised As Safe).[G41]

Herbal Use

Clove has been traditionally used as a carminative, anti-emetic, toothache remedy and counter-irritant.[G2,G41,G64]

Clove oil is stated to be a carminative, occasionally used in the treatment of flatulent colic[G54] and is commonly used topically for symptomatic relief of toothache.[G45]

Dosage

Clove 120–300 mg.[G44]

Clove oil 0.05–0.2 mL.[G44]

Pharmacological Actions

In vitro and animal studies

The anodyne and mild antiseptic properties documented for clove oil have been attributed to eugenol.[G41] Clove oil is stated to possess antihistaminic and antispasmodic properties.[G41] Eugenol, eugenol acetate and methyl acetate are reported to exhibit trypsin-potentiating activity.[G41]

Antibacterial, hypoglycaemic and potent CNS-depressant activities have been documented for *Syzygium cuminii* L., a related species cultivated in India.[1]

Clinical studies

A tincture of cloves (15% in 70% alcohol) was effective in treating athlete's foot.[G41]

Side-effects, Toxicity

None documented for the bud, leaf or stem of cloves. Clove oil is stated to be a dermal and mucous membrane irritant;[G58] contact dermatitis, cheilitis, and stomatitis have been reported for clove oil.[G51] The irritant nature of the oil can be attributed to the eugenol content. Eugenol is also stated to have sensitising properties.[G51] An LD_{50} (rat, by mouth) value for clove oil is stated as 2.65 g/kg body weight.[G22]

In humans, the accepted daily intake of eugenol is up to 2.5 mg/kg body weight.[G45]

Contra-indications, Warnings

None documented for the bud, leaf or stem. It is recommended that clove oil should be used with caution orally and should not be used on the skin.[G58] Repeated application of clove oil as a toothache remedy may result in damage to the gingival tissue.[G45] In view of the irritant nature of the volatile oil, concentrated clove oil is not suitable for internal use in large doses. Eugenol is a powerful inhibitor of platelet activity and it is recommended that caution be taken for patients on anticoagulant therapy.[G58]

Pregnancy and lactation   There are no known problems with the use of clove during pregnancy or lactation, provided that doses taken do not greatly exceed the amounts used in foods.

Pharmaceutical Comment

The pharmacological properties documented for cloves are associated with the volatile oil, in particular with eugenol which has local anaesthetic action. Cloves should not be taken in doses greatly exceeding those used in foods and caution should be exerted in patients taking anticoagulant or antiplatelet therapy.

References

See also General References G2, G3, G9, G15, G16, G22, G25, G31, G36, G37, G41, G43, G48, G51 and G64.

1   Chakraborty D *et al*. A new neuropsychopharmacological study of *Syzygium cuminii*. *Planta Med* 1986; **52**: 139–143.

Cohosh, Black

Species (Family)

Cimicifuga racemosa Nutt. (Ranunculaceae)

Synonym(s)

Actaea Racemosa Radix, Black Snakeroot, Cimicifuga, Macrotys Actaea

Part(s) Used

Rhizome, root

Pharmacopoeial and Other Monographs

BHC 1992[G6]
BHP 1996[G9]
BPC 1934[G10]
Complete German Commission E[G3]
Martindale 32nd edition[G43]
Mills and Bone[G50]
PDR for Herbal Medicines 2nd edition[G36]

Legal Category (Licensed Products)

GSL[G37]

Constituents[1,G6,G22,G41,G64]

Alkaloids Quinolizidine-type. N-Methylcytisine and other unidentified compounds.

Tannins Type unspecified. Tannic and gallic acids are usually associated with hydrolysable tannins.

Terpenoids Triterpene glycosides, principally the xylosides actein (aglycone: acetylacteol) and cimicifugoside (also known as cimigoside; aglycone: cimigenol),[2–8,G6] also 26-deoxycimicifugoside, cimiaceroside A, 27-deoxyactein),[9,10] cimiracemosides A–H,[9–11] and cimicifugosides H-3, H-4 and H-6.[12]

Other constituents Acetic acid, butyric acid, formic acid, hydroxycinnamic acid esters of fukiic and piscidic acids (fukinolic acid, cimicifugic acids A, B, E, F), caffeic acid, ferulic acid,[13] isoferulic acid, oleic acid, palmitic acid, salicylic acid, racemosin, formononetin,[3] phytosterols, cimicifugin 15–20%, acteina (resinous mixture) and volatile oil.

Food Use

In the USA, black cohosh is listed by the Food and Drugs Administration (FDA) as a 'Herb of Undefined Safety'.[G22] Black cohosh is not used in foods.

Herbal Use

Black cohosh is stated to possess antirheumatic, antitussive, sedative and emmenagogue properties. It has been used for intercostal myalgia, sciatica, whooping cough, chorea, tinnitus, dysmenorrhoea, uterine colic, and specifically for muscular rheumatism and rheumatoid arthritis.[G6,G7,G8,G32,G64] Modern use of black cohosh is focused on its use in treating peri- and postmenopausal symptoms.[1,14,G50]

Dosage

Dried rhizome/root 40–200 mg daily.[G6]

Liquid extract Ethanolic extracts equivalent to 40 mg dried rhizome/root daily.[G3,G50]

Tincture 0.4–2 mL (1 : 10 in 60% ethanol) daily.[G6]

Several clinical trials of black cohosh have used a standardised black cohosh extract (Remifemin; each 20 mg tablet contained 1 mg triterpene glycosides, calculated as 27-deoxyactein) 40 mg twice daily for up to 24 weeks.[15–17]

Pharmacological Actions

Several pharmacological activities, including hormonal, cardiovascular, circulatory and anti-inflammatory activities, have been documented for black cohosh and/or its constituents. The triterpene glycosides and flavonoids are considered to be the active components of black cohosh.[18,G56]

In vitro and animal studies

Hormonal activity A methanolic extract of the rhizome of black cohosh reduced the serum concentration of luteinising hormone (LH) in ovariectomised rats, and exhibited a binding affinity to oestrogen receptors in isolated rat uterus.[2] *In vivo*, the activity of the methanolic extract was significantly reduced following enzymatic hydrolysis of glucosides present.

Subsequent *in vitro* studies isolated three compounds with endocrine activity, including an isoflavone, formononetin. Formononetin was found to exhibit competitive oestrogen receptor activity, but did not cause a reduction in serum concentrations of LH.[2] Recent research found that formononenetin could not be detected in commercial preparations of black cohosh, although other flavonoids were present.[19]

In ovariectomised rats, administration of a lipophilic extract of black cohosh (140 mg by intraperitoneal injection for three days) led to a significant reduction in serum LH concentrations, compared with control ($p < 0.01$), whereas no effect was observed with a hydrophilic extract (216 mg intraperitoneally for three days).[16] Subsequent studies using fractions of the lipophilic extract demonstrated that constituents inhibited LH secretion and/or exhibited activity in an oestrogen receptor-binding assay.

In an *in vitro* study in oestrogen receptor-positive breast cancer cells, black cohosh extract did not stimulate cancer cell growth, i.e. it did not exhibit oestrogen-like effects, but at a concentration of 2.5 µg/mL led to a marked inhibition of breast cancer cell proliferation.[20]

Oestrogenic activity has been documented *in vitro* for fukinolic acid, a hydroxycinnamic acid ester of fukiic acid, in oestrogen-dependent MCF-7 cells (a breast cancer cell line).[13] Fukinolic acid at concentrations of 5×10^{-7} mol/L and 5×10^{-8} mol/L led to significantly increased cell proliferation (mean (standard deviation): +120 (6%) and +126 (5%), respectively, compared with control. These effects were reported to be equivalent to those of oestradiol at 10^{-10} mol/L. By contrast, in other *in vitro* studies, a methanol extract of black cohosh rhizomes and roots did not demonstrate oestrogenic activity in several assays, including binding affinity for oestrogen receptors α and β, stimulation of pS2 mRNA expression in S30 cells (S30 is a subclone of an oestrogen receptor-negative breast cancer cell line), and induction of alkaline phosphatase in an oestrogen receptor-positive endometrial adenocarcinoma cell line.[21]

Other activities Anti-inflammatory and analgesic activity for constituents of black cohosh has been documented following *in vitro* and *in vivo* studies (mice and rats).

In vitro, caffeic acid, fukinolic acid and cimicifugic acids A, B, E and F inhibited the activity of neutrophil elastase in a concentration-dependent manner.[22] (Raised plasma concentrations of neutrophil elastase are a typical feature of active inflammation. Neutrophil elastase contributes to the destruction of basement membranes during inflammation.) Caffeic acid inhibited the enzyme with an IC_{50} of 16 µg/mL (93 µmol/L), whereas fukinolic acid had an IC_{50} of 0.1 µg/mL (0.23 µmol/L), relative to controls. Of the cimicifugic acids, A and B were the strongest inhibitors of the enzyme, with IC_{50} values of 2.2 µmol/L and 11.4 µmol/L, respectively.

Compared with controls, a methanol extract, a butanol-soluble fraction and a water-soluble fraction obtained from *Cimicifuga* rhizome inhibited carrageenan-induced rat paw oedema by 73–76%, 80–84% and 46–54%, respectively, compared with controls, 30–120 minutes after injection of 0.1 mL carrageenan 1%.[23] The same fractions (100 mg/kg by intraperitoneal injection), compared with controls, demonstrated analgesic activity determined by significant reductions in acetic acid-induced writhing in mice, and the methanol extract and butanol-soluble fraction also displayed analgesic activity in a tail-flick test (demonstrated by increased latency time upon infrared light exposure). All three fractions (40 µg/mL) inhibited bradykinin and histamine receptor-mediated contractions of guinea-pig ileum, and all inhibited lipopolysaccharide-induced 6-keto prostaglandin $F_{1\alpha}$ ($PGF_{1\alpha}$) formation in macrophages. Incubation of macrophages with lipopolysaccharide and the water-soluble fraction 10 µg/mL almost completely blocked (99% inhibition) lipopolysaccharide-induced 6-keto-$PGF_{1\alpha}$ formation. Lipopolysaccharide-induced 6-keto-$PGF_{1\alpha}$ formation in macrophages is related to selective expression of cyclooxygenase 2 (COX-2). The inhibitory effects of fractions of *Cimicifuga* rhizome in this model, and their inhibitory effects on bradykinin and histamine receptor-mediated reactions are possible mechanisms for the observed anti-inflammatory and analgesic activities.

In vitro studies using rat aortic strips have investigated the vasoactive effects of constituents of *Cimicifuga* species.[24] Cimicifugic acid D and fukinolic acid (3×10^{-4} mol/L) caused a sustained relaxation of aortic strips precontracted with noradrenaline (norepinephrine) in preparations with or without endothelium. By contrast, cimicifugic acid C inversely caused a weak contraction, and fukiic acid and cimicifugic acids A, B and E showed no vasoactivity at the concentration tested.

A resinous component, termed acteina, has exhibited a hypotensive action in both unanaesthetised rabbits and anaesthetised cats. The effect in unanaesthetised dogs was found to be inconsistent.[25] An effective dose of acteina 1 mg/kg body weight was recorded, with maximum hypotension attained using 10 mg/kg. It was stated that acteina may act by an effect on the vasomotor centres.

Triterpene compounds in black cohosh have been shown to possess hypocholesterolaemic activity *in vivo*, and an inhibitory effect on phytohaemagglutin-induced proliferative response *in vitro*. These activities were thought to be linked to molecular characteristics between the identified triterpenes and intermediates in cholesterol biosynthesis.[26]

Triterpenoid constituents from several *Cimicifuga* species, including actein from *C. racemosa*, have been investigated for antimalarial activity against *Plasmodium falciparum in vitro*.[27] Cimicifugoside (isolated from *C. simplex*) and actein were among the compounds with potent antimalarial activity (EC_{50} 5.0 μmol/L and 10.0 μmol/L, respectively), although activity was 2- to 3-fold less than that of positive controls (quinine, chloroquine and pyrimethamine).

The root of a related species, *Cimicifuga dahurica*, has been reported to exhibit antibacterial activity towards Gram-positive (*Bacillus subtilis*, *Mycobacterium smegmatis*, *Staphylococcus aureus*), and Gram-negative (*Escherichia coli*, *Shigella flexneri*, *Shigella sonnei*) organisms.[28]

In ovariectomised rats, ethyl acetate-soluble fractions from the rhizome of the related species *Cimicifuga heracleifolia* and *C. foetida* administered orally at doses of 100 mg/kg/day for 42 days led to a significant increase in bone mineral density of the lumbar spine, compared with that in untreated ovariectomised control rats.[29]

Clinical studies

Clinical trials of extracts of black cohosh have investigated mainly its effects in women with peri- and/or postmenopausal symptoms.

Menopausal symptoms In a randomised, double-blind, placebo-controlled trial, 80 women (mean (standard deviation) age: 51.2 (3.1) years) with menopausal symptoms received standardised black cohosh extract (Remifemin; each 20-mg tablet contained 1 mg triterpene glycosides, calculated as 27-deoxyactein) 40 mg twice daily, conjugated oestrogens 0.625mg daily, or placebo, for 12 weeks.[15] At the end of the study, somatic and psychological symptoms, measured by the Kupperman Menopausal Index and the Hamilton Anxiety Scale, had improved significantly only in women who received black cohosh, compared with those who received oestrogen or placebo. Similarly, a significant increase in proliferation of vaginal epithelium was noted only in the black cohosh group. However, there is a view that the dose of oestrogen used in the study was too low to provide a useful comparison.

A randomised, double-blind, placebo-controlled trial involving 85 women with a history of breast cancer assessed the effects of black cohosh (no details of extract provided) one tablet twice daily for 60 days on the frequency and intensity of hot flushes.[30] Participants were stratified according to whether or not they were using tamoxifen. Both treatment and placebo groups reported decreases in the number and intensity of hot flushes, compared with baseline values. There were no statistically significant differences between the two groups, and subgroup analysis of tamoxifen users and non-users did not reveal any statistically significant differences. Changes in other parameters measured during the study (other menopausal symptoms, serum concentrations of follicle-stimulating hormone (FSH) and luteinising hormone (LH)) were also not statistically significant between groups.

In a placebo-controlled study involving 110 women with menopausal symptoms, black cohosh extract (Remifemin) two tablets daily for two months significantly reduced serum LH concentrations, compared with placebo ($p < 0.05$).[16] There was no significant difference between the two groups with respect to serum FSH concentrations.

Most other studies of black cohosh involving women with menopausal symptoms have an open and/or uncontrolled design and, therefore, do not provide an unbiased assessment of efficacy. Generally, these studies report significant improvements in menopausal symptoms, compared with baseline values, after at least four weeks' treatment. Some studies involved administration of black cohosh extract for up to 12 weeks. These studies have been summarised elsewhere.[1,18,G50] Details of two of these studies are provided below.

In an open study, 60 women with at least one intact ovary who had undergone hysterectomy and who were experiencing menopausal symptoms were randomised to receive oestriol (1 mg daily), conjugated oestrogens (1.25 mg daily), oestrogen–progestagen sequential therapy (dose not specified), or black cohosh extract (Remifemin) 40 mg twice daily, for 24 weeks.[17] At the end of the study, improvements in Kupperman Index scores were significantly lower, compared with baseline values, in all groups. There were no statistically significant differences between groups.

Another open, controlled study involving women with menopausal symptoms ($n = 60$) assessed the effects of black cohosh extract administered as a tincture (80 drops daily), compared with oestrogen (0.625 mg daily) or diazepam (2 mg daily), over a 12-week period.[31] Cytological responses (proliferation and maturation of vaginal epithelial cells) were observed for participants in the black cohosh and oestrogen groups, but not in the diazepam group. For all three groups, improvements in neurovegetative and psychological symptoms (e.g. self-assessed depression) were reported.

Other conditions   Black cohosh has been reported to cause peripheral vasodilatation and an increase in peripheral blood flow, following the administration of a resinous constituent, acteina (500 µg/kg body weight), to patients suffering from peripheral arterial disease.[25] The blood pressure of conscious individuals, both normotensive and hypertensive, was stated to be unaffected. The chemical composition of acteina is undefined.

In a randomised, double-blind trial, 82 patients with osteoarthritis or rheumatoid arthritis received a proprietary combination herbal preparation containing black cohosh 35 mg (other ingredients: white willow bark, guaiacum resin, sarsaparilla and poplar bark; Reumalex), or placebo, two tablets daily for two months.[32] At the end of the study, there was a small, but statistically significant improvement in pain symptoms (as assessed by the Arthritis Pain Scale) in the treatment group, compared with the placebo group ($p < 0.05$).

Side-effects, Toxicity

A review of the literature on black cohosh[18] describes a postmarketing surveillance study involving 629 women with menopausal symptoms who received standardised black cohosh extract as a tincture (80 drops daily) for 6–8 weeks.[33] Tolerability was rated as 'good' in 93% of patients; mild, transient gastrointestinal symptoms were noted in 7% of patients.

A randomised, double-blind, placebo-controlled trial involving 80 women with menopausal symptoms who received standardised black cohosh extract (Remifemin) 40 mg twice daily, conjugated oestrogens, or placebo, for 12 weeks reported that non-specific adverse events, such as headaches, not considered treatment-related occurred in all three groups.[15] Another controlled trial ($n = 60$) of the same extract reported that tolerability of black cohosh extract was 'good'.[17] In a randomised, double-blind trial involving 85 women with a history of breast cancer who received black cohosh (no details of extract provided) one tablet twice daily, or placebo, for 60 days, 10 adverse events occurred in the treatment group, compared with three in the placebo group.[30] Three events were considered serious (treatment group: hysterectomy, recurrence of breast cancer; placebo group: appendectomy) all of which occurred in women who were also receiving tamoxifen. Minor adverse events (including constipation, weight gain, cramping, indigestion, vaginal bleeding) were not thought to be treatment related.

Older reference texts state that overdose may produce symptoms of nausea, vomiting, dizziness, visual and nervous disturbances, together with reduced pulse rate and increased perspiration.[G22,G42,G49]

Contra-indications, Warnings

In vitro studies investigating the oestrogenic activity of extracts of black cohosh and their constituents report conflicting results (*see In vitro* and animal studies, Hormonal activity). Some studies have documented that certain constituents of black cohosh bind to oestrogen receptors,[2,16] and others have reported oestrogenic activity *in vitro* for fukinolic acid, a hydroxycinnamic acid ester of fukiic acid, in an oestrogen receptor-positive breast cancer cell line (MCF-7 cells).[13] These findings contrast with those of a previous *in vitro* study in oestrogen receptor-positive breast cancer cells, which reported that black cohosh extract did not stimulate cancer cell growth, i.e. it did not exhibit oestrogen-like effects, but at a concentration of 2.5 µg/mL led to a marked inhibition of breast cancer cell proliferation.[20]

There is a view that the therapeutic effects of black cohosh extract are not attributable to oestrogenic effects, and that there is clinical evidence, such as lack of vaginal cell proliferation, as well as *in vitro* evidence to support this view.[18] The German Commission E monograph states that there are no known contraindications to the use of black cohosh. Concern has been expressed that herbs with oestrogenic activity might stimulate breast cancer cell growth and oppose the effects of competitive oestrogen receptor antagonists, such as tamoxifen.[34] A randomised, double-blind, placebo-controlled trial involving 85 women with a history of breast cancer assessed the effects of black cohosh (no details of extract provided) on hot flushes (*see* Clinical studies, Menopausal symptoms).[30] Participants were stratified according to whether or not they were using tamoxifen. One woman receiving both black cohosh and tamoxifen experienced a recurrence of breast cancer, although it was reported that the woman had an increase in carcinoembryonic antigen when she entered the trial (this had not been reported to the referring physician).

Further study is required to establish whether black cohosh has oestrogenic activity. Herbal medicines with oestrogenic activity should be avoided in women with oestrogen-dependent tumours, such as breast cancer.[G50]

Pregnancy and lactation *In vitro* studies using rat uterus have indicated that black cohosh binds to uterine oestrogen receptors. Black cohosh has been used traditionally to assist labour. However, as there are insufficient data on the use of black cohosh during pregnancy and also during lactation, it is contra-indicated during these periods.[G49,G50,G56]

There is an isolated report of a child born with no spontaneous breathing and who subsequently experienced brain hypoxia and seizures following the oral administration of black cohosh and blue cohosh by a midwife in an attempt to induce labour in a woman who had had an uneventful pregnancy.[35] The report has been criticised as it did not provide any further details of the dose or formulation of the herbs, and as the authors of the report make several assumptions about the clinical activity of the herbs on the basis of studies in animals.[36]

Pharmaceutical Comment

The chemistry of black cohosh is well studied, although most of the documented information concerns the triterpene constituents. Most of the reputed traditional uses of black cohosh are not supported by data from experimental or clinical studies. One exception is the use of black cohosh in rheumatism and rheumatoid arthritis – there are data from *in vitro* and *in vivo* studies in rodents which indicate that black cohosh extracts have anti-inflammatory activity.[22,23] Other pharmacological actions have been observed in both animals and humans which provide supporting data for the hormonal activity of the herb. However, there are conflicting reports on the oestrogenic activity of black cohosh. As it is known that there are at least two types of oestrogen receptor, there is a view that research relating to the oestrogenic effects of black cohosh needs to be considered against this background.[1]

Little is known about the toxicity of black cohosh and excessive use should be avoided. It has been stated that the duration of use should not exceed three months.[G56] Further study is required to determine whether black cohosh has oestrogenic activity before definitive statements about its use in women with oestrogen-dependent tumours can be made.

There is evidence from one published, randomised clinical trial to indicate that black cohosh extract is more effective than placebo in the treatment of menopausal symptoms. However, another randomised clinical trial involving women with a history of breast cancer who were experiencing menopausal symptoms found no effect for an unspecified black cohosh extract on the frequency and intensity of hot flushes. There are supporting data for the effects of black cohosh extracts on menopausal symptoms from open, uncontrolled studies and from postmarketing surveillance studies that assessed effectiveness as well as safety. However, further randomised clinical trials are required to establish the effects of black cohosh in women with menopausal symptoms. There is also a lack of information on the toxicity of black cohosh.

References

See also General References G3, G5, G6, G9, G22, G31, G32, G36, G41, G42, G43, G49, G50, G56 and G64.

1 McKenna DJ *et al*. Black cohosh: efficacy, safety, and use in clinical and preclinical applications. *Altern Ther* 2001; 7: 93–100.
2 Jarry H, Harnischfeger G. Untersuchungen zur endokrinen wirksamkeit von inhaltsstoffen aus *Cimicifuga racemosa* 1. Einfluss auf die serumspiegel von hypophysenhormonen ovariektomierter ratten. *Planta Med* 1985; 51: 46–49.
3 Jarry H *et al*. Untersuchungen zur endokrinen wirksamkeit von inhaltsstoffen aus *Cimicifuga racemosa* 2. In vitro-bindung von inhaltsstoffen an östrogenrezeptoren. *Planta Med* 1985; 51: 316–319.
4 Linde H. Die inhaltsstoffe von Cimicifuga racemosa 2. Mitt.: zur struktur des acteins. *Arch Pharm* 1967; 300: 885–892.
5 Linde H. Die inhaltsstoffe von Cimicifuga racemosa 3. Mitt.: über die konstitution der ringe A, B and C des acteins. *Arch Pharm* 1967; 300: 982–992.
6 Linde H. Die inhaltsstoffe von Cimicifuga racemosa 4. Mitt.: actein: der ring D und seitenkette. *Arch Pharm* 1968; 301: 120–138.
7 Linde H. Die inhaltsstoffe von Cimicifuga racemosa 5. Mitt.: 27-desoxyacetylacteol. *Arch Pharm* 1968; 301: 335–341.
8 Radics L *et al*. Carbon-13 NMR spectra of some polycyclic triterpenoids. *Tetrahedron Lett* 1975; 48: 4287–4290.
9 Bedir E, Khan IA. Cimiracemoside A: a new cyclolanostanol xyloside from the rhizome of *Cimicifuga racemosa*. *Chem Pharm Bull* 2000; 48: 425–427.
10 Shao Y *et al*. Triterpene glycosides from *Cimicifuga racemosa*. *J Nat Prod* 2000; 63: 905–910.
11 Bedir E, Khan IA. A new cyclolanostanol arabinoside from the rhizome of *Cimicifuga racemosa*. *Pharmazie* 2001; 56: 268–269.
12 Sakurai N *et al*. Studies on the Chinese crude drug

'Shoma.' X. Three new trinor-9,19-cyclolanostanol xylosides, cimicifugosides H-3, H-4 and H-6, from Cimicifuga rhizome and transformation of cimicifugoside H-1 into cimicifugosides H-2, H-3 and H-4. *Chem Pharm Bull* 1995; **43**: 1475–1482.

13 Kruse SO *et al*. Fukiic and piscidic acid esters from the rhizome of *Cimicifuga racemosa* and the in vitro estrogenic activity of fukinolic acid. *Planta Med* 1999; **65**: 763–764.

14 Pepping J. Black cohosh: *Cimicifuga racemosa*. *Am J Health-Syst Pharm* 1999; **56**: 1400–1402.

15 Stoll W. (Phytopharmacon influences atrophic vaginal epithelium: double-blind study, *Cimicifuga* vs estrogenic substances). *Therapeuticon* 1987; **1**: 23–31.

16 Düker E-M *et al*. Effects of extracts from *Cimicifuga racemosa* on gonadotropin release in menopausal women and ovariectomized rats. *Planta Med* 1991; **57**: 420–424.

17 Lehman-Willenbrock E, Riedel H-H. Klinische und endokrinologische Untersuchungen zur Therapie ovarieller Ausfallserscheinungen nach Hysterektomie unter Belassung der Adnexe. *Z Gynäkol* 1988; **110**: 611–618.

18 Liske E. Therapeutic efficacy and safety of *Cimicifuga racemosa* for gynecologic disorders. *Adv Ther* 1998; **15**: 45–53.

19 Struck D *et al*. Flavones in extracts of *Cimicifuga racemosa*. *Planta Med* 1997; **63**: 289.

20 Nesselhut T *et al*. Untersuchungen zur proliferativen Potenz von Phytopharmaka mit östrogenähnlicher Wirkung bei Mammakarzinomzellen. *Arch Gynecol Obstet* 1993; **254**: 817–818.

21 Liu J *et al*. Evaluation of estrogenic activity of plant extracts for the potential treatment of menopausal symptoms. *J Agric Food Chem* 2001; **49**: 2472–2479.

22 Löser B *et al*. Inhibition of neutrophil elastase activity by cinnamic acid derivatives from *Cimicifuga racemosa*. *Planta Med* 2000; **66**: 751–753.

23 Kim S-J, Kim M-S. Inhibitory effects of Cimicifugae rhizoma extracts on histamine, bradykinin and COX-2 mediated inflammatory actions. *Phytother Res* 2000; **14**: 596–600.

24 Noguchi M *et al*. Vasoactive effects of cimicifugic acids C and D, and fukinolic acid in Cimicifuga rhizome. *Biol Pharm Bull* 1998; **21**: 1163–1168.

25 Genazzani E, Sorrentino L. Vascular action of acteina: active constituent of *Actaea racemosa* L. *Nature* 1962; **194**: 544–545.

26 Resing K, Fitzgerald A. Crystal data for 15-o-acetylacerinol and two related triterpenes isolated from Japanese *Cimicifuga* plants. *J Appl Crystallogr* 1978; **11**: 58.

27 Takahara M *et al*. Antimalarial activity and nucleoside transport inhibitory activity of the triterpenic constituents of *Cimicifuga* spp. *Biol Pharm Bull* 1998; **21**: 823–828.

28 Moskalenko SA. Preliminary screening of Far-Eastern ethnomedicinal plants for antibacterial activity. *J Ethnopharmacol* 1986; **15**: 231–259.

29 Li JX *et al*. Effects of Cimicifugae rhizoma on serum calcium and phosphate levels in low calcium dietary rats and on bone mineral density in ovariectomized rats. *Phytomedicine* 1996/97; **3**: 379–385.

30 Jacobson JS *et al*. Randomized trial of black cohosh for the treatment of hot flashes among women with a history of breast cancer. *J Clin Oncol* 2001; **19**: 2739–2745.

31 Warnecke G. Beeinflussung klimakterischer Beschwerden durch ein Phytotherapeutikum. Erfolgreiche Therapie mit Cimicifuga-Monoextrakt. *Med Welt* 1985; **36**: 871–874.

32 Mills SY *et al*. Effect of a proprietary herbal medicine on the relief of chronic arthritic pain: a double-blind study. *Br J Rheumatol* 1996; **35**: 874–878.

33 Stolze H. Der andere Weg, klimakterische Beschwerden zu behandeln. *Gyne* 1982; **3**: 14–16.

34 Boyle FM. Adverse interaction of herbal medicine with breast cancer treatment. *Med J Aust* 1997; **167**: 286.

35 Gunn TR, Wright IMR. The use of black and blue cohosh in labour. *N Z Med J* 1996; **109**: 410–411.

36 Baillie N, Rasmussen P. Black and blue cohosh in labour. *N Z Med J* 1997; **110**: 20–21.

Cohosh, Blue

Species (Family)

Caulophyllum thalictroides (L.) Mich. (Berberida-

Synonym(s)

Caulophyllum, Papoose Root, Squaw Root

Part(s) Used

Rhizome, root

Pharmacopoeial and Other Monographs

BHP 1983[G7]
PDR for Herbal Medicines 2nd edition[G36]

Legal Category (Licensed Products)

GSL[G37]

Constituents[G22,G41,G48,G64]

Alkaloids Quinolizidine and isoquinoline-types. Anagyrine, baptifoline, magnoflorine, methylcytisine (caulophylline). Other unidentified minor tertiary alkaloids.[1]

Saponins Caulosaponin and cauloside D yielding hederagenin on hydrolysis.[2]

Other constituents Citrullol, gum, resins, phosphoric acid, phytosterol and starch.

Other Caulophyllum species A related species, *C. robustum* Maxim., is rich in triterpene glycosides (caulosides A–G), most of which possess hederagenin as their aglycone.

Food Use

Blue cohosh is not used in foods.

Herbal Use

Blue cohosh is stated to possess antispasmodic, emmenagogue, uterine tonic and antirheumatic properties. Traditionally, it has been used for amenorrhoea, threatened miscarriage, false labour pains, dysmenorrhoea, rheumatic pains, and specifically for conditions associated with uterine atony.[G7,G64]

Dosage

Dried rhizome/root 0.3–1.0 g or by decoction three times daily.[G7]

Liquid extract 0.5–1.0 mL (1:1 in 70% alcohol) three times daily.[G7]

Pharmacological Actions

In vitro and animal studies

A blue cohosh extract exhibited stimulant properties on the isolated guinea-pig uterus, although subsequent *in vivo* studies in cats, dogs and rabbits demonstrated no uterine activity.[3] Antifertility actions documented in rats were reported to be caused by inhibition of ovulation[4] and by interruption of implantation.[5]

Smooth muscle stimulation has been documented for a crystalline glycoside constituent on the uterus (*in vitro*), the small intestine (*in vitro*), and the coronary blood vessels (*in vivo*) of various small mammals.[6] The glycoside was also reported to cause erythrolysis and to be of an irritant nature. An earlier study that used a crystalline glycoside identified as caulosaponin, reported a variety of actions including an oxytocic effect on the isolated rat uterus, constriction of coronary and carotid blood vessels, a toxic action on cardiac muscle, and a spasmogenic action on the isolated intestine.[6]

Methylcytisine is stated to have a nicotinic-like action, causing an elevation in blood pressure and stimulating both respiration and intestinal motility.[G60]

An alcoholic extract of the aerial parts of blue cohosh produced up to 55% inhibition of inflammation in the carrageenan rat paw test[7].

Side-effects, Toxicity

Powdered blue cohosh is stated to be irritant, especially to mucous membranes.[G51] The leaves and seeds are reported to contain methylcytisine and some glycosides that can cause severe stomach pains. Children have been poisoned by eating the bright blue bitter-tasting seeds.[G22] Caulosaponin is reported to be cardiotoxic, causing constriction of coronary blood vessels, to produce intestinal spasms, and to possess oxytocic properties.[G60]

Contra-indications, Warnings

Blue cohosh may interfere with existing therapy for angina, and may irritate gastrointestinal conditions. Excessive doses may cause a rise in blood pressure, because of the methylcytisine constituent and give rise to other symptoms of nicotine poisoning.

Pregnancy and lactation   Blue cohosh should not be taken in pregnancy; it is reputed to be an aborti-facient and to affect the menstrual cycle.[G30] Some texts give conflicting advice. It has been documented that blue cohosh should be avoided by pregnant women,[G22] only be taken once labour has commenced,[G49] only taken in small doses during the first trimester of pregnancy,[G7] or only be used under expert supervision.[G42]

Pharmaceutical Comment

Limited data are available on the chemistry of blue cohosh. Documented pharmacological actions support some of the reputed traditional uses, although many of these are not suitable indications for self-medication. No evidence regarding antirheumatic properties was located, although anti-inflammatory action has been documented for the aerial plant parts.

In view of the potential toxicity associated with blue cohosh, it should be used with caution.

References

See also General References G7, G10, G20, G22, G30, G31, G32, G36, G37, G41, G42, G48, G49, G51, G60 and G64.

1   Flom MS *et al*. Isolation and characterization of alkaloids from *Caulophyllum thalictroides*. *J Pharm Sci* 1967; **56**: 1515–1517.
2   Strigina LI *et al*. Cauloside D a new triterpenoid glycoside from *Caulophyllum robustum*. Maxim. Identification of cauloside A. *Phytochemistry* 1976; **15**: 1583–1586.
3   Pilcher JD *et al*. The action of various female remedies on the excised uterus of the guinea-pig. *Arch Intern Med* 1916; **18**: 557–583.
4   Chaudrasekhar K, Sarma GHR. Observations on the effect of low and high doses of Caulophyllum on the ovaries and the consequential changes in the uterus and thyroid in rats. *J Reprod Fertil* 1974; **38**: 236–237.
5   Chaudrasekhar K, Raa Vishwanath C. Studies on the effect of Caulophyllum on implantation in rats. *J Reprod Fertil* 1974; **38**: 245–246.
6   Ferguson HC, Edwards LD. A pharmacological study of a crystalline glycoside of *Caulophyllum thalictroides*. *J Am Pharm Assoc* 1954; **43**: 16–21.
7   Benoit PS *et al*. Biological and phytochemical evaluation of plants XIV. Anti-inflammatory evaluation of 163 species of plants. *Lloydia* 1976; **393**: 160–171.

Cola

Species (Family)

(i) *Cola nitida* A. Chev. (Sterculiaceae)
(ii) *Cola acuminata* Schott & Endl. and related species

Synonym(s)

Cola Seed, Guru Nut, Kola Nut
(ii) *Sterculia acuminata* Beauv.

Part(s) Used

Cotyledon

Pharmacopoeial and Other Monographs

BHC 1992[G6]
BHP 1996[G9]
BP 2001[G15]
Complete German Commission E[G3]
Martindale 32nd edition[G43]
PDR for Herbal Medicines 2nd edition[G36]
Ph Eur 2002[G28]

Legal Category (Licensed Products)

GSL[G37]

Constituents[G6,G22,G41,G48,G62,G64]

Alkaloids Xanthine-types. Caffeine (0.6–3.0%), theobromine (up to 0.1%).

Tannins Condensed type, catechins.

Other constituents Betaine, cellulose, enzyme, fats, a glucoside, protein, red pigment and sugars.

Food Use

Cola is listed by the Council of Europe as a natural source of food flavouring (cola and cola nut extract: category 4, with limits on caffeine) (*see* Appendix 23).[G17] Cola is commonly used in foods. In the USA,
it is listed as GRAS (Generally Recognised As Safe).[G41]

Herbal Use

Cola is stated to possess CNS stimulant, thymoleptic, antidepressant, diuretic, cardioactive and antidiarrhoeal properties. It has been used for depressive states, melancholy, atony, exhaustion, dysentery, atonic diarrhoea, anorexia, migraine and specifically for depressive states associated with general muscular weakness.[G6,G7,G8,G64]

Dosage

Powdered cotyledons 1–3 g or by decoction three times daily.[G6,G7]

Liquid Extract of Kola (BPC 1949) 0.6–1.2 mL (1 : 1 in 60% alcohol).

Tincture of Kola (BPC 1934) 1–4 mL (1 : 5 in 60% alcohol).

Pharmacological Actions

The xanthine constituents, caffeine and theobromine, are the active principles in cola. The pharmacological properties of caffeine are well documented and include stimulation of the CNS, respiratory system and skeletal muscle, cardiac stimulation, coronary dilatation, smooth muscle relaxation and diuresis.[G41] Cola-containing beverages are stated to provide active doses of caffeine.[G45]

Side-effects, Toxicity

Side-effects commonly associated with xanthine-containing beverages include sleeplessness, anxiety, tremor, palpitations and withdrawal headache.[G54]

Contra-indications, Warnings

Consumption of cola should be restricted in individuals with hypertension or cardiac disorders, because of the caffeine content.

Pregnancy and lactation It is generally recommended that caffeine consumption should be restricted during pregnancy, although conflicting reports have been documented regarding the association between birth defects and caffeine consumption. In view of this, excessive consumption of cola during pregnancy should be avoided. Caffeine is excreted in breast milk, but at concentrations too low to represent a hazard to breastfed infants.[G45] As with all xanthine-containing beverages, excessive consumption of cola by lactating mothers should be avoided.

Pharmaceutical Comment

The principal active constituent in cola is caffeine. The reputed herbal uses of cola can be attributed to the actions of caffeine, and precautions associated with other xanthine-containing beverages are applicable to cola.

References

See also General References G3, G6, G9, G11, G16, G22, G31, G36, G37, G41, G43, G48, G62 and G64.

Coltsfoot

Species (Family)

Tussilago farfara L. (Asteraceae/Compositae)

Synonym(s)

Farfara

Part(s) Used

Flower, leaf

Pharmacopoeial and Other Monographs

BHC 1992[G6]
BHP 1983[G7]
Complete German Commission E[G3]
Martindale 32nd edition[G43]
PDR for Herbal Medicines 2nd edition[G36]

Legal Category (Licensed Products)

GSL[G37]

Constituents[G2,G22,G48,G64]

Acids Caffeic acid, caffeoyltartaric acid, ferulic acid, gallic acid, *p*-hydroxybenzoic acid, and tannic acid (phenolic); malic acid and tartaric acid (aliphatic).[1]

Alkaloids Pyrrolizidine-type. Senkirkine 0.015% and senecionine (minor) (unsaturated)[2,3] and tussilagine (saturated).[4]

Carbohydrates Mucilage (water-soluble polysaccharides) 7–8% yielding various sugars following hydrolysis (e.g. arabinose, fructose, galactose, glucose, uronic acid and xylose); inulin (polysaccharide).[5]

Flavonoids Flavonols (e.g. kaempferol, quercetin) and their glycosides.[1]

Tannins Up to 17% (type unspecified).

Other constituents Bitter (glycoside), choline, paraffin (fatty acid), phytosterols (sitosterol, stigmasterol, taraxasterol), triterpene (amyrin), tussilagone (sesquiterpene)[6] and volatile oil.

Food Use

Coltsfoot is not commonly used as a food but it is listed by the Council of Europe as a source of natural food flavouring (category N4). This category indicates that although coltsfoot is permitted for use as a food flavouring, there are insufficient data available for an assessment of toxicity to be made.[G16]

Herbal Use

Coltsfoot is stated to possess expectorant, antitussive, demulcent and anticatarrhal properties. It has been used for asthma, bronchitis, laryngitis and pertussis.[G2,G7,G49,G64]

Dosage

Dried herb 0.6–2.0 g by decoction three times daily.[G6]

Liquid extract 0.6–2.0 mL (1:1 in 25% alcohol) three times daily.[G7]

Tincture 2–8 mL (1:5 in 45% alcohol) three times daily.[G7]

Syrup 2–8 mL (liquid extract 1:4 in syrup) three times daily.[G7]

Pharmacological Actions

In vitro and animal studies

Antibacterial activity has been documented for coltsfoot against various Gram-negative bacteria including *Staphylococcus aureus*, *Proteus hauseri*, *Bordetella pertussis*, *Pseudomonas aeruginosa* and *Proteus vulgaris*.[7–9]

Anti-inflammatory activity comparable to that of indomethacin, determined in Selye's experimental chronic inflammation test, has been attributed to water-soluble polysaccharides in coltsfoot.[10] Weak acute anti-inflammatory activity has been reported for coltsfoot when tested against carrageenan-induced rat paw oedema.[11,12]

Platelet-activating factor (PAF) is known to be involved in various inflammatory, respiratory and cardiovascular disorders. The aggregating action of PAF is known to be weaker if intracellular concentrations of calcium are low. A sesquiterpene, L-652,469, isolated from coltsfoot buds has been reported to be a weak inhibitor of both PAF receptor binding and calcium channel blocker binding to membrane vesicles.[13] This combination of actions was found to effectively block PAF-induced platelet aggregation. L-652,469 was also found to be active orally, inhibiting PAF-induced rat paw oedema.[13] Interestingly, L-652,469 was reported to interact with the cardiac calcium channel blocker receptor complex (dihydropyridine receptor), but was also found to be a calcium channel blocker.[13]

Tussilagone has been reported to be a potent cardiovascular and respiratory stimulant.[6,14] Dose-dependent pressor activity following intravenous injection has been observed in the cat, rat and dog.[14] The pressor effect is stated to be similar to that of dopamine, but without tachyphylaxis. A significant stimulation of respiration was also observed.[6] Cardiovascular and respiratory effects are thought to be mediated by peripheral and central mechanisms, respectively.[6]

Side-effects, Toxicity

Coltsfoot has been reported to be phototoxic in guinea-pig skin.[15]

Pyrrolizidine alkaloids with an unsaturated pyrrolizidine nucleus are known to be hepatotoxic in both animals and humans (see Comfrey). Of the pyrrolizidine alkaloids documented for coltsfoot, senecionine and senkirkine are unsaturated. Chronic hepatotoxicity has been described in rats following the incorporation of coltsfoot into their diet at concentrations ranging from 4 to 33%.[16] After 600 days, it was found that rats fed more than 4% coltsfoot had developed hepatic tumours (haemangioendothelial sarcoma) while none were observed in the control group. Furthermore, histological changes associated with pyrrolizidine alkaloid toxicity, such as centrilobular necrosis of the liver and cirrhosis, were observed in many of the rats who had ingested coltsfoot but who had not developed tumours.[16] The hepatotoxicity of coltsfoot was attributed to senkirkine, which is present at a concentration of only 0.015%, thus highlighting the dangers associated with chronic exposure to low concentrations of pyrrolizidine alkaloids.

Newborn rats have been found to be more susceptible than weanlings to the hepatotoxic effects of senkirkine despite lacking the hepatic microsomal enzymes required for the formation of the toxic pyrrolic metabolites.[17] Fatal hepatic veno-occlusive disease has been documented in a newborn infant whose mother had regularly consumed a herbal tea during pregnancy.[18] Analysis of the herbal tea revealed the presence of 10 different plants including coltsfoot and a *Senecio* species (known source of pyrrolizidine alkaloids, see Liferoot). The mother exhibited no signs of hepatic damage, suggesting an increased sensitivity of the fetal liver to pyrrolizidine alkaloid toxicity.

Pre-blooming coltsfoot flowers are reported to contain the highest concentration of alkaloids.[3] Considerable loss of both senkirkine and senecionine has been observed upon prolonged storage of the dried plant material.[3] Senkirkine and senecionine are both easily extracted into hot water and, therefore, would presumably be ingested in a herbal tea prepared from the fresh plant.[3] A cup of tea prepared from 10 g pre-blooming flowers has been estimated to contain a maximum of 70 μg senecionine and 1.4 mg senkirkine. Tea from the young leaves or mature plant would presumably contain considerably less alkaloids.[3] These concentrations are not considered to represent a health hazard compared to the known hepatotoxicity of senecionine (intravenous LD_{50} 64 mg/kg body weight, mice).[3] However, prolonged exposure to low concentrations of pyrrolizidine alkaloids has resulted in hepatotoxicity (see Comfrey).

Tussilagine LD_{50} (mice, intravenous injection) has been determined as 28.9 mg/kg.[14]

Contra-indications, Warnings

Excessive doses of coltsfoot may interfere with existing antihypertensive or cardiovascular therapy. In view of the known pyrrolizidine alkaloid content, excessive or prolonged ingestion should be avoided. In particular, herbal teas containing coltsfoot should be avoided.

Pregnancy and lactation Coltsfoot should not be taken during pregnancy or lactation in view of the toxicity associated with the pyrrolizidine alkaloid constituents. Coltsfoot is reputed to be an abortifacient.[G30]

Pharmaceutical Comment

The majority of the traditional uses associated with coltsfoot can be attributed to the mucilage content. However, coltsfoot also contains toxic pyrrolizidine alkaloids albeit at a low concentration. The risk of exposure to low concentrations of pyrrolizidine alkaloids is unclear although hepatotoxicity following prolonged exposure has been documented (see Comfrey). The regular or excessive consumption of coltsfoot, especially in the form of herbal teas, should therefore be avoided.

References

See also General References G2, G3, G6, G7, G11, G16, G18, G19, G22, G30, G31, G32, G36, G37, G43, G48, G49 and G64.

1 Didry N *et al.* Phenolic compounds from *Tussilago farfara. Ann Pharm Fr* 1980; **38**: 237–241.

2 Culvenor CCJ *et al.* The occurrence of senkirkine in *Tussilago farfara. Aust J Chem* 1976; **29**: 229–230.

3 Rosberger DF *et al.* The occurrence of senecione in *Tussilago farfara. Mitt Geb Lebensm Hyg* 1981; **72**: 432–436.

4 Röder E *et al.* Tussilagine – a new pyrrolizidine alkaloid from *Tussilago farfara. Planta Med* 1981; **41**: 99–102.

5 Haaland E. Water-soluble polysaccharides from the leaves of *Tussilago farfara* L. *Acta Chem Scand* 1969; **23**: 2546–2548.

6 Yi-Ping L, Wang Y-M. Evaluation of tussilagone: a cardiovascular-respiratory stimulant isolated from Chinese herbal medicine. *Gen Pharmacol* 1988; **19**: 261–263.

7 Didry N *et al.* Components and activity of *Tussilago farfara. Ann Pharm Fr* 1982; **40**: 75–80.

8 Didry N, Pinkas M. Antibacterial activity of fresh leaves of *Tussilago* spp. *Bull Soc Pharm (Lille)* 1982; **38**: 51–52.

9 Ieven M *et al.* Screening of higher plants for biological activities I. Antimicrobial activity. *Planta Med* 1979; **36**: 311–321.

10 Engalycheva E-I *et al.* Anti-inflammatory activity of polysaccharides obtained from *Tussilago farfara* L. *Farmatsiya* 1982; **31**: 37–40.

11 Benoit PS *et al.* Biological and phytochemical evaluation of plants. XIV. Antiinflammatory evaluation of 163 species of plants. *Lloydia* 1976; **39**: 160–171.

12 Mascolo N *et al.* Biological screening of Italian medicinal plants for anti-inflammatory activity. *Phytother Res* 1987; **1**: 28–31.

13 Hwang S-B *et al.* L-652,469 – a dual receptor antagonist of platelet activating factor and dihydropyridines from *Tussilago farfara* L. *Eur J Pharmacol* 1987; **141**: 269–281.

14 Wang Y-M. Pharmacological studies of extracts of *Tussilago farfara* L. II Effects on the cardiovascular system. *Acta Pharm Sin* 1979; **5**: 268–276.

15 Masaki H *et al.* Primary skin irritation and phototoxicity of plants extracts for cosmetic ingredients. *J Soc Cosmet Chem Jpn* 1984; **18**: 47–49.

16 Hirono I *et al.* Carcinogenic activity of coltsfoot, *Tussilago farfara* L. *Gann* 1976; **67**: 125–129.

17 Schoental R. Hepatotoxic activity of retrorsine, senkirkine and hydroxysenkirkine in newborn rats, and the role of epoxides in carcinogenesis by pyrrolizidine alkaloids and aflatoxins. *Nature* 1970; **227**: 401–402.

18 Roulet M *et al* Hepatic veno-occlusive disease in newborn infant of a woman drinking herbal tea. *J Pediatr* 1988; **112**: 433–436.

Comfrey

Species (Family)

Symphytum officinale L. (Boraginaceae)

Synonym(s)

Consolidae Radix, *Symphytum peregrinum* Ledeb., Symphytum Radix

Related species include Prickly Comfrey (*Symphytum asperum*), Quaker and Russian Comfrey (*Symphytum uplandicum*, hybrid of *S. officinale* × *S. asperum*)

Part(s) Used

Leaf, rhizome, root

Pharmacopoeial and Other Monographs

BHC 1992[G6]
BHP 1996[G9]
Complete German Commission E[G3]
Martindale 32nd edition[G43]
PDR® for Herbal Medicines 2nd edition[G36]

Legal Category (Licensed Products)

GSL (external use only)[G37]

Constituents[G2,G6,G22,G41,G48,G64]

Alkaloids Pyrrolizidine-type. 0.3%. Symphytine, symlandine, echimidine, intermidine, lycopsamine, myoscorpine, acetyllycopsamine, acetylintermidine, lasiocarpine, heliosupine, viridiflorine and echiumine.[1–5]

Carbohydrates Gum (arabinose, glucuronic acid, mannose, rhamnose, xylose); mucilage (glucose, fructose).

Tannins Pyrocatechol-type. 2.4%.

Triterpenes Sitosterol and stigmasterol (phytosterols), steroidal saponins and isobauerenol.

Other constituents Allantoin 0.75–2.55%, caffeic acid, carotene 0.63%, chlorogenic acid, choline, lithospermic acid, rosmarinic acid and silicic acid.

Food Use

Comfrey is occasionally used as an ingredient of soups and salads. It is listed by the Council of Europe as natural source of food flavouring (category N4). This category indicates that although comfrey is permitted for use as a food flavouring, insufficient data are available to assess toxicity.[G16]

Herbal Use

Comfrey is stated to possess vulnerary, cell-proliferant, astringent, antihaemorrhagic and demulcent properties. It has been used for colitis, gastric and duodenal ulcers, haematemesis, and has been applied topically for ulcers, wounds and fractures.[G2,G6,G7,G8,G49,G64]

Dosage

Dried root/rhizome 2–4 g in a decoction three times daily.[G7]

Root, liquid extract 2–4 mL (1:1 in 25% alcohol) three times daily.[G7]

Ointment symphytum root 10–15% root extractive in usual type ointment basis three times daily.[G7]

Dried leaf 2–8 g or by infusion three times daily.[G7]

Leaf, liquid extract 2–8 mL (1:1 in 25% alcohol) three times daily.[G7]

Pharmacological Actions

The classical pharmacology of pyrrolizidine alkaloids is overshadowed by the well-recognised toxicity of this class of compounds. Consequently, the majority of data documented for comfrey involve toxicity. Many useful reviews have been published on the toxicity of pyrrolizidine alkaloids in humans (*see below*).[5–11]

In vitro and animal studies

Wound-healing and analgesic activities have been documented in rats administered comfrey extract orally.[12] Percutaneous absorption of pyrrolizidine alkaloids obtained from comfrey is reported to be low in rats, with minimal conversion of the pyrrolizidine alkaloid N-oxides to the free pyrrolizidine alkaloids in the urine (reduction of the N-oxides is required before they can be metabolised into the reactive pyrrolic esters).[13,14]

Rosmarinic acid has been isolated from comfrey (S. officinale) as the main constituent with in vitro anti-inflammatory activity.[15] Biological activity was determined by inhibition of malonic dialdehyde formation in human platelets. Minor components, chlorogenic and caffeic acids, were not found to exhibit any significant activity. The pyrrolic esters have been reported to possess mild antimuscarinic activity, which is more pronounced in the non-hepatotoxic esters of saturated amino alcohols.[16] Conversely, the free amino alcohols are reported to exert indirect cholinomimetic action involving the release of acetylcholine from postganglionic sites in the guinea-pig ileum.[16]

Comfrey has been reported to stimulate the activity of the hepatic drug-metabolising enzyme aminopyrine N-demethylase in rats.[17]

A comfrey extract has been reported to enhance uterine tone in vitro.[18] The action of comfrey was reported to be weaker than that exhibited by German chamomile, calendula and plantain, but stronger than that shown by shepherd's purse, St. John's wort and uva-ursi.

Clinical studies

The antimuscarinic properties of certain pyrrolic esters have been utilised. Two non-hepatotoxic pyrrolizidine alkaloids, sarracine and platyphylline, have been used for the treatment of gastrointestinal hypermotility and peptic ulceration.[16]

Side-effects, Toxicity

Two reports of human hepatotoxicity associated with the ingestion of comfrey have been documented.[19,20] One case involved a 13-year-old boy who had been given a comfrey root preparation in conjunction with acupuncture to treat Crohn's disease.[19] The boy was diagnosed with veno-occlusive disease of the liver and the authors concluded comfrey to be the only possible causal factor of the liver disease. The second case involved a 49-year-old woman diagnosed with veno-occlusive disease.[20] She had been taking various food supplements including a herbal tea and comfrey-pepsin pills. Pyrrolizidine alkaloids were identified in both the tea (stated to contain ginseng) and the comfrey-pepsin pills. The authors estimated that over a period of six months the woman had ingested 85 mg of pyrrolizidine alkaloids, equivalent to 15 µg/kg body weight per day. This report high-

lighted the potential toxicity associated with chronic ingestion of relatively small amounts of pyrrolizidine alkaloids.

The toxicity of pyrrolizidine alkaloids is well recognised. Pyrrolizidine alkaloids with an unsaturated pyrrolizidine nucleus are metabolised in the liver to toxic pyrrole metabolites.[8] Acute toxicity results in hepatic necrosis, whereas chronic toxicity typically results in veno-occlusive disease characterised by the presence of greatly enlarged liver cells.[8,10]

Reports of human hepatotoxicity associated with pyrrolizidine alkaloid ingestion have been documented.[5,8–10,21–30] Many of these reports have resulted from crop (and subsequently flour and bread) contamination with Crotalaria, Heliotropium and Senecio species and from the use of pyrrolizidine-containing plants in medicinal 'bush' teas. In addition, pyrrolizidine alkaloid poisoning has been associated with the use of herbal teas in Europe and the United States.[20,25–27] The diagnosis of veno-occlusive disease in a newborn infant who subsequently died highlights the susceptibility of the fetus to pyrrolizidine alkaloid toxicity.[30] In this case, the mother had consumed a herbal tea as an expectorant during pregnancy. The tea, which was purchased from a pharmacy in Switzerland, was analysed and found to contain pyrrolizidine alkaloids. The mother did not exhibit any signs of hepatotoxicity.

Interestingly, liver function tests in 29 chronic comfrey users have been reported to show no abnormalities.[31]

The hepatotoxicity of pyrrolizidine alkaloids is well documented in animals.[5] In addition, carcinogenicity has been described in rats fed a diet supplemented with comfrey.[32] The mutagenicity of comfrey has been attributed to lasiocarpine,[23] which is known to be mutagenic and carcinogenic. However, other workers have reported a lack of mutagenic activity for comfrey following assessment using direct bacterial test systems (Ames), host mediated assay (Legator), liver microsomal assay and the micronucleus technique.[33,34]

Contra-indications, Warnings

In view of the hepatotoxic properties documented for the pyrrolizidine alkaloid constituents, comfrey should not be taken internally. The topical application of comfrey-containing preparations to broken skin should be avoided.

Pregnancy and lactation The safety of comfrey has not been established. In view of the toxicity associated with the alkaloid constituents, comfrey should not be taken during pregnancy or lactation.

Pharmaceutical Comment

Comfrey is characterised by its pyrrolizidine alkaloid constituents. The hepatotoxicity of these compounds is well known, and cases of human poisoning involving comfrey have been documented. Human hepatotoxicity with pyrrolizidine-containing plants is well documented, particularly following the ingestion of *Crotalaria*, *Heliotropium* and *Senecio* species. Comfrey has traditionally been used topically for treating wounds. Percutaneous absorption of pyrrolizidine alkaloids present in comfrey is reported to be low, although application of comfrey preparations to the broken skin should be avoided.

Licensed herbal products intended for internal use are not permitted to contain comfrey.

The inclusion of comfrey in products intended for topical application is permitted, provided the preparation is only applied to the unbroken skin and that its use is restricted to ten days or less at any one time.

As a result of a report by the Committee on Toxicity of Chemicals in Food to the Food Advisory Committee and the Ministry of Agriculture, Fisheries and Food, the health food trade voluntarily withdrew all products, such as tablets and capsules, and advice was issued that the root and leaves should be labelled with warnings against ingestion. It was considered that comfrey teas contained relatively low levels of pyrrolizidine alkaloids and did not need any warning labels.[35]

References

See also General References G2, G3, G6, G9, G10, G16, G18, G19, G22, G29, G31, G32, G36, G37, G41, G43, G48, G49, G56 and G64.

1 Culvenor CCJ *et al*. Structure and toxicity of the alkaloids of Russian comfrey (*Symphytum × uplandicum* Nyman), a medicinal herb and item of human diet. *Experientia* 1980; **36**: 377–379.

2 Smith LW, Culvenor CCJ. Hepatotoxic pyrrolizidine alkaloids. *J Nat Prod* 1981; **44**: 129–152.

3 Huizing HJ. Phytochemistry, systematics and biogenesis of pyrrolizidine alkaloids of *Symphytum* taxa. *Pharm Weekbl (Sci)* 1987; **9**: 185–187.

4 Mattocks AR. Toxic pyrrolizidine alkaloids in comfrey. *Lancet* 1980; **ii**: 1136–1137.

5 Pyrrolizidine alkaloids. *Environmental Health Criteria 80*. Geneva: WHO, 1988.

6 Abbott PJ. Comfrey: assessing the low-dose health risk. *Med J Aust* 1988; **149**: 678–682.

7 Awang DVC. Comfrey. *Can Pharm J* 1987; **120**: 101–104.

8 McLean EK. The toxic actions of pyrrolizidine (Senecio) alkaloids. *Pharmacol Rev* 1970; **22**: 429–483.

9 Huxtable RJ. Herbal teas and toxins: novel aspects of pyrrolizidine poisoning in the United States. *Perspect Biol Med* 1980; **24**: 1–14.

10 Mattocks AR. *Chemistry and Toxicology of Pyrrolizidine Alkaloids*. London: Academic Press, 1986.

11 Jadhav SJ *et al*. Pyrrolizidine alkaloids: A review. *J Food Sci Technol* 1982; **19**: 87–93.

12 Goldman RS *et al*. Wound healing and analgesic effect of crude extracts of *Symphytum officinale*. *Fitoterapia* 1985; **6**: 323–329.

13 Brauchli J *et al*. Pyrrolizidine alkaloids from *Symphytum offinale* L. and their percutaneous absorption in rats. *Experientia* 1982; **38**: 1085–1087.

14 Brauchli J *et al*. Pyrrolizidine alkaloids in *Symphytum officinale* L. and their dermal absorption in rats. *Experientia* 1981; **37**: 667.

15 Gracza L *et al*. Biochemical-pharmacological investigations of medicinal agents of plant origin, I: Isolation of rosmarinic acid from *Symphytum officinale* L. and its anti-inflammatory activity in an *in-vitro* model. *Arch Pharm (Weinheim)* 1985; **318**: 1090–1095.

16 Culvenor CCJ. Pyrrolizidine alkaloids: some aspects of the Australian involvement. *Trends Pharmacol Sci* 1985; **6**: 18–22.

17 Garrett BJ *et al*. Consumption of poisonous plants (*Senecio jacobaea*, *Symphytum officinale*, *Pteridium aquilinum*, *Hypericum perforatum*) by rats: Chronic toxicity, mineral metabolism, and hepatic drug-metabolizing enzymes. *Toxicol Lett* 1982; **10**: 183–188.

18 Shipochliev T. Extracts from a group of medicinal plants enhancing the uterine tonus. *Vet Med Nauki* 1981; **18**: 94–98.

19 Weston CFM *et al*. Veno-occlusive disease of the liver secondary to ingestion of comfrey. *Br Med J* 1987; **295**: 183.

20 Ridker PM *et al*. Hepatic venocclusive disease associated with the consumption of pyrrolizidine-containing dietary supplements. *Gastroenterology* 1985; **88**: 1050–1054.

21 Anderson C. Comfrey toxicity in perspective. *Lancet* 1981; **i**: 944.

22 Huxtable RJ *et al*. Toxicity of comfrey-pepsin preparations. *N Engl J Med* 1986; **315**: 1095.

23 Furmanowa M *et al*. Mutagenic effects of aqueous extracts of *Symphytum officinale* L. and of its alkaloidal fractions. *J Appl Toxicol* 1983; **3**: 127–130.

24 Ridker PM, McDermott WV. Comfrey herb tea and hepatic veno-occlusive disease. *Lancet* 1989; **i**: 657–658.

25 Lyford CL *et al*. Hepatic veno-occlusive disease originating in Ecuador. *Gastroenterology* 1976; **70**: 105–108.

26 Kumana CR *et al*. Herbal tea induced hepatic veno-occlusive disease: quantification of toxic alkaloid exposure in adults. *Gut* 1985; **26**: 101–104.

27 Stillman AE *et al*. Hepatic veno-occlusive disease due to pyrrolizidine (Senecio) poisoning in Arizona. *Gastroenterology* 1977; **73**: 349–352.

28 McGee JO'D *et al*. A case of veno-occlusive disease of the liver in Britain associated with herbal tea consumption. *J Clin Pathol* 1976; **29**: 788–794.

29 Datta DV *et al*. Herbal medicines and veno-occlusive disease in India. *Postgrad Med J* 1978; **54**: 511–515.

30 Roulet M *et al*. Hepatic veno-occlusive disease in newborn infant of a woman drinking herbal tea. *J Pediatr* 1988; **112**: 433–436.

31 Anderson PC, McLean AEM. Comfrey and liver damage. *Hum Toxicol* 1989; **8**: 55–74.

32 Hirono I *et al*. Carcinogenic activity of *Symphytum officinale*. *J Natl Cancer Inst* 1978; **61**: 865–869.

33 Lim-Sylianco CY *et al*. Mutagenicity studies of aqueous extracts from leaves of comfrey (*Symphytum officinale* Linn). *NRCP Res Bull* 1977; **32**: 178–191.

34 White RD *et al*. An evaluation of acetone extracts from six plants in the Ames mutagenicity test. *Toxicol Lett* 1983; **15**: 23–31.

35 Food Safety Directive. FSD Information Bulletin May 1993; 2, and Food Sense Factsheet No. 14, May 1993.

Corn Silk

Species (Family)

Zea mays L. (Gramineae)

Synonym(s)

Stigma Maydis, Zea

Part(s) Used

Stigma, style

Pharmacopoeial and Other Monographs

BHC 1992[G6]
BHP 1996[G9]
PDR for Herbal Medicines 2nd edition[G36]

Legal Category (Licensed Products)

Corn silk is not included in the GSL.[G37]

Constituents[G2,G6,G40,G41,G44,G49,G64]

Amines 0.05%. Type not specified, although hordenine is listed for the genus *Zea*.

Fixed oils 1.85–2.25%. Contain glycerides of linoleic, oleic, palmitic and stearic acids.

Saponins 3% (unspecified).

Tannins Up to 11.5–13% (unspecified).

Other constituents Allantoin, bitter glycosides (1%), cryptoxanthin, cyanogenetic compound (unidentified),[1] flavone, gum, phytosterols (e.g. sitosterol, stigmasterol), pigments, resin, vitamins (C and K).

Food Use

Corn silk is listed as a natural source of food flavouring (category N2). This category indicates that corn silk can be added to foodstuffs in small quantities, with a possible limitation of an active principle (as yet unspecified) in the final product. In the USA, corn silk is listed as GRAS (Generally Recognised As Safe).[G41] The fruits are classified as category N1 with no restriction on their use.[G16] Corn (maize) oil and flour are commonly used in cooking.

Herbal Use

Corn silk is stated to possess diuretic and stone-reducing properties. It has been used for cystitis, urethritis, nocturnal enuresis, prostatitis, and specifically for acute or chronic inflammation of the urinary system.[G2,G6,G7,G8,G64]

Dosage

Dried style/stigma 4–8 g or by infusion three times daily.[G6,G7]

Liquid Extract of Maize Stigmas (BPC 1923) 4–8 mL.

Tincture 5–15 mL (1 : 5 in 25% alcohol) three times daily.[G6,G7]

Syrup of Maize Stigmas (BPC 1923) 8–15 mL.

Pharmacological Actions

In vitro and animal studies

Corn silk is stated to possess cholagogue, diuretic, hypoglycaemic, and hypotensive activities in laboratory animals.[2,G41] Utilising aqueous extracts, a methanol-insoluble fraction has been reported to exhibit diuretic activity in rabbits,[G41] and an isolated crystalline component has been documented to have a hypotensive action and to stimulate uterine contraction in rabbits.[3] The latter two actions were thought to involve a cholinergic mechanism. The action of corn silk extract on experimental periodontolysis in hamsters has been documented.[4]

Cryptoxanthin is stated to possess vitamin A activity,[G48] and tannins are known to possess astringent properties.

Clinical studies

It has been stated that an aqueous extract is strongly diuretic in humans,[G41] and that clinical studies have indicated corn silk to be effective in kidney and other diseases.[G41] No further information on human studies was located to support these statements.

Side-effects, Toxicity

Allergic reactions including contact dermatitis and urticaria have been documented for corn silk, its pollen and for starch derived from corn silk.[G51] Cornstarch is considered to be a known allergen.[G51] The toxicity of a methanol-insoluble fraction of an aqueous corn silk extract has been reported to be low in rabbits. The effective intravenous dose for a diuretic action was documented as 1.5 mg/kg body weight compared to the lethal intravenous dose of 250 mg/kg.[G41] Corn silk contains an unidentified toxic principle,[1,2] and is listed as being capable of producing a cyanogenetic compound.[1]

Contra-indications, Warnings

Corn silk may cause an allergic reaction in susceptible individuals. Excessive doses may interfere with hypoglycaemic drug therapy (*in vivo* hypoglycaemic activity has been documented) or with hypertensive or hypotensive therapy (*in vivo* hypotensive activity reported), and prolonged use may result in hypokalaemia because of the diuretic action.

Pregnancy and lactation Corn silk has been documented to stimulate uterine contractions in rabbits. In view of this, doses of corn silk greatly exceeding amounts used in foods should not be taken during pregnancy or lactation.

Pharmaceutical Comment

Limited information is available on the constituents of corn silk. Extracts have been reported to exhibit diuretic actions in both humans and animals, thus justifying the reputed herbal uses. However, no additional data were located to support these reported actions. In view of the lack of toxicity data, excessive use of corn silk should be avoided.

References

See also General References G2, G6, G9, G10, G16, G36, G37, G40, G41, G48, G49, G51 and G64.

1 Seigler DS. Plants of the northeastern United States that produce cyanogenic compounds. *Economic Bot* 1976; **30**: 395–407.
2 Bever BO, Zahnd GR. Plants with oral hypoglycaemic action. *Q J Crude Drug Res* 1979; **17**: 139–196.
3 Hahn SJ. Pharmacological action of Maydis stigma. *K'at'ollik Taehak Uihakpu Nonmunjip* 1973; **25**: 127–141.
4 Chaput A *et al*. Action of *Zea mays* L. unsaponifiable titre extract on experimental periodontolysis in hamsters. *Med Hyg (Geneve)* 1972; **30**: 1470–1471.

Couchgrass

Species (Family)

Agropyron repens (L.) Beauv. (Gramineae)

Synonym(s)

Agropyron, Dogs Grass, Quackgrass, Triticum, *Triticum repens* L., Twitchgrass

Part(s) Used

Rhizome

Pharmacopoeial and Other Monographs

BHP 1996[G9]
BP 2001[G15]
Complete German Commission E[G3]
Martindale 32nd edition[G43]
PDR for Herbal Medicines 2nd edition[G36]
Ph Eur 2002[G28]
WHO volume 1 1999[G63]

Legal Category (Licensed Products)

GSL (Agropyron)[G37]

Constituents[G2,G7,G40,G41,G53,G64]

Carbohydrates Fructose, glucose, inositol, mannitol, mucilaginous substances (10%), pectin, triticin.

Cyanogenetic glycosides Unspecified.

Flavonoids Tricin and other unidentified flavonoids.

Saponins No details documented.

Volatile oils 0.05%. Agropyrene (95%). Presence of agropyrene has been disputed,[1] with the oil reported to consist mainly of the monoterpenes carvacrol, *trans*-anethole, carvone, thymol, menthol, menthone and *p*-cymene and three sesquiterpenes.

Other constituents Fixed oil, vanillin glucoside.

Food Use

Couchgrass is listed by the Council of Europe as a natural source of food flavouring (category N2). This category indicates that couchgrass can be added to foodstuffs in small quantities, with a possible limitation of an active principle (as yet unspecified) in the final product.[G16] In the USA, couchgrass is listed as GRAS (Generally Recognised As Safe).[G41]

Herbal Use

Couchgrass is stated to possess diuretic properties. It has been used for cystitis, urethritis, prostatitis, benign prostatic hypertrophy, renal calculus, lithuria, and specifically for cystitis with irritation or inflammation of the urinary tract.[G2,G7,G64]

Dosage

Dried rhizome 4–8 g or in decoction three times daily.[G7]

Liquid extract 4–8 mL (1:1 in 25% alcohol) three times daily.[G7]

Tincture 5–15 mL (1:5 in 40% alcohol) three times daily.[G7]

Pharmacological Actions

In vitro and animal studies

Couchgrass is stated to exhibit diuretic and sedative activities in rats and mice, respectively.[G41] Broad antibiotic activity has been documented for agropyrene and its oxidation product.[G41] An ethanolic extract was found to exhibit only weak inhibition (14%) of carrageenan-induced inflammation in the rat paw.[2]

Couchgrass has been reported to be phytotoxic with flavonoid components implicated as the active constituents.[3]

Side-effects, Toxicity

None documented for couchgrass. An unspecified cyanogenetic glycoside has been reported as a constituent of couchgrass, although no further details were located.[G7]

Contra-indications, Warnings

In view of its reputed diuretic action, excessive or prolonged use of couchgrass should be avoided since this may result in hypokalaemia.

Pregnancy and lactation In view of the limited pharmacological and toxicological data, the use of couchgrass during pregnancy and lactation should be avoided.

Pharmaceutical Comment

Limited chemical data are available for couchgrass and little scientific evidence was located to justify the traditional herbal uses. Agropyrene is regarded as the main active principle in couchgrass on account of its antibiotic effect, although the presence of agropyrene in the volatile oil has been disputed.[1] In view of the lack of toxicity data, excessive ingestion should be avoided.

References

See also General References G2, G3, G9, G10, G15, G16, G31, G36, G37, G40, G41, G43, G48, G53 and G64.

1 Boesel R, Schilcher H. Composition of the essential oil of *Agropyrum repens* rhizome. *Planta Med* 1989; **55**: 399–400.
2 Mascolo N. Biological screening of Italian medicinal plants for anti-inflammatory activity. *Phytother Res* 1987; **1**: 28–29.
3 Weston LA *et al.* Isolation, characterization and activity of phytotoxic compounds from quackgrass [*Agropyron repens* (L.) Beauv.]. *J Chem Ecol* 1987; **13**: 403–421.

Cowslip

Species (Family)

Primula veris L. (Primulaceae)

Synonym(s)

Paigle, Peagle, Primula, *Primula officinalis* (L.) Hill.

Part(s) Used

Flower

Pharmacopoeial and Other Monographs

BHP 1983[G7]
Complete German Commission E (Primrose flower)[G3]
ESCOP 1997[G52]
PDR for Herbal Medicines 2nd edition[G36]

Legal Category (Licensed Products)

GSL[G37]

Constituents[G2,G40,G49,G59,G62,G64]

Carbohydrates Arabinose, galactose, galacturonic acid, glucose, rhamnose, xylose and water-soluble polysaccharide (6.2–6.6%).

Flavonoids Apigenin, isorhamnetin, kaempferol, luteolin and quercetin.[1]

Phenols Glycosides primulaveroside (primulaverin) and primveroside.

Quinones Primin and other quinone compounds.

Saponins Primula acid in sepals but saponins absent from other parts of the flower.

Tannins Condensed (e.g. proanthocyanidin B2), pseudotannins (e.g. epicatechin, epigallocatechin).[1]

Other constituents Silicic acid and volatile oil (0.1–0.25%).

Other plant parts Saponins have been documented for the underground parts.[1] 'Primulic acid' is a collective term for the saponin mixture.[2] Primulic

acid A glycoside (5–10%) yields primulagenin A as aglycone together with arabinose, galactose, glucose, glucuronic acid, rhamnose and xylose.[3,4] The saponin content of the roots is stated to peak at two years.[5] After five years of storage the saponin content was reported to have decreased by 45%.

Food Use

Cowslip is not commonly used in foods. A related species, *Primula eliator*, is listed by the Council of Europe as a natural source of food flavouring (category N2). This category indicates that *Primula eliator* can be added to foodstuffs, provided that the concentration of coumarin does not exceed 2 mg/kg.[G16] Coumarins, however, are not documented as constituents of *Primula veris*, the subject of this monograph.

Herbal Use

Cowslip is stated to possess sedative, antispasmodic, hypnotic, mild diuretic, expectorant and mild aperient properties. It has been used for insomnia, nervous excitability, hysteria and specifically for anxiety states associated with restlessness and irritability.[G2,G7,G64]

Dosage

Dried flowers 1–2 g as an infusion three times daily.[G7]

Liquid extract 1–2 mL (1:1 in 25% alcohol) three times daily.[G7]

Pharmacological Actions

In vitro and animal studies

The saponin fraction has been reported to cause an initial hypotension followed by a long-lasting hypertension in anaesthetised animals.[6]

In vitro, the saponins have been documented to inhibit prostaglandin (PG) synthetase, but to a lesser extent than aspirin because of insignificant protein binding; to exhibit a slight anti-inflammatory effect against carrageenan rat paw oedema; to contract isolated rabbit ileum; and to possess analgesic and antigranulation activity.[6]

Flavonoid and tannin constituents have been documented for cowslip. A variety of activities has been reported for flavonoids including anti-inflammatory and antispasmodic effects. The tannins are known to be astringent.

Side-effects, Toxicity

Allergic contact reactions to related *Primula* species have been documented; quinone compounds are stated to be the allergenic principles with primin described as a strong contact allergen.[7] Two positive patch test reactions to cowslip have been recorded, although allergenicity was not proven.[G51] An LD$_{50}$ value (mice, intraperitoneal injection) for the saponin fraction is documented as 24.5 mg/kg body weight compared to a value of 9.5 mg/kg for reparil (aescin). Haemolytic activity has been reported for the saponins, and an aqueous extract of cowslip is stated to contain saponins that are toxic to fish. Saponins are stated to be irritant to the gastrointestinal tract.

The toxicity of cowslip seems to be associated with the saponin constituents. However, these compounds have only been documented for the underground plant parts, and not for the flowers which are the main plant parts used in the UK.

Contra-indications, Warnings

Cowslip may cause an allergic reaction in sensitive individuals. Excessive doses may interfere with hypo- or hypertensive therapy or cause gastrointestinal irritation.

Pregnancy and lactation The safety of cowslip has not been established. In view of the lack of toxicity data, use of cowslip during pregnancy and lactation should be avoided.

Pharmaceutical Comment

The chemistry of cowslip is not well documented and it is unclear whether saponins reported as constituents of the underground plant parts are also present in the flowers. Little pharmacological information has been documented to justify the herbal uses of cowslip. In view of the lack of toxicity data, excessive use of cowslip should be avoided.

References

See also General References G2, G3, G7, G15, G16, G36, G37, G40, G44, G49, G51, G52, G59, G62 and G64.

1 Karl C *et al.* Die flavonoide in den blüten von Primula officinalis. *Planta Med* 1981; **41**: 96–99.
2 Grecu L, Cucu V. Saponine aus *Primula officinalis* und *Primula elatior*. *Planta Med* 1975; **27**: 247–253.
3 Kartnig T, Ri CY. Dünnschichtchromatographische untersuchungen an den zuckerkomponenten der saponine aus den wurzeln von *Primula veris* und *P. elatior*. *Planta Med* 1973; **23**: 379–380.
4 Grecu L, Cucu V. Primulic acid aglycone from the roots of *Primula officinalis*. *Farmacia (Bucharest)* 1975; **23**: 167–170.
5 Jentzsch K *et al.* Saponin level in the radix of *Primula veris*. *Sci Pharm* 1973; **41**: 162–165.
6 Cebo B *et al.* Pharmacological properties of saponin fractions from Polish crude drugs. *Herb Pol* 1976; **22**: 154–162.
7 Hausen BM. On the occurrence of the contact allergen primin and other quinoid compounds in species of the family of Primulaceae. *Arch Dermatol Res* 1978; **261**: 311–321.

Cranberry

Species (Family)

Vaccinium macrocarpon Ait, *Vaccinium oxycoccus* (Ericaceae)

Synonym(s)

Large Cranberry (*V. macrocarpon*) is the species grown for commercial purposes.[1] *V. oxycoccus* is European Cranberry, Mossberry and Small Cranberry.

Part(s) Used

Fruit (whole berries)

Pharmacopoeial and Other Monographs

Martindale 32nd edition[G43]

Legal Category (Licensed Products)

Cranberry is not included in the GSL.[G37]

Constituents

Acids Citric, malic, quinic and benzoic acids are present.[2]

Carbohydrates Fructose and oligosaccharides.

Phenolics Anthocyanins and proanthocyanidins.

Other constituents Trace glycoside has been isolated from *V. oxycoccus*.[3] Cranberries are also a good source of fibre. Cranberry juice cocktail contains more carbohydrate than do products (i.e. soft or hard gelatin capsules) based on cranberry powder (prepared from rapidly dried fruits), whereas the latter contain more fibre.[2] Alkaloids (N-methylazatricyclo type) have been isolated from the leaves.[4]

Food Use[G32]

Cranberries are commonly used in foods;[5] cranberry juice cocktail (containing approximately 25% cranberry juice) is widely available.[2,5] Cranberry is listed by the Council of Europe as a natural source of food flavouring (fruit: category 1) (*see* Appendix 23).[G17]

Herbal Use[G32]

Cranberry juice and crushed cranberries have a long history of use in the treatment and prevention of urinary tract infections.[1] Traditionally, cranberries have also been used for blood disorders, stomach ailments, liver problems, vomiting, loss of appetite, scurvy and in the preparation of wound dressings.[5]

Dosage

The doses used in clinical trials of cranberry for prevention of urinary tract infections have been variable. One study used 300 mL cranberry juice cocktail (containing 30% cranberry concentrate) daily for six months.[6]

Pharmacological Actions

Documented activity for cranberry is mainly of its use in the prevention and treatment of urinary tract infections; its role in urinary tract infection has been reviewed.[1]

Initially it was thought that the antibacterial effect of cranberry juice was due to its ability to acidify urine and, therefore, to inhibit bacterial growth. However, recent work has focused on the effects of cranberry in inhibiting bacterial adherence and on determining anti-adhesion agents in cranberry juice. Bacterial adherence to mucosal surfaces is considered to be an important step in the development of urinary tract infections;[7] it is facilitated by fimbriae (proteinaceous fibres on the bacterial cell wall) which produce adhesins that attach to specific receptors on uroepithelial cells.[8]

In vitro and animal studies

In *in vitro* studies using human urinary tract isolates of *Escherichia coli*, cranberry cocktail (which contains fructose and vitamin C in addition to cranberry juice) inhibited bacterial adherence to uroepithelial cells by 75% or more in over 60% of the clinical isolates.[9] In addition, urine from mice fed cranberry juice significantly inhibited *E. coli* adherence to uroepithelial cells when compared with urine from control mice.[9] However, these studies did not define the bacteria tested in terms of the type of fimbriae they might have expressed (specific fimbriae mediate bacterial adherence to cells).

Irreversible inhibition of adherence of urinary isolates of *E. coli* expressing type 1 and type P fimbriae has been demonstrated with cranberry juice cocktail.[10] It was thought that fructose might be responsible for the inhibition of type 1 fimbriae[10] and an unidentified high molecular weight substance responsible for type P fimbriae inhibition.[11] Further *in vitro* studies in which cranberry juice was added to the growth medium of P-fimbriated *E. coli* duplicated immediate inhibition of adherence, but also showed the loss of fimbriae with cellular elongation after long-term exposure; such changed bacteria are unable to adhere to urothelium.[12]

Proanthocyanidins extracted from cranberries have been shown to inhibit the adherence of P-fimbriated *E. coli* to uroepithelial cell surfaces at concentrations of 10–50 µg/mL, suggesting that proanthocyanidins may be important for the stated effects of cranberry in urinary tract infections.[13]

The effects of a high molecular weight constituent of cranberry juice on adhesion of bacterial strains found in the human gingival crevice have also been investigated.[14] A non-dialysable material derived from cranberry juice concentrate used at concentrations of 0.6–2.5 mg/mL reversed the interspecies adhesion of 58% of 84 bacterial pairs. Gram-negative dental plaque bacteria appeared to be more sensitive to the inhibitory effects of the cranberry constituent on adhesion.[14]

Crude extracts of cranberry have been reported to exhibit potential anticarcinogenic activity *in vitro* as demonstrated by inhibition of the induction of ornithine decarboxylase (ODC) by the tumour promoter phorbol 12-myristate 13-acetate (TPA).[15] The greatest activity appeared to be in the polymeric proanthocyanidin fraction which had an IC_{50} for ODC activity of 6.0 µg. The anthocyanidin fraction and the ethyl acetate extract were either inactive or relatively weak inhibitors of ODC activity.

A cranberry extract with a polyphenolic content of 1548 mg gallic acid equivalents per litre inhibited low-density lipoprotein (LDL) oxidation *in vitro*.[16]

Cranberry juice has demonstrated marked *in vitro* antifungal activity against *Epidermophyton floccosum* and against several *Microsporum* and *Trichophyton* species, but had no effect against *Candida albicans*.[17] Benzoic acid and/or other low molecular weight constituents of cranberry juice were reported to be responsible for the fungistatic action.

Clinical studies

Clinical trials investigating the use of cranberries for the treatment[18] and prevention[19] of urinary tract infections have been subject to Cochrane systematic reviews; both of these systematic reviews sought to include all randomised or quasi-randomised controlled trials.[18,19]

Prevention of urinary tract infections Four trials[6,20–22] were included in a systematic review of cranberries for prevention of urinary tract infections; three trials compared the effectiveness of cranberry juice versus placebo or water and one trial compared cranberry capsules with placebo.[19] Three of the four trials reported beneficial effects for cranberry compared with placebo on at least one of the outcomes (number of symptomatic or asymptomatic urinary tract infections, side-effects, adherence to therapy). However, the methodological quality of the trials was found to be poor and the reliability of the results questionable. It was stated that 'on the basis of the available evidence, cranberry juice cannot be recommended for the prevention of urinary tract infections in susceptible populations'.[19]

The largest study of cranberry juice for the prevention of urinary tract infections was a double-blind, placebo-controlled trial involving 153 women (mean age 78.5 years) randomised to receive 300 mL cranberry juice cocktail ($n = 72$) or an indistinguishable placebo ($n = 81$) daily for six months.[6] The odds of experiencing bacteriuria with pyuria were significantly lower in cranberry-treated subjects than in those who received a placebo beverage ($p = 0.004$). A randomised, controlled, crossover study was conducted involving 38 persons (mean age 81 years) who had had hospital treatment and were waiting to be transferred to a nursing home.[21] Subjects received cranberry juice (15 mL) mixed with water or water alone twice daily for four weeks before crossing over to the alternative regimen. Seventeen participants completed the study and, of the seven from whom data were suitable for comparison, there were fewer occurrences of bacteriuria during the period of treatment with cranberry juice.[21]

The role of cranberry in the prevention of urinary tract infections in younger women has been explored in a randomised, double-blind, placebo-controlled, crossover trial involving 19 non-pregnant, sexually active women aged 18–45 years.[22] Participants received capsules containing 400 mg cranberry solids daily (exact dose not stated) or placebo for three months before crossing over to the alternative regimen. Ten subjects completed the six-month study period. Of the 21 incidents of urinary tract infection recorded among these participants, significantly fewer occurred during periods of treatment with cranberry than with placebo ($p < 0.005$).[22]

A randomised, physician-blind, crossover study investigated the efficacy of cranberry cocktail (30% cranberry concentrate) (15 mL/kg/day) for six months in 40 children (age range 1.4–18 years, mean age 9.35 years) with neuropathic bladder and managed by clean intermittent catheterisation; water was used as a control.[20] No benefit was reported for cranberry compared with control.

A randomised, double-blind, placebo-controlled, crossover trial of the effects of consumption of cranberry concentrate on the prevention of bacteriuria and symptomatic urinary tract infection has been carried out in children (n = 15) with neurogenic bladder receiving clean intermittent catheterisation.[23] Children drank 2 oz of cranberry concentrate or placebo daily for three months before changing to the alternative regimen. At the end of the study, the number of urinary tract infections occurring under each regimen was identical (n = 3). There was no significant difference between cranberry treatment and placebo with regard to the number of collected urine samples testing positively for a pathogen (75% of samples for both cranberry and placebo) (p = 0.97). It was concluded that cranberry concentrate had no effect on the prevention of bacteriuria in the population studied.[23]

Treatment of urinary tract infections Although several trials investigating the effectiveness of cranberry juice and cranberry products for treating urinary tract infections were found, none of these trials met all the inclusion criteria for systematic review.[18] Two of the studies found[24,25] did report a beneficial effect with cranberry products, although both contained methodological flaws and no firm conclusions can be drawn from these studies.[18] Thus, it was stated that 'at the present time, there is no evidence to suggest that cranberry juice or other cranberry products are effective in treating urinary tract infections' (*see* Pharmaceutical Comment).[18]

Other studies Early studies involving the administration of large amounts of cranberry juice to human subjects reported reductions in mean urinary pH values.[26,27] A crossover study involving eight subjects with multiple sclerosis reported that administration of cranberry juice and ascorbic acid was more effective than orange juice and ascorbic acid in acidifying the urine. However, neither treatment consistently maintained a urinary pH lower than 5.5, the pH previously determined as necessary for maintaining bacteriostatic urine.[28] Inhibition of bacterial adherence (*see* In vitro and animal studies) has been observed with urine from 22 human subjects who had ingested cranberry cocktail 1–3 hours previously.[9] Protection against bacterial adhesion has also been reported in a study involving urine collected from ten healthy male volunteers who had ingested

water, ascorbic acid (500 mg twice daily for 2.5 days) or cranberry (400 mg three times daily for 2.5 days) supplements.[29] Urine samples were used to determine uropathogen adhesion to silicone rubber in a parallel plate flow chamber; urine obtained after ascorbic acid or cranberry supplementation reduced the initial deposition rates and numbers of adherent *E. coli* and *Enterococcus faecalis*, but not *Pseudomonas aeruginosa*, *Staphylococcus epidermidis* or *C. albicans*.

Other preliminary studies have explored the use of cranberry juice in reducing urine odours,[30] in improving peristomal skin conditions in urostomy patients[31] and in reducing mucus production in patients who have undergone entero-uroplasty.[32]

The ingestion of cranberry juice by subjects with hypochlorhydria due to omeprazole treatment or atrophic gastritis has been shown to result in increased protein-bound vitamin B_{12} absorption, although the clinical benefit of ingesting cranberry juice along with a meal (i.e. with the buffering action of food) remains to be determined.[33] Possible mechanisms by which the ingestion of an acidic drink such as cranberry juice could result in improved protein-bound vitamin B_{12} absorption include increased release of vitamin B_{12} from protein by direct action of acid on the vitamin B_{12}–protein bond and a pH-sensitive bacterial binding activity of vitamin B_{12} that is altered in an acidic environment.[33]

Side-effects, Toxicity

None documented for cranberry, although diarrhoea is possible if large quantities are consumed.[G31] One study has reported that no subjects withdrew because of undesirable side-effects,[22] although this study involved only a small number (n = 19) of patients. A systematic review of cranberry products for the prevention of urinary tract infections reported that the drop-out rates in the four studies included [6,20–22] were high (20–55%).[19] In one of these studies, of 17 withdrawals during cranberry treatment (a further two occurred during the control period), nine participants gave the taste of cranberry as the reason for withdrawal.[20]

It has been claimed that ingesting large amounts of cranberry juice may result in the formation of uric acid or oxalate stones secondary to a constantly acidic urine and because of the high oxalate content of cranberry juice.[1] However, it has also been stated that the role of cranberry juice as a urinary acidifier has not been well established.[34] The use of cranberry juice in preventing the formation of stones which develop in alkaline urine, such as those comprising magnesium ammonium phosphate and calcium carbonate, has been described.[26]

Contra-indications, Warnings

The calorific content of cranberry juice should be borne in mind. Patients with diabetes who wish to use cranberry juice should be advised to use sugar-free preparations. Patients using cranberry juice should be advised to drink sufficient fluids in order to ensure adequate urine flow.[G31] Although a constituent of cranberry juice has been reported to have potential for altering the subgingival microbiota, some commercially available cranberry juice cocktails may not be suitable for oral hygiene purposes because of their high dextrose and fructose content.[14]

It has been stated that cranberry should be used with caution in patients with benign prostatic hypertrophy or urinary obstruction, because there is the theoretical possibility that cranberry may enhance the elimination of drugs excreted in urine.[G31] Interference with dipstick tests for glucose and haemoglobin in urine has been reported in a study involving 28 patients who had drunk 100 or 150 mL of low-sugar or regular cranberry juice daily for seven weeks;[35] ascorbic acid in cranberry juice was reported to be the component responsible for interference resulting in negative test results.

Pregnancy and lactation   There are no known problems with the use of cranberry during pregnancy. Doses of cranberry greatly exceeding the amounts used in foods should not be taken during pregnancy and lactation.

Pharmaceutical Comment

Limited chemical information is available for cranberry. Documented *in vitro* and animal studies provide supporting evidence for a mechanism of action for cranberry in preventing urinary tract infections. However, little is known about the specific active constituent(s); proanthocyanidins have been reported to be important.[13]

Preliminary clinical trials of cranberry for the prevention of urinary tract infections have generally been uncontrolled and/or involved only small numbers of patients. The validity of the results of a controlled trial involving relatively large numbers of (female only) patients[6] was questioned because of methodological shortcomings in the study design, particularly the method of randomisation.[36,37] Other controlled studies claiming to involve random assignment to treatment[20–22] either did not employ true randomisation[21] or the method of randomisation was not stated.[20,22] In addition, these four controlled studies[6,20–22] differed in the formulations of cranberry, doses and treatment periods used. Therefore, clinical studies do not provide compelling evidence for the efficacy of cranberry in the prevention of urinary tract infections, nor do they provide evidence that it is not efficacious. However, the findings do indicate that the area warrants further investigation. Cochrane systematic reviews of cranberry for the treatment and prevention of urinary tract infections have stated that, at present, there is no reliable evidence to suggest that cranberry juice or other cranberry products are effective.[18,19] It has also been stated that properly randomised, double-blind, placebo-controlled, parallel group trials using appropriate outcome measures are needed in order to determine the efficacy of cranberry products in the prevention and treatment of urinary tract infections.[18,19] Prevention trials should be of at least 6-months' duration in order to take into account the natural course of the illness.[19]

Patients wishing to use cranberry for urinary tract infections should be advised to consult a pharmacist, doctor or other suitably trained health care professional for advice.

References

See also General References G31 and G43.

1   Kingwatanakul P, Alon US. Cranberries and urinary tract infection. *Child Hosp Q* 1996; **8**: 69–72.
2   Hughes BG, Lawson LD. Nutritional content of cranberry products. *Am J Hosp Pharm* 1989; **46**: 1129.
3   Jankowski K, Paré JRJ. Trace glycoside from cranberries (*Vaccinium oxycoccus*). *J Nat Prod* 1983; **46**: 190–193.
4   Jankowski K. Alkaloids of cranberries V. *Experientia* 1973; **29**: 1334–1335.
5   Siciliano AA. Cranberry. *Herbalgram* 1996; **38**: 51–54.
6   Avorn J *et al.* Reduction of bacteriuria and pyuria after ingestion of cranberry juice. *JAMA* 1994; **271**: 751–754.
7   Reid G, Sobel JD. Bacterial adherence in the pathogenesis of urinary tract infection: a review. *Rev Infect Dis* 1987; **9**: 470–487.
8   Beachey EH. Bacterial adherence: adhesin–receptor interactions mediating the attachment of bacteria to mucosal surface. *J Infect Dis* 1981; **143**: 325–345.
9   Sobota AE. Inhibition of bacterial adherence by cranberry juice: potential use for the treatment of urinary tract infections. *J Urol* 1984; **131**: 1013–1016.
10 Zafiri D *et al.* Inhibitory activity of cranberry juice

on adherence of type 1 and type P fimbriated *Escherichia coli* to eucaryotic cells. *Antimicrob Agents Chemother* 1989; **33**: 92–98.

11 Ofek I *et al*. Anti-*Escherichia coli* adhesin activity of cranberry and blueberry juices. *Adv Exp Med Biol* 1996; **408**: 179–183.

12 Ahuja S *et al*. Loss of fimbrial adhesion with the addition of *Vaccinium macrocarpon* to the growth medium of P-fimbriated *Escherichia coli*. *J Urol* 1998; **159**: 559–562.

13 Howell AB *et al*. Inhibition of the adherence of P fimbriated *Escherichia coli* to uroepithelial-cell surfaces by proanthocyanidin extracts from cranberries. *N Engl J Med* 1998; **339**: 1085–1086.

14 Weiss EI *et al*. Inhibiting interspecies coaggregation of plaque bacteria with a cranberry juice constituent. *J Am Dent Assoc* 1998; **129**: 1719–1723.

15 Bomser J *et al*. *In vitro* anticancer activity of fruit extracts from *Vaccinium* species. *Planta Med* 1996; **62**: 212–216.

16 Wilson T *et al*. Cranberry extract inhibits low density lipoprotein oxidation. *Life Sci* 1998; **62**: 381–386.

17 Swartz JH, Medrek TF. Antifungal properties of cranberry juice. *Appl Microbiol* 1968; **16**: 1524–1527.

18 Jepson RG *et al*. Cranberries for treating urinary tract infections (Cochrane Review). In: *The Cochrane Library, Issue 1, 2000*. Oxford: Update Software.

19 Jepson RG *et al*. Cranberries for preventing urinary tract infections (Cochrane Review). In: *The Cochrane Library, Issue 1, 2000*. Oxford: Update Software.

20 Foda MM *et al*. Efficacy of cranberry in prevention of urinary tract infection in a susceptible pediatric population. *Can J Urol* 1995; **2**: 98–102.

21 Haverkorn MJ, Mandigers J. Reduction of bacteriuria and pyuria using cranberry juice (letter). *JAMA* 1994; **272**: 590.

22 Walker EB *et al*. Cranberry concentrate: UTI prophylaxis. *J Family Pract* 1997; **45**: 167–168.

23 Schlager TA *et al*. Effect of cranberry juice on bacteriuria in children with neurogenic bladder receiving intermittent catheterization. *J Pediatr* 1999; **135**: 698–702.

24 Papas PN *et al*. Cranberry juice in the treatment of urinary tract infections. *Southwest Med* 1966; **47**: 17–20.

25 Rogers J. Pass the cranberry juice. *Nurs Times* 1991; **87**: 36–37.

26 Kahn HD *et al*. Effect of cranberry juice on urine. *J Am Diet Assoc* 1967; **51**: 251–254.

27 Kinney AB, Blount M. Effect of cranberry juice on urinary pH. *Nurs Res* 1979; **28**: 287–290.

28 Schultz A. Efficacy of cranberry juice and ascorbic acid in acidifying the urine in multiple sclerosis subjects. *J Commun Health Nurs* 1984; **1**: 159–169.

29 Habash MB *et al*. The effect of water, ascorbic acid, and cranberry derived supplementation on human urine and uropathogen adhesion to silicone rubber. *Can J Microbiol* 1999; **45**: 691–694.

30 DuGan CR, Cardaciotto PS. Reduction of ammoniacal urine odors by sustained feeding of cranberry juice. *J Psych Nurs* 1966; **8**: 467–470.

31 Tsukada K *et al*. Cranberry juice and its impact on peri-stomal skin conditions for urostomy patients. *Ostomy/Wound Manage* 1994; **40**: 60–67.

32 Rosenbaum TP *et al*. Cranberry juice helps the problem of mucus production in entero-uroplasties. *Neurol Urodynamics* 1989; **8**: 344–345.

33 Saltzman JR *et al*. Effect of hypochlorhydria due to omeprazole treatment or atrophic gastritis on protein-bound vitamin B_{12} absorption. *J Am Coll Nutr* 1994; **13**: 584–591.

34 Soloway MS, Smith RA. Cranberry juice as a urine acidifier. *JAMA* 1988; **260**: 1465.

35 Kilbourn JP. Interference with dipstick tests for glucose and hemoglobin in urine by ascorbic acid in cranberry juice. *Clin Chem* 1987; **33**: 1297.

36 Hopkins WJ *et al*. Reduction of bacteriuria and pyuria using cranberry juice (letter). *JAMA* 1994; **272**: 589.

37 Katz LM. Reduction of bacteriuria and pyuria using cranberry juice (letter). *JAMA* 1994; **272**: 589.

Damiana

Species (Family)

Turnera diffusa Willd. var.*aphrodisiaca* Urb. (Bigno-Turneraceae) and related species indigenous to Texas and Mexico.

Synonym(s)

Damiana aphrodisiaca, Turnera, *Turnera aphrodisiaca* L.F. Ward, *Turnera microphyllia* Desv.

Part(s) Used

Leaf, stem

Pharmacopoeial and Other Monographs

BHC 1992[G6]
BHP 1996[G9]
Martindale 32nd edition[G43]
PDR for Herbal Medicines 2nd edition[G36]

Legal Category (Licensed Products)

GSL[G37]

Constituents[G6,G22,G40,G41,G64]

Carbohydrates Gum 13.5%, starch 6%, sugars.

Cyanogenetic glycosides Tetraphyllin B.[1]

Phenolic glycoside Arbutin (up to 0.7%).[2]

Tannins 3.5%. Type unspecified.

Volatile oils 0.5–1.0%. At least 20 components including 1,8-cineole (11%), *p*-cymene (2%), α- and β-pinene (2%), thymol, α-copaene, δ-cadinene and calamene. The presence of 1,8-cineole and *p*-cymene has been disputed.[2]

Other constituents Acids (fatty, plant), alkanes (e.g. hexacosanol-1 and triacontane), damianin (7%) (a bitter principle), flavone, β-sitosterol, resin (6.5%).[3]

Food Use

Damiana is used in foods and is listed by the Council of Europe as a natural source of food flavouring (category N2). This category indicates that damiana can be added to foodstuffs in small quantities with a possible limitation of an active principle (as yet unspecified) in the final product.[G16] In the USA, damiana is approved for food use.[G41]

Herbal Use

Damiana is stated to possess antidepressant, thymoleptic, mild purgative, stomachic and reputedly aphrodisiac properties.[4] It has been used for depression, nervous dyspepsia, atonic constipation, coital inadequacy, and specifically for anxiety neurosis with a predominant sexual factor.[G6,G7,G8,G64]

Dosage

Dried leaf 2–4 g or by infusion three times daily.[G6,G7]

Liquid Extract of Damiana (BPC 1934) 2–4 mL.

Pharmacological Actions

In vitro and animal studies

Hypoglycaemic activity has been reported in mice following both oral and intraperitoneal administration of damiana.[5] An ethanolic extract was stated to exhibit CNS-depressant activity although no other experimental details were available.[6]

Antibacterial activity against *Escherichia coli*, *Proteus mirabilis*, *Pseudomonas aeruginosa* and *Staphylococcus aureus* has been documented for a mixed herbal preparation, with some of the activity attributed to damiana.[7] The same herbal preparation was also reported to inhibit acetylcholine-induced spasm of the isolated guinea-pig ileum, although none of the antispasmodic activity was attributed to damiana.[7]

Arbutin is stated to be responsible for the urinary antiseptic properties (*see* Uva-ursi). However, the arbutin content of damiana is much less than that quoted for uva-ursi (0.7% and 5 to 18%, respectively).

The roots of various *Turnera* species have exhibited utero-activity.[G30]

Clinical studies

A herbal preparation containing damiana as one of the ingredients was reported to have a favourable effect on the symptoms of irritable bladder associated with functional and neurohormonal disorders, and on bacterial bladder infections.[7]

Side-effects, Toxicity

Tetanus-like convulsions and paroxysms resulting in symptoms similar to those of rabies or strychnine poisoning have been described in one individual following the ingestion of approximately 200 g damiana extract; cyanide poisoning was considered to be a possible cause. No other reported side-effects for damiana were located.

High doses of arbutin (e.g. 1 g) are considered to be toxic, although the concentration of arbutin documented for damiana (1 g arbutin is equivalent to more than 100 g plant material) is probably too low to warrant concerns over safety.

Contra-indications, Warnings

Excessive use should be avoided because of the presence of cyanogenetic glycosides and arbutin; damiana may interfere with existing hypoglycaemic therapy.

Pregnancy and lactation The safety of damiana has not been established. In view of the lack of toxicity data and possible cyanogenetic constituents, doses greatly exceeding amounts used in foods should not be taken during pregnancy or lactation.

Pharmaceutical Comment

There is limited chemical information available on damiana. There has been little documented evidence to justify the herbal uses, and the reputation of damiana as an aphrodisiac is unproven.[7,8] In view of the lack of toxicity data and reported cyanogenetic and arbutin constituents, excessive use of damiana should be avoided.

References

See also General References G6, G9, G10, G16, G22, G30, G31, G32, G36, G37, G40, G41, G43 and G64.

1 Spencer KC, Siegler DS. Tetraphyllin B from *Turnera diffusa*. *Planta Med* 1981; **43**: 175–178.
2 Auterhoff H, Häufel H-P. Inhaltsstoffe der damiana-droge. *Arch Pharm* 1968; **301**: 537–544.
3 Domínguez XA, Hinojosa M. Mexican medicinal plants. XXVIII Isolation of 5-hydroxy-7,3′,4′-trimethoxy-flavone from *Turnera diffusa*. *Planta Med* 1976; **30**: 68–71.
4 Braun JK, Malone MH. Legal highs. *Clin Toxicol* 1978; **12**: 1–31.
5 Pérez RM *et al*. A study of the hypoglycemic effect of some Mexican plants. *J Ethnopharmacol* 1984; **12**: 253–262.
6 Jiu J. A survey of some medical plants of Mexico for selected biological activity. *Lloydia* 1966; **29**: 250–259.
7 Westendorf J. Carito-In-vitro-Untersuchungen zum Nachweis spasmolytischer und kontraktiler Einflüsse. *Therapiewoche* 1982; **32**: 6291–6297.
8 Lowry TP. Damiana. *J Psychoactive Drugs* 1984; **16**: 267–268.

Dandelion

Species (Family)

Taraxacum officinale Weber (Asteraceae/Compositae)

Synonym(s)

Lion's Tooth, *Taraxacum palustre* (Lyons) Lam & DC., *Leontodon taraxacum* L., Taraxacum

Part(s) Used

Leaf, root

Pharmacopoeial and Other Monographs

BHC 1992[G6]
BHP 1996[G9]
Complete German Commission E[G3]
ESCOP 1996[G52]
Martindale 32nd edition[G43]
PDR for Herbal Medicines 2nd edition[G36]

Legal Category (Licensed Products)

GSL[G37]

Constituents[G2,G6,G8,G22,G41,G48,G52,G57,G64]

Acids Caffeic acid, *p*-hydroxyphenylacetic acid, chlorogenic acid,[1] cichoric acid, monocaffeyl tartaric acids[2] linoleic acid, linolenic acid, oleic acid and palmitic acid.

Coumarins Cichoriin and aesculin.[2]

Flavonoids Luteolin-7-glucoside and luteolin-7-diglucosides.[2]

Minerals Potassium 4.5% in leaf, 2.45% in root.[3]

Resin Undefined bitter complex (taraxacin).

Terpenoids Sesquiterpene lactones taraxinic acid (germacranolide) esterified with glucose,[4] and eudesmanolides.[5]

Vitamins Vitamin A 14 000 iu/100 g leaf (compared with 11 000 iu/100 g carrots).

Other constituents Carotenoids, choline, inulin, pectin, phytosterols (e.g. sitosterol, stigmasterol, taraxasterol, homotaraxasterol), sugars (e.g. fructose, glucose, sucrose), triterpenes (e.g. β-amyrin, taraxol, taraxerol).

Food Use

Dandelion is used as a food, mainly in salads and soups. The roasted root and its extract have been used as a coffee substitute.[G41] Dandelion is listed by the Council of Europe as a natural source of food flavouring (category N2). This category indicates that dandelion can be added to foodstuffs in small quantities, with a possible limitation of an active principle (as yet unspecified) in the final product.[G16] In the USA, dandelion is listed as GRAS (Generally Recognised As Safe).[G41]

Herbal Use[G2,G4,G6,G7,G8,G32,G43,G52,G54,G56,G60,G64]

Dandelion is stated to possess diuretic, laxative, cholagogue and antirheumatic properties. It has been used for cholecystitis, gallstones, jaundice, atonic dyspepsia with constipation, muscular rheumatism, oliguria, and specifically for cholecystitis and dyspepsia. The German Commission E approved use of root and herb for disturbance of bile flow, stimulation of diuresis, loss of appetite and dyspepsia.[G3] Root is used in combination with celandine herb and artichoke for epigastric discomfort due to functional disorders of the biliary system.[G3]

Dosage

Dried leaf 4–10 g or by infusion three times daily.[G6,G7]

Leaf, liquid extract 4–10 mL (1 : 1 in 25% alcohol) three times daily.[G6,G7]

Leaf tincture 2–5 mL.[G3]

Leaf, fresh juice 5–10 mL.[G52]

Dried root 2–8 g or by infusion or decoction three times daily.[G6,G7]

Root, tincture 5–10 mL (1 : 5 in 45% alcohol) three times daily.[G6,G7]

Liquid Extract of Taraxacum (BPC 1949) 2–8 mL.

Juice of Taraxacum (BPC 1949) 4–8 mL.

Pharmacological Actions

In vitro and animal studies

A diuretic effect in rats and mice has been documented for dandelion extracts, following oral administration.[6] Herb extracts were found to produce greater diuresis than root extracts; a dose of 50 mL (equivalent to 2 g dried herb/kg body weight) produced an effect comparable to that of frusemide 80 mg/kg. By contrast, no significant increases in urine volume or sodium excretion were observed in mice following oral administration of either leaf or root extracts, or of purified fractions.[3] Similarly, oral and intravenous administration of an ethanolic extract of dandelion root failed to produce a diuretic effect in laboratory animals.[7]

Moderate anti-inflammatory activity against carrageenan-induced rat paw oedema has been documented for a dandelion root extract.[8] An 80% ethanol extract of root (100 mg/kg orally) inhibited oedema by 43% in the carrageenan-induced rat paw oedema test at 3 hours.[7]

Bile secretion was doubled in dogs by a decoction of fresh root (equivalent to 5 g dried plant); similar activity has been observed for rats.[G52]

Hypoglycaemic activity has been described in normal, but not in diabetic rabbits, following oesophageal administration of dandelion.[9] Doses greater than 500 mg/kg produced a significant blood glucose concentration which had returned to normal after 24 hours. The maximum decrease produced by a dose of 2 g/kg was reported to be 65% of the effect produced by tolbutamide 500 mg/kg. Sulphonylureas (e.g. tolbutamide) act by stimulating pancreatic beta-cells and a similar mechanism was proposed for dandelion.

In vitro antitumour activity has been documented for an aqueous extract of dandelion, given by intraperitoneal injection, in the tumour systems ddY-Ehrlich and C3H/He-MM46.[10] The mechanism of action was thought to be similar to that of tumour polysaccharides such as lentinan.

Clinical studies

There is a lack of well-designed clinical studies investigating the effects of dandelion.

Side-effects, Toxicity

Contact allergic reactions to dandelion have been documented[11,G51] and animal studies have reported dandelion to have a weak sensitising capacity.[12] Sesquiterpene lactones are thought to be the allergenic principles in dandelion.[4] These compounds contain an exocyclic α-methylene β-lactone moiety, which is thought to be a prerequisite for allergenic activity of sesquiterpene lactones.

The acute toxicity of dandelion appears to be low, with LD_{50} values (mice, intraperitoneal injection) estimated at 36.8 g/kg and 28.8 g/kg for the root and herb, respectively.[6] No visible signs of toxicity were observed in rabbits administered dandelion 3, 4, 5 and 6 g/kg body weight by mouth for up to seven days.[9] In addition, no behavioural changes were recorded.

Contra-indications, Warnings

Treatment with dandelion is contraindicated for patients with occlusion of bile duct, gall bladder empyema and obstructive ileus.[G3,G52] Dandelion may precipitate an allergic reaction in susceptible individuals, although no reports following the ingestion of dandelion have been documented. Dandelion may potentiate the action of other diuretics and may interfere with existing hypoglycaemic activity.

Pregnancy and lactation There are no known problems with the use of dandelion during pregnancy, provided that doses do not greatly exceed the amounts used in foods.

Pharmaceutical Comment

Dandelion is a well-known traditional herbal remedy, although limited scientific information, particularly clinical research, is available to justify the reputed uses. Several investigations have failed to demonstrate significant diuretic effects in laboratory animals and have proposed that any diuretic activity is due to the high potassium content of the leaf and root. Dandelion has also been used in foods for many years. Animal studies indicate dandelion to be of low toxicity. However, excessive ingestion of dandelion, particularly in amounts exceeding those normally consumed in foods, should be avoided.

References

See also General References G2, G3, G5, G6, G9, G11, G16, G19, G20, G22, G29, G31, G32, G36, G37, G41, G43, G48, G51, G52, G54, G56, G57, G60 and G64.

1 Clifford MN *et al*. The chlorogenic acids content of coffee substitutes. *Food Chem* 1987; **24**: 99–107.

2 Williams CA *et al*. Flavonoids, cinnamic acids and coumarins from the different tissues and medicinal preparations of *Taraxacum officinale*. *Phytochem* 1996; **42**: 121–127.

3 Hook I *et al*. Evaluation of dandelion for diuretic activity and variation in potassium content. *Int J Pharmacog* 1993; **31**: 29–34.

4 Hausen BM. Taraxinsäure-1′-O-β-D-glucopyranosid, das kontaktallergen des löwenzahns (*Taraxacum officinale* Wiggers). *Dermatosen* 1982; **30**: 51–53.

5 Hänsel R *et al*. Sequiterpenlacton-β-d-glucopyranoside sowie ein neues eudesmanolid aus *Taraxacum officinale*. *Phytochem* 1980; **19**: 857–861.

6 Rácz-Kotilla *et al*. The action of *Taraxacum officinale* extracts on the body weight and diuresis of laboratory animals. *Planta Med* 1974; **26**: 212–217.

7 Tita B *et al*. *Taraxacum officinale* W.: Pharmacological effect of ethanol extract. *Pharmacol Res* 1993; **27**: 23–24.

8 Mascolo N *et al*. Biological screening of Italian medicinal plants for anti-inflammatory activity. *Phytother Res* 1987; **1**: 28–29.

9 Akhtar MS *et al*. Effects of *Portulaca oleracae* (kulfa) and *Taraxacum officinale* (dhudhal) in normoglycaemic and alloxan-treated hyperglycaemic rabbits. *J Pak Med Assoc* 1985; **35**: 207–210.

10 Baba K *et al*. Antitumor activity of hot water extract of dandelion, *Taraxacum officinale* – correlation between antitumor activity and timing of administration. *Yagugaku Zasshi* 1981; **101**: 538–543.

11 Hausen BM, Schulz KH. Allergische kontaktdermatitis durch löwenzahn (*Taraxacum officinale* Wiggers). *Dermatosen* 1978; **26**: 198.

12 Davies MG, Kersey PJW. Contact allergy to yarrow and dandelion. *Contact Dermatitis* 1986; **14**: 256–257.

Devil's Claw

Species (Family)

Harpagophytum procumbens DC. (Pedaliaceae)

Synonym(s)

Harpagophytum, Grapple Plant, Wood Spider

Part(s) Used

Secondary root tuber

Pharmacopoeial and Other Monographs

BHC 1992[G6]
BHP 1996[G9]
BP 2001[G15]
Complete German Commission E[G3]
ESCOP 1996[G52]
Martindale 32nd edition[G43]
PDR for Herbal Medicines 2nd edition[G36]
Ph Eur 2002[G28]

Legal Category (Licensed Products)

Devil's claw is not included in the GSL.[G37]

Constituents[G2,G6,G62]

Carbohydrates Fructose, galactose, glucose and *myo*-inositol (monosaccharides), raffinose, stachyose (46%) and sucrose (oligosaccharides).[1]

Iridoids Harpagide, 8-O-(p-coumaroyl)-harpagide, harpagoside, procumide, 6'-O-(p-coumaroyl)-procumbide, and procumboside (glucosides).[2] Pharmacopoeial standard: not less than 1.2% harpagoside, calculated with reference to the dried drug.[G15,G25]

Phenols Acetoside and isoacetoside (glycosides), and a bioside.[3]

Other constituents Amino acids and flavonoids (kaempferol, luteolin).

Other plant parts The flower, stem and ripe fruit are reported to be devoid of harpagoside; the leaf contains traces of iridoids.[4]

Food Use

Devil's claw is not used in foods.

Herbal Use

Devil's claw is stated to possess anti-inflammatory, antirheumatic, analgesic, sedative and diuretic properties. Traditionally, it has been used as a stomachic and a bitter tonic, and for arthritis, gout, myalgia, fibrositis, lumbago, pleurodynia and rheumatic disease.[G2,G6,G7,G8,G32,G64] Modern use of devil's claw is focused on its use in the treatment of rheumatic and arthritic conditions, and low back pain.

Dosage

Painful arthrosis and tendonitis

1.5–3 g dried tuber as a decoction, three times daily; 1–3 g drug or equivalent aqueous or hydroalcoholic extracts;[G52] liquid extract 1–3 mL (1 : 1, 25% ethanol) three times daily.[G6]

Loss of appetite or dyspepsia

Dried tuber 0.5 g as a decoction, three times daily.[G6]

Tincture 1 mL (1 : 5, 25% ethanol) three times daily.[G6]

Clinical trials of devil's claw root extracts for the treatment of low back pain have tested doses ranging from 600 to 2400 mg daily, orally, in two or three divided doses (equivalent to up to 100 mg harpagoside (depending on the concentration of the extract)).[5–7] In a clinical trial in osteoarthritis, participants received capsules containing powdered cryoground devil's claw root 2610 mg daily.[8] Other clinical trials in arthrosic conditions have used daily doses of devil's claw of 2.4 g dried tuber and 2.46 g hydroalcoholic extract.[9] Clinical trials in various rheumatic conditions have used daily doses of devil's claw of 0.75–2 g dried tuber and 1.23 g aqueous extract in two or three divided doses.[9]

Pharmacological Actions

The active constituents of devil's claw are widely held to be the iridoid glucosides although, of these, it has not been definitively established whether harpagoside is the most important pharmacologically active constituent of the whole extract. Other compounds present in the root may contribute to the pharmacological activities of devil's claw.[9,10] It has also been suggested that harpagogenin, formed by *in vivo* acid hydrolysis of harpagoside, may have biological activity.[11]

In vitro and animal studies

Animal studies using aqueous extracts of devil's claw have suggested that the extract may be inactivated by passage through the acid environment of the stomach.[10,12] One study compared the anti-inflammatory activities of aqueous devil's claw extract administered by different routes. Intraperitoneal and intraduodenal administration led to a significant reduction in the carrageenan-induced rat paw oedema test, but there was no effect following oral administration.[12] In another study, aqueous devil's claw extract pretreated with hydrochloric acid to mimic acid conditions in the stomach showed no activity in pharmacological models of pain and inflammation.[10]

Transformation of the iridoids harpagide, harpagoside and 8-O-(p-coumaroyl)-harpagide into the pyridine monoterpene alkaloid aucubinine B, chemically or by human intestinal bacteria *in vitro*, has been documented.[13,14] However, it is not known if aucubinine B is formed *in vivo* by intestinal bacteria and, therefore, whether it contributes to the pharmacological activity of devil's claw.[14]

Animal studies of the anti-inflammatory activity of devil's claw have reported conflicting results. Activity differs depending on the route of administration of devil's claw, and the model of inflammation, whether acute or subacute.

Weak anti-inflammatory activity has been reported in rats following intravenous administration of devil's claw extract.[15] Anti-inflammatory activity of harpagoside has been demonstrated in experimental models, including the croton oil-induced granuloma pouch test, and for harpagogenin, the aglucone of harpagoside, in the croton oil-induced granuloma pouch test and in formalin-induced arthritis in rats.[16] Dried aqueous extract of devil's claw administered by intraperitoneal injection demonstrated significant activity in the carrageenan-induced oedema test in rats, an acute model of inflammation.[10] The effect on oedema was dose dependent for doses of devil's claw extract 100–400 mg/kg, and reached a maximum 3 hours after carrageenan injection. Other studies in rats have reported significant reductions in oedema using the same model following pretreatment with intraperitoneal[12,17] and intraduodenal, but not oral, dried aqueous extract of devil's claw.[12] Other studies have reported that dried aqueous extract of devil's claw administered orally had no effect on carrageenan- or *Mycobacterium butyricum*-induced oedema in rat paw.[18,19] In addition, oral dried aqueous extract of devil's claw had no significant effect in adjuvant-induced arthritis in rats.[18] By contrast, in these studies, both indomethacin and aspirin displayed significant anti-inflammatory activity.[18,19]

Analgesic activity has also been documented for devil's claw in animal studies. Pretreatment with dried aqueous devil's claw extract at doses of 100 mg/kg and above, administered intraperitoneally, resulted in peripheral analgesic activity demonstrated by a significant reduction in the number of writhings induced by acetic acid in mice.[10] However, no effect was observed in the hotplate test, indicating a lack of central analgesic activity with devil's claw extract. The peripheral analgesic properties of intraperitoneal dried aqueous extract of devil's claw have been confirmed in other studies for doses of 400 mg/kg and above.[17] These studies also reported peripheral analgesic and anti-inflammatory properties for the related species *Harpogophytum zeyheri*.[17]

A clear mechanism of action for the purported anti-inflammatory effects of devil's claw has yet to be established. *In vitro*, devil's claw (100 mg/mL) had no significant effect on prostaglandin (PG) synthetase activity, whereas indomethacin (316 µg/mL) and aspirin (437 µg/mL) caused 50% inhibition of this enzyme.[19] In other *in vitro* studies in human whole blood samples, devil's claw extracts and fractions of extracts were tested for their effects on thromboxane B_2 (TXB_2) and leukotriene (LT) biosynthesis.[20] TXB_2 is an end-product of arachidonic acid metabolism by the cyclooxygenase 1 (COX-1) pathway. Inhibition appeared to be dependent on the harpagoside content of the extracts or fractions.[20] Harpagoside (100 µmol/L), but not harpagide (100 µmol/L), inhibited calcium ionophore A23187-stimulated release of TXB_2 from human platelets.[21] However, harpagoside and harpagide had no significant inhibitory effect on calcium ionophore A23187-stimulated release of PGE_2 and LTC_4 from mouse peritoneal macrophages.[21] *In vitro* inhibition of tumour-necrosis-factor-α (TNF-α) synthesis in lipopolysaccharide-stimulated human monocytes by a hydroalcoholic extract of devil's claw (SteiHap 69) has also been documented.[22]

Crude methanolic extracts of devil's claw have been shown to be cardioactive *in vitro* and *in vivo* in animals. A protective action against ventricular arrhythmias induced by aconitine, calcium chloride, epinephrine (adrenaline)/chloroform and reperfusion has been reported for devil's claw given intraperitoneally or added to the reperfusion medium.[23,24] The crude extract was found to exhibit greater activity than pure harpagoside.[24] In isolated rabbit heart, low concentrations of a crude methanolic extract had mild negative chronotropic and positive inotropic effects,[23] whereas high concentrations caused a marked negative inotropic effect with reduction in coronary blood flow.[23] In anaesthetised dogs, harpagoside administered orally by gavage caused a decrease in mean aortic pressure and arterial and pulmonary capillary pressure.[25]

In vitro, harpagoside has been shown to decrease the contractile response of smooth muscle to acetylcholine and barium chloride on guinea-pig ileum and rabbit jejunum.[26] Harpagide was found to increase this response at lower concentrations, but antagonised it at higher concentrations.[26] On the basis of these studies in isolated smooth muscle, it was suggested that the constituents of devil's claw may influence mechanisms regulating calcium influx.[26]

Methanolic extracts have also exhibited hypotensive properties in normotensive rats, causing a decrease in arterial blood pressure following oral doses of 300 mg/kg and 400 mg/kg body weight.[23]

Devil's claw extracts possess weak antifungal activity against *Penicillium digitatum* and *Botrytis cinerea*.[27]

Clinical studies

Pharmacokinetics There is little published information on the pharmacokinetics of devil's claw extract in humans. A pharmacokinetic study involving a small number of healthy male volunteers ($n = 3$) measured plasma harpagoside concentrations after oral administration of devil's claw extract (WS1531 containing 9% harpagoside) 600, 1200 and 1800 mg as film-coated tablets.[20] Maximal plasma concentrations of harpagoside were reached after 1.3–1.8 hours, and were 8.2 ng/mL and 27.8 ng/mL for doses of harpagoside of 108 and 162 mg, respectively (corresponding to 1200 and 1800 mg devil's claw extract, respectively). Other studies involving small numbers of healthy male volunteers indicated that the half-life ranged between 3.7 and 6.4 hours. Other results suggested that there may be low oral absorption or a considerable first-pass effect with devil's

claw extract, although this needs further investigation.[20]

Pharmacodynamics A study involving healthy volunteers investigated the effects on eicosanoid production of orally administered devil's claw (four 500-mg capsules of powder, containing 3% glucoiridoids, daily for 21 days).[28] No statistically significant differences on PGE_2, TXB_2, 6-keto-$PGF_{1\alpha}$ and LTB_4 were observed following the period of devil's claw administration, compared with baseline values. By contrast, in a subsequent study involving whole blood samples taken from healthy male volunteers, a biphasic decrease in basal cysteinyl-leukotriene (Cys-LT) biosynthesis, compared with baseline values, was observed following oral administration of devil's claw extract (WS1531 containing 9% harpagoside) 600, 1200 and 1800 mg as film-coated tablets.[20]

Therapeutic activity The efficacy and effectiveness of devil's claw has been investigated in more than 10 clinical studies involving patients with rheumatic and arthritic conditions, and low back pain.[9,29] These studies have involved different methodological designs, including several uncontrolled studies, and different preparations of devil's claw, including crude drug and aqueous extracts. These studies have been summarised elsewhere,[9,29,G56] and several are discussed in detail below.

A randomised, double-blind, placebo-controlled study involving 118 patients with acute exacerbations of chronic low back pain investigated the effects of devil's claw extract 800 mg three times daily (equivalent to 50 mg harpagoside daily) for four weeks.[7] There was no statistically significant difference between the devil's claw and placebo groups in the primary outcome measure – consumption of the opioid analgesic tramadol over weeks 2–4 of the study – among the 109 patients who completed the study. This was an unusual choice of primary outcome measure as it gives no direct indication of the degree of pain experienced by participants. There was a trend towards improvement in a modified version of the Arhus Low Back Pain Index (a measure of pain, disability and physical impairment) for devil's claw recipients compared with placebo recipients, although this did not reach statistical significance. A greater proportion of patients in the devil's claw group were pain-free at the end of the study, although this was only a secondary outcome measure.

On the basis of these findings, a subsequent randomised, double-blind, placebo-controlled trial involving 197 patients with exacerbations of low back pain tested the effects of two doses of devil's claw (WS1531) extract against placebo.[6] Participants received devil's claw extract 600 mg or 1200 mg daily (equivalent to 50 mg and 100 mg harpagoside daily, respectively), or placebo, for four weeks. There was a statistically significant difference ($p = 0.027$) between devil's claw and placebo with respect to the primary outcome measure – the number of patients who were pain-free without tramadol for at least five days during the last week of the study. However, numbers of patients who were pain-free were low (3, 6 and 10 for placebo, devil's claw 600 mg daily and devil's claw 1200 mg daily, respectively). Furthermore, this is a non-standard outcome measure. Arhus Low Back Pain Index scores improved significantly in all three groups, compared with baseline values, although there was no statistically significant difference between groups.

In a randomised, double-blind, placebo-controlled study involving patients with non-specific low back pain, 65 participants received devil's claw extract (LI-174, Rivoltan), or placebo, 480 mg twice daily (equivalent to 24 mg harpagoside daily) for four weeks.[5] There was a significant improvement ($p < 0.001$) in visual analogue scale (VAS) scores for muscle pain in the devil's claw group, but not the placebo group, compared with baseline values, after two and four weeks' treatment. Differences in VAS scores between the two groups were statistically significant after four weeks' treatment ($p < 0.001$). Significant differences between the two groups in favour of devil's claw after four weeks' treatment were also observed with several other parameters, including muscle stiffness and muscular ischaemic pain.

A randomised, double-blind trial has compared the efficacy of devil's claw extract with that of diacerein in 122 patients with osteoarthritis of the knee and hip.[8] Participants received powdered cryo-ground devil's claw (Harpadol) 2.61 g daily, or diacerein 100 mg daily, for four months.

VAS scores for spontaneous pains improved significantly in both groups, compared with baseline values, and there were no differences between devil's claw and diacerein with respect to VAS scores.

In a placebo-controlled study involving 89 patients with rheumatic complaints, devil's claw recipients (who received powdered crude drug 2 g daily for two months) showed significant improvements in sensitivity to pain and in motility (as measured by the finger-to-floor distance), compared with placebo recipients.[30]

Open, uncontrolled studies involving patients with rheumatic and arthritic disorders report conflicting results for the effectiveness of devil's claw. One study involved 13 patients with arthritis, rheumatoid arthritis or psoriatic arthropathy who received tablets of devil's claw aqueous extract 1.23 g daily for six weeks in addition to their conventional drug treatment. There were no significant changes after 6 and 12 weeks in pain, early morning stiffness, and the Ritchie Articular Index (a method of assessing joint tenderness), compared with baseline values.[31] By contrast, other open uncontrolled studies of devil's claw involving patients with rheumatic disorders (who received devil's claw powder 1.5 g daily for 60 days)[32] or arthrosis (who received devil's claw aqueous extract, containing 2.5% iridoid glycosides, 3–9 g daily for 6 months)[33] reported improvements in pain and 'complaints' at the end of the treatment period compared with baseline values.

Another study involved 45 patients with osteo- or rheumatoid arthritis who received devil's claw root extract 2.46 g daily for two weeks in addition to non-steroidal anti-inflammatory drug (NSAID) treatment, followed by devil's claw extract alone, for four weeks.[34] It was reported that there were no statistically significant changes in pain intensity and duration of morning stiffness during the period of treatment with devil's claw extract alone. In subgroups of patients with rheumatoid arthritis and those with osteoarthritis, small decreases were observed in concentrations of C-reactive protein and creatinine, respectively. The design of this study in terms of the treatment regimen (NSAID followed by devil's claw extract without a washout period), however, renders the results difficult to interpret.

Side-effects, Toxicity

Randomised, placebo-controlled trials involving patients with rheumatic and arthritic conditions who have received devil's claw extracts or powdered drug at approximately recommended doses for four weeks have reported mild, transient gastrointestinal symptoms (such as diarrhoea, flatulence) in a small proportion (less than 10%) of devil's claw recipients.[5–7] No serious adverse events were reported, although one patient withdrew from one study because of tachycardia.[7] In an open, uncontrolled study, one patient withdrew after four days' treatment with devil's claw aqueous extract 1.23 g daily because of several symptoms, including frontal headache, tinnitus, anorexia and loss of taste.[31]

In a randomised, controlled trial comparing devil's claw extract with diacerein in patients with osteoarthritis, numbers of patients ending the study prematurely because of suspected adverse drug reactions were 8 and 14 for devil's claw and diacerein recipients, respectively.[8] In total, 26 diacerein recipients and 16 devil's claw recipients reported one or more adverse events ($p = 0.042$). The numbers of adverse events attributed to the treatment was significantly lower for devil's claw than for diacerein (10 versus 21; $p = 0.017$). The most frequently reported adverse event, diarrhoea, occurred in 8.1% and 26.7% of devil's claw and diacerein recipients, respectively.

There is an isolated report of conjunctivitis, rhinitis and respiratory symptoms in a 50-year-old woman who had experienced chronic occupational exposure to devil's claw.[35]

The mechanism of action of devil's claw remains unclear, in particular, whether it has significant effects on the mediators of acute inflammation. Data from *in vitro* and clinical studies in this regard do not yet give a clear picture (*see In vitro* and animal studies and Clinical studies, Pharmacodynamics). It has been stated that adverse effects associated with the use of NSAIDs are unlikely to occur with devil's claw, even during long-term treatment.[G50,G52] While there are no documented reports of gastrointestinal bleeding or peptic ulcer associated with the use of devil's claw, the latter statement requires confirmation. Use of devil's claw in gastric and duodenal ulcer is contraindicated, although this appears to be because of the drug's bitter properties.[G50]

Acute and subacute toxicity tests in rodents have demonstrated low toxicity of devil's claw extracts. In a study in mice, the acute oral lethal dose (LD) LD_0 and LD_{50} were greater than 13.5 g/kg body weight.[19] In rats, clinical, haematological and gross pathological findings were unremarkable following administration of devil's claw extract 7.5 g/kg by mouth for seven days. Hepatic effects (liver weight, and concentrations of microsomal protein and several liver enzymes) were not observed following oral treatment with devil's claw extract 2 g/kg for seven days.[19] Other studies in mice have reported acute oral acute intravenous LD_0 values of greater than 4.64 g/kg and greater than 1 g/kg, respectively.[15] For an extract containing harpagoside 85%, acute oral LD_0, acute intravenous LD_0 and acute intravenous LD_{50} values were greater than 4.64 g/kg, 395 mg/kg and 511 mg/kg, respectively.[15]

Contra-indications, Warnings

Devil's claw is stated to be contra-indicated in gastric and duodenal ulcers,[G3,G52] and in gallstones should be used only after consultation with a physician.[G3] On the basis of pharmacological evidence of devil's claw's cardioactivity, the possibility of excessive doses interfering with existing treatment for cardiac

disorders or with hypo/hypertensive therapy should be considered.

Pregnancy and lactation It has been stated that devil's claw has oxytocic properties,[36] although the reference gives no further details and the basis for this statement is not known. In addition, there is no further evidence to substantiate the statement. However, given the lack of data on the effects of devil's claw taken during pregnancy and lactation, its use should be avoided during these periods.

Pharmaceutical Comment

The chemistry of devil's claw has been well documented. The iridoid constituents are thought to be responsible for the reputed anti-inflammatory activity of devil's claw, although it is not known precisely which of these are the most important for pharmacological activity, and the importance of other compounds. There is conflicting evidence from *in vitro*, animal and human studies regarding the anti-inflammatory activity of devil's claw and possible mechanisms of action. Several randomised trials using devil's claw extracts standardised on harpagoside content have reported superiority over placebo for some aspects of low back pain and rheumatic complaints. However, some studies used non-standard outcome measures and carried out several post-hoc analyses. Further studies have used recognised, predefined outcome measures to establish the therapeutic value of standardised devil's claw extracts in patients with arthritic and rheumatic conditions.

On the basis of randomised controlled trials involving patients with arthritic and rheumatic disorders, devil's claw extracts appear to have a favourable short-term adverse effect profile when taken in recommended doses. Mild, transient gastrointestinal effects, such as diarrhoea and flatulence, may occur. Chronic toxicity studies and clinical experience with prolonged use are lacking, so the effects of long-term use are not known. On this basis, and in view of the possible cardioactivity of devil's claw, devil's claw should not be used for long periods of time at doses higher than recommended. Further studies involving large numbers of patients are required.

Some commercial extracts of devil's claw root may have been prepared not only from the roots of *H. procumbens*, but also from the roots of *H. zeyheri*, which are similar macroscopically.[17] However, the two species differ in the concentration of the constituents harpagoside and 8-O-*p*-coumaroyl-harpagide. On this basis it has been stated that the species can be distinguished chemically by determining the ratio harpagoside:8-O-*p*-coumaroyl-harpagide. The ratio is stated to be near one for *H. zeyheri* and between 20 and 38 for *H. procumbens* which has a low 8-O-*p*-coumaroyl-harpagide content.[17] While this ratio may be sufficient for chemotaxonomic differentiation, it may not be adequate for quality control.[37] Other studies have demonstrated that the harpagoside content of several powdered dry extracts of devil's claw from different manufacturers varies, and that each extract has a unique profile of other constituents.[38]

References

See also General References G2, G3, G5, G6, G9, G15, G25, G31, G32, G36, G43, G49, G50, G52, G56, G62 and G64.

1 Ziller KH and Franz G. Analysis of the water-soluble fraction from the roots of *Harpagophytum procumbens*. *Planta Med* 1979; **37**: 340–348.

2 Kikuchi T *et al*. New iridoid glucosides from *Harpagophytum procumbens* DC. *Chem Pharm Bull* 1983; **31**: 2296–2301.

3 Burger JFW *et al*. Iridoid and phenolic glycosides from *Harpagophytum procumbens*. *Phytochemistry* 1987; **26**: 1453–1457.

4 Czygan FC, Krueger A. Pharmaceutical biological studies of the genus harpagophytum. Part 3 Distribution of the iridoid glycoside harpagoside in the different organs of *Harpagophytum procumbens* and *Harpagophytum zeyheri*. *Planta Med* 1977; **31**: 305–307.

5 Göbel H *et al*. *Harpagophytum* extract LI 174 (Devil's claw) for treating non-specific back pain. Effects on sensory, motor and vascular muscle response. *Schmerz* 2001; **15**: 10–18.

6 Chrubasik S *et al*. Effectiveness of *Harpagophytum* extract WS 1531 in the treatment of exacerbation of low back pain: a randomized, placebo-controlled, double-blind study. *Eur J Anaesthesiol* 1999; **16**: 118–129.

7 Chrubasik S *et al*. Effectiveness of *Harpagophytum procumbens* in treatment of acute low back pain. *Phytomedicine* 1996; **3**: 1–10.

8 Chantre P *et al*. Efficacy and tolerance of *Harpagophytum procumbens* versus diacerhein in treatment of osteoarthritis. *Phytomedicine* 2000; **7**: 177–183.

9 Wegener T. Devil's claw: from African traditional remedy to modern analgesic and antiinflammatory. *Herbalgram* 2000; **50**: 47–54.

10 Lanhers M-C *et al*. Anti-inflammatory and analgesic effects of an aqueous extract of *Harpagophytum procumbens*. *Planta Med* 1992; **58**: 117–123.

11 Vanhaelen M *et al*. Biological activity of *Harpagophytum procumbens*. 1. Preparation and structure of Harpagogenin. *J Pharm Belg* 1981 **36**: 38–42.

12 Soulimani R *et al*. The role of stomachal digestion on the pharmacological activity of plant extracts, using as an example extracts of *Harpagophytum procumbens*. *Can J Physiol Pharmacol* 1994; **72**: 1532–1536.

13 Baghdikian B *et al*. Two new pyridine monoterpene alkaloids by chemical conversion of a commercial extract of *Harpagophytum procumbens*. *J Nat Prod* 1999; **62**: 211–213.

14 Baghdikian B *et al*. Formation of nitrogen-containing metabolites from the main iridoids of *Harpagophytum procumbens* and *H. zeyheri* by human intestinal bacteria. *Planta Med* 1999; **65**: 164–166.

15 Erdös A *et al*. Beitrag zur pharmakologie und toxikologie verschiedener extrakte, sowie des harpagosids aus *Harpagophytum procumbens* DC. *Planta Med* 1978; **34**: 97–108.

16 Sticher O. Plant mono-, di- and sesquiterpenoids with pharmacological and therapeutical activity. In: Wagner H, Wolff P, eds. *New Natural Products with Pharmacological, Biological or Therapeutical Activity*. Berlin: Springer Verlag, 1977: 137–176.

17 Baghdikian B *et al*. An analytical study, anti-inflammatory and analgesic effects of *Harpagophytum procumbens* and *Harpagophytum zeyheri*. *Planta Med* 1997; **63**: 171–176.

18 McLeod DW *et al*. Investigations of *Harpagophytum procumbens* (devil's claw) in the treatment of experimental inflammation and arthritis in the rat. *Br J Pharmacol* 1979; **66**: P140.

19 Whitehouse LW *et al*. Devil's claw (*Harpagophytum procumbens*): no evidence for anti-inflammatory activity in the treatment of arthritic disease. *Can Med Assoc J* 1983; **129**: 249–251.

20 Loew D *et al*. Investigations on the pharmacokinetic properties of *Harpagophytum* extracts and their effects on eicosanoid biosynthesis in vitro and ex vivo. *Clin Pharmacol Ther* 2001; **69**: 356–364.

21 Benito PB *et al*. Effects of some iridoids from plant origin on arachidonic acid metabolism in cellular systems. *Planta Med* 2000; **66**: 324–328.

22 Fiebich BL *et al*. Inhibition of TNF-α synthesis in LPS-stimulated primary human monocytes by *Harpagophytum* extract SteiHap 69. *Phytomedicine* 2001; **8**: 28–30.

23 Circosta C *et al*. A drug used in traditional medicine: *Harpagophytum procumbens* DC. II. Cardiovascular activity. *J Ethnopharmacol* 1984; **11**: 259–274.

24 Costa de Pasquale R *et al*. A drug used in traditional medicine: *Harpagophytum procumbens* DC. III. Effects on hyperkinetic ventricular arrhythmias by reperfusion. *J Ethnopharmacol* 1985; **13**: 193–199.

25 Occhiuto F, De Pasquale A. Electrophysiological and haemodynamic effects of some active principles of *Harpagophytum procumbens* DC. in the

dog. *Pharmacological Res* 1990; **22**: 72–73.

26 Occhiuto F *et al.* A drug used in traditional medicine: *Harpagophytum procumbens* DC. IV. Effects on some isolated muscle preparations. *J Ethnopharmacol* 1985; **13**: 201–208.

27 Guérin J-C, Réveillère H-P. Activité antifongique d'extraits végétaux à usage thérapeutique. II. Étude de 40 extraits sur 9 souches fongiques. *Ann Pharmaceut Fr* 1985; **43**: 77–81.

28 Moussard C *et al.* A drug used in traditional medicine, *Harpagophytum procumbens*: no evidence for NSAID-like effect on whole blood eicosanoid production in human. *Prostaglandins Leukot Essent Fatty Acids* 1992; **46**: 283–286.

29 Wegener T, Wiedenbrück R. Die Teufelskralle (*Harpagophytum procumbens* DC.)in der Therapie rheumatischer Erkrankungen. *Z Phytother* 1998; **19**: 284–294.

30 Lecomte A, Costa JP. Harpagophytum dans l'arthrose: étude en double insu contre placebo. *Le Magazine* 1992; 27–30.

31 Grahame R, Robinson BV. Devil's claw (*Harpagophytum procumbens*): pharmacological and clinical studies. *Ann Rheum Dis* 1981; **40**: 632.

32 Pinget M, Lecomte A. Die Wirkung der 'Harpa-gophytum Arkocaps' bei degenerativem Rheuma. *Naturheilpraxis* 1992; **50**: 267–269.

33 Bélaiche P. Étude clinique de 630 cas d'arthrose traités par le nébulisat aqueux d'*Harpagophytum procumbens* (Radix). *Phytothérapy* 1982; **1**: 22–28.

34 Szczepański L. (Efficacy and tolerability of 'Pago-sid' (*Harpagophytum procumbens* root extract) in the treatment of rheumatoid arthritis and osteoarthritis). *Reumatologia* 2000; **38**: 67–73.

35 Altmeyer N *et al.* Conjonctivite, rhinite et asthme rythmés par l'exposition professionelle à l'*Harpagophytum*. *Arch Mal Prof Med Trav Soc* 1992; **53**: 289–291.

36 Abramowitz M. Toxic reactions to plant products sold in health food stores. *Med Lett Drugs Ther* 1979; **21**: 29–30.

37 Eich J *et al.* HPLC analysis of iridoid compounds of *Harpagophytum* taxa: quality control of pharmaceutical drug material. *Pharmac Pharmacol Lett* 1998; **8**: 75–78.

38 Chrubasik S *et al.* Zum Harpagosidehalt verschiedener Trockenextraktpulver aus *Harpagophytum procumbens*. *Forsch Komplementärmed* 1996; **3**: 6–11.

Drosera

Species (Family)

Drosera rotundifolia L. (Droserceae)

Synonym(s)

Sundew

Part(s) Used

Herb

Pharmacopoeial and Other Monographs

BHP 1983[G7]
Complete German Commission E (Sundew)[G3]
Martindale 32nd edition[G43]
PDR for Herbal Medicines 2nd edition (Sundew)[G36]

Legal Category (Licensed Products)

Drosera is not included in the GSL.[G37]

Constituents[G2,G40,G48,G53,G64]

Flavonoids Kaempferol, myricetin, quercetin and hyperoside.[1]

Quinones Plumbagin,[2] hydroplumbagin glucoside[3] and rossoliside (7-methyl-hydrojuglone-4-glucoside).[4]

Other constituents Carotenoids, plant acids (e.g. butyric acid, citric acid, formic acid, gallic acid, malic acid, propionic acid), resin, tannins (unspecified) and ascorbic acid (vitamin C).

Food Use

Drosera is not used in foods.

Herbal Use

Drosera is stated to possess antispasmodic, demulcent and expectorant properties. It has been used for bronchitis, asthma, pertussis, tracheitis, gastric ulceration and specifically for asthma and chronic bronchitis with peptic ulceration or gastritis.[G2,G7,G64]

Dosage

Dried plant 1–2 g or by infusion three times daily.[G7]

Liquid extract 0.5–2.0 mL (1:1 in 25% alcohol) three times daily.[G7]

Tincture 0.5–1.0 mL (1:5 in 60% alcohol) three times daily.[G7]

Pharmacological Actions

In vitro and animal studies

Drosera is reported to prevent acetylcholine- or histamine-induced bronchospasm, and to relax acetylcholine- or barium chloride-induced spasm of the isolated intestine.[5] Drosera is stated to possess antitussive properties and has been reported to prevent coughing induced by excitation of the larynx nerve in the rabbit.[5] These antispasmodic actions have been attributed to the naphthoquinone constituents.[G53]

Antimicrobial properties have also been documented for the naphthoquinones.[6] *In vivo*, plumbagin is reported to exert a broad spectrum of activity against Gram-positive and Gram-negative bacteria, influenza viruses, pathogenic fungi, and parasitic protozoa. *In vitro*, a plumbagin solution (1:50 000) was reported to exhibit activity against staphylococci, streptococci and pneumococci (Gram-positive bacteria), but to lack activity against *Haemophilus pertussis* (Gram-negative bacteria).[5] Plumbagin administered orally to mice for five days, was found to be ineffective against *Lamblia muris* and tuberculosis infection. *Microsporum* infections in guinea-pigs were treated successfully by local applications of 0.25–0.5% solutions (in 40% alcohol) or of 1% emulsions.[6]

An aqueous drosera extract was reported to possess pepsin-like activity.[G53]

In vitro, drosera extracts and plumbagin, in concentrations of 0.01–1.0 mg/mL, have been documented to exert a cytotoxic or immunosuppressive effect in human granulocytes and lymphocytes.[2] Lower concentrations were reported to exhibit immunostimulating properties. Plumbagin possesses chemotherapeutic properties, but is irritant when administered at therapeutic doses.[6]

Side-effects, Toxicity

None documented for drosera. Plumbagin is stated to be an irritant principle[G51] and an LD_{50} (mice, intraperitoneal injection) has been reported to be 15 mg/kg body weight.[G48]

Cytotoxic properties have been documented for drosera and plumbagin (*see In vitro* and animal studies).

Contra-indications, Warnings

None documented.

Pregnancy and lactation   The safety of drosera has not been established. In view of the lack of toxicity data, the use of drosera during pregnancy and lactation should be avoided.

Pharmaceutical Comment

Limited chemical information is available for drosera. Documented animal studies support some of the herbal uses. Reported immunostimulant and immunosuppressant activities may warrant further research into the pharmacological activities of drosera. In view of the lack of chemical and toxicity data, excessive use of drosera should be avoided.

References

See also General References G2, G3, G7, G31, G36, G37, G40, G43, G45, G48, G51, G53 and G64.

1   Ayuga C *et al*. Contribución al estudio de flavonoides en *D. rotundifolia* L. *An R Acad Farm* 1985; **51**: 321–326.
2   Wagner H *et al*. Immunological investigations of naphthoquinone-containing plant extracts, isolated quinones and other cytostatic compounds in cellular immunosystems. *Phytochem Soc Eur Symp* 1986; 43.
3   Vinkenborg J *et al*. De aanwezigheid van hydro-plumbagin-glucoside in *Drosera rotundifolia*. *Pharm Weekbl* 1969; **104**: 45–49.
4   Sampara-Rumantir N. Rossoliside. *Pharm Weekbl* 1971; **106**: 653–664.
5   Oliver-Bever B. *Plants in Tropical West Africa*. Cambridge University Press: Cambridge, 1986: 129.
6   Vichkanova SA *et al*. Chemotherapeutic properties of plumbagin. In: Aizenman BE, ed. *Fitontsidy Mater Soveshch, 6th 1969*. Kiev: Naukova Dumka, 1972: 183–185.

Echinacea

Species (Family)

(i) *Echinacea angustifolia* (DC.) Hell. (Asteraceae/Compositae)
(ii) *Echinacea pallida* (Nutt.) Britt.
(iii) *Echinacea purpurea* Moensch.

Synonym(s)

Black Sampson, Coneflower
(i) *Brauneria angustifolia*
(ii) *Brauneria pallida* (Nutt.) Britt.

Part(s) Used

Rhizome, root

Pharmacopoeial and Other Monographs

BHC 1992[G6]
BHP 1996[G9]
Complete German Commission E[G3]
ESCOP 1999[G52]
Martindale 32nd edition[G43]
Mills and Bone[G50]
PDR for Herbal Medicines 2nd edition[G36]
WHO volume 1 1999[G63]

Legal Category (Licensed Products)

GSL[G37]

Constituents[1–5,G2,G6,G39,G40,G48,G53,G64]

Alkaloids Saturated pyrrolizidine-type. Isotussilagine and tussilagine 0.006% in *Echinacea angustifolia* and *Echinacea purpurea*.[1]

Amides Alkylamides, at least 20, especially isobutylamides of C_{11}–C_{16} straight-chain fatty acids;[2–6] echinacein, an unsaturated amide reported to be identical with neoherculin and α-sanshool.

Carbohydrates High molecular weight polysaccharides, echinacin (polysaccharide component), inulin and sugars (fructose, glucose, pentose).[7–9]

Glycosides Caffeic acid derivatives (e.g. echinacoside 0.5–1.0%).[4,10,11] Cynarin (quinic acid deriva-

tive) is reported to be specific to *E. angustifolia* and is stated to be the first documented isolation of cynarin from the genus *Echinacea*.

Polyenes Polyacetylenes are reported to be specific to *E. pallida*. However, polyacetylenes have also been documented for both *E. angustifolia* and *E. purpurea*.[4,12,13]

Terpenoids Sesquiterpene lactone esters (germacrane- or guaiane-type skeleton) isolated from *E. purpurea*[14] have subsequently been attributed to *Parthenium integrifolium*,[15] a known adulterant of *E. purpurea*.

Other constituents Betaine (carotenoid), fatty acids, phytosterol, resin and volatile oil (alkylketones main constituents in *E. pallida*).

Other plant parts The aerial parts of *E. purpurea* have been reported to contain amides (highly unsaturated), germacrene (a sesquiterpene) alcohol, a labdane derivative, methyl *p*-hydroxycinnamate and vanillin.

Food Use

Echinacea is not used in foods.

Herbal Use

Echinacea is stated to possess antiseptic, antiviral and peripheral vasodilator properties. Traditionally, it has been used for furunculosis, septicaemia, nasopharangeal catarrh, pyorrhoea, tonsillitis, and specifically for boils, carbuncles and abscesses.[1,G2,G6,G7,G8,G64] It is under investigation for its immunostimulant action.

Dosage

Dried root/rhizome 1 g or by infusion or decoction three times daily.[G6,G7]

Liquid extract 0.25–1.0 mL (1 : 1 in 45% alcohol) three times daily.[G6,G7]

Tincture 1–2 mL (1 : 5 in 45% alcohol) three times daily.[G6,G7]

Pharmacological Actions[16–20]

In vitro and animal studies

In vivo immunostimulant activity in mice has been documented for echinacea, indicated by phagocytosis enhancement and by an increase in the serum elimination of carbon particles (carbon clearance test).[7,21] Documented in vitro immunostimulant activity, indicated by phagocytosis enhancement and by stimulation of TNF (tumour necrosis factor) secretion in human macrophages and lymphocytes, is stated to be indicative of non-specific T cell activation.[7,22]

Immunostimulant activity has been associated with polysaccharide fractions (PSF) and polyacetylene fractions (PCF) in both in vivo and in vitro studies.[23] However, no direct influence on T lymphocytes and only a moderate induction of B lymphocyte proliferation were reported for a PSF, from E. purpurea, that was found to selectively induce macrophage cytotoxicity against tumour targets in vitro.

Phagocytosis enhancement in vitro has also been reported for non-volatile sesquiterpene esters isolated from E. purpurea,[14] and tissue culture experiments have yielded immunologically active polysaccharides.[24]

In vitro antiviral activity has been described for alcoholic and aqueous echinacea extracts.[25] Incubation of mouse cells with the extracts was stated to result in 24 hour resistance to influenza, herpes and vesicular (pox) viruses.[25] Documented immunostimulant and antiviral properties are thought to be partly mediated via the binding of the PSF to carbohydrate receptors on the cell surface of T cell lymphocytes, resulting in non-specific T cell activation (e.g. interferon production, lymphokine (TNF) secretion).[26,27]

In vivo anti-inflammatory activity has been reported for the PSF in the carrageenan rat paw oedema test and in the croton oil mouse ear test, with the PSF administered intravenously and topically, respectively.[8] The isolated PSF was stated to be twice as active as the total aqueous extract in the carrageenan test, and to be about half as active as indomethacin in the croton oil test.

In addition, an aqueous echinacea extract was reported to be more effective in the croton oil test than benzydamine, a topical non-steroidal anti-inflammatory drug. When an echinacea leaf extract was administered orally to rats, it was stated to be devoid of anti-inflammatory activity in the carrageenan test.[28]

A long-chain alkene from E. angustifolia is stated to possess significant antitumour activity in vivo, inhibiting the growth of Walker tumours in rats and lymphocytic leukaemia (P388) in mice.[29]

Antibacterial activity against Escherichia coli, Proteus mirabilis, Pseudomonas aeruginosa and Staphylococcus aureus has been demonstrated for a multi-herbal preparation containing echinacea and other herbal ingredients, with slight activity against Staphylococcus aureus and Proteus mirabilis attributed to echinacea.[30]

The same preparation exhibited in vitro antispasmodic activity against acetylcholine-induced spasm of the isolated guinea-pig ileum. Echinacea was one of two components to which the main antispasmodic activity was attributed.[30]

Echinacin, a polysaccharide extract, has been used experimentally as an antagonist of hyaluronidase.[31] The wound-healing properties documented for echinacea have been attributed to echinacin (polysaccharide extract), which is said to inhibit the action of hyaluronidase via formation of a stable hyaluronic acid–polysaccharide complex and to stimulate fibroblast cell growth.[G2]

Echinacea is stated to have some cortisone-like activity.[31]

Clinical studies

Echinacea has been used for its non-specific action on cell-mediated immunity. A single 2-mL subcutaneous injection (stated as equivalent to 0.1 g of press sap) followed by a free interval of one week was reported to stimulate cell-mediated immunity, whereas daily administration of the injection was stated to have a depressant effect on cell-mediated immunity.[30]

A multi-herbal preparation containing echinacea as one of the ingredients was reported to have a favourable effect on the symptoms of irritable bladder associated with functional and neurohormonal disorders, and on bacterial bladder infections. Contributions of the individual ingredients to the overall efficacy of the preparations were assessed in animal experiments (see In vitro and animal studies).[30]

Numerous trials have been undertaken with the commercial preparations Echinacin (fresh juice of the aerial parts) and Esberitox (a mixture of Echinacea purpurea, Echinacea angustifolia, Baptisia tinctoria and Thuja occidentalis). The majority of these trials, which utilised intravenous injections and small groups of patients, were not randomised and controlled double-blind trials. The clinical conditions studied have included infections and wound-healing, polyarthritis, influenza, colds, upper respiratory tract infections, eczema, psoriasis, urogenital infections, allergies, candidiasis, gynaecological infections, chronic osteomyelitis and chronic skin ulcers.[18]

Side-effects, Toxicity

Echinacea is stated to have produced positive patch test reactions in four patients with a previous history of plant dermatitis.[G51] Trace amounts of echinacin (polysaccharide extract) placed on the tongue are stated to produce excessive salivation and an intense burning paralytic effect on the tongue and on the mucous membranes of the lips and mouth. The roots are stated to produce a similar but milder effect.[G39]

Pyrrolizidine alkaloids with an unsaturated pyrrolizidine nucleus are reported to be hepatotoxic in both animals and humans (*see* Comfrey). The alkaloids isotussilagine and tussilagine have been documented for echinacea; they possess a saturated pyrrolizidine nucleus and are not thought to be toxic.

In vivo antitumour activity and *in vitro* stimulation of TNF secretion have been reported for echinacea. TNF is one of a group of polypeptide inflammatory mediators which have been collectively termed cytokines (produced by various cell types) or lymphokines (produced by lymphocytes).[G45] TNF is stated to be produced mainly by lymphocytes and macrophages. In addition to its antitumour effects, TNF is stated to be a mediator of cachexia and the manifestations of endotoxic shock. Concern has been expressed over the possible toxicity of TNF.[G45]

Contra-indications, Warnings

None documented. Echinacea may interfere with immunosuppressive therapy.

Pregnancy and lactation   The safety of echinacea has not been established. In view of the lack of toxicity data, excessive use of echinacea during pregnancy should be avoided.

Pharmaceutical Comment

The chemistry of echinacea is well documented.[1–20] *E. angustifolia* and *E. pallida* are described under the same monograph heading in the BHP 1983, although it has been proposed that the two species are in fact chemically dissimilar. *E. purpurea* and *E. angustifolia* both contain amides as their major lipophilic constituents, but of differing structural types.[4,5] By contrast, the lipophilic fraction of *E. pallida* is characterised by polyacetylenes and contains only very low concentrations, if any, of amides.[4,5]

Commercial echinacea samples may contain one or more of the three *Echinacea* species mentioned above, and the reported presence of polyenes in commercial samples of *E. angustifolia* is thought to result from sample contamination with *E. pallida*.[4]

The polyene components are stated to be susceptible to auto-oxidation resulting in the formation of artefacts during storage. It has therefore been recommended that the roots should be stored full-size and that extracts should be kept in solution.[4,G2]

Documented scientific evidence from animal studies supports some of the uses for echinacea as well as the more recent interest in immunostimulant properties.[16–20] Reported pharmacological activities seem to be mainly associated with polyene and high molecular weight polysaccharide constituents. Further well-designed clinical studies using standardised preparations and larger numbers of patients are required in order to verify the efficacy of echinacea.

In view of the lack of toxicity data, excessive use of echinacea should be avoided.

References

See also General References G2, G3, G5, G6, G7, G8, G9, G18, G30, G31, G32, G34, G36, G37, G39, G40, G43, G45, G48, G50, G52, G53, G56 and G64.

1   Bauer R *et al*. Alkamides from the roots of *Echinacea angustifolia*. *Phytochemistry* 1989; **28**: 505–508.
2   Wagner H *et al*. Immunostimulating polysaccharides (heteroglycans) of higher plants. *Arzneimittelforschung* 1985; **35**: 1069–1075.
3   Tubaro A *et al*. Anti-inflammatory activity of a polysaccharide fraction of *Echinacea angustifolia*. *J Pharm Pharmacol* 1987; **39**: 567–569.
4   Protsch A, Wagner H. Structural analysis of a 4-O-methylgluconoarabinoxylan with immunostimulating activity from *Echinacea purpurea*. *Phytochemistry* 1987; **26**: 1989–1993.
5   Becker H *et al*. Structure of echinoside. *Z Naturforsch* 1982; **37c**: 351–353.
6   Becker H, Hsieh WC. Cichoric acid and its derivatives from Echinacea species. *Z Naturforsch* 1985; **40c**: 585–587.
7   Schulte KE *et al*. Das Vorkommen von Polyacetylen-Verbindungen in *Echinacea purpurea* Mnch. und *Echinacea angustifolia* DC. *Arzneimittelforschung* 1967; **17**: 825–829.
8   Bauer R *et al*. Two acetylenic compounds from *Echinacea pallida* roots. *Phytochemistry* 1987; **26**: 1198–1200.
9   Bauer R *et al*. Structure and stereochemistry of new sesquiterpene esters from *Echinacea purpurea*. *Helv Chim Acta* 1985; **68**: 2355–2358.
10 Bauer R *et al*. Nachweis einer Verfälschung von *Echinacea purpurea* (L.) Moench mit *Parthenium integrifolium* L. *Dtsch Apoth Ztg* 1987; **127**: 1325.
11 Bauer R, Wagner H. *Echinacea. Ein Handbuch für*

Ärzte, Apotheker und andere Naturwissenschaftler. Stuttgart: Wissenschaftliche Verlagsgesellschaft, 1990: 182.

12   Bauer R, Wagner H. Echinacea – Der Sonnenhut – Stand der Forschung. *Z Phytother* 1988; **9**: 151–159.

13   Hobbs C. In: Miovich M, ed. *The Echinacea Handbook*, Portland, Oregon: Eclectic Medical Publications, 1989: 118.

14   Hobbs C. Echinacea – a literature review. *Herbalgram* 1994; **30**: 33–47.

15   Houghton PJ. Echinacea. *Pharm J* 1994; **253**: 342–343.

16   Röder E *et al.* Pyrrolizidine in *Echinacea angustifolia* DC und *Echinacea purpurea* M. *Arzneimittelforschung* 1984; **124**: 2316–2317.

17   Jacobson M. The structure of echinacein, the insecticidal component of American coneflower roots. *J Org Chem* 1967; **32**: 1646–1647.

18   Bohlman F, Hoffmann M. Further amides from *Echinacea purpurea*. *Phytochemistry* 1983; **22**: 1173–1175.

19   Bauer R *et al.* Analysis of *Echinacea pallida* and *E. angustifolia* roots. *Planta Med* 1988; **54**: 426–430.

20   Bauer R, Remiger P. TLC and HPLC analysis of alkamides in *Echinacea* drugs. *Planta Med* 1989; **55**: 367–371.

21   Bauer R *et al.* Immunologische *in-vivo* und *in-vitro* Untersuchungen mit *Echinacea* Extracten. *Arzneimittelforschung* 1988; **38**: 276–281.

22   Vömel T. Der einfluss eines pflanzelischen Immunostimulans auf die Phagozytose von Erythozyten durch das retikulohistozytäre System der isoliert perfundierten Rattenleber. *Arzneimittelforschung* 1985; **35**: 1437–1439.

23   Stimpel M *et al.* Macrophage activation and induction of macrophage cytotoxicity by purified polysaccharide fractions from the plant *Echinacea purpurea*. *Infect Immun* 1984; **46**: 845–849.

24   Wagner H *et al.* Immunologically active polysaccharides of *Echinacea purpurea* cell cultures. *Phytochemistry* 1988; **27**: 119–126.

25   Wacker A, Hilbig W. Virus inhibition by *Echinacea purpurea*. *Planta Med* 1978; **33**: 89–102.

26   Mose J. Effect of echinacin on phagocytosis and natural killer cells. *Med Welt* 1983; **34**: 1463–1467.

27   Wagner H *et al.* Immunostimulating polysaccharides (heteroglycans) of higher plants – preliminary communications. *Arzneimittelforschung* 1984; **34**: 659–660.

28   Tragni E *et al.* Evidence from two classical irritation tests for an anti-inflammatory action of a natural extract, echinacea B. *Food Chem Toxic* 1985; **23**: 317–319.

29   Voaden DJ, Jacobson M. Tumour inhibitors. 3. Identification and synthesis of an oncolytic hydrocarbon from American coneflower roots. *J Med Chem* 1972; **15**: 619–623.

30   Westendorf J. Carito® – *in-vitro* Untersuchungen zum Nachweiss spasmolytischer und kontraktiler Einflüsse. *Therapiewoche* 1982; **32**: 6291–6297.

31   Busing K. Hyaluronidasehemmung durch echinacin. *Arzneimittelforschung* 1952; **2**: 467–469.

Elder

Species (Family)

Sambucus nigra L. (Caprifoliaceae)

Synonym(s)

Black Elder, European Elder, Sambucus
  Sambucus canadensis L. refers to American Elder

Part(s) Used

Flower

Pharmacopoeial and Other Monographs

BHC 1992[G6]
BHP 1996[G9]
BP 2001[G15]
Complete German Commission E[G3]
Martindale 32nd edition[G43]
PDR for Herbal Medicines 2nd edition[G36]
Ph Eur 2002[G28]

Legal Category (Licensed Products)

GSL[G37]

Constituents[G2,G6,G41,G62,G64]

Flavonoids Flavonols (kaempferol, quercetin), quercetin glycosides (1.5–3.0%) including hyperoside, isoquercitrin and rutin.

Triterpenes α- and β-amyrin, oleanolic and ursolic acids.

Volatile oils 0.3%. 66% fatty acids (primarily linoleic, linolenic and palmitic) and 7% alkanes (C_{19}, C_{21}, C_{23} and C_{25}). Numerous other constituent types have been identified including ethers and oxides, ketones, aldehydes, alcohols and esters.[1]

Other constituents Chlorogenic acid, tannin, mucilage, plastocynin (protein),[2] pectin and sugar.

Other plant parts *Leaf* Sambunigrin (0.042%), prunasin, zierin and holocalin (cyanogenetic glycosides),[3] choline, flavonoids (rutin, quercetin), sterols (sitosterol, stigmasterol, campesterol), triterpenes (α-

and β-amyrin palmitates, oleanolic and ursolic acids), alkanes, fatty acids, tannins and others.[G41]

Bark Lectin (mol. wt 140 000) rich in asparagine/aspartic acid, glutamine/glutamic acid, valine and leucine,[4] phytohaemagglutinin,[5] triterpenoids (α-amyrenone, α-amyrin, betulin, oleanolic acid, β-sitosterol).[6]

Food Use

Elder is listed by the Council of Europe as a source of natural food flavouring (categories N1 and N2). Category N1 refers to the fruit and indicates that there are no restrictions on quantities used. Category N2 refers to the restrictions on the concentrations of hydrocyanic acid that are permitted, namely 1 mg/kg in beverages and foods, 1 mg/kg for every per cent proof of alcoholic beverages, 5 mg/kg in stone fruit juices, 25 mg/kg in confectionery and 50 mg/kg in marzipan.[G16] In the USA, the flowers have a regulatory status of GRAS (Generally Recognised As Safe).[G41]

Herbal Use

Elder is stated to possess diaphoretic and anticatarrhal properties. Traditionally, it has been used for influenza colds, chronic nasal catarrh with deafness and sinusitis.[G8] Elder is also stated to act as a diuretic, laxative and local anti-inflammatory agent.[G2,G6,G7,G8,G41,G49,G64]

Dosage

Dried flower 2–4 g by infusion three times daily.[G6,G7]

Liquid extract 2–4 mL (1:1 in 25% alcohol) three times daily.[G6,G7]

Pharmacological Actions

In vitro and animal studies

Elder is stated to possess diuretic and laxative properties.[G41]

  Moderate (27%) anti-inflammatory action in carrageenan-induced rat paw oedema has been documented for an elder preparation given one hour before carrageenan (100 mg/kg, by mouth).[7] Indomethacin as a control exhibited 45% inhibition at a dose of 5 mg/kg.[7]

An infusion made from the flowers of elder, St. John's wort herb and root of soapwort (*Saponaria officinalis*) has exhibited antiviral activity against influenza types A and B (*in vivo* and *in vitro*) and herpes simplex virus type 1 (*in vitro*).[8]

A diuretic effect in rats exceeding that exerted by theophylline has been reported for elder.[9] An infusion and extracts rich in potassium and in flavonoids all caused diuresis. Greatest activity was exerted by the combined potassium- and flavonoid-rich extracts.

In vitro antispasmodic activity (rat ileum, rabbit/guinea-pig intestine) and spasmogenic activity (rat uterus) have been reported for lectins isolated from elder.[10]

A lectin isolated from elder bark was found to be a lactose-specific haemagglutinin with a slightly higher affinity for erythrocytes from blood group A.[4] Unlike many other plant lectins, the lectin did not inhibit protein synthesis.[4] The carbohydrate-binding properties of a lectin isolated from elder bark have been studied.[11]

Phytohaemagglutinins are biologically active extracts isolated from various plants and represent a class of lectin. They are associated with haemagglutination and mitogenic, antigenic and immunosuppressant properties.[5] *In vitro*, phytohaemagglutinin has been found to stimulate production of an interferon-like substance in human leukocytes.[G45]

Hepatoprotective activity against carbon tetrachloride-induced toxicity has been reported for triterpenes isolated from *Sambucus formosana* Nakai.[12]

Clinical studies

None documented for elder. Phytohaemagglutinin extracts have been used clinically to treat drug-induced leucopenia and some types of anaemia.[5] The blastogenic response of lymphocytes to phytohaemagglutinin has been used extensively as a measure of immunocompetence.[G45]

Side-effects, Toxicity

No reported side-effects specifically for elder were located. Human poisoning has occurred with *Sambucus* species.[13] The roots, stems and leaves and, much less so, the flowers and unripe berries, are stated to contain a poisonous alkaloid and cyanogenic glycoside causing nausea, vomiting and diarrhoea.[13] The flowers and ripe fruit are stated to be edible without harm.[13]

The effects of a lectin isolated from elder bark on mammalian embryonic and fetal development has been studied.[5] The lectin exerted mainly a toxic effect and, to a lesser degree, a teratogenic effect when administered subcutaneously to pregnant mice. In view of the high doses administered, the authors stated that the results did not indicate a potential hazard to human fetuses exposed to lectins.[5]

Contra-indications, Warnings

Excessive or prolonged use may result in hypokalaemia in view of the documented diuretic effect. Plant parts other than the flowers are reported to be poisonous and should not be ingested.

Pregnancy and lactation The safety of elder taken during pregnancy has not been established. In view of the lack of toxicity data, the use of elder during pregnancy and lactation should be avoided.

Pharmaceutical Comment

Phytochemical details have been documented for elder, with flavonoids and triterpenes representing the main biologically active constituents. Anti-inflammatory, antiviral and diuretic effects have been observed in *in vivo* studies, thus supporting the herbal uses of elder. No documented studies in humans were found. Potentially toxic compounds have been reported for the bark (lectins) and the leaves (cyanogenetic glycosides); the flowers are suitable for use as a herbal remedy.

References

See also General References G2, G3, G5, G6, G9, G11, G15, G16, G28, G31, G36, G37, G41, G43, G48, G49, G56, G62 and G64.

1   Toulemonde B, Richard HMJ. Volatile constituents of dry elder (*Sambucus nigra* L.) flowers. *J Agric Food Chem* 1983; **31**: 365–370.
2   Scawen MD *et al.* The amino-acid sequence of plastocyanin from *Sambucus nigra* L. (elder). *Eur J Biochem* 1974; **44**: 299–303.
3   Jensen SR, Nielsen BJ. Cyanogenic glucosides in *Sambucus nigra* L. *Acta Chem Scand* 1973; **27**: 2661–2685.
4   Broekaert WF *et al.* A lectin from elder (*Sambucus nigra* L.) bark. *Biochem J* 1984; **221**: 163–169.
5   Paulo E. Effect of phytohaemagglutinin (PHA) from the bark of *Sambucus nigra* on embryonic and foetal development in mice. *Folia Biol (Kraków)* 1976; **24**: 213–222.

6   Lawrie W *et al.* Triterpenoids in the bark of elder (*Sambucus nigra*). *Phytochemistry* 1964; **3**: 267–268.

7   Mascolo N *et al.* Biological screening of Italian medicinal plants for anti-inflammatory activity. *Phytother Res* 1987; **1**: 28.

8   Serkedjieva J *et al.* Antiviral activity of the infusion (SHS-174) from flowers of *Sambucus nigra* L., aerial parts of *Hypericum perforatum* L., and roots of *Saponaria officinalis* L. against influenza and herpes simplex viruses. *Phytother Res* 1990; **4**: 97.

9   Rebuelta M *et al.* Étude de l'effet diurétique de différentes préparations des fleurs du *Sambucus nigra* L. *Plant Méd Phytothér* 1983; **17**: 173–181.

10   Richter A. Changes in the motor activity of smooth muscles of the rat uterus *in vitro* as the effect of phytohaemagglutinins from *Sambucus nigra*. *Folia Biol* 1973; **21**: 33–48.

11   Shibuya N *et al.* The elderberry (*Sambucus nigra* L.) bark lectin recognizes the Neu5Ac(α2–6)Gal/GalNAc sequence. *J Biol Chem* 1987; **262**: 1596–1601.

12   Lin C-N, Tome W-P. Antihepatotoxic principles of *Sambucus formosana*. *Planta Med* 1988; **54**: 223–224.

13   Hardin JW, Arena JM, eds. *Human Poisoning from Native and Cultivated Plants*, 2nd edn. North Carolina: Duke University Press, 1974.

Elecampane

Species (Family)

Inula helenium L. (Asteraceae/Compositae)

Synonym(s)

Alant, *Aster helenium* (L.) Scop., *Aster officinalis* All., *Helenium grandiflorum* Gilib., Horseheal, Inula, Scabwort, Yellow Starwort

An elecampane extract has been referred to as helenin. Alantolactone is also known as elecampane camphor, alant camphor, helenin and inula camphor.[G45]

Part(s) Used

Rhizome, root

Pharmacopoeial and Other Monographs

BHC 1992[G6]
BHP 1996[G9]
Martindale 32nd edition[G43]
PDR for Herbal Medicines 2nd edition[G36]

Legal Category (Licensed Products)

GSL[G37]

Constituents[G2,G6,G41,G64]

Carbohydrates   Inulin (up to 44%), mucilage.

Terpenoids   β- and γ-sitosterols, stigmasterol and damaradienol (sterols), friedelin.

Volatile oils   1–4%. Mainly contains sesquiterpene lactones including alantolactone, isoalantolactone and dihydroalantolactone (eudesmanolides), alantic acid and azulene.

Other constituents   Resin.

Food Use

Elecampane is listed by the Council of Europe as a natural source of food flavouring (category N2). This category indicates that elecampane can be added to foodstuffs in small quantities, with a possible limitation of an active principle (as yet unspecified) in the final product.[G16]

In the USA, elecampane is only approved for use in alcoholic beverages.[G41]

Herbal Use

Elecampane is stated to possess expectorant, antitussive, diaphoretic and bactericidal properties. Traditionally, it has been used for bronchial/tracheal catarrh, cough associated with pulmonary tuberculosis and dry irritating cough in children.[G2,G6,G7,G8,G64]

Alantolactone has been used as an anthelmintic in the treatment of roundworm, threadworm, hookworm and whipworm infection.[G44,G45]

Dosage

Rhizome/root   1.5–4.0 g or by decoction three times daily.[G6,G7]

Liquid extract   1.5–4.0 mL (1:1 in 25% alcohol) three times daily.[G6,G7]

Alantolactone   300 mg daily for two courses of 5 days, with an interval of 10 days. Children, 50–200 mg daily.[G44]

Pharmacological Actions

In vitro and animal studies

Elecampane infusion has exhibited a pronounced sedative effect in mice.[G41] Alantolactone has been reported to exhibit hypotensive, hyperglycaemic (large doses) and hypoglycaemic (smaller doses) actions in animals.[G41] Antibacterial properties have also been documented. Alantolactone and iso-alantolactone have been reported to exhibit high bactericidal and fungicidal properties *in vitro*.[G41]

The volatile oil has been reported to exert a potent smooth muscle relaxant effect *in vitro* on guinea-pig ileal and tracheal muscle.[1]

Various activities have been documented for *Inula racemosa*: an extract lowered plasma insulin and glucose concentrations in rats 75 minutes after oral administration,[2] counteracted adrenaline-induced hyperglycaemia in rats,[2] exhibited negative inotropic and chronotropic effects on the frog heart,[2] and provided a preventative and curative action against experimentally induced myocardial infarction in rats.[3] Pretreatment was found to be most effective.[3]

Sesquiterpene lactones with antitumour activity have been isolated from *Helenium microcephalum*.[4,5]

Clinical studies

Alantolactone has been used as an anthelmintic in the treatment of roundworm, threadworm, hookworm and whipworm infection.[G44,G45]

Inula racemosa has been reported to prevent ST-segment depression and T-wave inversion in patients with proven ischaemic heart disease,[2] and to have a beneficial effect on angina pectoris.[6]

Side-effects, Toxicity

Elecampane has been reported to cause allergic contact dermatitis.[G51] Sensitising properties have been documented for the volatile oil,[G51,G58] and for alantolactone and isoalantolactone.[7] *In vitro* cytotoxicty has been reported for alantolactone and isoalantolactone.[8]

Contraindications, Warnings

Elecampane may cause an allergic reaction, particularly in individuals with an existing allergy or sensitivity to other plants in the Asteraceae family. Elecampane may interfere with existing hypoglycaemic and antihypertensive treatment.

Pregnancy and lactation The safety of elecampane taken during pregnancy has not been established. In view of the lack of toxicity data, the use of elecampane during pregnancy and lactation should be avoided.

Pharmaceutical Comment

The pharmacological actions documented for elecampane seem to be attributable to the sesquiterpene lactone constituents, in particular alantolactone and isoalantolactone. The demulcent action of mucilage and reported *in vivo* antispasmodic activity of the volatile oil support the traditional uses of this remedy

in coughs. In addition, alantolactone has been utilised as an anthelmintic. A number of interesting cardiovascular activities have been documented for a related species, *I. racemosa*. Whether the constituents responsible for these actions are also present in elecampane is unclear. In view of the paucity of toxicity data for elecampane, excessive or prolonged use should be avoided.

References

See also General References G2, G6, G9, G16, G31, G36, G37, G41, G43, G48, G51, G58 and G64.

1 Reiter M, Brandt W. Relaxant effects on tracheal and ileal smooth muscles of the guinea pig. *Arzneimittelforschung* 1985; **35**: 408–414.

2 Tripathi YB *et al.* Assessment of the adrenergic beta-blocking activity of *Inula racemosa*. *J Ethnopharmacol* 1988; **23**: 3–9.

3 Patel V *et al.* Effect of indigenous drug (puskarmula) on experimentally induced myocardial infarction in rats. *Act Nerv Super (Praha)* 1982; (Suppl 3): 387–394.

4 Sims D *et al.* Antitumor agents 37. The isolation and structural elucidation of isohelenol, a new antileukemic sesquiterpene lactone, and isohelenalin from *Helenium microcephalum*. *J Nat Prod* 1979; **42**: 282–286.

5 Imakura Y *et al.* Antitumor agents XXXVI: Structural elucidation of sesquiterpene lactones microhelenins-A, B, and C, microlenin acetate, and plenolin from *Helenium microcephalum*. *J Pharm Sci* 1980; **69**: 1044–1049.

6 Tripathi SN *et al.* Beneficial effect of *Inula racemosa* (pushkarmoola) in angina pectoris: a preliminary report. *Indian J Physiol Pharmacol* 1984; **28**: 73–75.

7 Stampf JL *et al.* The sensitising capacity of helenin and two of its main constituents the sesquiterpene lactones alantolactone and isoalantolactone: a comparison of epicutaneous and intradermal sensitising methods in different strains of guinea pig. *Contact Dermatitis* 1982; **8**: 16–24.

8 Woerdenbag HJ. In vitro cytotoxicity of sesquiterpene lactones from *Eupatorium cannabinum* L. and semi-synthetic derivatives from eupatoriopicrin. *Phytother Res* 1988; **2**: 109–114.

Ephedra

Species (Family)

Ephedra sinica Stapf., *E. equisetina*, *E. intermedia*, *E. geriardiana*, *E. major* and other *Ephedra* species that contain ephedrine (Ephedraceae)

Synonym(s)

Cao Ma Huang (Chinese Ephedra), Herba Ephedrae, Ma Huang. Ephedra (and some other herbs) has also been referred to as 'herbal ecstasy'.

Part(s) Used

Aerial parts

Pharmacopoeial and Other Monographs

Complete German Commission E[G3]
Martindale 32nd edition[G43]
PDR for Herbal Medicines 2nd edition[G36]
WHO volume 1 1999[G63]

Legal Category (Licensed Products)

Ephedra is not included in the GSL.[G37]

Ephedra is included in Parts II and III of SI 2130.[1] This allows supply of ephedra (maximum dose of 600 mg and a maximum daily dose of 1800 mg) following a one-to-one consultation with a practitioner.

Ephedrine and pseudoephedrine are not included on the GSL. Both are prescription-only medicines (POM), but can be supplied through pharmacies at certain permitted doses, as follows. Ephedrine for internal preparations: maximum dose 30 mg, maximum daily dose 60 mg; nasal preparations, ephedrine 2%. Pseudoephedrine hydrochloride for internal preparations: maximum dose 60 mg, maximum daily dose 240 mg; prolonged-release preparations: maximum dose 120 mg, maximum daily dose 240 mg. Pseudoephredine sulfate for internal preparations: maximum dose 60 mg, maximum daily dose 180 mg.

Constituents

Alkaloids 0.5–2.0%. Mainly (−)-ephedrine (30–90% in most species, except *E. intermedia*) and (+)-pseudoephedrine, also (−)-norephedrine, (+)-nor-pseudoephedrine, (−)-methylephedrine and (+)-methylpseudoephedrine.[2,G63]

Volatile oil Mainly terpenoids (e.g. α-terpineol, limonene, tetramethylpyrazine, terpinen-4-ol, linalol).[3]

Other constituents Tannins (catechin, gallic acid), ephedrans (glycans) and acids (citric, malic, oxalic).

Roots

Alkaloids Ephedroxane, ephedradines A to D, feruloylhistamine and maokonine.[4]

Flavonoids A flavonoflavonol (ephedrannin A), bis-flavonols (mahuannins A to D).[4]

Food Use

Ephedra is not used in foods.

Herbal Use

Ephedra has traditionally been used for the treatment of bronchial asthma, hayfever, coughs and colds, fever, urticaria, enuresis, narcolepsy, myasthenia gravis, chronic postural hypotension and rheumatism.[G32,G34,G36,G49,G54,G63,G64]

It is stated to have vasoconstricting, bronchodilating and central stimulating properties.[G56] Modern interest in ephedra is focused on its use in cough and bronchitis,[G56] and in nasal congestion due to hayfever, allergic rhinitis, common cold and sinusitis.[G63] There is also interest in the potential of ephedra as an appetite suppressant.

Dosage

Herb 1.2–2.3 g cut herbs containing approximately 1.3% (13 mg/g) total alkaloids.[G4]

Extract Adults: 15–30 mg alkaloids (maximum daily dose 300 mg), calculated as ephedrine.[G56]

Tincture 6–8 mL (1 : 4) three times daily.[G36]

In 1997, the US Food and Drugs Administration (FDA) proposed restrictions on the use of ephedra, although these restrictions have not, to date, been implemented. The FDA proposals included a restriction on the maximum dose of ephedrine: 8 mg taken every 6 hours to a maximum daily dose of 24 mg for no more than seven days.[5,G56]

Pharmacological Actions

The pharmacological properties of ephedra are due to the presence of ephedrine, pseudoephedrine and other ephedra alkaloids (see Constituents). Ephedrine and pseudoephedrine are sympathomimetic agents that have direct and indirect effects on both α- and β-adrenoceptors, as well as stimulating the central nervous system (CNS).[G43,G63] Pseudoephedrine is stated to have less pressor activity and fewer CNS effects than ephedrine.[G43]

In vitro and animal studies

Pharmacological activities documented for ephedrine and/or pseudoephedrine in vitro or in vivo (animals) include smooth muscle relaxant, cardiovascular, anti-inflammatory, immunomodulatory, CNS stimulatory and antimicrobial effects. The pharmacology of ephedra and its constituent alkaloids has been reviewed.[4,6–8]

Ephedrine and pseudoephedrine have been stated to have a relaxant effect on bronchial smooth muscle in isolated rabbit lung and bronchi.[6] Relaxant effects on gastrointestinal smooth muscle have also been noted.[4,6]

Ephedrine has been shown to cause vasoconstriction and to have hypertensive effects in several animal models.[4,6] Maokonine, a constituent of ephedra root, has been reported to be have hypertensive effects in anaesthetised rats.[9] By contrast, other constituents of ephedra roots, such as ephedrannin A and feruloylhistamine, have been reported to have hypotensive activity.[10,11] An aqueous extract of ephedra and its alkaloid fraction increased blood pressure, heart rate and blood glucose concentration in anaesthetised dogs following intravenous administration.[12]

Anti-inflammatory activity has been documented for ephedrine and pseudoephedrine in carrageenan-induced hind-paw oedema in mice.[13] Oral administration of ephedrine and pseudoephedrine also inhibited hind-paw oedema induced by histamine, serotonin, bradykinin and prostaglandin E_1. Crude extracts of ephedra have been reported to inhibit complement in vitro.[14] Further investigation, using an aqueous extract of E. sinica leaves, showed that the complement-inhibiting component of ephedra inhibited the classical complement pathway in sera from several species, including human, pig, guinea-pig, rat and rabbit.[14]

In vitro antibacterial activity against several species, including Staphylococcus aureus, has been reported.[6]

In vitro studies have assessed the cytotoxicity of extracts of ephedra prepared under various conditions (e.g. using ground or unground material boiled for 0.5 or 2 hours) against a range of cell lines, including a human hepatoblastoma cell line (HepG2,), a mouse neuroblastoma cell line (Neuro-2a) and a mouse fibroblastoma cell line.[15] Ephedrine and ephedra extracts prepared from ground material appeared to be significantly more cytotoxic in these cell lines than did preparations from unground material. Also, Neuro-2a cells were more sensitive to ephedra extracts than were the other cell lines tested. Findings of this in vitro work also indicated that ephedra contains toxins other than ephedrine, as IC_{50} values were lower (i.e. indicating greater cytotoxicity) for ephedra extracts than for ephedrine alone.

Clinical studies

Pharmacokinetics Ephedrine and pseudoephedrine are readily absorbed from the gastrointestinal tract and are excreted, largely unchanged, in the urine.[G43] Small amounts of metabolites following hepatic metabolism may be produced. The half-lives of ephedrine and pseudoephedrine range from 3 to 6 hours and from 5 to 8 hours, respectively, depending on urinary pH.[G43]

In a study involving 12 healthy volunteers aged 23–40 years, four capsules of an ephedra product were administered twice, 9 hours apart. Each capsule contained ephedra 375 mg (E. sinica), with a mean (standard deviation (SD)) ephedrine content of 4.84 (0.45) mg.[16] The half-life was reported to be 5.2 hours, maximum plasma concentration (C_{max}) was 81.0 ng/mL, the time to reach C_{max} (t_{max}) was 3.9 hours, and clearance was 24.3 L/hour.

In a randomised, crossover study, 10 healthy volunteers received ephedrine 25 mg or one of three ephedrine-containing nutritional supplements on one day during different phases of the study, each with a one-week washout period.[17] Following single-dose administration of ephedrine 25 mg, mean (SD) half-life, C_{max}, t_{max} and clearance were found to be 5.37 (1.67) hours, 86.5 (15.4) ng/mL, 2.81 (1.35) hours and 28.5 (5.92) L/hour, respectively.

Therapeutic effects The pharmacological properties of ephedrine and pseudoephedrine in humans have been documented and include cardiovascular, bronchodilator and CNS stimulant effects.[G43,G63]

Ephedrine is stated to raise blood pressure by increasing cardiac output and also by peripheral vasoconstriction. Ephedrine relaxes bronchial smooth muscle, reduces intestinal tone and motility, relaxes the bladder wall and reduces the activity of the uterus. Ephedrine is a CNS stimulant; this has led to its investigation for use in assisting weight loss.

A randomised, double-blind, placebo-controlled trial assessed the effects of a herbal combination preparation which included ephedra and other herbal ingredients.[18] In the study, 67 overweight to obese individuals (body mass index 29–35 kg/m^2) received the ephedra-containing preparation, or placebo, for eight weeks. Among the 48 participants who completed the study (24 in each group), a greater mean (SD) weight loss was noted for the treatment group, compared with the placebo group (4.0 (3.4) kg versus 0.8 (2.4) kg, respectively; $p < 0.006$).

Side-effects, Toxicity

The most common adverse effects of ephedrine and pseudoephedrine are tachycardia, anxiety, restlessness and insomnia.[G43] Tremor, dry mouth, impaired circulation to the extremities, hypertension and cardiac arrhythmias may also occur with ephedrine, and skin rashes and urinary retention have been reported for pseudoephedrine.[G43] There are isolated reports of hallucinations in children following use of pseudoephedrine.[G43]

In the US, adverse effects have been reported following self-treatment with products containing ephedra alkaloids marketed for several uses, including as an aid to weight loss, to increase athletic performance, and as an alternative to illegal drugs of abuse.[19,G43] A review assessed 140 reports of adverse events related to the use of products containing ephedra alkaloids, usually combined with caffeine, submitted to the US FDA between June 1997 and March 1999.[19] The main reasons for use of these products were weight loss (59%) and to increase athletic performance (16%); the reason for use was unknown in 17% of cases. Thirty-one per cent of cases ($n = 43$) were considered to be 'definitely' or 'probably' related to the use of products containing ephedra alkaloids, and a further 31% ($n = 44$) were judged to be 'possibly' related; for 29 cases, insufficient information was available to assess causation, and 24 cases were deemed to be 'unrelated' to use of these products. In several cases, individuals were thought to be ingesting up to 60 mg ephedra alkaloids daily. Of the 87 cases where causality was assessed, cardiovascular symptoms (mainly hypertension, palpitations, tachycardia) were the most com-

mon adverse events (47%). The most common CNS events were stroke ($n = 10$) and seizures ($n = 7$). Where events were 'definitely' or 'probably' related ($n = 43$), clinical outcomes were death (three cases), permanent impairment (seven) and ongoing treatment (four); a full recovery occurred in 29 cases.[19]

In a randomised, double-blind, placebo-controlled trial of a herbal supplement containing ephedra (72 mg/day) and guarana (240 mg/day), as well as other herbal ingredients, 23% ($n = 8$) of participants in the treatment group withdrew from the study because of adverse events (e.g. dry mouth, insomnia, headache) that may have been treatment-related; there were no withdrawals among placebo recipients.[18]

There are isolated reports of myocarditis,[20] exacerbation of autoimmune hepatitis,[21] acute hepatitis,[22] nephrolithiasis[23] and psychiatric complications[24] associated with the use of ephedra-containing products. There is a report of sudden death associated with ephedrine toxicity in a 23-year-old man.[25] Several other reports also document psychosis and renal calculi following chronic use or misuse of ephedrine.[G18]

In a study involving 12 normotensive adults who ingested four capsules each containing 375 mg powdered ephedra, followed by four more capsules nine hours later, a statistically significant increase in heart rate, compared with baseline values, was noted in six participants, although effects on blood pressure were variable.[16]

A study involving 47 dogs who were considered to have accidentally ingested herbal products containing ephedra and guarana reported that most dogs (80%) developed clinical signs of toxicosis, within eight hours of ingestion, which persisted for up to 48 hours.[26] Hyperactivity, tremors, seizures and behaviour changes were reported in 83% of dogs; other signs and symptoms included vomiting, tachycardia and hyperthermia.

Contra-indications, Warnings

Ephedra is stated to be contra-indicated in coronary thrombosis, diabetes, glaucoma, heart disease, hypertension, thyroid disease, phaeochromocytoma and enlarged prostate.[G63] Another source states that ephedrine (and, therefore, ephedrine-containing products) should be used with caution in patients with diabetes, ischaemic heart disease, hypertension, hyperthyoidism, renal impairment and angle-closure glaucoma, and that in patients with prostate enlargement, ephedrine may increase difficulty with micturition.[G43] It has been recommended to reduce the dose or discontinue treatment if nervousness, tremor, sleeplessness, loss of appetite or nausea occur with use of ephedra preparations.[G63]

Ephedrine-containing products should be avoided in patients receiving monoamine oxidase inhibitors as concomitant treatment may lead to a hypertensive crisis.[G43] Ephedrine should also be avoided or used with caution in patients undergoing anaesthesia with cyclopropane, halothane or other volatile anaesthetics. There may be an increased risk of arrhythmias in patients receiving ephedrine together with cardiac glycosides, quinidine or tricyclic antidepressants, and there is an increased risk of vasoconstrictor or pressor effects in patients receiving ergot alkaloids or oxytocin.[G43]

There is a report of a professional sportsman who tested positive for norpseudoephedrine after having consumed a liquid herbal product listing ephedra as one of the 15 ingredients.[27]

Pregnancy and lactation There are no reliable data on the use of ephedra during pregnancy and lactation. The safety of ephedra during pregnancy and lactation has not been established and its use should be avoided.

Pharmaceutical Comment

The activities of ephedra are due to the presence of the ephedra alkaloids; of these, the pharmacological effects of ephedrine and pseudoephedrine are most well-documented and support their modern uses. There is less information on the pharmacological effects of ephedra extracts and clinical trials, in particular, are generally lacking.

In view of the safety concerns regarding the use of ephedra products, individuals wishing to use these products should be advised to consult an appropriately trained health care professional. Pharmacists and other health care professionals should be aware that ephedra may be included in unlicensed herbal products and food supplements under the name Ma Huang. Such products will not include reference to ephedra in the labelling.

References

See also General References G5, G18, G29, G31, G32, G34, G36, G43, G49, G54, G56, G63 and G64.

1 Medicines Act 1968, Statutory Instrument 1977 No. 2130 (Retail Sale of Supply of Herbal Remedies) Order, 1977.
2 Dewick P. *Medicinal Natural Products. A Biosynthetic Approach*. Wiley: Chichester, 1997.
3 Miyazawa M *et al*. Volatile components of *Ephedra sinica* Stapf. *Flavour Fragrance J* 1997; 12: 15–17.
4 Tang W, Eisenbrand G. *Chinese Drugs of Plant Origin. Chemistry, Pharmacology and Use in Traditional and Modern Medicine*. Berlin: Springer-Verlag, 1992: 481–490.
5 Blumenthal M. Ephedra update: industry coalition asks FDA to adopt national labeling guidelines on ephedra; offers co-operative research with NIH. *Herbal Gram* 2000; 50: 64–65.
6 Chang H-M, But PP-H, eds. *Pharmacology and Applications of Chinese Materia Medica*, vol 2. Singapore: World Scientific Publishing, 1987: 1119–1124.
7 Kalix P. The pharmacology of psychoactive alkaloids from Ephedra and Catha. *J Ethnopharmacol* 1991; 32: 201–208.
8 Bowman WC, Rand MJ. *Textbook of Pharmacology*, 2nd edn. Oxford: Blackwell, 1980.
9 Tamada M *et al*. Maokonine, hypertensive principle of *Ephedra* roots. *Planta Med* 1978; 34: 291–293.
10 Hikino H *et al*. Structure of feruloylhistamine, a hypotensive principle of *Ephedra* roots. *Planta Med* 1983; 48: 108–110.
11 Hikino H *et al*. Structure of ephedrannin A, a hypotensive principle of *Ephedra* roots. *Tetrahedron Lett* 1982; 23: 673–676.
12 Harada M, Nichimura M. Contribution of alkaloid fraction to pressor and hyperglycemic effect of crude ephedra extract in dogs. *J Pharm Dyn* 1981; 4: 691–699.
13 Kasahara Y *et al*. Antiinflammatory actions of ephedrines in acute inflammations. *Planta Med* 1985; 51: 325–331.
14 Ling M *et al*. A component of the medicinal herb ephedra blocks activation in the classical and alternative pathways of complement. *Clin Exp Immunol* 1995; 102: 582–588.
15 Lee MK *et al*. Cytotoxicity assessment of Ma-huang (Ephedra) under different conditions of preparation. *Toxicol Sci* 2000; 56: 424–430.
16 White LM *et al*. Pharmacokinetics and cardiovascular effects of ma-huang (*Ephedra sinica*) in normotensive adults. *J Clin Pharmacol* 1997; 37: 116–122.
17 Gurley BJ *et al*. Ephedrine pharmacokinetics after the ingestion of nutritional supplements containing *Ephedra sinica* (ma huang). *Ther Drug Monitoring* 1998; 20: 439–445.
18 Boozer CN *et al*. An herbal supplement containing Ma-Huang-Guarana for weight loss: a randomised, double-blind trial. *Int J Obesity* 2001; 25: 316–324.
19 Haller CA, Benowitz NL. Adverse cardiovascular and central nervous system events associated with dietary supplements containing ephedra alkaloids. *N Engl J Med* 2000; 343: 1833–1838.

20 Zaacks SM *et al*. Hypersensitivity myocarditis associated with ephedra use. *J Toxicol Clin Toxicol* 1999; **37**: 485–489.

21 Borum ML. Fulminant exacerbation of autoimmune hepatitis after the use of Ma Huang. *Am J Gastroenterol* 2001; **96**: 1654–1655.

22 Nadir A *et al*. Acute hepatitis associated with the use of a Chinese herbal product, ma-huang. *Am J Gastroenterol* 1996; **91**: 1436–1438.

23 Powell T *et al*. Ma-Huang strikes again: ephedrine nephrolithiasis. *Am J Kidney Dis* 1998; **32**: 153–159.

24 Jacobs KM, Hirsch KA. Psychiatric complications of Ma-huang. *Psychosomatics* 2000; **41**: 58–62.

25 Theoharides TC. Sudden death of a healthy college student related to ephedrine toxicity from a ma huang-containing drink. *J Clin Psychopharmacol* 1997; **17**: 437–439.

26 Ooms TG *et al*. Suspected caffeine and ephedrine toxicosis resulting from ingestion of an herbal supplement containing guarana and ma huang in dogs: 47 cases (1997–1999). *J Am Vet Med Assoc* 2001; **218**: 225–229.

27 Ros JJJW *et al*. A case of positive doping associated with a botanical food supplement. *Pharm World Sci* 1999; **21**: 44.

Eucalyptus

Species (Family)

Eucalyptus globulus Labill. (Myrtaceae)

Synonym(s)

Fevertree, Gum Tree, Tasmanian Bluegum

Part(s) Used

Leaf

Pharmacopoeial and Other Monographs

BHP 1996[G9]
BP 2001[G15]
Complete German Commission E[G3]
Martindale 32nd edition[G43]
PDR for Herbal Medicines 2nd edition[G36]
Ph Eur 2002[G28]

Legal Category (Licensed Products)

GSL[G37]

Constituents[G2,G22,G41,G48,G64]

Flavonoids Eucalyptrin, hyperoside, quercetin, quercitrin and rutin.

Volatile oils 0.5–3.5%. Eucalyptol (cineole) 70–85%. Others include monoterpenes (e.g. α-pinene, β-pinene, *d*-limonene, *p*-cymene, α-phellandrene, camphene, γ-terpinene) and sesquiterpenes (e.g. aromadendrene, alloaromadendrene, globulol, epiglobulol, ledol, viridiflorol), aldehydes (e.g. myrtenal) and ketones (e.g. carvone, pinocarvone).

Other constituents Tannins and associated acids (e.g. gallic acid, protocatechuic acid), caffeic acid, ferulic acids, gentisic acid, resins and waxes

Food Use

Eucalyptus is listed by the Council of Europe as a natural source of food flavouring (leaves, flowers and preparations: category N4, with limits on eucalyptol) (*see* Appendix 23).[G17] Both eucalyptus and eucalyptol (cineole) are used as flavouring agents in many food products.[G41] In the USA, eucalyptus is approved for food use and eucalyptol is listed as a synthetic flavouring agent.[G41]

Herbal Use

Eucalyptus leaves and oil have been used as an antiseptic, febrifuge and expectorant.[G2,G41,G64]

Dosage

Eucalyptol (cineole BPC 1973) 0.05–0.2 mL.

Eucalyptus Oil (BPC 1973) 0.05–0.2 mL.

Fluid extract 2–4 g.

Oil for local application 30 mL oil to 500 mL lukewarm water.

Pharmacological Actions

In vitro and animal studies

Hypoglycaemic activity in rabbits has been documented for a crude leaf extract rich in phenolic glycosides. Purification of the extract resulted in a loss of activity.[G41] Expectorant and antibacterial activities have been reported for eucalyptus oil and for eucalyptol.[G41] Various *Eucalyptus* species have been shown to possess antibacterial activity against both Gram-positive and Gram-negative organisms. Gram-positive organisms were found to be the most sensitive, particularly *Bacillus subtilis* and *Micrococcus glutamious*.[1]

In vitro antiviral activity against influenza type A has been documented for quercitrin and hyperoside.[G41]

Clinical studies

Eucalyptus oil oil has been taken orally for catarrh, used as an inhalation and applied as a rubefacient.[G45] A plant preparation containing tinctures of various herbs including eucalyptus has been used successfully in the treatment of chronic suppurative otitis.[2] The efficacy of the preparation was attributed to the antibacterial and anti-inflammatory actions of the herbs included.

Side-effects, Toxicity

Externally, eucalyptus oil is stated to be generally non-toxic, non-sensitising and non-phototoxic.[G58] Undiluted eucalyptus oil is toxic and should not be taken internally. A dose of 3.5 mL has proved fatal.[G45] Symptoms of poisoning with eucalyptus oil include epigastric burning, nausea and vomiting, dizziness, muscular weakness, miosis, a feeling of suffocation, cyanosis, delirium and convulsions.

Contra-indications, Warnings

Eucalyptus may interfere with existing hypoglycaemic therapy. Eucalyptus oil should be diluted before internal or external use.

Pregnancy and lactation   Eucalyptus oil should not be taken internally during pregnancy.

Pharmaceutical Comment

Eucalyptus is characterised by its volatile oil components. Antiseptic and expectorant properties have been attributed to the oil, in particular to the principal component eucalyptol. The undiluted oil is toxic if taken internally. Essential oils should not be applied to the skin unless they are diluted with a carrier vegetable oil.

References

See also General References G2, G3, G9, G15, G16, G19, G22, G28, G31, G36, G37, G41, G43, G48, G58 and G64.

1 Kumar A *et al*. Antibacterial properties of some *Eucalpytus* oils. *Fitoterapia* 1988; **59**: 141–144.
2 Shaparenko BA *et al*. On use of medicinal plants for treatment of patients with chronic suppurative otitis. *Zh Ushn Gorl Bolezn* 1979; **39**: 48–51.

Euphorbia

Species (Family)

Euphorbia hirta L. (Euphorbiaceae)

Synonym(s)

Euphorbia capitata Lam., *Euphorbia pilulifera* L., Pillbearing Spurge, Snakeweed

Part(s) Used

Herb

Pharmacopoeial and Other Monographs

BHP 1983[G7]

Legal Category (Licensed Products)

GSL[G37]

Constituents[G41,G48,G64]

Flavonoids Leucocyanidin, quercetin, quercitrin and xanthorhamnin.

Terpenoids α- and β-Amyrin, taraxerol and esters, friedelin; campesterol, sitosterol and stigmasterol (sterols).

Other constituents Choline, alkanes, inositol, phenolic acids (e.g. ellagic, gallic, shikimic), sugars and resins.

Food Use

Euphorbia is not used in foods.

Herbal Use

Euphorbia is stated to be used for respiratory disorders, such as asthma, bronchitis, catarrh and laryngeal spasm. It has also been used for intestinal amoebiasis.[G7,G64]

Dosage

Herb 120–300 mg or as an infusion.[G7]

Liquid Extract of Euphorbia (BPC 1949) 0.12–0.3 mL.

Euphorbia Tincture (BPC 1923) 0.6–2.0 mL.

Pharmacological Actions

In vitro and animal studies

Euphorbia has been reported to have antispasmodic and histamine-potentiating properties.[G41] Smooth muscle relaxing and contracting activities have been exhibited by euphorbia *in vitro* (guinea-pig ileum) and have been attributed to shikimic acid and to choline, respectively.[1]

In vivo antitumour activities have been documented for euphorbia.[G41]

Antibacterial activity *in vitro* versus both Gram-positive and Gram-negative bacteria has been documented for euphorbia.[2] Stem extracts were slightly more active than leaf extracts. *In vitro* amoebicidal activity versus *Entamoeba histolytica* has been reported for a euphorbia decoction.[3]

Side-effects, Toxicity

None documented for euphorbia. Carcinogenic properties in mice have been reported for shikimic acid, although no mutagenic activity was observed in the Ames assay.[G41]

Contra-indications, Warnings

None documented.

Pregnancy and lactation The safety of euphorbia has not been established. Euphorbia has been reported to cause both contraction and relaxation of smooth muscle. In view of the lack of pharmacological and toxicity data, the use of euphorbia during pregnancy and lactation should be avoided.

Pharmaceutical Comment

There is little published information concerning euphorbia, although documented actions observed in animals do support the traditional herbal uses. There is a lack of information concerning toxicity, although the documented constituents of euphorbia do not indicate any obvious toxic component. Nevertheless, excessive or prolonged ingestion should be avoided.

References

See also General References G7, G10, G31, G37, G41, G44, G48 and G64.

1 El-Naggar L *et al*. A note on the isolation and identification of two pharmacologically active constituents of *Euphorbia pilulifera*. *Lloydia* 1978; **41**: 73–75.

2 Ajao AO *et al*. Antibacterial activity of *Euphorbia hirta*. *Fitoterapia* 1985; **56**: 165–167.

3 Basit N *et al*. In vitro effect of extracts of *Euphorbia hirta* Linn. on *Entamoeba histolytica*. *Riv Parasitol* 1977; **38**: 259–262.

Evening Primrose

Species (Family)

Oenothera species including *Oenothera biennis* L. (Onagraceae)

Synonym(s)

King's Cureall

Part(s) Used

Seed oil

Pharmacopoeial and Other Monographs

Martindale 32nd edition[G43]
Mills and Bone[G50]
PDR for Herbal Medicines 2nd edition[G36]

Legal Category (Licensed Products)

Evening primrose is not included in the GSL.[G37] Gamolenic acid is a prescription-only medicine.

Constituents

Fixed oils   14%. cis-Linoleic acid (LA) 72% (65–80%), cis-gammalinolenic acid (gamolenic acid, GLA) 2–16%, oleic acid 9%, palmitic acid 7% and stearic acid (3%).[1–5]

Food Use

Evening primrose root has been used as a vegetable with a peppery flavour.[5] The seed oil has been used as a food supplement for many years. LA and gamolenic acid are both essential fatty acids (EFAs), with LA representing the main EFA in the diet, whilst gamolenic acid is found in human milk, in oats and barley, and in small amounts in a wide variety of common foods.[4,5]

Herbal Use

An infusion of the whole plant is reputed to have sedative and astringent properties, and has traditionally been used for asthmatic coughs, gastrointestinal disorders, whooping cough and as a sedative painkiller.[5] Externally, poultices were reputed to ease bruises and to speed wound-healing.[5]

Evening primrose oil (EPO) is licensed for the treatment of atopic eczema, and cyclical and non-cyclical mastalgia. Other conditions in which evening primrose oil is used include premenstrual syndrome, psoriasis, multiple sclerosis, hypercholesterolaemia, rheumatoid arthritis, Raynaud's phenomenon, Sjögren's syndrome, postviral fatigue syndrome, asthma and diabetic neuropathy.[1–3,5]

Dosage

Recommended doses for evening primrose oil are specific to the condition being treated.

Daily doses for a licensed evening primrose oil product are 6–8 g (adults) and 2–4 g (children) in atopic eczema.[6] In cyclical and non-cyclical mastalgia, a daily dose of 3 to 4 g is recommended. These doses are based on a standardised gamolenic acid content of 8%. No special precautions are noted for the elderly. The oil may be swallowed directly, mixed with milk or another liquid, or taken with food.

A patient may need to receive evening primrose oil for a period of three months before a clinical response is observed.[3,6]

Pharmacological Actions

The pharmacological actions of evening primrose oil have been reviewed.[1–3,5]

The actions of evening primrose oil are attributable to the essential fatty acid content of the oil and to the involvement of these compounds in prostaglandin biosynthetic pathways.

Gamolenic acid and its metabolite dihomo-gamma-linolenic acid (DGLA) are precursors of both the inflammatory prostaglandin E_2 (PGE$_2$) series via arachidonic acid (AA), and of the less inflammatory prostaglandin E_1 (PGE$_1$) series. Actions attributed to PGE$_1$ include anti-inflammatory, immunoregulatory and vasodilatory properties, inhibition of platelet aggregation and cholesterol biosynthesis, hypotension and elevation of cyclic AMP (inhibits phospholipase A_2, *see below*).[1–3]

Dietary supplementation with gamolenic acid has been noted to have a favourable effect on the DGLA : AA ratio. Although an increase in arachidonic acid concentrations is also seen, this is much smaller and less consistent compared to the increase seen for DGLA.[3] Contributory factors to this negative effect on arachidonic acid are PGE_1 and 15-hydroxy-DGLA. The latter inhibits conversion of arachidonic acid to inflammatory lipoxygenase metabolites including leukotrienes, whilst PGE_1 inhibits the enzyme phospholipase A_2 which is required for the mobilisation of arachidonic acid from phospholipid membrane stores.[3] In addition, DGLA desaturation to arachidonic acid is a rate-limiting step in humans and proceeds very slowly.[3]

Gamolenic acid is not normally obtained directly from dietary sources and the body relies on metabolic conversion from dietary LA. This conversion is readily saturable and is considered to be the rate-limiting step in the production of gamolenic acid. A reduced rate of LA conversion to gamolenic acid has been observed in a number of clinical situations including ageing, diabetes, cardiovascular disorders and high cholesterol concentrations, high alcohol intake, viral infections, cancer, nutritional deficits, atopic eczema and premenstrual syndrome.[1–3] Direct dietary supplementation with gamolenic acid effectively bypasses this rate-limiting conversion step and has a beneficial effect on the ratio of inflammatory:noninflammatory prostaglandin compounds.

Evening primrose oil represents a good source of both LA and, more importantly, of gamolenic acid. Numerous papers have been published on the biochemical rationale for the therapeutic uses of evening primrose oil and on its efficacy in various disease states associated with low concentrations of gamolenic acid. The use of evening primrose oil in various disease states which include atopic eczema, premenstrual syndrome including mastalgia, diabetic neuropathy, rheumatoid arthritis, Sjögren's syndrome, cardiovascular, renal, hepatic and gastrointestinal disorders, viral infections, endometriosis, schizophrenia, alcoholism, Alzheimer's disease and cancers has been reviewed.[3]

Atopic eczema   An inherited slow rate of 6-desaturation (LA to gamolenic acid conversion) has been documented in this condition. Normal or elevated concentrations of LA are associated with reduced concentrations of their metabolites. Randomised, double-blind, placebo-controlled trials have shown gamolenic acid to produce a highly significant improvement in all features of atopic eczema, especially in itch.[1–3,7,8] The requirement for topical and oral steroids, histamines and antibiotics was also reduced.[3] However, attention has been drawn to the conflicting evidence of clinical trials on evening primrose oil. Two large trials have not shown evidence of benefit[10,11] whereas other trials have resulted in benefits, particularly for patients with moderate or severe eczema.[12,13] Adequate doses of evening primrose oil for treatment of atopic eczema are 160–320 mg of gamolenic acid daily in children aged 1–12 years and 320–480 mg in adults for three months.[9]

Cyclical/non-cyclical mastalgia PGE_1 is thought to modulate the action of prolactin. Abnormal concentrations may result in an excessive peripheral action of prolactin.[3]

Several placebo-controlled studies have demonstrated that gamolenic acid is better than placebo in the treatment of both premenstrual syndrome and breast pain.[1–3,14] Overall, cyclical mastalgia responds better than non-cyclical to all treatments (danazol, bromocriptine, evening primrose oil).

Premenstrual syndrome   The use of evening primrose oil for the treatment of premenstrual syndrome has been rationalised on the grounds that hypersensitivity to prolactin is due to low levels of PGE_1.[15] High levels of linoleic acid and low levels of gammalinolenic acid have been observed for patients with premenstrual syndrome. Several clinical studies have been reported and the conclusions vary from no beneficial effects being observed to marked improvements.[1–3,16]

Diabetic neuropathy   Diabetes has been associated with reduced ability to desaturate essential fatty acids, with deficits resulting in abnormal neuronal membrane structure. Animal studies have shown that diabetic neuropathy can be either prevented or reversed by the provision of gamolenic acid as evening primrose oil. In humans, a double-blind, placebo-controlled trial has demonstrated reversal of diabetic neuropathy by gamolenic acid.[17]

Multiple sclerosis   The results of clinical trials on the use of evening primrose oil for the treatment of multiple sclerosis are contradictory.[1,2] Patients with recent onset or less severe forms of the disease are more likely to respond. Linoleic acid may have a beneficial effect on the severity and duration of relapses and on the progression of the disease.[1] It is suggested that linoleic acid is involved in the immunosuppressive effect at the cellular level and may be of use when combined with a low animal fat/high polyunsaturated fat diet.[2]

Rheumatoid arthritis   A randomised, double-blind trial has demonstrated a significant improvement in subjective symptoms of rheumatoid arthritis (RA) (indicated by a reduction in required non-steroidal anti-inflammatory drug treatment) in the active group receiving evening primrose oil compared with the placebo group. However, no objective changes were observed in any of the biochemical indicators of RA.[1–3]

Sjögren's syndrome This disease is associated with the loss of secretions from exocrine glands throughout the body, but especially from the salivary and lacrimal glands. One of the features of EFA deficiency is exocrine gland atrophy. Placebo-controlled trials have shown a modest improvement in tear flow together with relief of lethargy, a prominent feature of the syndrome.[1,3]

Coronary heart disease Abnormal intake and metabolism of EFAs (both *n*-3 and *n*-6) are thought to be important risk factors for coronary heart disease (CHD), resulting in enhanced cholesterol and triglyceride biosynthesis, enhanced platelet aggregation and elevated blood pressure. Dietary supplementation with foods or oils rich in LA (*n*-6) or in marine (*n*-3) EFAs have been found to decrease significantly the risk of CHD, although it is considered that an optimum balance between *n*-3 and *n*-6 EFAs may well be important.[1–3,18] gamolenic acid has been reported to decrease blood pressure and platelet aggregation in both animal and human studies.[3]

Renal disease Renal tissue is especially rich in EFAs, and prostaglandins of the E series are believed to be important in maintaining adequate renal blood flow. Administration of gamolenic acid to animals has been reported to prevent or attenuate renal damage. A single placebo-controlled trial involving postrenal transplant patients demonstrated better graft survival rate for the group receiving evening primrose oil (45 patients) compared with the placebo group (44 patients).[3]

Liver disease PGE_1 has been administered to patients with liver failure, and has been observed to exert some cytoprotective effect and to maintain the normal function of the liver. There is little experience of gamolenic acid supplementation in liver disease.[17]

Gastrointestinal disorders A double-blind placebo-controlled crossover trial has indicated a beneficial effect of evening primrose oil on irritable bowel syndrome exacerbated by premenstrual syndrome. A beneficial effect superior to that of fish oil or placebo has been reported for evening primrose oil in ulcerative colitis. A protective effect of gamolenic acid against gastric ulceration has yet to be shown in humans.[3]

Viral infections/postviral fatigue A single placebo-controlled study has demonstrated significant beneficial effects in patients with well-defined postviral fatigue (PVF) receiving evening primrose oil compared with those receiving placebo. Symptoms arrested were muscle weakness, aches and pains, lack of concentration, exhaustion, memory loss, depression, dizziness and vertigo.[1,3]

Endometriosis A placebo-controlled trial has shown that gamolenic acid in combination with eicosapentaenoic acid (*n*-3 EFA metabolite) reduced symptoms of endometriosis in 90% women, whereas 90% of the placebo group reported no relief from symptoms.[3]

Schizophrenia It is believed that EFAs, in particular PGE_1, antagonise the excessive central dopaminergic activity that is thought to be a possible cause of schizophrenia. Low concentrations of LA in plasma phospholipids have been observed in populations of schizophrenics from Ireland, England, Scotland, Japan and the USA. It is thought that a poor recovery rate from the disease is associated with the presence of saturated fats in the diet, but not with unsaturated fats. Various open and placebo-controlled trials of gamolenic acid and DGLA supplementation have reportedly produced mixed results. Administration of evening primrose oil with co-factors known to be important in EFA metabolism (zinc, pyridoxine, niacin and vitamin C) enhanced the improvements in memory loss, schizophrenic symptoms and tardive dyskinesia that were observed in evening primrose oil-treated compared with placebo-treated patients.[1–3]

Alcoholism Evening primrose oil has been documented to reduce symptoms in the first three weeks of withdrawal, indicated by a reduced requirement for tranquillisers, and to significantly improve the rate of return to normal liver function. However, in the longer term, evening primrose did not affect the relapse rate.[3]

Dementia Alzheimer's disease and other forms of dementia are associated with low serum concentrations of EFAs. A single placebo-controlled trial in patients with Alzheimer's disease reported improvements in cerebral function in the evening primrose oil group compared with the placebo group.

Hyperactivity in children Hyperactive children tend to have abnormal levels of essential fatty acids. No improvements in behavioural patterns and no changes in blood fatty acids were observed in one trial with evening primrose oil.[2]

Cancer *In vitro* studies have observed that malignant cells die following exposure to gamolenic acid and related fatty acids at concentrations that are non-lethal to normal cells. *In vitro* studies have shown gamolenic acid to inhibit the growth of various human cancer cell lines, and *in vivo* studies have described an inhibitory effect of gamolenic acid on tumour growth. Human studies are currently ongoing to assess the impact of gamolenic acid supplementation in various human cancers.[3]

Side-effects, Toxicity

Evening primrose oil appears to be well tolerated with very few side-effects reported, despite it being available for many years in a number of countries as a food supplement.[3] Mild gastrointestinal effects, indigestion, nausea and softening of stools and headache have occasionally occurred.[3,5] It has been noted that there may be an increased risk of temporal lobe epilepsy in schizophrenic patients being treated with epileptogenic drugs such as phenothiazines.[6] In cases of overdosage, symptoms of loose stools and abdominal pain have been noted. No special treatment is required.[6]

Toxicity studies have indicated evening primrose oil to be non-toxic.[3] The two principal components in evening primrose oil are LA and gamolenic acid. LA is commonly ingested as part of the diet. It has been estimated that the concentration of gamolenic acid provided by evening primrose oil is comparable to that metabolised in the body from normal dietary LA.[4] In addition, it has been calculated that a breastfed infant receives a higher proportion (mg/kg) of LA and gamolenic acid from human milk compared to that received from evening primrose oil.[4]

Contra-indications, Warnings

Evening primrose oil may have the potential to make manifest undiagnosed temporal lobe epilepsy, especially in schizophrenic patients and/or those who are already receiving known epileptogenic drugs such as phenothiazines.[6] No epileptic events have been reported in patients not being treated with phenothiazines.[6]

Pregnancy and lactation Animal studies have indicated evening primrose oil to be non-teratogenic.[6] However, data on the safety of evening primrose oil during human pregnancy are not available and therefore the risk of taking evening primrose oil during pregnancy should be carefully considered against the perceived benefit to the patient. Both LA and gamolenic acid are normally present in breast milk (*see* Side-effects, Toxicity) and therefore it is reasonable to assume that evening primrose oil may be taken while breast feeding.

Pharmaceutical Comment

Interest in the seed oil of the evening primrose plant lies in its essential fatty acid content, in particular in the linoleic acid (LA) and gamolenic acid (GLA) content. Both of these compounds are prostaglandin precursors and dietary gamolenic acid supplementation has been shown to increase the ratio of non-inflammatory to inflammatory prostaglandin compounds.

The use of evening primrose oil in various disease states associated with low gamolenic acid concentrations has been extensively investigated and a vast body of published literature is available. The beneficial effects of evening primrose oil in treating atopic eczema and mastalgia (cyclical/non-cyclical) have been recognised with product licences granted to evening primrose oil-containing preparations for these indications.[6] However, doubt has also been expressed over the effectiveness of evening primrose oil in eczema.[2,9,10,11,19] Alternative natural oil sources such as blackcurrant or borage (*see* Borage) that offer a higher gamolenic acid yield compared to evening primrose oil have been identified, although these oils have not been found to exhibit the same biological effects as those observed for evening primrose oil.[3]

Evening primrose oil is reported to be virtually non-toxic with only minor adverse effects such as headache and nausea occasionally associated with its use. The range of potential uses for evening primrose oil is extensive and results of further human studies are awaited to establish its efficacy in various therapeutic conditions.

References

See also General References G5, G29, G32, G36, G43, G50, G56 and G64.

1 Li Wan Po A. Evening primrose oil. *Pharm J* 1991; **246**: 670–676.
2 Barber HJ. Evening primrose oil: a panacea? *Pharm J* 1988; **240**: 723–725.
3 Horrobin DF. Gammalinolenic acid: an intermediate in essential fatty acid metabolism with potential as an ethical pharmaceutical and as a food. *Rev Contemp Pharmacother* 1990; **1**: 1–45.
4 Carter JP. Gamma-linolenic acid as a nutrient. *Food Technol* 1988; 72.

5   Briggs CJ. Evening primrose. *Rev Pharm Can* 1986; **119**: 249–254.

6   Anon. Data Sheet Compendium 1994–95, 1520-1. Efamast, Epogam, Epogam Paediatric (Searle).

7   Lovell CR *et al.* Treatment of atopic eczema with evening primrose oil. *Lancet* 1981; **1**: 278.

8   Schalin-Karrila M *et al.* Evening primrose oil in the treatment of atopic eczema: effect on clinical status, plasma phospholipid fatty acids and circulating blood prostaglandins. *Br J Dermatol* 1987; **117**: 11–19.

9   McHenry PM *et al.* Management of atopic eczema. *BMJ* 1995; **310**: 843–847.

10 Bamford JTM *et al.* Atopic eczema unresponsive to evening primrose oil (linolenic and gamma-linolenic acids). *J Am Acad Dermatol* 1985; **13**: 959–965

11 Berth-Jones J, Graham-Brown RAC. Placebo-controlled trial of essential fatty acid supplementation in atopic dermatitis. *Lancet* 1993; **341**: 1557–1560.

12 Wright S, Burton JL. Oral evening primrose seed oil improves atopic eczema. *Lancet* 1982; **ii**: 1120–1122.

13 Stewart JCM *et al.* Treatment of severe and moderately severe atopic dermatitis with evening primrose oil (Epogam); a multicentre study. *J Nutr Med* 1991; **2**: 9–15.

14 Pye JK *et al.* Clinical experience of drug treatments for mastalgia. *Lancet* 1985; **ii**: 373–377.

15 Brush MG. Efamol (evening primrose oil) in the treatment of the premenstrual syndrome. In: Horrobin DF, ed. *Clinical Uses for Essential Fatty Acids.* Buffalo, New York: Eden Press, 1982: 155.

16 Horrobin DF. The role of essential fatty acids and prostaglandins in the premenstrual syndrome. *J Reprod Med* 1983; **28**: 465–468.

17 Jamal GA *et al.* Gamma–linolenic acid in diabetic neuropathy. *Lancet* 1986; **i**: 1098.

18 Horrobin DF, Manku MS. How do polyunsaturated fatty acids lower plasma cholesterol levels?. *Lipids* 1983; **18**: 558–562.

19 Anon. Gamolenic acid in atopic eczema: Epogam. *Drug Ther Bull* 1990; **28**: 69–70.

Eyebright

Species (Family)

Euphrasia species including
(i) *Euphrasia brevipila* Burnat & Gremli
(ii) *Euphrasia officinalis* L.
(iii) *Euphrasia rostkoviana* Hayne (Scrophulariaceae)

Synonym(s)

Euphrasia

Part(s) Used

Herb

Pharmacopoeial and Other Monographs

BHP 1983[G7]
Mills and Bone[G50]
PDR for Herbal Medicines 2nd edition[G36]

Legal Category (Licensed Products)

Eyebright is not included in the GSL.[G37]

Constituents[G2,G22,G40,G64]

Unless otherwise stated, constituents listed are for *E. officinalis*.

Acids Caffeic acid, ferulic acid.[1]

Alkaloids Unidentified tertiary alkaloids, choline, steam volatile bases[1]

Amino acids Glycine, leucine and valine.

Flavonoids Four compounds (unidentified). Quercetin and rutin stated to be absent.[1] Quercetin, quercitrin and rutin have been documented for *E. rostkoviana*.

Iridoids Aucubin 0.05%. Additional glycosides have been reported for related *Euphrasia* species including catalpol, euphroside, eurostoside, geniposide, ixoroside and mussaenoside for *E. rostkoviana*.[2–5]

Phenethyl glycosides Dehydroconiferyl alcohol-4-β-D-glucoside[3] and eukovoside (3,4-dihydroxy-4-phe-

nethyl-*O*-α-L-rhamnoside(13)-4-*O*-isoferuoyl-β-D-glucoside)[4] from *E. rostkoviana*.

Tannins About 12%. Condensed and hydrolysable; gallic acid is among the hydrolysis products.[1]

Volatile oils About 0.2%. Seven major and numerous minor components, mainly unidentified; four of the major compounds are thought to be aldehydes or ketones.[1]

Other constituents Bitter principle, β-carotene, phytosterols (e.g. β-sitosterol, stigmasterol),[1] resin, carbohydrates (e.g. arabinose, glucose, galactose) and vitamin C.

Food Use

Eyebright is listed by the Council of Europe as a natural source of food flavouring (category N3). This category indicates that eyebright can be added to foodstuffs in the traditionally accepted manner, although there is insufficient information available for an adequate assessment of potential toxicity.[G16]

Herbal Use

Eyebright is stated to possess anticatarrhal, astringent and anti-inflammatory properties. Traditionally it has been used for nasal catarrh, sinusitis and specifically for conjunctivitis when applied locally as an eye lotion.[G2,G7,G64]

Dosage

Dried herb 2–4 g or by infusion three times daily.[G7]

Liquid extract 2–4 mL (1 : 1 in 25% alcohol) three times daily.[G7]

Tincture 2–6 mL (1 : 5 in 45% alcohol) three times daily.[G7]

Pharmacological Actions

In vitro and animal studies

None documented for eyebright. Caffeic acid is bacteriostatic,[1] and a purgative action in mice has been documented for iridoid glycosides.[6] The purgative action of aucubin is approximately 0.05 times the potency of sennosides, with onset of diarrhoea stated to occur more than 6 hours after aucubin administration.[6] Tannins are known to possess astringent properties.

Side-effects, Toxicity

It has been stated that 10–60 drops of eyebright tincture could induce toxic symptoms including mental confusion and cephalalgia, raised pressure in the eyes with lachrymation, pruritus, redness, swelling of the eyelid margins, dim vision, photophobia, weakness, sneezing, nausea, toothache, constipation, cough, dyspnoea, insomnia, polyuria and diaphoresis.[G22]

Contra-indications, Warnings

The use of eyebright for ophthalmic application has been discouraged.[G60]

Pregnancy and lactation   The safety of eyebright has not been established. In view of the lack of pharmacological and toxicity data, the use of eyebright during pregnancy and lactation should be avoided.

Pharmaceutical Comment

Limited information is available regarding the constituents of eyebright and it is unclear which *Euphrasia* species is most commonly utilised. In addition, eyebright is also used as a common name for plants other than *Euphrasia* species. Little scientific information was found to justify the reputed herbal uses, although tannin constituents would provide an astringent effect. The use of home-made preparations for ophthalmic purposes should be avoided. Little is known regarding the toxicity of eyebright and, in view of the reported presence of unidentified alkaloids, it should be used with caution avoiding excessive doses.

References

See also General References G2, G7, G16, G22, G31, G32, G36, G37, G40, G44, G50, G60 and G64.

1   Harkiss KJ, Timmins P. Studies in the Scrophulariaceae Part VIII. Phytochemical investigation of *Euphrasia officinalis. Planta Med* 1973; **23**: 342–347.
2   Sticher O, Salama O. Iridoid glucosides from *Euphrasia rostkoviana. Planta Med* 1981; **42**: 122–123.
3   Salama O *et al.* A lignan glucoside from *Euphrasia rostkoviana. Phytochemistry* 1981; **20**: 2003–2004.
4   Sticher O *et al.* Structure analysis of eukovoside, a new phenylpropanoid glycoside from *Euphrasia rostkoviana. Planta Med* 1982; **45**: 159.
5   Salama O, Sticher O. Iridoidglucoside von *Euphrasia rostkoviana* 4. Mitteilung über Euphrasia-Glykoside. *Planta Med* 1983; **47**: 90–94.
6   Inouye H *et al.* Purgative activities of iridoid glycosides. *Planta Med* 1974; **25**: 285–288.

False Unicorn

Species (Family)

Chamaelirium luteum (L.) A. Gray (Liliaceae)

Synonym(s)

Blazing Star, *Chamaelirium carolianum* Wild., Helonias, *Helonias dioica* Pursh., *Helonias lutea* Ker-Gawl., Starwort, *Veratrum luteum* L.

Part(s) Used

Rhizome, root

Pharmacopoeial and Other Monographs

BHP 1996[G9]
Martindale 32nd edition[G43]
PDR for Herbal Medicines 2nd edition[G36]

Legal Category (Licensed Products)

GSL[G37]

Constituents[G40,G48,G64]

Limited chemical information is available on false unicorn. It is stated to contain a steroidal saponin glycoside, chamaelirin, and another glycoside helonin.

Food Use

False unicorn is not used in foods.

Herbal Use

False unicorn is stated to possess an action on the uterus. Traditionally it has been used for ovarian dysmenorrhoea, leucorrhoea and specifically for amenorrhoea. It is reported to be useful for vomiting of pregnancy and threatened miscarriage.[G7,G8,G64]

Dosage

Dried rhizome/root 1–2 g or by infusion three times daily.[G7]

Liquid extract 1–2 mL (1 : 1 in 45% alcohol) three times daily.[G7]

Tincture 2–5 mL (1 : 5 in 45% alcohol) three times daily.[G7]

Pharmacological Actions

None documented.

Side-effects, Toxicity

No reported side-effects or documented toxicity studies were located. It is stated that large doses of false unicorn may cause nausea and vomiting.[G7]

Contra-indications, Warnings

None documented.

Pregnancy and lactation The safety of false unicorn has not been established. In view of the lack of phytochemical, pharmacological and toxicity data, and its reputed action as a uterine tonic, the use of false unicorn during pregnancy and lactation should be avoided.

Pharmaceutical Comment

The chemistry of false unicorn is poorly documented and no scientific evidence was located to justify the herbal uses. In view of this and the lack of toxicity data, the use of false unicorn should be avoided.

References

See General References G9, G31, G36, G37, G40, G43, G48 and G64.

Fenugreek

Species (Family)

Trigonella foenum-graecum L. (Leguminosae)

Synonym(s)

Bockshornsame

Part(s) Used

Seed

Pharmacopoeial and Other Monographs

BHP 1996[G9]
BP 2001[G15]
Complete German Commission E[G3]
Martindale 32nd edition[G43]
PDR for Herbal Medicines 2nd edition[G36]
Ph Eur 2002[G28]

Legal Category (Licensed Products)

GSL[G37]

Constituents[G2,G41,G48,G64]

Alkaloids Pyridine-type. Gentianine, trigonelline (up to 0.13%), choline (0.05%).

Proteins and amino acids Protein (23–25%) containing high quantities of lysine and tryptophan. Free amino acids include 4-hydroxyisoleucine (0.09%), histidine, lysine and arginine.

Flavonoids Flavone (apigenin, luteolin) glycosides including orientin and vitexin, quercetin (flavonol).

Saponins 0.6–1.7%. Glycosides yielding steroidal sapogenins diosgenin and yamogenin (major), with tigogenin, neotigogenin, gitogenin, neogitogenin, smilagenin, sarsasapogenin, yuccagenin;[1] fenugreekine, a sapogenin-peptide ester involving diosgenin and yamogenin;[2] trigofoenosides A–G (furostanol glycosides).[3–6]

Other constituents Coumarin,[7] lipids (5–8%),[8] mucilaginous fibre (50%),[8] vitamins (including nicotinic acid) and minerals.

Food Use

Fenugreek is listed by the Council of Europe as a natural source of food flavouring (category N2). This category indicates that fenugreek can be added to foodstuffs in small quantities, with a possible limitation of an active principle (as yet unspecified) in the final product.[G16] In the USA, fenugreek extracts are permitted in foods at concentrations usually below 0.05%. In addition, fenugreek is listed as GRAS (Generally Recognised As Safe) in the USA.

Herbal Use

Fenugreek is stated to possess mucilaginous demulcent, laxative, nutritive, expectorant and orexigenic properties, and has been used topically as an emollient and vulnerary. Traditionally, it has been used in the treatment of anorexia, dyspepsia, gastritis and convalescence, and topically for furunculosis, myalgia, lymphadenitis, gout, wounds and leg ulcers.[G2,G7,G22,G64]

Dosage

Seed 1–6 g or equivalent three times daily.[G49]

Pharmacological Actions

In vitro and animal studies

Hypocholesterolaemic activity has been reported for fenugreek in rats[9,G41] and alloxan-diabetic dogs.[10] Activity has been attributed to the fibre and saponin fractions, and not to lipid or amino acid fractions.[9,10] Studies have reported a reduction in cholesterol but not triglyceride concentrations,[9] or in both cholesterol and triglyceride concentrations, but without significant alterations in high-density lipoprotein (HDL) and low-density lipoprotein (LDL) concentrations.[10]

Hypoglycaemic activity has been observed in rabbits, rats and dogs, and attributed to the defatted seed fraction (DSF),[8] trigonelline, nicotinic acid and coumarin.[7,11] Oral administration of DSF reduced hyperglycaemia in four alloxan-diabetic dogs, and reduced the response to an oral glucose tolerance test in eight normal dogs, whereas the lipid fraction had no effect on serum glucose and insulin concentrations.[8] The high fibre content (50%) of DSF was thought to contribute to its antidiabetic effect although the initial rate of glucose absorption was not affected.[8] Nicotinic acid and coumarin were reported to be the major hypoglycaemic components of fenugreek seeds, following administration to normal and alloxan-diabetic rats.[7] The hypoglycaemic action exhibited by coumarin was still significant 24 hours post administration.[7] In addition, a slight antidiuretic action was noted for coumarin.[7] Trigonelline inhibited cortisone-induced hyperglycaemia in rabbits if administered (250 mg/kg) concomitantly or two hours before, but not two hours after, cortisone.[11] In addition, trigonelline exhibited significant hypoglycaemic activity in alloxan-diabetic rats (50 mg/kg), lasting 24 hours.[11]

A stimulant action on the isolated uterus (guinea-pig), especially during late pregnancy, has been noted for both aqueous and alcoholic extracts.[G41] An aqueous extract is stated to increase the number of heart beats in the isolated mammalian heart.[G41]

In vitro antiviral activity against vaccinia virus has been reported for fenugreekine, which also possesses cardiotonic, hypoglycaemic, diuretic, antiphlogistic and antihypertensive properties.[2]

Clinical studies

A transient hypoglycaemic effect was observed in 5 of 10 diabetic patients who received 500 mg oral trigonelline whilst fasting.[11] Increasing the dose did not increase this effect, and 500 mg ingested three times a day for five days did not alter the diurnal blood glucose concentration.[11] Hypoglycaemic activity in healthy individuals has been reported for whole seed extracts, with slightly lesser activity exhibited by gum isolate, extracted seeds and cooked seeds.[12] The addition of fenugreek to an oral glucose tolerance test reduced serum glucose and insulin concentrations. Chronic ingestion (21 days) of extracted seeds (25 g seeds daily incorporated into two meals) by non-insulin-dependent diabetics improved plasma glucose and insulin responses (no control group), and reduced 24-hour urinary glucose concentrations.[12] Furthermore, in two diabetic insulin-dependent subjects, daily administration of 25 g fenugreek seed powder reduced fasting plasma-glucose profile, glycosuria and daily insulin requirements (56–20 units) after eight weeks. A significant reduction in serum cholesterol concentrations in diabetic patients was also noted.[12]

Side-effects, Toxicity

No reported side-effects were located for fenugreek. Acute toxicity values (LD_{50}) documented for fenugreek alcoholic seed extract are 5 g/kg (rat, oral) and 2 g/kg (rabbit, dermal).[13] The alcoholic seed extract is reported to be non-irritating and non-sensitising to human skin and non-phototoxic (mice, pigs).[13] Coumarin is a toxic seed component.[7] Acute LD_{50} (rat, oral) values per kilogram documented for various seed constituents are 5 g (trigonelline), 8.8 g (nicotinic acid), 7.4 g (nicotinamide) and 0.72 g (coumarin).[7]

Contra-indications, Warnings

Hypoglycaemic activity has been reported for fenugreek, which may therefore interfere with existing hypoglycaemic therapy. Caution is advisable in patients receiving monoamine oxidase inhibitor (MAOI), hormonal or anticoagulant therapies in view of amine, steroidal saponin and coumarin constituents, respectively, although their clinical significance is unclear. Cardioactivity has been documented *in vitro*. The absorption of drugs taken concomitantly with fenugreek may be affected (high mucilaginous fibre content).

Pregnancy and lactation   Fenugreek is reputed to be oxytocic[G22] and *in vitro* uterine stimulant activity has been documented. In view of this, and the documented pharmacologically active components, the use of fenugreek during pregnancy and lactation in doses greatly exceeding those normally encountered in foods is not advisable.

Pharmaceutical Comment

Fenugreek seeds contain a high proportion of mucilaginous fibre, together with various other pharmacologically active compounds including steroidal and amine components. The majority of the traditional uses of fenugreek are probably attributable to the mucilage content. In addition, hypocholesterolaemic and hypoglycaemic actions have been documented for fenugreek in both laboratory animals and humans. The mechanism by which fenugreek exerts these actions is unclear. Proposed theories include a reduction in carbohydrate absorption by the mucilaginous fibre,[12] and an effect on cholesterol metabolism, cholesterol absorption and bile acid excretion by the saponin components.[8] Toxicity studies indicate fenugreek seeds to be relatively non-toxic, although the presence of pharmacologically active constituents would suggest that excessive ingestion is inadvisable.

References

See also General References G2, G3, G9, G11, G15, G16, G22, G28, G31, G32, G36, G37, G40, G41, G43, G48, G49 and G64.

1 Gupta RK *et al*. Minor steroidal sapogenins from fenugreek seeds, *Trigonella foenum-graecum. J Nat Prod* 1986; **49**: 1153.
2 Ghosal S *et al*. Fenugreekine, a new steroidal sapogenin-peptide ester of *Trigonella foenum-graecum. Phytochemistry* 1974; **13**: 2247–2251.
3 Gupta RK *et al*. Two furostanol saponins from *Trigonella feonum-graecum. Phytochemistry* 1986; **25**: 2205–2207.
4 Varshney IP *et al*. Saponins from *Trigonella foenum-graucum* leaves. *J Nat Prod* 1984; **47**: 44–46.
5 Gupta RK *et al*. Furostanol glycosides from *Trigonella foenum-graecum* seeds. *Phytochemistry* 1984; **23**: 2605–2607.
6 Gupta RK *et al*. Furostanol glycosides from *Trigonella foenum-graecum* seeds. *Phytochemistry* 1985; **24**: 2399–2401.
7 Shani J *et al*. Hypoglycaemic effect of *Trigonella foenum graecum* and *Lupinus termis* (Leguminosae) seeds and their major alkaloids in alloxan-diabetic and normal rats. *Arch Int Pharmacodyn Ther* 1974; **210**: 27–37.
8 Ribes G *et al*. Hypocholesterolaemic and hypotriglyceridaemic effects of subfractions from fenugreek seeds in alloxan diabetic dogs. *Phytother Res* 1987; **1**: 38–42.
9 Ribes G *et al*. Effects of fenugreek seeds on endocrine pancreatic secretions in dogs. *Ann Nutr Metab* 1984; **28**: 37–43.
10 Sharma RD. An evaluation of hypocholesterolemic factor of fenugreek seeds (*T. foenum graecum*) in rats. *Nutr Rep Int* 1986; **33**: 669–677.
11 Mishkinsky J *et al*. Hypoglycaemic effect of trigonelline. *Lancet* 1967; **2**: 1311–1312.
12 Sharma RD. Effect of fenugreek seeds and leaves on blood glucose and serum insulin responses in human subjects. *Nutr Res* 1986; **6**: 1353–1364.
13 Opdyke DLJ. Fenugreek absolute. *Food Cosmet Toxicol* 1978; **16**(Suppl.): 755–756.

Feverfew

Species (Family)

Tanacetum parthenium (L.) Schultz Bip. (Asteraceae/Compositae)

Synonym(s)

Altamisa, *Chrysanthemum parthenium* (L.) Bernh., *Leucanthemum parthenium* (L.) Gren & Godron, *Pyrethrum parthenium* (L.) Sm.

Part(s) Used

Leaf, aerial parts

Pharmacopoeial and Other Monographs

BHC 1992[G6]
BHP 1996[G9]
ESCOP 1996[G52]
Martindale 32nd edition[G43]
Mills and Bone[G50]
PDR for Herbal Medicines[G36]
USP24/NF19[G61]

Legal Category (Licensed Products)

Feverfew is not included in the GSL.[G37]

Constituents[G6,G22,G49,G64]

Terpenoids Sesquiterpene lactones: germacranolides (GE), guaianolides (GU) and eudesmanolides (EU). The structural feature common to all three types is an α-unsaturated γ-lactone moiety, and examples of each type include parthenolide, 3-β-hydroxy-parthenolide, costunolide, 3-β-hydroxycostunolide, artemorin, 8-α-hydroxyestafiatin and chrysanthemonin (novel dimeric nucleus) (GE); artecanin, chrysanthemin A (canin) and B (stereoisomers), chrysanthemolide, partholide, two chlorine-containing sesquiterpene lactones (GU); magnolialide, reynosin, santamarine, 1-β-hydroxyarbusculin and 5-β-hydroxyreynosin (EU).[1–5]

Volatile oils (0.02–0.07%). Various monoterpene and sesquiterpene components (e.g. camphor, borneol, α-pinene derivatives, germacrene, farnesene and their esters).

Other constituents Pyrethrin, flavonoids, tannins (type unspecified) and melatonin.[6]

Food Use

Feverfew is not generally used in foods.

Herbal Use[G6,G8,G32,G43,G49,G52,G64]

Feverfew has traditionally been used in the treatment of migraine, tinnitus, vertigo, arthritis, fever, menstrual disorders, difficulty during labour, stomachache, toothache and insect bites. Modern use of feverfew is focused on its effects in the prevention and treatment of migraine.

Dosage

Limited information is available regarding the traditional dose of feverfew. The doses that have been recommended for migraine prophylaxis are as follows.

Leaf (fresh) 2.5 leaves daily with or after food.

Leaf (freeze-dried) 50 mg daily with or after food.

Aerial parts (dried) 50–200 mg daily; equivalent to 0.2–0.6 mg parthenolide daily.[G6,G52]

Clinical trials of feverfew for the prevention of migraine have assessed the effects of, for example, 143 mg of a dried alcoholic extract of feverfew daily (equivalent to 0.5 mg parthenolide),[7] and capsules containing powdered feverfew leaf 50 mg daily,[8,9] for one to six months.

Pharmacological Actions

In vitro and animal studies

Feverfew extracts have been documented to inhibit platelet aggregation and prostaglandin, thromboxane and leukotriene production, although feverfew has also been reported to have no effect on cyclooxygenase (the mechanism by which non-steroidal anti-inflammatory drugs inhibit prostaglandin production).[10–12] Instead, feverfew is thought to act by inhibiting the enzyme phospholipase A_2, which facilitates the release of arachidonic acid from the phospholipid cellular membrane.[11–13] The clinical significance of this action has been questioned.[14] In addition, *in vitro* experiments have shown that feverfew extracts inhibit the interaction of human platelets with collagen substrates.[15,16] Feverfew has been shown to inhibit granule secretion in blood platelets and neutrophils, which has been associated with the aetiology of migraine and rheumatoid arthritis, respectively.[17] Feverfew was also found to inhibit the release of vitamin B_{12}-binding protein from polymorphonuclear leukocytes, but to be ineffective against platelet and polymorphonucleocyte secretion induced by calcium ionophore A2318.[17] Sesquiterpene lactone constituents of feverfew containing an α-methylene butyrolactone unit are thought to be responsible for the antisecretory activity.[18] Their inhibitory effect on platelet aggregation is thought to involve neutralisation of sulfhydryl groups on specific enzymes of proteins that are necessary for platelet aggregation and secretion.[19] A similar mode of action has been proposed for the inhibitory action of feverfew on polymorphonuclocyte secretion.[20] In addition, feverfew extracts have been reported to produce a dose-dependent inhibition of anti-IgE-induced histamine release from mast cells.[21] The authors concluded that the mechanism of action of the feverfew extract was different to that of both cromoglycate and quercetin.

Parthenolide markedly interfered with contractile and relaxant mechanisms in blood vessels.[G52] An aqueous extract of feverfew administered intravenously significantly inhibited collagen-induced bronchoconstriction in guinea-pigs.[G52]

The presence of large numbers of lymphocytes and monocytes in the synovium is considered to be of significance in rheumatoid arthritis.[22] Feverfew extract and parthenolide have been documented to inhibit mitogen-induced proliferation of human peripheral blood mononuclear cells and mitogen-induced prostaglandin E_2 (PGE_2) production by synovial cells.[22] The feverfew extract and parthenolide also proved to be cytotoxic to mitogen-treated peripheral blood mononuclear cells and the authors considered that this cytotoxicity was responsible for the actions observed.[22] *In vitro* studies using crude feverfew extracts and parthenolide have documented other activities that may contribute to the reported anti-inflammatory effects of feverfew. Pretreatment of human synovial fibroblasts with feverfew extract and with purified parthenolide inhibited cytokine-induced expression of intercellular adhesion molecule 1 (ICAM-1) expression.[23] A reduction in T cell adhesion to the treated fibroblasts also occurred. In other *in vitro* studies, parthenolide inhibited lipopolysaccharide-induced interleukin-12 (IL-12) produc-

tion by mouse macrophages in a concentration-dependent manner.[24] Parthenolide has also been shown to inhibit promoter activity of the inducible nitric oxide synthase gene in a human monocyte cell line, THP-1, in a concentration-dependent manner.[25] (Excessive nitric oxide production in inflammatory cells is thought to be a causative factor in cellular injury in inflammatory disease.) Anti-inflammatory activity of feverfew has also been attributed to the presence of flavonoids, e.g. santonin.[26]

Anti-inflammatory properties have also been documented for feverfew extract and parthenolide *in vivo*. Oral administration of feverfew extract (10, 20 and 40 mg/kg) reduced carrageenan-induced oedema in rat paw in a dose-dependent manner.[27] Intraperitoneal parthenolide (1 and 2 mg/kg) also demonstrated anti-inflammatory effects in this model.

Parthenolide has been documented to have cytotoxic activity in Eagle's 9KB carcinoma of the nasopharynx cell culture system, the activity being associated with the presence of an α-methylene-γ-lactone moiety in the molecule.[28] *In vitro*, parthenolide has been shown to inhibit growth of mouse fibrosarcoma (MN-11) and human lymphoma (TK6) cell lines.[29] The effect appeared to be reversible.

Antinociceptive properties have been reported for feverfew and parthenolide *in vivo*. Oral administration of feverfew extract (10, 20 and 40 mg/kg) and intraperitoneal administration of parthenolide (1 and 2 mg/kg) led to reductions in acetic acid-induced writhing in mice.[27]

Antimicrobial properties against Gram-positive bacteria, yeasts and filamentous fungi *in vitro* have been documented for parthenolide.[30] Gram-negative bacteria were not affected.

Clinical studies

Migraine Several placebo-controlled clinical trials have assessed the effects of preparations of feverfew in the prevention of migraine.[7–9,31]

A randomised, double-blind, placebo-controlled trial involved 17 patients who had been successfully controlling their migraine by eating raw feverfew leaves for at least three months.[8] Patients either continued to receive feverfew (50 mg daily) or were given placebo for six periods of four weeks. The authors reported that the placebo group experienced a significant increase in the frequency and severity of headache. Those given feverfew showed no change. It was suggested that the placebo group was in fact suffering withdrawal symptoms from feverfew and a 'post-feverfew syndrome' was described (*see* Side-effects, Toxicity).

Another study, a randomised double-blind, placebo-controlled, crossover trial involved 72 adults who had experienced migraine for more than two years and who had at least one attack per month.[31] The only concurrent medication allowed was the oral contraceptive pill. Patients completed a one-month, single-blind, placebo run-in phase, followed by four months' administration of placebo/active and four months' crossover. It was reported that patients experienced a 24% reduction in the number of attacks during feverfew treatment (one capsule daily; 70–114 mg feverfew equivalent to 2.19 µg parthenolide) although the duration of each individual attack was not significantly affected. Patients allocated to the active and then placebo group did not experience the withdrawal symptoms documented in another study,[8] although patients involved in the previous study had used feverfew over a longer period of time.

In a randomised, double-blind, placebo-controlled trial, 57 patients received capsules of dried, powdered feverfew leaves (parthenolide 0.2%) 100 mg daily for 60 days (open-label phase), followed by randomisation to feverfew or placebo (ground parsley) for 30 days then crossover to the other arm for 30 days.[9] There was no washout between crossover. At the end of the open-label phase (i.e. during which all participants received feverfew), there was a significant reduction in pain intensity and symptoms, such as vomiting and sensitivity to light, compared with baseline values ($p < 0.001$). At the end of the double-blind, crossover phase, it was reported that pain intensity was significantly lower during feverfew administration, compared with placebo administration ($p < 0.01$).

Thus, these three studies reported beneficial effects for feverfew, as demonstrated by fewer and/or less severe migraine episodes and/or reductions in pain intensity, compared with placebo.[8,9,31] However, one double-blind, placebo-controlled trial involving 50 feverfew-naïve patients who experienced migraine attacks at least once a month reported no difference in the number of migraine attacks between placebo recipients and participants who received capsules containing a dried alcoholic extract of feverfew equivalent to 0.5 mg parthenolide daily for nine months.[7] Another randomised, double-blind, placebo-controlled, crossover trial involving 20 patients with migraine assessed the effects of feverfew 100 mg daily for two months on serotonin uptake and platelet activity.[32] This trial found no effect for feverfew in the prevention of migraine attacks and also reported that feverfew administration had no effect on the uptake of serotonin by platelets.

The authors of a Cochrane systematic review of six randomised, double-blind, placebo-controlled trials (the five studies mentioned above, plus one another) concluded that although data suggest that feverfew preparations are superior to placebo in preventing migraine, further well-designed clinical trials are required to establish the beneficial effects of feverfew for migraine prophylaxis.[33]

Rheumatoid arthritis A double-blind, placebo-controlled, non-crossover trial studying the use of feverfew in rheumatoid arthritis has also been documented.[34] Forty-one female patients with inflammatory joint symptoms inadequately controlled by non-steroidal anti-inflammatory drugs were given either one feverfew capsule (70–86 mg equivalent to 2–3 µmol parthenolide) daily, or one placebo capsule, for six weeks. Current non-steroidal therapy was maintained. It was concluded that patients in the trial had experienced no additional benefit from feverfew.[34] The authors commented that while concomitant non-steroidal anti-inflammatory drug therapy has been stated to reduce the effectiveness of feverfew, the majority of rheumatoid arthritis sufferers will use feverfew to supplement existing therapy.

Side-effects, Toxicity

Randomised, double-blind, placebo-controlled trials have documented the following adverse effects during feverfew administration, although most effects were also reported (sometimes more frequently) during placebo administration: mouth ulcers (reported more frequently during placebo administration in one study[31]), sore mouth, abdominal pain and indigestion, diarrhoea, flatulence, nausea, dizziness and skin rash.[7,8,31] On balance, adverse effects reported for feverfew are mild and transient, are similar to those reported during placebo administration and occur with a similar frequency.

A 'post-feverfew syndrome' has been described on stopping feverfew administration[8] (*see* Clinical studies) with symptoms such as nervousness, tension headaches, insomnia, stiffness/pain in joints and tiredness.

The onset of side-effects with feverfew is reported to vary, with symptoms becoming apparent within the first week of treatment, or appearing gradually over the first two months.

Sesquiterpene lactones that contain an α-methylene butyrolactone ring are known to cause allergic reactions.[35,G51] Compounds with this structure are present in feverfew and reports of contact dermatitis have been documented.[36–39] No documented allergic reactions following oral ingestion were located.

An LD_{50} value for feverfew has not been estimated. No adverse effects were reported for rats and guinea-pigs receiving feverfew at doses 100 and 150 times the human daily dose, respectively.[40] No chronic toxicity studies have been reported. However, detailed haematological analysis of 60 feverfew users, some of whom had used feverfew for more than one year, did not show any significant differences when compared with analysis of controls.[40] A human toxicity study has investigated whether the sesquiterpene lactones in feverfew induce chromosomal or other changes in normal human cells of individuals who have taken the herb.[41] The study compared 30 chronic female feverfew users (leaves, tablets or capsules taken daily for more than 11 consecutive months) with matched non-users. The results of lymphocyte cultures established from blood samples taken over a period of several months were stated to indicate that feverfew affects neither the frequency of chromosomal aberrations nor the frequency of sister chromatid exchanges in the circulating peripheral lymphocytes.

Contra-indications, Warnings

Feverfew is contra-indicated in individuals with a known hypersensitivity to other members of the family Compositae (Asteraceae), such as chamomile, ragweed and yarrow. Feverfew should not be ingested by individuals who develop a rash on contact with the plant.

Feverfew should only be considered as a treatment for migraine that has proved unresponsive to conventional forms of medication. Although traditionally recommended as a remedy for rheumatic conditions, self-medication with feverfew should not be undertaken without first consulting a doctor.

Pregnancy and lactation Feverfew is contra-indicated during pregnancy. It is reputed to be an abortifacient and to affect the menstrual cycle. It is documented to modify menstrual flow, cause abortion in cattle and induce uterine contraction in full-term women.[G30]

Pharmaceutical Comment

Feverfew is characterised by the sesquiterpene lactone constituents, in particular by parthenolide which is thought to be the main active component. *In vitro* studies provide some evidence to support the reputation of feverfew as a herb used to treat migraine and arthritis. Clinical studies have suggested that feverfew may be a useful prophylactic remedy against

migraine,[42,43] although further research is deemed necessary to establish the benefits.[33] It has been recommended that feverfew should only be used by sufferers who have proved unresponsive to conventional forms of migraine treatment. Those using feverfew as a remedy for migraine should preferably do so under medical supervision.

Results of a study that investigated the usefulness of feverfew in treating rheumatoid arthritis were less encouraging: feverfew provided no additional benefit when added to existing non-steroidal anti-inflammatory treatment. Feverfew products currently available are unlicensed and vary in their recommended daily doses.[44] Furthermore, variation between the stated and actual amount of feverfew in commercial products (based on their ability to inhibit platelet secretion) has been reported.[16]

References

See also General References G5, G6, G9, G18, G19, G22, G29, G31, G32, G36, G43, G49, G50, G51, G52, G55, G61 and G64.

1 Stefanovic M *et al.* Sesquiterpene lactones from the domestic plant species *Tanacetum parthenium* L. (Compositae). *J Serb Chem Soc* 1985; **50**: 435–441.

2 Bohlmann F, Zdero C. Sesquiterpene lactones and other constituents from *Tanacetum parthenium*. *Phytochemistry* 1982: **21**: 2543–2549.

3 Osawa T, Taylor D. Revised structure and stereochemistry of chrysartemin B. *Tetrahedron Lett* 1977; **13**: 1169–1172.

4 Hylands DM, Hylands PJ. New sesquiterpene lactones from feverfew. *Phytochem Soc Eur Symp* 1986: 17.

5 Wagner H *et al.* New chlorine-containing sesquiterpene lactones from *Chrysanthemum parthenium*. *Planta Med* 1988; **54**: 171–172.

6 Murch SJ *et al.* Melatonin in feverfew and other medicinal plants. *Lancet* 1997; **350**: 1598–1599.

7 De Weerdt CJ, Bootsma HPR, Hendriks H. Herbal medicines in migraine prevention. Randomized double-blind placebo-controlled crossover trial of a feverfew preparation. *Phytomedicine* 1996; **3**: 225–230.

8 Johnson ES *et al.* Efficacy of feverfew as prophylactic treatment of migraine. *BMJ* 1985; **291**: 569–573.

9 Palevitch D *et al.* Feverfew (*Tanacetum parthenium*) as a prophylactic treatment for migraine: a double-blind placebo-controlled study. *Phytother Res* 1997; **11**: 508–511.

10 Collier HOJ *et al.* Extract of feverfew inhibits prostaglandin biosynthesis. *Lancet* 1980; **ii**: 922–973.

11   Makheja AM, Bailey JM. The active principle in feverfew. *Lancet* 1981; ii, 1054.

12   Capasso F. The effect of an aqueous extract of *Tanacetum parthenium* L. on arachidonic acid metabolism by rat peritoneal leucocytes. *J Pharm Pharmacol* 1986; **38**: 71–72.

13   Makheja AM, Bailey JM. A platelet phospholipase inhibitor from the medicinal herb feverfew (*Tanacetum parthenium*). *Prostaglandins Leukot Med* 1982: **8**: 653–660.

14   Biggs MJ *et al*. Platelet aggregation in patients using feverfew for migraine. *Lancet* 1982; ii: 776.

15   Loesche W *et al*. Feverfew – an antithrombotic drug? *Folia Haematol* 1988; **115**: 181–184.

16   Groenewegen WA, Heptinstall S. Amounts of feverfew in commercial preparations of the herb. *Lancet* 1986; i: 44–45.

17   Heptinstall S *et al*. Extracts of feverfew inhibit granule secretion in blood platelets and polymorphonuclear leucocytes. *Lancet* 1985; i: 1071–1073.

18   Groenewegen WA *et al*. Compounds extracted from feverfew that have anti-secretory activity contain an α-methylene butyrolactone unit. *J Pharm Pharmacol* 1986; **38**: 709–712.

19   Heptinstall S *et al*. Extracts of feverfew may inhibit platelet behaviour via neutralization of sulphydryl groups. *J Pharm Pharmacol* 1987; **39**: 459–465.

20   Lösche W *et al*. Inhibition of the behaviour of human polynuclear leukocytes by an extract of *Chrysanthemum parthenium*. *Planta Med* 1988; **54**: 381–384.

21   Hayes NA, Foreman JC. The activity of compounds extracted from feverfew on histamine release from rat mast cells. *J Pharm Pharmacol* 1987; **39**: 466–470.

22   O'Neill LAJ *et al*. Extracts of feverfew inhibit mitogen-induced human peripheral blood mononuclear cell proliferation and cytokine mediated responses: a cytotoxic effect. *Br J Clin Pharmac* 1987; **23**: 81–83.

23   Piela-Smith TH, Liu X. Feverfew extracts and the sesquiterpene lactone partenolide inhibit intercellular adhesion molecule-1 expression in human synovial fibroblasts. *Cell Immunol* 2001; **209**: 89–96.

24   Kang BY *et al*. Inhibition of interleukin-12 production in lipopolysaccharide-activated mouse macrophages by parthenolide, a predominant sesquiterpene lactone in *Tanacetum parthenium*: involvement of nuclear factor-kappa-B. *Immunol Lett* 2001; **77**: 159–163.

25   Fukuda K *et al*. Inhibition by parthenolide of phorbol ester-induced transcriptional activation of inducible nitric oxide synthase gene in a human monocyte cell line THP-1. *Biochem Pharmacol* 2000; **60**: 595–600.

26   Williams CA *et al*. A biologically active lipophilic flavonol from *Tanacetum parthenium*. *Phytochemistry* 1995; **38**: 267–270.

27   Jain NK, Kulkarni SK. Antinociceptive and anti-inflammatory effects of *Tanacetum parthenium* L. extract in mice and rats. *J Ethnopharmacol* 1999; **68**: 251–259.

28   Berry MI. Feverfew faces the future. *Pharm J* 1984; **232**: 611–614.

29   Ross JJ *et al*. Low concentrations of the feverfew component parthenolide inhibit in vitro growth of tumor lines in a cytostatic fashion. *Planta Med* 1999; **65**: 126–129.

30   Blakeman JP, Atkinson P. Antimicrobial properties and possible role in host–pathogen interactions of parthenolide, a sesquiterpene lactone isolated from glands of *Chrysanthemum parthenium*. *Physiol Plant Pathol* 1979; **15**: 183–192.

31   Murphy JJ *et al*. Randomised double-blind, placebo-controlled trial of feverfew in migraine prevention. *Lancet* 1988; ii: 189–192.

32   Kuritzky A *et al*. Feverfew in the treatment of migraine: its effects on serotonin uptake and platelet activity. *Neurology* 1994; 44(Suppl 2): A201.

33   Pittler MH *et al* Feverfew for preventing migraine (Cochrane Review). In: *The Cochrane Library*, Issue 3, 2001. Oxford: Update Software.

34   Pattrick M *et al*. Feverfew in rheumatoid arthritis: a double blind, placebo controlled study. *Ann Rheum Dis* 1989; **48**: 547–549.

35   Rodríguez E *et al*. The role of sesquiterpene lactones in contact hypersensitivity to some North and South American species of feverfew (*Parthenium* – Compositae). *Contact Dermatitis* 1977; **3**: 155–162.

36   Burry J. Compositae dermatitis in South Australia: Contact dermatitis from *Chrysanthemum parthenium*. *Contact Dermatitis* 1980; **6**: 445.

37   Mitchell JC *et al*. Allergic contact dermatitis caused by *Artemisia* and *Chrysanthemum* species. The role of sesquiterpene lactones. *J Invest Dermatol* 1971; **56**: 98–101.

38   Schmidt RJ, Kingston T. Chrysanethemum dermatitis in South Wales; diagnosis by patch testing with feverfew (*Tanacetum parthenium*) extract. *Contact Dermatitis* 1985; **13**: 120–127.

39   Mensing H *et al*. Airborne contact dermatitis. *Der Hautarzt* 1985; **36**: 398–402.

40   Johnson S. *Feverfew*. London: Sheldon Press, 1984.

41   Johnson ES *et al*. Investigation of possible genetoxic effects of feverfew in migraine patients. *Hum Toxicol* 1987; **6**: 533–534.

42   Awang DVC. Feverfew fever – a headache for the consumer. *Herbalgram* 1993; **29**: 34–36.

43   Berry M. Feverfew. *Pharm J* 1994; **253**: 806–808.

44   Baldwin CA *et al*. What pharmacists should know about feverfew. *Pharm J* 1987; **239**: 237–238.

Figwort

Species (Family)

Scrophularia nodosa L. (Scrophulariaceae)

Synonym(s)

Common Figwort, Scrophularia

Part(s) Used

Herb

Pharmacopoeial and Other Monographs

BHP 1983[G7]
PDR for Herbal Medicines 2nd edition[G36]

Legal Category (Licensed Products)

Figwort is not included in the GSL.[G37]

Constituents[G62,G64]

Amino acids Alanine, isoleucine, leucine, lysine, phenylalanine, threonine, tyrosine and valine.[1]

Flavonoids Diosmetin, diosmin and acacetin rhamnoside.[2]

Iridoids Aucubin, acetylharpagide, harpagide, harpagoside, isoharpagoside, procumbid and a catalpol glycoside.[3–5] Figwort is stated to have the same qualitative iridoid composition as devil's claw, but about half the content of harpagoside.

Acids Various acids including caffeic acid, cinnamic acid, ferulic acid, sinapic acid and vanillic acid, present as both esters and glycosides.[6,7]

Food Use

Figwort is not used in foods.

Herbal Use

Figwort is stated to act as a dermatological agent and a mild diuretic, and to increase myocardial contraction. Traditionally, it has been used for chronic skin disease, and specifically for eczema, psoriasis and pruritus.[G7,G64]

Dosage

Dried herb 2–8 g by infusion.[G7]

Liquid extract 2–8 mL (1 : 1 in 25% alcohol).[G7]

Tincture 2–4 mL (1 : 10 in 45% alcohol).[G7]

Pharmacological Actions

In vitro and animal studies

The iridoid glycosides aucubin and catalpol have been documented to exert a purgative action in mice.[8] Cardioactive properties and anti-inflammatory activity have been claimed for harpagide and the other iridoid constituents (*see* Devil's Claw).[G62]

Clinical studies

None documented. The iridoids are stated to be bitter principles.[G62]

Side-effects, Toxicity

None documented.

Contra-indications, Warnings

Figwort should be avoided in ventricular tachycardia.[G7]

Pregnancy and lactation The safety of figwort has not been established. In view of the lack of pharmacological and toxicity data, use of figwort during pregnancy and lactation should be avoided.

Pharmaceutical Comment

The chemistry of figwort is well studied and it is stated to be an acceptable substitute for devil's claw (*Harpagophytum procumbens*) with the same qualitative composition of bitter principles but half the content of harpagoside.[G62] Little scientific evidence was located to justify the herbal uses. In view of the lack of toxicity data and possible cardioactive properties, excessive use of figwort should be avoided.

References

See also General References G7, G31, G36, G37, G62 and G64.

217

1 Toth L *et al*. Amino acids in Scrophulariaceae species. *Bot Kozl* 1977; **64**: 43–52.

2 Marczal G *et al*. Flavonoids as biologically active agents and their occurrence in the Scrophulariaceae family. *Acta Pharm Hung* 1974: **44**(Suppl.): 83–90.

3 Swann K, Melville C. Iridoid content of some *Scrophularia* species. *J Pharm Pharmacol* 1972; **24**: 170P.

4 Swiatek L. Iridoid glycosides in the Scrophulariaceae family. *Acta Pol Pharm* 1973; **30**: 203–212.

5 Weinges K, Von der Eltz H. Natural products from medicinal plants. XXIII. Iridoid glycosides from *Scrophularia nodosa* L. *Justus Liebigs Ann Chem* 1978; **12**: 1968–1973.

6 Swiatek L. Phenolic acids of underground parts of *Scrophularia nodosa*. *Pol J Pharmacol Pharm* 1973; **25**: 461–464.

7 Swiatek L. Pharmacobotanical investigations of some Scrophulariaceae species. *Diss Pharm Pharmacol* 1970; **22**: 321–328.

8 Inouye H *et al*. Purgative activities of iridoid glucosides. *Planta Med* 1974; **25**:285–288.

Frangula

Species (Family)

Rhamnus frangula L. (Rhamnaceae)

Synonym(s)

Alder Buckthorn, *Frangula alnus* Mill.

Part(s) Used

Bark

Pharmacopoeial and Other Monographs

BHC 1992[G6]
BHP 1996[G9]
BP 2001[G15]
Complete German Commission E (Buckthorn)[G3]
ESCOP 1997[G52]
Martindale 32nd edition[G43]
PDR for Herbal Medicines 2nd edition[G36]
Ph Eur 2002[G28]

Legal Category (Licensed Products)

GSL[G37]

Constituents[G2,G6,G22,G41,G48,G59,G62,G64]

Anthraquinones 3–7%. Frangulosides as major components including frangulin A and B (emodin glycosides) and glucofrangulin A and B (emodin diglycosides); emodin derivatives including emodin dianthrone and its monorhamnoside, palmidin C (*see* Rhubarb) and its monorhamnoside, emodin glycoside; also glycosides of chrysophanol and physcione, and various free aglycones.

Other constituents Flavonoids and tannins.

Food Use

Frangula is listed by the Council of Europe as a natural source of food flavouring (category N4). While this category recognises the use of frangula as a flavouring agent, it indicates that there is insufficient information available to classify it further into categories N1, N2, or N3.[G16]

Herbal Use

Frangula is stated to possess mild purgative properties and has been used traditionally for constipation.[G2,G6,G7,G8,G64]

The Committee on Proprietary Medicinal Products (CPMP) has adopted a core SPC (Summary of Product Characteristics) for frangula. The core SPC includes indications for short-term use of frangula in cases of occasional constipation.[1]

Dosage

Dried bark 0.5–2.5 g.[G6]

Liquid extract 2–5 mL (1 : 1 in 25% alcohol) three times daily.[G7]

Pharmacological Actions

The pharmacological activity of frangula can be attributed to the anthraquinone glycoside constituents. The laxative action of these compounds is well recognised (*see* Senna).

Side-effects, Toxicity[G20]

See Senna for side-effects and toxicity associated with anthraquinones.

The CPMP core SPC for frangula includes the following information.[1] There are no studies on single dose toxicity, on repeated dose toxicity, on reproductive toxicity or on carcinogenicity. Different frangula extracts were shown to be genotoxic in several *in vitro* systems (bacterial mutation, chromosomal aberration and DNA-repair in mammalian cells). No increases in mutations were observed in a gene mutation assay with mammalian cells. For emodin, the main laxative principle of frangula, signs of a genotoxic potential were observed in several systems (bacteria and mammalian cells *in vitro*). Other anthraquinone constituents also gave positive results in limited experiments.

Contra-indications, Warnings

See Senna for contra-indications and warnings associated with anthraquinones.

The CPMP core SPC for frangula states the following contraindications and warnings.[1]

Contra-indications Not to be used in cases of intestinal obstruction and stenosis, atony, inflammatory colon diseases (e.g. Crohn's disease, ulcerative colitis), appendicitis, abdominal pain of unknown origin, severe dehydration states with water and electrolyte depletion.

Precautions As with all laxatives, frangula bark should not be given when any undiagnosed acute or persistent abdominal symptoms are present. If laxatives are needed every day, the cause of the constipation should be investigated. Long-term use of laxatives should be avoided. Use for more than two weeks requires medical supervision. Chronic use may cause pigmentation of the colon (pseudomelanosis coli) which is harmless and reversible after drug discontinuation.

Abuse, with diarrhoea and consequent fluid and electrolyte losses, may cause: dependence, with possible need for increased dosages, disturbance of the water and electrolyte (mainly hypokalaemia) balance, an atonic colon with impaired function. Intake of anthranoid containing laxatives exceeding short-term use may result in an aggravation of constipation.

Hypokalaemia can result in cardiac and neuromuscular dysfunction, especially if cardiac glycosides, diuretics or corticosteroids are taken. Chronic use may result in albuminuria and haematuria.

In chronic constipation, stimulant laxatives are not an acceptable alternative to a changed diet.

Interaction with other medicaments and other forms of interaction. Hypokalaemia (resulting from long-term laxative abuse) potentiates the action of cardiac glycosides and interacts with antiarrhythmic drugs and drugs which induce reversion to sinus rhythm (e.g. quinidine). Concomitant use with other drugs inducing hypokalaemia (e.g. thiazide diuretics, adrenocorticosteroids and liquorice root) may enhance electrolyte imbalance.

Pregnancy and lactation The use of stimulant laxatives, particularly unstandardised preparations, is not generally recommended during pregnancy (*see* Senna).

The CPMP core SPC for frangula includes the following information on use during pregnancy and lactation.

Pregnancy Frangula is not recommended during pregnancy.[1]

There are no reports of undesirable or damaging effects during pregnancy and on the foetus when used at the recommended dosage schedule. However, experimental data concerning a genotoxic risk of several anthranoids, e.g. emodine and physcione, and frangula extract are not counterbalanced by sufficient studies to eliminate a possible risk.[1]

Lactation Frangula is not recommended during breast feeding, as there are insufficient data on the excretion of its metabolites in breast milk. Excretion of the active principles of frangula in breast milk has not been investigated. However, small amounts of active metabolites (e.g. rhein) from other anthranoids are known to be excreted in breast milk. A laxative effect in breastfed babies has not been reported.[1]

Pharmaceutical Comment

The chemistry of frangula is characterised by the anthraquinone glycoside constituents. The laxative action of these compounds is well recognised and supports the herbal use of frangula as a laxative. The use of non-standardised anthraquinone-containing preparations should be avoided, since their pharmacological effect will be variable and unpredictable. In particular, the use of products containing combinations of anthraquinone laxatives should be avoided.

References

See also General References G2, G3, G6, G9, G11, G15, G16, G20, G22, G28, G29, G36, G37, G41, G43, G48, G52, G62 and G64.

1 European Commission, CPMP Guidelines on Information on Medicinal Products: Core Summary of Product Characteristics for Frangulae Cortez, February 1994.

FUCUS

Species (Family)

Fucus vesiculosus L. and other *Fucus* species (Fuca-

Synonym(s)

Black Tang, Bladderwrack, Kelp, Kelpware, Rock-weed, Seawrack

Brown seaweeds refer to species of *Fucus*, *Ascophyllum*, *Laminaria* and *Macrocystis*. 'Kelps' refer to species of *Laminaria* and *Macrocystis*, although kelp is often used in reference to species of *Fucus*.

Part(s) Used

Thallus (whole plant)

Pharmacopoeial and Other Monographs

BHC 1992[G6]
BHP 1996[G9]
BP 2001[G15]
Martindale 32nd edition[G43]
PDR for Herbal Medicines 2nd edition[G36]
Ph Eur 2002[G28]

Legal Category (Licensed Products)

GSL[G37]

Constituents[G2,G6,G64]

Carbohydrates Polysaccharides: alginic acid (algin) as the major component; fucoidan and laminarin (sulfated polysaccharide esters).[1]

Iodine Content of various *Laminaria* species has been reported as 0.07–0.76% of dry weight.[2]

Other constituents Various vitamins and minerals, particularly ascorbic acid (vitamin C) (0.013–0.077% of fresh material).[2]

Food Use

Seaweeds are commonly included in the diet of certain populations. The gelling properties of alginic acid, the major polysaccharide in brown seaweeds, including fucus, are extensively utilised in the dairy and baking industries to improve texture, body and smoothness of products.[1] Fucus is listed by the Council of Europe as a natural source of food flavouring (category N2). This category indicates that fucus can be added to foodstuffs in small quantities, with a possible limitation of an active principle (as yet unspecified) in the final product.[G16]

Herbal Use

Fucus is stated to possess antihypothyroid, anti-obesic and antirheumatic properties. Traditionally, it has been used for lymphadenoid goitre, myxoedema, obesity, arthritis and rheumatism.[G2,G6,G7,G8,G64]

Dosage

Dried thallus 5–10 g or infusion three times daily.[G6,G7]

Liquid extract 4–8 mL (1:1 in 25% alcohol) three times daily.[G6,G7]

Pharmacological Actions

There is a paucity of information documented specifically for *Fucus vesiculosus*, although pharmacological activities are recognised for individual constituents and other brown seaweed species.

Alginic acid is a hydrophilic colloidal substance that swells to approximately 25–35 times its original bulk in an alkaline environment and as such exerts a bulk laxative action.[3] It is stated to compare favourably with the carboxylic type of cation exchange resins. The colloidal properties of alginates have been utilised in wound dressings and skin grafts.[3]

Anticoagulant properties have been documented for brown seaweeds.[3] The glucose polymer laminarin has been identified as the anticoagulant principle in a Laminaria species.[4] A fucoidan fraction has been isolated from *Fucus vesiculosus* with 40–50% blood anticoagulant activity of heparin.[5]

The iodine content of seaweeds is well recognised. The low incidence of goitre amongst maritime people has been attributed to the inclusion of seaweeds in their diet.[3,4] Similarly, the traditional use of *Fucus vesiculosus* in 'slimming teas' is thought to be attributable to the effect of iodine on hypothyroidism.[4]

Extracts of various brown seaweeds including *Ascophyllum nodosum* and *Fucus vesiculosus* have been reported to exhibit a high *in vitro* inhibitory activity towards mammalian digestive enzymes (α-amylase, trypsin and lipase) isolated from the porcine pancreas.[6] Activity was attributed to high molecular weight (30 000–100 000) polyphenols.[6]

Inhibitory effects of laminarin sulfate on lipidaemia and atherosclerosis (*in vivo*, rabbit) have been partially attributed to the *in vitro* inhibition of lipid synthesis observed in cultured chick aortic cells.[7]

Hypotensive activity observed in rats intravenously administered extracts of commercial seaweed (*Laminaria* species) preparations has been attributed to their histamine content.[8] However, histamine concentrations varied considerably between preparations, and authentic specimens of the *Laminaria* species were devoid of histamine.

Kelp extracts have antiviral activity[9] and laminarin is reported to have exhibited some tumour-inhibiting actions.[1]

Side-effects, Toxicity

Hyperthyroidism has been associated with the ingestion of kelp and is attributable to the iodine content in the plant.[10,11] Typical symptoms of hyperthyroidism (weight loss, sweating, fatigue, frequent soft stools) were exhibited by a 72-year-old woman following ingestion of a commercial kelp product for six months.[10] Laboratory tests confirmed the hyperthyroidism although no pre-existing evidence of thyroid disease was found and the condition resolved in six months following discontinuation of the tablets. Analysis of the kelp tablets reported an iodine content of 0.7 mg/tablet representing a daily intake of 2.8–4.2 mg iodine.[10] Clinically evident hyperthyroidism developed in an otherwise healthy woman following the daily ingestion of six 200-mg kelp tablets.[11] Symptoms gradually resolved on cessation of therapy.

The association between halogen salts and acneiform eruptions is well established.[12] Ingestion of kelp products has been associated with the worsening of pre-existing acne and the development of acneiform eruptions, which improved following withdrawal of the tablets.[12]

The ability of marine plants to accumulate heavy metals and other toxic elements is recognised, and the uptake of various radioactive compounds by seaweeds has been reported.[3,13,14] Fifteen samples of kelp-containing dietary supplements have been analysed for their iodine and arsenic contents.[15] The levels of arsenic were low in all but one product. The iodine levels varied widely, even between different samples of the same product, and in some products the iodine levels were high in relation to safe daily intake.

Brown algae (*Ascophyllum nodosum* and *Fucus vesiculosus*) have been found to be capable of synthesising volatile halogenated organic compounds (VHOCs).[16] VHOCs are considered to be troublesome pollutants because land plants and animals have difficulty in degrading the compounds which consequently persist in terrestrial ecosystems.[16] VHOCs released into the seawater predominantly contain bromine with iodine-containing compounds showing a slower rate of turnover.[16] Concentration of iron by brown seaweeds has been attributed to fucoidan, and alginic acid exhibits a high specificity for the binding of strontium.[13] Elevated urinary arsenic concentrations (138 and 293 μg/24 hour) in two female patients have been associated with the ingestion of kelp tablets. Subsequent analysis of the arsenic content of various kelp preparations revealed concentrations ranging from 16 to 58 μg/g product.[17,18] The botanical source of the kelp in the products was not stated.[18]

Ascophyllum nodosum is commonly added to animal foodstuffs as a source of vitamin and minerals, with beneficial results reported for dairy cattle, sheep, pigs and poultry.[13] Feeding studies using *A. nodosum* have highlighted an atypical toxic response for rabbits compared with that of rats and pigs.[13,19] Addition of *A. nodosum* to the diet of rabbits (at 5–10%) caused a severe drop in haemoglobin content, serum iron concentrations and packed cell volume, leading to weight loss and death in two-thirds of the animals.[13] No differences in renal and liver function, and in lipid metabolism were found between test and control animals.[13] Similar, but much milder, toxicity has also been observed in rabbits fed *Fucus serratus*.[19] Subsequent studies incorporating *A. nodosum* into the feed of rats and pigs failed to demonstrate the toxic effects observed in rabbits.[19] The toxic components in *A. nodosum* have been reported to be non-extractable with chloroform, ethanol, water and 20% sodium carbonate solution, remaining in the insoluble residue.[19]

Contra-indications, Warnings

The iodine content in kelp may cause hyper- or hypothyroidism and may interfere with existing treatment for abnormal thyroid function. In view of this, ingestion of kelp preparations by children is inadvisable. The iodine content in kelp has also been associated with acneiform eruptions and aggravation of pre-existing acne. In general, brown seaweeds are known to concentrate various heavy metals and other toxic elements. Elevated urinary arsenic concentrations have been traced to the ingestion of kelp tablets. Prolonged ingestion of kelp may reduce gastrointestinal iron absorption (binding properties of fucoidan), resulting in a slow reduction in haemoglobin, packed cell volume and serum iron concentrations. Prolonged ingestion may also affect absorption of sodium and potassium ions (alginic acid) and cause diarrhoea.

Pregnancy and lactation The safe use of kelp products during pregnancy and lactation has not been established. In view of the potential actions on the thyroid gland and possible contamination with toxic elements, the use of kelp should be avoided.

Pharmaceutical Comment

Kelp is a generic term that strictly speaking refers to *Laminaria* and *Macrocystis* species of brown seaweeds, although in practice it may be used in reference to other species of brown algae including *Nereocystis* and *Fucus*. The species *Fucus vesiculosus* is reported to be commonly used in the preparation of kelp products.[G60] The principal constituents of seaweeds are polysaccharides. For brown seaweeds the major polysaccharide is alginic acid (algin). Fucoidan, present in all brown algae, is thought to refer to a number of related polysaccharide esters whose main sugar component is fucose. The traditional uses of kelp in obesity and goitre are presumably attributable to the iodine content, although the self-diagnosis and treatment of these conditions with a herbal remedy is not suitable. There have been no documented studies supporting the traditional use of kelp in rheumatic conditions. In view of the iodine content and potential accumulation of toxic elements, excessive ingestion of kelp is inadvisable. Doubt over the quality of commercial seaweed preparations has been reported.[10]

References

See also General References G2, G6, G9, G11, G15, G16, G21, G28, G36, G37, G43, G48, G60 and G64.

1 Wood CG. Seaweed extracts. A unique ocean resource. *J Chem Ed* 1974; **51**: 449–452.
2 Algae as food for man. In: Chapman VJ, ed. *Seaweeds and their Uses*. London: Methuen, 1970: 115.
3 Whistler RL, ed. *Industrial Gums*, 2nd edn. New York: Academic Press, 1973: 13.
4 Burkholder PR. Drugs from the sea. *Armed Forces Chem J* 1963; **17**: 6, 8, 10, 12–16.
5 Doner LW. Fucoidan. In: Whistler RL, ed. *Industrial Gums*, 2nd edn. New York: Academic Press, 1973: 115–121.
6 Barwell CJ *et al.* Inhibitors of mammalian digestive enzymes in some species of marine brown algae. *Br Phycol J* 1983; **18**: 200.
7 Murata K. Suppression of lipid synthesis in cultured aortic cells by laminaran sulfate. *J Atheroscl Res* 1969; **10**: 371–378.
8 Funayama S, Hikino H. Hypotensive principle of Laminaria and allied seaweeds. *Planta Med* 1981; **41**: 29–33.
9 Kathan RH. Kelp extracts as antiviral substances. *Ann N Y Acad Sci* 1965; **130**: 390–397.
10 Shilo S, Hirsch HJ. Iodine-induced hyperthyroidism in a patient with a normal thyroid gland. *Postgrad Med J* 1986; **62**: 661–662.
11 Smet PAGM de *et al.* Kelp in herbal medicines: hyperthyroidism. *Ned Tijdschr Geneeskd* 1990; **134**: 1058–1059.
12 Harrell BL, Rudolph AH. Kelp diet: A cause of acneiform eruption. *Arch Dermatol* 1976; **112**: 560.
13 Blunden G, Jones RT. Toxic effects of *Ascophyllum nodosum* as a rabbit food additive. In: *Food – Drugs from the Sea Proceedings 1972*. Washington: Marine Technology Society, 1972: 267–293.
14 Hodge VF *et al.* Rapid accumulation of plutonium and polonium on giant brown algae. *Health Phys* 1974; **27**: 29–35.
15 Norman JA *et al.* Human intake of arsenic and iodine from seaweed-based food supplements and health foods available in the UK. *Food Additives Contaminants* 1987; **5**: 103–109.
16 Halocarbons. Natural pollution by algal seaweeds. *Chem Br* 1985: 513–514.
17 Walkiw O, Douglas DE. Health food supplements prepared from kelp – a source of elevated urinary arsenic. *Can Med Assoc J* 1974; **111**: 1301–1302.
18 Walkiw O, Douglas DE. Health food supplements prepared form kelp – a source of elevated urinary arsenic. *Clin Toxicol* 1975; **8**: 325–331.
19 Jones RT *et al.* Effects of dietary *Ascophyllum nodosum* on blood parameters of rats and pigs. *Botanica Marina* 1979; **22**: 393–394.

Fumitory

Species (Family)

Fumaria officinalis L. (Fumariaceae)

Synonym(s)

Fumitory

Part(s) Used

Herb

Pharmacopoeial and Other Monographs

BHC 1992[G6]
BHP 1996[G9]
Complete German Commission E[G3]
Martindale 32nd edition[G43]
PDR for Herbal Medicines 2nd edition[G36]

Legal Category (Licensed Products)

GSL[G37]

Constituents[G2,G6,G40,G64]

Alkaloids Isoquinoline-type. Protopines including protopine (fumarine) as the major alkaloid and cryptopine,[1,2] protoberberines including aurotensine, stylopine, sinactine and N-methylsinactine,[3] spirobenzylisoquinolines including fumaritine, fumaricine and fumariline,[4,5] benzophenanthridines including sanguinarine,[6] and indenobenzazepines including fumaritridine and fumaritrine.[6,7]

Flavonoids Glycosides of quercetin including isoquercitrin, rutin and quercetrin-3,7-diglucoside-3-arabinoglucoside.[8,9]

Acids Chlorogenic, caffeic and fumaric acids.[8]

Other constituents Bitter principles, mucilage and resin.

Food Use

Fumitory is listed by the Council of Europe as a natural source of food flavouring (category N3). This category indicates that fumitory can be added to foodstuffs in the traditionally accepted manner, although there is insufficient information available for an adequate assessment of potential toxicity.[G16]

Herbal Use

Fumitory is stated to possess weak diuretic and laxative properties and to act as a cholagogue. Traditionally, it has been used to treat cutaneous eruptions, conjunctivitis (as an eye lotion) and, specifically, chronic eczema.[G2,G6,G7,G8,G64]

Dosage

Herb 2–4 g or by infusion three times daily.[G6,G7]

Liquid extract 2–4 mL (1:1 in 25% alcohol) three times daily.[G6,G7]

Tincture 1–4 mL (1:5 in 45% alcohol) three times daily.[G6,G7]

Pharmacological Actions

In vitro and animal studies

The herb had no effect on normal choloresis but it modified bile flow which was artificially increased or decreased.[10] Antispasmodic activity on smooth muscle has been reported.[11] Extracts inhibited formation of gall-bladder calculi in animals.[12] The major alkaloid protopine has antihistaminic,[13] hypotensive, bradycardic and sedative activities in small doses,[14] whereas larger doses cause excitation and convulsions.[14] Bactericidal activity against the Gram-positive organisms *Bacillus anthracis* and *Staphylococcus* have been reported.[14]

Clinical studies

Clinical studies involving 105 patients with biliary disorders claimed favourable results.[15]

Side-effects, Toxicity

No reported side-effects or documented toxicity studies were located, although possible adverse effects include raised intraocular pressure and oedema.[16]

Contra-indications, Warnings

Hypotensive actions have been documented in animal studies.

Pregnancy and lactation The safety of fumitory during pregnancy and lactation has not been established. In view of lack of pharmacological and toxicity data, the use of fumitory during pregnancy and lactation should be avoided.

Pharmaceutical Comment

Fumitory is characterised by isoquinoline alkaloids which represent the principal active ingredients. Animal studies support some of the traditional uses, but it should not be used in home-made ophthalmic preparations. In view of the active constituents and the lack of safety data, excessive ingestion of fumitory should be avoided.

References

See also General References **G2, G3, G6, G9, G16, G31, G36, G37, G43, G56** and **G64.**

1 Sener B. Turkish species of *Fumaria* L. and their alkaloids. VII Alkaloids from *Fumaria officinalis* L. and *F. cilicica* Hansskn. *Gazi Univ Eczacilik Fak Derg* 1985; **2**: 45–49.

2 Hermansson J, Sandberg F. Alkaloids of *Fumaria officinalis. Acta Pharm Suec* 1973; **10**: 520–522.

3 Mardirossian ZH *et al.* Alkaloids of *Fumaria officinalis. Phytochemistry* 1983; **22**: 759–761.

4 MacLean DB *et al.* Structure of three minor alkaloids of *Fumaria officinalis. Can J Chem* 1969; **47**: 3593–3599.

5 Murav'eva DA *et al.* Isolation of fumaritine from *Fumaria officinalis. Khim Farm Zh* 1974; **8**: 32–34.

6 Forgacs P *et al.* Alcaloides des Papavéracées II: Composition chimique de dix-sept espèces de *Fumaria. Plantes Med Phytother* 1986; **20**: 64–81.

7 Forgacs P *et al.* Composition chimique des Fumariacées. Alcaloides de quatorze espèces de *Fumaria. Plantes Med Phytother* 1982; **16**: 99–115.

8 Massa V *et al.* Sur les pigments phenoliques du *Fumaria officinalis* L. *Trav Soc Pharm Montpellier* 1971; **31**: 233–236.

9 Torck M *et al.* Flavonoids of *Fumaria officinalis* L. *Ann Pharm Fr* 1971; **29**: 591–596.

10 Boucard M, Laubenheimer B. Action du nébulisat de fumeterre sur le débit bilaire du rat. *Therapie* 1966; **21**: 903–911.

11 Reynier M *et al.* Action du nébulisat de fumeterre officinal sur la musculature lisse. Contribution à l'étude du mécanisme de son activité thérapeutique. *Trav Soc Pharm Montpellier* 1977; **37**: 85–102.

12 Lagrange E, Aurousseau M. Effect of spray-dried product of *Fumaria officinalis* on experimental gall bladder lithiasis in mice. *Ann Pharm Fr* 1973; **31**: 357–362.

13 Abdul Habib Dil. Activité anti-histaminique de la fumarine. *Therapie* 1973; **28**: 767–774.

14 Preininger V. The pharmacology and toxicology of the papaveraceae alkaloids. In: RHF Manske, ed. *The Alkaloids XV.* London: Academic Press, 1975: 207–261.

15 Fiegel G. Die amphocholoretische Wirkung der *Fumaria officinalis. Z Allgemeinmed Landarzt* 1971; **34**: 1819–1820.

16 Anderson LA, Phillipson JD. Herbal medicine, education and the pharmacist. *Pharm J* 1986; **236**: 303–305.

Garlic

Species (Family)

Allium sativum L. (Amaryllidaceae/Liliaceae)

Synonym(s)

Ajo, Allium

Part(s) Used

Bulb (clove)

Pharmacopoeial and Other Monographs

BHP 1996[G9]
BP 2001[G15]
BPC 1949[G11]
Complete German Commission E[G3]
ESCOP 1997[G52]
Martindale 32nd edition[G43]
Mills and Bone[G50]
PDR for Herbal Medicines 2nd edition[G36]
Ph Eur 2002[G28]
WHO year volume 1[G63]

Legal Category (Licensed Products)

GSL[G37]

Constituents[1–3,G6,G41,G52,G56,G64]

Enzymes Allinase, peroxidases, myrosinase and others (e.g. catalases, superoxide dismutases, arginases, lipases).[2,3]

Volatile oils 0.1–0.36%. Sulfur-containing compounds including alliin, compounds produced enzymatically from alliin including allicin (diallyl thiosulfinate), allylpropyl disulfide, diallyl disulfide, diallyl trisulfide; ajoene and vinyldithiines (secondary products of alliin produced non-enzymatically from allicin); S-allylmercaptocysteine (ASSC) and S-methylmercaptocysteine (MSSC); terpenes include citral, geraniol, linalool, α- and β-phellandrene.

Other constituents Proteins (e.g. glutamyl peptides), amino acids (e.g. arginine, glutamic acid, asparagic acid, methionine, threonine), minerals, vitamins, trace elements, lipids, prostaglandins (A_2, D_2, E_2, $F_{1\alpha}$, F_2).[2,4]

Allicin and other sulfur-containing compounds are formed from alliin by the enzyme alliinase when garlic is crushed or chopped. (Alliin and alliinase are separated while the cells of a garlic bulb are intact, but crushing and chopping damage the cells of the bulb, allowing alliin and alliinase to come into contact with each other.[G56]) It is considered that 1 mg alliin is equivalent to 0.45 mg allicin.[G52] Commercial garlic preparations are often standardised on content of sulfur-containing constituents, particularly to alliin, or on allicin yield.

Garlic powder contains not less than 0.45% allicin calculated with reference to the dried drug.[G28]

Food Use

Garlic is used extensively as a food and as an ingredient in foods. It is listed by the Council of Europe as a natural source of food flavouring (category N1). This category indicates that there are no restrictions on the use of garlic in foods.[G16] In the USA, garlic is listed as GRAS (Generally Recognised As Safe).[G41]

Herbal Use

Garlic is stated to possess diaphoretic, expectorant, antispasmodic, antiseptic, bacteriostatic, antiviral, hypotensive and anthelmintic properties, and to be a promoter of leukocytosis. Traditionally, it has been used to treat chronic bronchitis, respiratory catarrh, recurrent colds, whooping cough, bronchitic asthma, influenza and chronic bronchitis.[G2,G6,G32,G34,G49,G64] Modern use of garlic and garlic preparations is focused on their reputed antihypertensive, anti-atherogenic, antithrombotic, antimicrobial, fibrinolytic, cancer preventive and lipid-lowering effects.

Dosage

Dried bulb 2–4 g three times daily;[G6] fresh garlic 4 g daily.[G3]

Tincture 2–4 mL (1 : 5 in 45% alcohol) three times daily.[G6]

Oil   0.03–0.12 mL three times daily.[G6]

Juice of Garlic   (BPC 1949) 2–4 mL.[G11]

Syrup of Garlic   (BPC 1949) 2–8 mL.[G11]

Clinical trials assessing the effects of garlic powder tablets on various parameters, including total serum cholesterol concentrations, triglyceride concentrations, blood pressure, platelet aggregation, vascular resistance, fibrinolysis and measures of peripheral arterial occlusive disease, have generally involved the administration of doses of 600–900 mg daily for 4–24 weeks.[G56] For prophylaxis of atherosclerosis, ESCOP (European Scientific Co-operative on Phytotherapy) states a dosage 0.5–1.0 g dried garlic powder daily (approximately equivalent to alliin 6–10 mg and allicin 3–5 mg).[G52]

Pharmacological Actions

In vitro and animal studies

Many pharmacological properties have been documented for garlic and its constituents *in vitro* and *in vivo* (animals), including antihypertensive, lipid-lowering, anti-atherogenic, antithrombotic, fibrinolytic, antioxidant, anticarcinogenic, antitumorigenic, immunomodulatory and antimicrobial activities. The pharmacological properties of garlic are attributed mainly to its sulfur-containing compounds. An extensive review of the pharmacological properties of garlic and its constituents is beyond the scope of this monograph, although several studies are described in brief below. The pharmacological activities of garlic and its constituents have been summarised in many reviews.[3,5–21,G5,G56]

Pharmacokinetics   The available literature on the metabolism and pharmacokinetics of the constituents of garlic in animals has been reviewed.[3,G18]

In an *ex vivo* study, allicin showed a marked first-pass clearance effect in isolated perfused rat liver.[3] In rats, alliin and allicin were administered orally at doses of 8 mg/kg.[22] Absorption of alliin and allicin was complete after 10 minutes and 30–60 minutes, respectively. The mean total urinary and faecal excretion of allicin after 72 hours was 85.5% of the dose. No unchanged alliin or allicin was detected in urine, suggesting rapid and extensive metabolism of these constituents.[3] Pharmacokinetic studies of the garlic constituent *S*-allyl-L-cysteine administered orally to rats at doses of 12.5, 25 and 50 mg/kg have reported bioavailability of 64%, 77% and 98%, respectively.[23] Peak plasma concentrations of *S*-allyl-L-cysteine occurred at one hour, and the

half-life of *S*-allyl-L-cysteine was 2.33 hours following oral administration of 50 mg/kg to rats.

Anti-atherosclerotic and cholesterol- and lipid-lowering effects   The effects of garlic and its constituents on cholesterol biosynthesis *in vitro* and in animal models of hypercholesterolaemia are well documented.[3]

Several *in vitro* studies have shown that garlic and its sulfur-containing constituents inhibit cholesterol biosynthesis in cultured hepatocytes.[24–28] In other *in vitro* studies, garlic extracts were shown to inhibit fatty acid and triglyceride synthesis.[29,30]

The step(s) in the cholesterol biosynthetic pathway inhibited by garlic, and the constituents of garlic causing inhibition have not been definitively established. Several mechanisms of action for the effects of garlic constituents on cholesterol and lipid synthesis have been proposed, including inhibition of hydroxymethylglutaryl-CoA (HMG-CoA) reductase activity and other enzymes, such as lanosterol-14-demethylase, involved in cholesterol biosynthesis.[3] Other proposed mechanisms include reduction in triacylglycerol biosynthesis via a reduction in tissue concentrations of NADPH, increase in hydrolysis of triacylglycerols via increased lipase activity and inactivation of enzymes involved in lipid synthesis via an interaction with enzyme thiol groups.[6,8,31] More recently, fresh garlic extract and the constituents *S*-allylcysteine, diallyl trisulfide and diallyl disulfide were shown to inhibit human squalene monooxygenase, an enzyme catalysing a step in cholesterol biosynthesis.[32] Another *in vitro* study reported that *S*-allylcysteine, *S*-propylcysteine and *S*-ethylcysteine inhibit triglyceride biosynthesis in part by decreasing *de novo* fatty acid synthesis via inhibition of fatty acid synthase.[30]

The anti-atherogenic, anti-atherosclerotic and cholesterol- and lipid-lowering effects of garlic and its constituents have been documented in several animal models (e.g. rabbits, rats, chickens, pigs) of atherosclerosis, hypercholesterolaemia and hyperlipidaemia.[3] For example, a reduction in both blood and tissue lipid concentrations in hypercholesterolaemic animals fed a diet supplemented with dried garlic powder, garlic oil, or allicin has been documented.[6,33] Garlic has also been reported to reduce hepatic triglyceride and cholesterol concentrations in rats, and to reduce aortic lipid deposition and atheromatous lesions in rabbits fed a high-fat diet.[6] Several studies have reported hypolipidaemic effects for garlic oil following administration to rats and rabbits fed a fat-rich diet to induce hyperlipidaemia.[3] Administration of aged garlic extract to rabbits fed a 1% cholesterol-enriched diet for six weeks reduced the surface area of the thoracic aorta covered by fatty streaks (atherosclerosis) and significantly reduced aortic arch cholesterol, although plasma cholesterol concentrations were not reduced.[34] Allicin administration has been reported to reduce significantly the formation of fatty streaks in mice fed a cholesterol-rich diet, compared with control mice (no allicin treatment).[35]

The cholesterol-lowering effect of garlic is thought to be dose-related; proposed mechanisms of action include inhibition of lipid synthesis and increased excretion of neutral and acidic sterols.[6,8] An *in vitro* study reported that aged garlic extract may exert its anti-atherogenic effects via inhibition of smooth muscle proliferation and phenotypic change, and by an effect on lipid accumulation in the artery wall.[34,]

Antithrombotic and fibrinolytic activities Antithrombotic activity is well documented for garlic in both *in vitro* and *in vivo* (animal) studies.[3] Antithrombotic effects have been documented for fresh garlic, garlic powder and garlic oils.[3]

Increased serum fibrinogen concentrations together with a decrease in blood coagulation time and fibrinolytic activity are associated with a high-fat diet and enhance thrombosis.[6] Garlic has been shown to have a beneficial effect on all of these parameters. Garlic has been shown to inhibit platelet aggregation[36,37] caused by several inducers such as ADP, collagen, arachidonic acid, adrenaline (epinephrine) and calcium ionophore A23187.[38] Antiplatelet activity has been documented for garlic in *in vitro* studies using human platelets.[5,39]

Several mechanisms have been proposed by which garlic is thought to exert an anti-aggregatory action. These include inhibition of thromboxane synthesis via cyclooxygenase and lipoxygenase inhibition,[8] inhibition of membrane phospholipase activity and incorporation of arachidonic acid into platelet membrane phospholipids,[40] intraplatelet mobilisation of calcium uptake and inhibition of calcium uptake into platelets.[38] Garlic oil has been reported to reduce artificial surface adhesion of platelets *in vitro*.[41] Certain garlic constituents also affect processes preceding platelet aggregation, such as activation of platelets.[3]

Garlic is thought to contain more than one inhibitor of platelet aggregation and release; allicin is considered to be the major inhibitor.[3,42] Other studies have investigated the role of ajoene (a secondary degradation product of alliin) as an inhibitor of platelet aggregation and release.[3,43] Ajoene inhibits platelet aggregation caused by various inducers.[44,45] Its action is noted to be dose-dependent and reversible both *in vitro* and *in*

vivo.[43] It has been suggested that this latter feature may be of clinical significance in instances where a rapid inhibition of platelet aggregation is required with subsequent reversal, such as chronic haemodialysis and coronary bypass surgery.[43] It has been proposed that ajoene exerts its anti-aggregatory effect by altering the platelet membrane via an interaction with sulfhydryl groups.[46] The inhibitory action of ajoene on granule release from platelets is thought to involve alteration of the microviscosity in the inner part of the plasma membrane.[47] Ajoene is reported to synergistically potentiate the anti-aggregatory action of prostacyclin, forskolin, indomethacin and dipyridamole,[48] and to potentiate the inhibitory action of prostaglandin I_2 (PGI_2) on platelet aggregation.[21] Approximately 96% inhibition of prostaglandin synthetase and 100% inhibition of lipoxygenase has been described for ajoene *in vitro*.[40] Structure–activity investigations suggested that an allylic structure in the open disulfide ring is required for activity.[40]>

Antioxidant effects Antioxidant properties have been documented for garlic *in vitro* and *in vivo* (animals).[3] Garlic constituents inhibit the formation of free radicals, support endogenous radical-scavenging mechanisms, enhance cellular antioxidant enzymes (e.g. superoxide dismutase, catalase, glutathione peroxidase), protect low-density lipoprotein from oxidation by free radicals, and inhibit the activation of the oxidant-induced transcription factor nuclear factor kappa B (NF-κB).[3,18]

Garlic powder was reported to inhibit the production of superoxide by phorbol ester-activated human granulocytes *in vitro* (IC_{50} 390 µg/mL),[49] whereas alliin did not inhibit superoxide production in this model. It was suggested that allicin may be the constituent of garlic responsible for the observed oxygen-radical scavenging properties. *In vitro*, aged garlic extract and S-allylcysteine inhibited low-density lipoprotein oxidation and protected pulmonary artery endothelial cells against injury induced by oxidised low-density lipoprotein.[50] In subsequent studies using bovine pulmonary artery endothelial cells and murine macrophages, it was shown that aged garlic extract inhibited oxidised low-density lipoprotein-induced release of peroxides.[51] *In vivo* studies have reported reductions in liver lipid peroxidation and inhibition of ethanol-induced mitochondrial lipid peroxidation in rats fed garlic oil.[3]

The antioxidant properties are of interest in relation to the antiarteriosclerotic, antihepatotoxic and anticancer effects of garlic and its constituents. For example, oxidation of low-density lipoprotein plays an important role in the initiation and progression of atherosclerosis.[50]

Antihypertensive effects Several studies involving animal models (e.g. dogs, rats) of hypertension have reported hypotensive effects of garlic preparations.[3] A hypotensive effect in dogs administered garlic extract has been documented; prior administration of antagonists to known endogenous hypotensive substances such as histamine, acetylcholine, serotonin and kinins did not affect the hypotensive effect.[52] Spontaneously hypertensive rats fed standardised dry garlic powder 1 mg/kg for nine months exhibited lower blood pressure than control rats (150 versus 205 mmHg, respectively).[53] By contrast, an ethanolic extract of garlic (1–2 g and 4–8 g daily) fed to spontaneously hypertensive rats did not lead to a reduction in blood pressure.[54]

Anticarcinogenic and antitumorigenic activities Many *in vitro* and animal studies have documented anticancer activities of garlic and its constituents.[3,14,15] These studies indicate that allicin, allicin-derived compounds and other compounds unrelated to allicin contribute to the anticancer effects of garlic.

In several animal models, garlic has been shown to inhibit carcinogenesis and to protect against the development of experimentally induced tumours.[3,14,15] For example, aged garlic extract significantly inhibited the growth of Sarcoma-180 and LL/2 lung carcinoma cells transplanted into mice.[55] Garlic powder and its constituents *S*-allyl-cysteine and diallyl disulfide inhibited *N*-methyl-*N*-nitrosourea-induced mammary carcinogenesis in rats,[56] and fresh garlic (250 mg/kg orally, three times weekly) suppressed 4-nitroquinoline-1-oxide–induced carcinogenesis in rat tongue.[57] Inhibition of benzo[*a*]pyrene-induced neoplasia of the forestomach and lung in female mice has been documented for four allyl group-containing derivatives in garlic.[58] Structure–activity requirements underlined the importance of the unsaturated allyl groups for activity. Saturated analogues containing propyl instead of allyl groups were devoid of activity.

In vitro studies using human tumour cell lines have reported that garlic powder and garlic extract inhibited the growth of a human lymphatic leukaemia cell line (CCRF CEM) in a concentration-dependent manner at concentrations down to 30 µg/mL.[59] Also, a combination of garlic extract and garlic powder inhibited the growth of human hepatoma (HepG2,) cells and human colorectal carcinoma (Caco2) cells in a concentration-dependent manner,

although no activity was observed on these tumour cell lines with garlic extract or powder alone.[59] Synthetic diallyl disulfide inhibited tumour cell growth in four human breast cancer cell lines.[60] Growth inhibition occurred regardless of oestrogen receptor status.

Evidence indicates that there are several mechanisms by which garlic and its constituents may exert anticancer effects, such as inhibition of carcinogen formation, modulation of carcinogen metabolism, inhibition of mutagenesis and genotoxicity, increased apoptosis and inhibition of angiogenesis.[20]

Garlic has been shown to inhibit the synthesis of *N*-nitroso compounds (there is a view that *N*-nitroso compounds are possible carcinogens for humans).[14] Also, in rats pretreated with dimethylbenz[*a*]anthracene (DMBA) and fed a diet supplemented with garlic powder, the occurrence of DNA adducts in mammary tissue was significantly inhibited, compared with control.[61] (DMBA initiates and promotes cancer, and alkylation of DNA is thought to be an important step in carcinogenesis.) Dietary garlic has also been shown to suppress the occurrence of DNA adducts caused by *N*-nitroso compounds.[62]

Another possible explanation is that garlic constituents may modify drug-metabolising enzymes, which would have the effect of altering the bioactivation of carcinogens.[14] Glutathione-*S*-transferase activity has been shown to increase in rat and mouse tissues after administration of garlic powder or its sulfur-containing constituents.[3,14,15] Certain garlic constituents, e.g. diallyl sulfide, may depress the activity of some hepatic cytochrome P450 (CYP) enzymes, such as CYP2E1 and CYP2A6,[3,14,15,63] although other studies have shown that garlic constituents induce the activity of other CYP enzymes.[3,17] In rats, the antimutagenic properties of sulfur-containing compounds from garlic, e.g. diallyl disulfide and diallyl sulfide, against the carcinogens styrene oxide and 4-nitroquinoline-1-oxide and a benzo[*a*]pyrene compound have been shown to be associated with induction of phase II enzymes.[64]

A study in mice with transitional cell carcinoma (TCC) of the bladder reported that injection of liquid extract of garlic at the site of tumour transplantation led to a significant reduction in the incidence of TCC in this model.[65] Furthermore, garlic extract together with suicide-gene therapy significantly inhibited tumour growth (as determined by evidence of apoptosis following histomorphological and immunohistochemical studies) compared with control (no gene therapy).

Effects of garlic constituents on the immune system have been documented *in vitro* and *in vivo*; these effects may contribute, at least in part, to the anticancer effects of garlic (*see* Immunomodulatory activity).

Immunomodulatory activity Immunostimulant activity has been described for a high molecular weight protein fraction obtained from an aged garlic extract.[66] The fraction was found to strongly stimulate mice peritoneal macrophages *in vitro*, and to stimulate carbon clearance in mice *in vivo*. It has been suggested that garlic may suppress tumour cell growth by the stimulation of immunoresponder cells.[55,66,67]

In vitro and/or *in vivo* (animal) studies have found that garlic has several immune-enhancing effects, such as stimulation of lymphocyte proliferation and macrophage phagocytosis, induction of macrophage- and lymphocyte-infiltration into transplanted tumours, and stimulation of interferon-γ release.[67] Other effects on the immune system documented for garlic and/or its constituents include increased natural killer cell activity and increased interleukin-2 production by garlic fractions *in vitro*,[68] and increased numbers of antibody-forming cells in mice spleens following administration of standardised garlic powder.[3] Other studies demonstrated that, *in vitro*, aged garlic extract, compared with control, enhanced the proliferation of spleen cells in a concentration-dependent manner, increased production of cytokines (including interleukin-2 and tumour necrosis factor α) and enhanced natural killer cell activity of a T cell fraction of mouse splenic cells against YAC-1 after incubation for 24 hours.[55] Also, compared with control, aged garlic extract significantly inhibited the growth of sarcoma-180 and LL/2 lung carcinoma cells transplanted into mice, and significant increases in natural killer cell activity of spleen were observed in splenic cells from sarcoma-bearing mice treated with aged garlic extract, compared with those from control mice.[55,69]

Antimicrobial activity Antimicrobial activity (including antibacterial, antiviral, antifungal, antiprotozoal and antiparasitic activites) is well documented for garlic.[3,7] The *in vitro* antimicrobial activity of garlic is considered to be mainly due to allicin.[3]

In vitro studies have demonstrated that bacteria sensitive to garlic include species from *Staphylococcus*, *Escherichia*, *Proteus*, *Salmonella*, *Providencia*, *Citrobacter*, *Klebsiella*, *Hafnia*, *Aeromonas*, *Vibrio* and *Bacillus* genera.[7,70] In these studies, *Pseudomonas aeruginosa* was found not to be sensitive to garlic.[7,70] *In vitro* studies have also shown that allicin has significant antibacterial activity against several species, including *Bacillus subtilis*, *Staphylococcus aureus*, *Staphylococcus faecalis*, *Escherichia coli*, *Proteus mirabilis*, *Salmonella typhi* and *Vibrio cholerae*.[70]

In other *in vitro* studies, garlic oil and four diallyl sulfide constituents, including diallyl disulfide, showed activity against antibiotic-resistant *Pseudomonas aeruginosa* and *Klebsiella pneumoniae*,[71] and against *S. aureus*, methicillin-resistant *S. aureus*, *Candida* spp. and *Aspergillus* spp.[72] Garlic has also been documented to inhibit growth in 30 strains (consisting of 17 species) of mycobacteria, including *Mycobacterium tuberculosis*.[73] *In vitro*, both aqueous garlic extract and ethanolic garlic extract inhibited the growth of *M. avium* complex (MAC) strains isolated from patients with or without acquired immune deficiency syndrome (AIDS).[74] Aqueous garlic extract at concentrations of 2–5 mg/mL inhibited the growth of clinical isolates of *Helicobacter pylori* from patients with chronic gastritis or duodenal ulcer.[75] The minimum inhibitory concentration to inhibit 90% of growth (MIC_{90}) was 5 mg/mL. Sulfur-containing compounds from garlic (diallyl sulfide and diallyl disulfide, produced from alliin) were shown to decrease growth of *H. pylori* isolates from patients with peptic ulcer.[76] It has been proposed that garlic inhibits bacterial cell growth by primarily inhibiting RNA synthesis.[77]

Broad-spectrum activity against fungi has been documented for garlic including the genera *Microsporum*, *Epidermophyton*, *Trichophyton*, *Rhodotorula*, *Torulopsis*, *Trichosporon*, *Cryptococcus neoformans* and *Candida*, including *Candida albicans*.[7]

Garlic extract has been reported to be more effective than nystatin against pathogenic yeasts, especially *Candida albicans*.[7] Inhibition of lipid synthesis is thought to be an important factor in the anticandidal activity of garlic, with a disulfide-containing component such as allicin thought to be the main active component.[78] Garlic has been found to inhibit the growth and toxin production of *Aspergillus parasiticus*.[79]

Allicin produced from synthetic alliin with alliinase isolated from garlic cloves inhibited the destruction of baby hamster kidney cells by trophozoites of the protozoan parasite *Entamoeba histolytica in vitro*.[80] Allicin also inhibited the cysteine proteinase activities of intact *E. histolytica* trophozoites. *In vitro* activity against *Giardia intestinalis* has also been documented for whole garlic extract (IC_{50}

0.3 mg/mL) and for several of its constituents, particularly allyl alcohol and allyl mercaptan (IC_{50} 7 μg/mL and 37 μg/mL, respectively).[81]

In vitro antiviral activity against parainfluenza type 3, herpes simplex type 1 and influenza B has been documented.[82,83] Activity was attributed to allicin or an allicin derivative. Garlic was reported to be ineffective towards coxsackie B1 virus.[84]

Antihepatotoxic effects Antihepatotoxic activity *in vitro* and *in vivo* has been reported for garlic and its constituents.[3] Garlic oil[85] and some of its constituents, namely alliin, S-allylmercaptocysteine (ASSC) and S-methylmercaptocysteine (MSSC) reduced carbon tetrachloride (CCl_4)- and galactosamine-induced hepatotoxicity *in vitro*.[85] Other *in vitro* studies have shown that S-allylcysteine, S-propylcysteine and S-allylmercaptocysteine neutralised CCl_4-induced hepatotoxicity, and that S-allylcysteine and S-allylmercaptocysteine prevent liver damage induced by hepatotoxins in acute hepatitis in mice.[3,86]

An *in vitro* study in rat hepatocytes found that diallyl sulfide (0.5 and 2 mmol/L) and diallyl disulfide (0.5 and 1 mmol/L) protected against DNA damage induced by aflatoxin B_1, compared with control.[87] In this model, diallyl sulfide and diallyl disulfide appeared to exert a hepatoprotective effect via increased activity of glutathione-S-transferase and glutathione peroxidase activity.

Other activities Garlic oil and juice have been reported to protect against isoprenaline-induced myocardial necrosis in rats.[88] Oral administration of garlic extract 100, 200 or 400 mg/kg to rats given oral lead acetate 5 mg/kg daily for six weeks was found to reduce tissue lead concentrations, compared with those in control rats.[89] A diet containing 2% aged garlic extract was reported to protect against intestinal damage induced by oral methotrexate and 5-fluorouracil administered to rats for 4–5 days, compared with a control diet.[90]

A study in senescence-accelerated mice found that S-allylcysteine, present in aged garlic extract, administered in the diet for eight months (40 mg/kg/diet daily) significantly attenuated the decrease in the conditioned avoidance response, compared with a diet lacking S-allylcysteine.[91] It was suggested that the findings indicate that dietary supplementation with S-allylcysteine may reduce age-related learning disabilities and cognitive disorders in senescence-accelerated mice.

Hypoglycaemic activity has been documented for an alcoholic garlic extract following oral administration to rabbits (dose equivalent to 50 g dry garlic powder). Fifty-nine per cent activity compared to that of 500 mg tolbutamide was observed.[92]

Garlic has been documented to cause both smooth muscle relaxation and contraction.[37,52,84] Garlic oil has been reported to depress gastrointestinal movements induced by charcoal meal and castor oil.[84] In mice, garlic has also inhibited acetylcholine- and PGE_2-induced contraction of the rat gastric fundus, with the most active components exhibiting the weakest antiplatelet aggregatory activity.[37] Garlic has also elicited contractions on the rat uterus and the guinea-pig ileum *in vitro*.[52] Both actions were blocked by flufenamic acid, but not by atropine or cyproheptadine, indicating a prostaglandin-like mode of action.

In vitro, ajoene was found to inhibit the release of lipopolysaccharide-induced prostaglandin E_2 in macrophages in a concentration-dependent manner.[93] This effect was reported to be due to inhibition of cyclooxygenase 2 (COX-2) activity by ajoene.

Clinical studies

Pharmacokinetics The available literature on the metabolism and pharmacokinetics of the constituents of garlic in humans has been reviewed.[3,94,G18]

Addition of allicin to fresh whole blood results in conversion of allicin to allyl mercaptan and other compounds produced from allicin, such as diallyl trisulfide and ajoene, have also been shown to form allyl mercaptan in blood.[3] Sulfur-containing compounds, such as diallyl disulfide, diallyl sulfide, dimethyl sulfide and mercapturic acids, have been isolated and identified in human urine following the ingestion of garlic.[3,95] A subsequent study detected N-acetyl-S-allyl-L-cysteine (allylmercapturic acid) in the urine of volunteers (n = 6) who had ingested two garlic tablets containing 100 mg garlic extract (Kwai).[96] The mean (standard deviation) elimination half-life of allylmercapturic acid was estimated to be 6 (1.3) hours.

It has been reported that the flavour of human breast milk is altered when lactating women consume foods containing sulfur-containing compounds, such as garlic (*see* Contra-indications, Warnings; Pregnancy and lactation).[97] Also, garlic ingestion by pregnant women significantly alters the odour of their amniotic fluid (*see* Contra-indications, Warnings; Pregnancy and lactation),[98] suggesting that the odorous components of garlic are present. Evidence for this comes from a placebo-controlled study involving 10 healthy pregnant women undergoing routine amniocentesis. The odour of samples of amniotic fluid from women who ingested capsules containing garlic extract was judged to be 'stronger' or more 'garlic-like' than that of samples from women who had ingested placebo capsules.

Pharmacodynamics Several of the pharmacological activities documented for garlic and its constituents *in vitro* and *in vivo* (animals) have also been reported in clinical studies (*see* Clinical studies, Therapeutic effects).

Numerous studies have assessed the effects of the administration of garlic preparations in hypercholesterolaemia.[3] Many, but not all, of these studies have documented the effects of garlic administration in lowering serum cholesterol and triglyceride concentrations. Clinical studies have also documented fibrinolytic activity associated with garlic administration and effects on platelet function.[99,100]

Therapeutic effects

Anti-atherosclerotic and cholesterol- and lipid-lowering effects Numerous studies have investigated the effects of garlic preparations in lowering raised serum cholesterol concentrations, and the findings of these studies have been reviewed in several meta-analyses.[101–104]

A meta-analysis of five randomised, placebo-controlled trials involving mostly patients with serum cholesterol concentrations greater than 5.17 mmol/L who received preparations of garlic extract at doses of 600–1000 mg daily for 8–24 weeks reported that garlic significantly reduced total serum cholesterol concentrations by about 9% (net reduction over placebo), compared with placebo ($p < 0.001$).[101] Another meta-analysis included 16 trials involving patients with a range of disorders (such as hyperlipidaemia, coronary heart disease and hypertension) as well as healthy volunteers, and compared garlic preparations (e.g. fresh garlic, garlic oil, garlic extract, dried garlic powder) with garlic-free diet, placebo or other agents (two studies used bezafibrate or a reserpine/diuretic combination as the comparator treatment).[102] This analysis reported a mean difference of -0.77 mmol/L (95% confidence interval (CI) -0.65, -0.89) in reduction of total serum cholesterol concentrations between garlic recipients and those receiving placebo or a garlic-free diet (net reduction over placebo: 12%). Analysis of data from the eight trials that assessed garlic powder preparations indicated that garlic powder administration significantly reduced serum triglyceride concentrations, compared with placebo (net reduction: 13%). It was stated, however, that several trials had methodological flaws, and that there was not enough evidence to recommend garlic as an effective lipid-lowering agent for routine use. The results of a subsequent randomised placebo-controlled trial involving 115 patients with moderate hyperlipidaemia (which showed no difference between garlic and placebo)[103] were included in a re-analysis[103] of the meta-analysis described above.[102] This analysis showed that the effect of garlic in reducing serum cholesterol concentrations remained statistically significant, compared with placebo, but that the size of the effect was reduced.

Several randomised, double-blind, placebo-controlled trials[105–108] have been published since the meta-analyses described above. One of these studies[105] has been criticised for its choice of garlic preparation.[109]

Several of these trials[105–107] were included in the most recent meta-analysis of randomised clinical trials of garlic preparations involving patients with hypercholesterolaemia.[104] This meta-analysis included 13 randomised, double-blind, placebo-controlled trials of garlic monopreparations involving 796 patients with coronary heart disease ($n = 1$ trial), hyperlipoproteinaemia (2), hypercholesterolaemia (7), hypertension (1), familial hyperlipidaemia in children (1) and healthy volunteers (1). Ten of the trials assessed the effects of a standardised garlic powder preparation (Kwai) at doses of 600–900 mg daily for 8–24 weeks; the other three trials tested garlic oil or spray dried powder. Ten trials reported differences favouring garlic over placebo in the reduction of total serum cholesterol concentrations, although these differences were statistically significant in only three studies. Overall, meta-analysis indicated a significant difference in the reduction of total cholesterol concentrations favouring garlic over placebo (-0.41 mmol/L; 95% CI -0.66 mmol/L, -0.15 mmol/L; $p < 0.01$), equivalent to a net reduction in total cholesterol concentrations of 5.8%. It was stated that although these findings indicated that garlic is more beneficial than placebo in reducing serum cholesterol concentrations, the size of the effect is small. Furthermore, several studies had methodological limitations.[104]

Another randomised, double-blind, placebo-controlled trial has been published since the meta-analysis described above. This study assessed the effects of garlic powder (tablets) 500 mg and 1000 mg daily, or placebo, for 12 weeks in 53 patients with moderate hypercholesterolaemia (baseline low-density lipoprotein cholesterol (LDL-C) 130–190 mg/dL).[108] At the end of the study there were no significant differences in the absolute mean change in LDL-C between the three groups (mean (SD) values were: 0.0 (4.3) mg/dL, 1.4 (4.8) mg/dL and -10.1 (6.8) mg/dL for the placebo, garlic powder 500 mg and garlic powder 1000 mg groups, respectively).

Another meta-analysis, which aimed to summarise the evidence for the effects of garlic on several cardiovascular-related factors, considered 45 randomised controlled trials of at least four weeks' duration.[110] It was reported that after one and three months, garlic treatment may lead to small reductions in total cholesterol concentrations (0.03–0.45 mmol/L and 0.32–0.66 mmol/L, respectively). However, no effect was noted for pooled six-month data. Changes in cholesterol concentrations were paralleled by changes in low-density lipoprotein and triglyceride concentrations.

A randomised, double-blind, placebo-controlled trial explored the anti-atherosclerotic effect of garlic powder 900 mg daily for 48 months in 280 patients with advanced atherosclerotic plaques and an established risk factor for arteriosclerosis (e.g. high systolic blood pressure, hypercholesterolaemia, diabetes mellitus, smoking).[111] It was reported that continuous garlic intake significantly reduced the increase in arteriosclerotic plaque volume, compared with placebo. However, the robustness of the findings of this study is difficult to assess independently as no exact *p*-value is given.

A Cochrane systematic review of garlic for the treatment of peripheral arterial occlusive disease identified only one eligible randomised, placebo-controlled trial.[112] The trial involved 78 participants with peripheral arterial occlusive disease (lower limb atherosclerosis) who received garlic, or placebo, for 12 weeks. At the end of the study, the difference in the increase in pain-free walking distance between the two groups was found to be statistically non-significant.

An open study involved 101 healthy adults aged 50–80 years who had taken a standardised garlic powder preparation at a dose of at least 300 mg daily for at least two years and 101 age- and sex-matched subjects.[113] Measures of the elastic properties of the aorta were compared for the two groups. Pulse-wave velocity and elastic vascular resistance were reported to be reduced significantly in the garlic group, compared with the control group. These findings suggest that long-term use of garlic powder to attenuate age-related increases in aortic stiffness is worth further study.

Antithrombotic and fibrinolytic effects Several placebo-controlled studies have documented fibrinolytic effects for garlic preparations in clinical studies involving patients with coronary heart disease, hyperlipidaemia and hypercholesterolaemia, and healthy volunteers.[3] Several studies involved the administration of ether-extracted garlic oil 20 mg daily for up to 90 days, whereas several others involved the administration of garlic powder 600–1500 mg daily for up to 28 days. Most, but not all, of these studies reported significant increases in fibrinolytic activity in garlic recipients, compared with placebo recipients.

An open, uncontrolled study explored the effects of garlic consumption (one fresh chopped clove daily for 16 weeks) in eight healthy male volunteers.[114] After 16 weeks, garlic consumption was reported to reduce significantly serum thomboxane B_2 and cholesterol concentrations, compared with baseline values.

Antioxidant effects Blood samples from 31 individuals who participated in a randomised, placebo-controlled trial involving 115 patients with moderate hyperlipidaemia who received a standardised garlic powder preparation 900 mg daily for six months (which showed no difference between garlic and placebo)[103] were analysed to explore the effects of garlic treatment on the resistance of low-density lipoprotein to oxidation.[115] There were no significant differences between garlic and placebo recipients in low-density lipoprotein composition. Thus, garlic administration did not reduce the susceptibility of low-density lipoprotein to oxidation. This finding contrasts with some of the results of a double-blind, placebo-controlled study involving 23 patients with coronary artery disease who received a standardised garlic powder preparation (Kwai tablets) 300 mg three times daily, or placebo, for four weeks.[116] The study reported that garlic powder administration reduced the atherogenicity of low-density lipoprotein. At the end of the study, the ability of low-density lipoprotein to induce intracellular cholesterol accumulation was decreased by 38%, compared with baseline values. Decreases in the susceptibility of low-density lipoprotein to oxidation and in low-density lipoprotein-stimulated cell proliferation (an indicator of low-density lipoprotein atherogenicity) were also documented.

The effects of standardised garlic powder tablets (Sapec; alliin 1.3%, allicin 0.6%) 900 mg daily for two months on oxidative stress status were explored in an open, uncontrolled study involving 25 healthy volunteers.[117] At the end of the study, a reduction in serum malondialdehyde concentrations was observed, compared with baseline values. It was stated that this finding indicates that standardised garlic powder may have antioxidant activity in humans.

Antihypertensive effects A meta-analysis of randomised controlled trials of garlic preparations assessed the evidence for the effects of garlic on blood pressure.[118] Eight trials involving 415 participants were included in the review, all of which had tested the effects of an allicin-standardised garlic powder preparation (Kwai tablets) at doses of 600–900 mg daily for 4–52 weeks. Overall, the absolute change in mean systolic blood pressure was 7.7 mmHg greater for the garlic group, compared with the placebo group (95% CI 4.3–11.0). However, only three trials specifically involved subjects with hypertension and, as reported by other meta-analyses of trials of garlic preparations, several trials had methodological limitations. Thus, it was stated that there was insufficient evidence to recommend garlic treatment for routine management of hypertension.

Another overview of trials reported that the effects of garlic treatment on blood pressure are 'insignificant'.[110]

Anticancer effects The protective effects of garlic consumption against various different cancers (including colon, stomach, larynx, breast and endometrial) have been explored in several epidemiological studies, and their findings have been summarised.[3,119] Most, but not all, of these studies suggest that garlic consumption may have a protective effect, particularly against cancers of the gastrointestinal tract.[3,119] However, the findings should be interpreted cautiously, as bias and/or confounding cannot be excluded, and there are other methodological issues, for example, most studies did not distinguish between consumption of raw or cooked garlic.

Antimicrobial effects An epidemiological study comprising a dietary interview and measurement of serum *H. pylori* antibodies was conducted among 214 adults in a low-risk area of Shandong Province in China.[120] The findings suggested a protective effect of garlic consumption against *H. pylori* infection.

An open, uncontrolled study involving 34 patients with tinea pedis explored the effectiveness of ajoene cream (0.4% w/w).[121] After seven days' treatment, complete cure of the infection was recorded for 27 (79%) participants. The remaining seven patients experienced complete cure after a further seven days' treatment. All patients were evaluated for recurrence of infection 90 days after the end of treatment; all found to be infection free as determined by negative cultures for the fungus.

Other effects A reduction in blood sugar concentrations and an increase in insulin have been observed following allylpropyl disulfide administration to normal volunteers, whereas another study reported that garlic exhibits hypoglycaemic actions in diabetic

patients but not in controls.[5] It has also been reported that garlic can prevent tolbutamide- and adrenaline-induced hyperglycaemia.[5]

A randomised, placebo-controlled, crossover trial involving 100 Swedish participants working in a tick-endemic area found that administration of garlic powder 1200 mg daily for eight weeks resulted in fewer tick bites than did placebo administration.[122]

An open, uncontrolled study involving 15 patients with hepatopulmonary syndrome explored the effects of treatment with capsules containing a standardised garlic powder preparation for at least six months.[123] Improvements in arterial oxygenation and symptoms were documented for several participants. The effects of garlic powder treatment in patients with hepatopulmonary syndrome require further study.

Side-effects, Toxicity[G19,G58]

Side-effects Garlic is generally considered to be non-toxic.[8,124] Adverse effects that have been documented in humans include a burning sensation in the mouth and gastrointestinal tract, nausea, diarrhoea and vomiting.[8]

A meta-analysis of 13 randomised, double-blind, placebo-controlled trials of garlic monopreparations, 10 of which assessed the effects of a standardised garlic powder preparation (Kwai) at doses of 600–900 mg daily for 8–24 weeks (*see* Clinical studies, Therapeutic effects, Anti-atherosclerotic and cholesterol- and lipid-lowering effects) reported that few adverse events were documented in the included trials.[104] The frequency and nature of adverse events reported for garlic were similar to those for placebo. The most common adverse events reported were 'garlic breath', body odour and gastrointestinal symptoms.

The allergenic potential of garlic is well recognised, and allergens have been identified as diallyl disulfide, allylpropyl sulfide and allicin (the latter may be an irritant).[125] A garlic antigen in the serum of affected patients has also been identified.[43] Cases of contact dermatitis resulting from occupational exposure to garlic have been reported.[43,126,G51] A case of garlic allergy associated with ingestion of raw or cooked garlic has been documented.[127] There is an isolated report of multifaceted dermatitis artefacta associated with local application of garlic by a 19-year-old individual.[128] Garlic burns following local application of garlic have also been documented.[129,130]

Garlic may enhance existing anticoagulant therapy; a potential interaction between garlic and warfarin has been documented.[131,132] Case reports have suggested that garlic supplementation may increase the risk of bleeding in patients undergoing surgery.[G21]

Toxicity Erratic pulse rates, abnormal ECGs, weight loss, lethargy and weakness, soft faeces, dehydration and tender skin on fore and hindlimbs have been observed in spontaneously hypertensive rats administered garlic extract at 0.25 and 0.5 mL/kg every 6 hours for 28 days.[133] The effects were most pronounced in animals receiving doses two or three times a day. Conversely, acute toxicity studies for garlic extract in mice and rats have reported LD_{50} values for various routes of administration (by mouth, intraperitoneal injection, intravenous injection) as all greater than 30 mL/kg.[124] Early studies, in 1944, reported LD_{50} values for allicin in mice as 120 mg/kg (subcutaneous injection) and 60 mg/kg (intravenous injection).[43] Results of chronic toxicity studies are stated to be conflicting.[43] High doses are reported to cause anaemia due to both decreased haemoglobin synthesis and haemolysis.[43] A chronic toxicity study in rats given a garlic extract (2 g/kg) five times a week for six months, reported no toxic symptoms.[134] High doses were found to decrease food consumption slightly, but did not inhibit weight gain. There were no significant differences in urinary, haematological or serological examinations, and no toxic symptoms in histopathological examinations. Genotoxicity studies using the micronucleus test have reported both positive[135] and negative[136] findings. No evidence of mutagenicity has been reported when assessed using the Ames and Ree assay.[135]

Slight cytotoxic signs have been observed at high doses in Hep2 and Chinese hamster embryo primary cultured cells.[135]

The literature relating to the toxicity of garlic has been reviewed.[3,G19,G20]

Contra-indications, Warnings

In view of the pharmacological actions documented for garlic, therapeutic doses of garlic may interfere with existing hypoglycaemic and anticoagulant therapies. There may be an increased risk of bleeding with use of garlic supplements in patients undergoing surgery.[G21] Garlic may potentiate the antithrombotic effects of anti-inflammatory drugs such as aspirin, and may be synergistic with eicosapentaenoic acid (EPA) in fish oils.[8] Gastrointestinal irritation may occur particularly if the clove is eaten raw by individuals not accustomed to ingesting garlic.

A study involving healthy volunteers detected *N*-acetyl-*S*-allyl-L-cysteine (allylmercapturic acid) in their urine following ingestion of garlic tablets (*see*

Clinical studies, Pharmacokinetics).[96] As allylmercapturic acid is used as a biomarker for monitoring human exposure to allylhalides and other chemicals leading to allylmercapturic acid excretion, it was suggested that garlic consumption may interfere with and confound this monitoring process.

Pregnancy and lactation Garlic is reputed to act as an abortifacient and to affect the menstrual cycle, and is also reported to be utero-active.[G30] *In vitro* uterine contraction has been documented.[84]

Studies have shown that consumption of garlic by lactating women alters the odour of their breast milk and the suckling behaviour of their infants.[97] Further evidence for this comes from a blinded, placebo-controlled study involving 30 nursing women.[137] The results indicated that infants who had no prior exposure to garlic odour in their mothers' milk spent more time breast feeding after their mothers ingested garlic capsules than did infants whose mothers had repeatedly consumed garlic. Findings from a placebo-controlled study involving 10 healthy pregnant women undergoing routine amniocentesis indicate that the odorous components of garlic can be found in amniotic fluid following garlic consumption.[98] The odour of samples of amniotic fluid from women who ingested capsules containing garlic extract was judged to be 'stronger' or more 'garlic-like' than that of samples from women who had ingested placebo capsules. The effects of *in utero* exposure to garlic odour and on the neonate's behaviour towards exposure to garlic-flavoured human breast milk are not known.

There are no experimental or clinical reports on adverse effects during pregnancy or lactation.[G19] In view of this, doses of garlic greatly exceeding amounts used in foods should not be taken during pregnancy and lactation.

Pharmaceutical Comment

There is a vast scientific literature on the chemistry, pharmacology and clinical properties of garlic. Experimental studies have focused mainly on the cardiovascular and anticancer effects of garlic and its constituents, as well as its antimicrobial properties. Clinical studies have investigated mainly the anti-atherosclerotic and cholesterol- and lipid-lowering effects of garlic preparations. Generally, these studies report beneficial results for garlic, although the evidence at present is insufficient to recommend garlic as routine treatment for hypercholesterolaemia. *In vitro* and animal studies provide supporting evidence for some of the clinical properties of garlic and its constituents.

Garlic is characterised by its sulfur-containing constituents. Pharmacological activities documented for garlic are also associated with these compounds. It is recognised that allicin, the unstable compound formed by enzymatic action of allinase on alliin when the garlic clove is crushed, is required for the antimicrobial activity that has been demonstrated by garlic. However, serum concentrations of allicin achieved in humans following oral ingestion of garlic are unclear. The hypolipidaemic and antithrombotic actions documented for garlic have been attributed to many of the degradation products of alliin.

One of the difficulties in comparing studies that have investigated the efficacy of garlic, is establishing the concentration of active principles present in the garlic preparations used. It has been reported that the percentage of active constituents in fresh garlic may vary by a factor of 10.[43] Many commercial garlic preparations are standardised on content of sulfur-containing constituents, particularly to alliin, or on allicin yield. Dried garlic powder contains both alliin and allinase and therefore has an allicin-releasing potential. Garlic preparations produced by heat or solvent extraction processes are stated to contain alliin but to be devoid of allinase and therefore have no allicin releasing potential.[43] Garlic oil macerates and steam distillation products are rich in secondary alliin metabolites, such as ajoene. However, it is unclear to what extent these secondary compounds are formed in the body following the ingestion of garlic and whether, therefore, these products exhibit the pharmacological actions of fresh garlic.[43]

Fermented garlic preparations are considered to be practically devoid of the active sulfur-containing compounds.[43] Many 'odourless' garlic preparations are available: obviously one should establish if these products are odourless due to the formulation of the product or because they are devoid of the odoriferous, active principles. Further randomised controlled clinical trials with standardised preparations are required to establish the true usefulness of garlic in reducing serum lipids, blood pressure, platelet aggregation and exerting an antimicrobial effect. Therapeutic doses of garlic should not be given to those whose blood clots slowly and caution is recommended for patients on anticoagulant therapy.[G58]

References

See also General References G3, G5, G6, G9, G16, G18, G19, G20, G21, G28, G31, G32, G36, G41, G43, G50, G51, G52, G56, G58, G61, G63 and G64.

1 Block E. The chemistry of garlic and onions. *Sci Am* 1985; **252**: 114–119.

2 Sendl A. *Allium sativum* and *Allium ursinum*: Part 1. Chemistry, analysis, history, botany. *Phytomedicine* 1995; **4**: 323–339.

3 Koch HP, Lawson LD, eds. *Garlic. The Science and Therapeutic Application of* Allium sativum L. *and Related Species*, 2nd edn. Baltimore, Maryland: Williams and Wilkins, 1996.

4 Al-Nagdy SA *et al.* Evidence for some prostaglandins in *Allium sativum* extracts. *Phytother Res* 1988: **2**: 196–197.

5 Ernst E. Cardiovascular effects of garlic (*Allium sativum*): a review. *Pharmatherapeutica* 1987; **5**: 83–89.

6 Lau BHS *et al. Allium sativum* (garlic) and atherosclerosis: a review. *Nutr Res* 1983; **3**: 119–128.

7 Adetumbi M, Lau BHS. *Allium sativum* (garlic) – a natural antibiotic. *Med Hypoth* 1983; **12**: 227–237.

8 Fulder S. Garlic and the prevention of cardiovascular disease. *Cardiol Pract* 1989; **7**: 30–35.

9 Pizzorno JE, Murray MT. *A Textbook of Natural Medicine*. Seattle, WA: John Bastyr College Publications, 1985 (looseleaf).

10 Hamon NW. Garlic and the genus *Allium*. *Can Pharm J* 1987; **120**: 493–498.

11 Fenwick GR, Hanley AB. The genus *Allium*. *CRC Crit Rev Food Sci Nutr* 1985; **22**: 199–376 and **23**: 1–73.

12 McElnay JC, Li Wan Po A. Garlic. *Pharm J* 1991; **246**: 324–326.

13 Reuter HD. *Allium sativum* and *Allium ursinum*: Part 2. Pharmacology and medicinal application. *Phytomedicine* 1995; **2**: 73–91.

14 Milner JA, Garlic: its anticarcinogenic and antitumorigenic properties. *Nutr Rev* 1996; **54**: S82–S86.

15 Lea MA. Organosulfur compounds and cancer. In: *American Institute for Cancer Research. Dietary Phytochemicals in Cancer Prevention and Treatment*. New York: Plenum Press, 1996.

16 Ali M *et al.* Garlic and onions: their effect on eicosanoid metabolism and its clinical relevance. *Prostaglandins Leukot Essent Fatty Acids* 2000; **62**: 55–73.

17 Yang CS *et al.* Mechanisms of inhibition of chemical toxicity and carcinogenesis by diallyl sulfide (DAS) and related compounds from garlic. *J Nutr* 2001; **131**(Suppl.3): S1041–S1045.

18 Borek C. Antioxidant health effects of aged garlic extract. *J Nutr* 2001; **131**(Suppl.3): S1010–S1015.

19 Yeh Y-Y, Liu L. Cholesterol-lowering effect of garlic extracts and organosulfur compounds: human and animal studies. *J Nutr* 2001; **131**(Suppl.3): S989–S993.

20 Le Bon A-M, Siess M-H. Organosulfur compounds

from *Allium* and the chemoprevention of cancer. *Drug Metab Drug Interact* 2001; **17**: 51–79.

21 Afzal M *et al*. Garlic and its medicinal potential. *Inflammopharmacology* 2000; **8**: 123–148.

22 Lachmann G *et al*. Untersuchungen zur Pharmakokinetik der mit 35S markierten Knoblauchinhaltsstoffe Alliin, Allicin und Vinyldithiine. *Arzneimittelforschung* 1994; **44**: 734–743.

23 Nagae S *et al*. Pharmacokinetics of the garlic compound *S*-allylcysteine. *Planta Med* 1994; **60**: 214–217.

24 Qureshi AA *et al*. Inhibition of cholesterol and fatty acid biosynthesis in liver enzymes and chicken hepatocytes by polar fractions of garlic. *Lipids* 1983; **18**: 343–348.

25 Gebhardt R. Multiple inhibitory effects of garlic extracts on cholesterol biosynthesis in hepatocytes. *Lipds* 1993; **28**: 613–619.

26 Gebhardt R *et al*. Inhibition of cholesterol biosynthesis by allicin and ajoene in rat hepatocytes and Hep G2 cells. *Biochim Biophys Acta* 1994; **1213**: 57–62.

27 Gebhardt R. Amplification of palmitate-induced inhibition of cholesterol biosynthesis in cultured rat hepatocytes by garlic-derived organosulfur compounds. *Phytomedicine* 1995; **2**: 29–34.

28 Gebhardt R, Beck H. Differential inhibitory effects of garlic-derived organosulfur compounds on cholesterol biosynthesis in primary rat hepatocytes. *Lipids* 1996; **31**: 1269–1276.

29 Yeh Y-Y, Yeh S-M. Garlic reduces plasma lipids by inhibiting hepatic cholesterol and triacylglycerol synthesis. *Lipids* 1994; **29**: 189–193.

30 Liu L, Yeh Y-Y. Water-soluble organosulfur compounds of garlic inhibit fatty acid and triglyceride synthesis in cultured rat hepatocytes. *Lipids* 2001; **36**: 395–400.

31 Adoga GI. The mechanism of the hypolipidemic effect of garlic oil extract in rats fed on high sucrose and alcohol diets. *Biochem Biophys Res Commun* 1987; **142**: 1046–1052.

32 Gupta N, Porter TD. Garlic and garlic-derived compounds inhibit human squalene monooxygenase. *J Nutr* 2001; **131**: 1662–1667.

33 Kamanna VS, Chandrasekhara N. Effect of garlic (*Allium sativum* Linn.) on serum lipoproteins and lipoprotein cholesterol levels in Albino rats rendered hypercholesterolemic by feeding cholesterol. *Lipids* 1982; **17**: 483–488.

34 Campbell JH *et al*. Molecular basis by which garlic suppesses atherosclerosis. *J Nutr* 2001; **131**(Suppl.3): S1006–S1009.

35 Abramowitz D. Allicin-induced decrease in formation of fatty streaks (atherosclerosis) in mice fed a cholesterol-rich diet. *Coronary Artery Dis* 1999; **10**: 515–519.

36 Boullin DJ. Garlic as a platelet inhibitor. *Lancet* 1981; i: 776–777.

37 Gaffen JD *et al*. The effect of garlic extracts on contractions of rat gastric fundus and human platelet aggregation. *J Pharm Pharmacol* 1984; **36**: 272–274.

38 Srivastava KC, Winslows JB. Evidence for the mechanism by which garlic inhibits platelet aggregation. *Prostaglandins Leukot Med* 1986; **22**: 313–321.

39 Apitz-Castro A *et al*. Effects of garlic extract and of three pure components isolated from it on human platelet aggregation, arachidonate metabolism, release reaction and platelet ultrastructure. *Thromb Res* 1983; **32**: 155–169.

40 Wagner H *et al*. Effects of garlic constituents on arachidonate metabolism. *Planta Med* 1987; **53**: 305–306.

41 Sharma CP, Nirmala NV. Effects of garlic extract and of three pure components isolated from it on human platelet aggregation, arachidonate metabolism, release reaction and platelet ultrastructure – comments. *Thromb Res* 1985; **37**: 489–490.

42 Mohammad SF, Woodward SC. Characterization of a potent inhibitor of platelet aggregation and release reaction isolated from *Allium sativum* (garlic). *Thromb Res* 1986; **44**: 793–806.

43 Symposium on the chemistry, pharmacology and medicinal applications of garlic. *Cardiol Pract* 1989; **7**: 1–15.

44 Srivastava KC, Tyagi OD. Effects of a garlic-derived principle (ajoene) on aggregation and arachidonic acid metabolism in human blood platelets. *Prostaglandins Leukot Essent Fatty Acids* 1993; **49**: 587–595.

45 Jamaluddin MP *et al*. Ajoene inhibition of platelet aggregation: possible mediation by a hemoprotein. *Biochem Biophys Res Commun* 1988; **153**: 479–486.

46 Block E *et al*. Antithrombotic organosulfur compounds from garlic: structural, mechanistic, and synthetic studies. *J Am Chem Soc* 1986; **108**: 7045–7055.

47 Rendu F *et al*. Ajoene, the antiplatelet compound derived from garlic, specifically inhibits platelet release reaction by affecting the plasma membrane internal microviscosity. *Biochem Pharmacol* 1989; **38**: 1321–1328.

48 Apitz-Castro R *et al*. Ajoene. The antiplatelet principle of garlic, synergistically potentiates the antiaggregatory action of prostacyclin, forskolin, indomethacin and dypiridamole on human platelets. *Thromb Res* 1986; **42**: 303–311.

49 Siegers C-P *et al*. Effects of garlic preparations on superoxide production by phorbol ester activated granulocytes. *Phytomedicine* 1999; **6**: 13–16.

50 Ide N, Lau BHS. Garlic compounds protect vascular endothelial cells from oxidised low

density lipoprotein-induced injury. *J Pharm Pharmacol* 1997; **49**: 908–911.

51 Ide N, Lau BHS. Aged garlic extract attentuates intracellular oxidative stress. *Phytomedicine* 1999; **6**: 125–131.

52 Rashid A, Khan HH. The mechanism of hypotensive effect of garlic extract. *J Pak Med Ass* 1974; **35**: 357–362.

53 Jacob J *et al*. Antihypertensive und Kardioprotektive Effekte von Knoblaucherpulver (*Allium sativum*). *Med Welt* 1991; **42**: 39–41.

54 Kiviranta J *et al*. Effects of onion and garlic extracts on spontaneously hypertensive rats. *Phytother Res* 1989; **3**: 132–135.

55 Kyo E *et al*. Immunomodulation and antitumour activities of aged garlic extract. *Phytomedicine* 1998; **5**: 259–267.

56 Schaffer EM *et al*. Garlic and associated allyl sulfur components inhibit *N*-methyl-*N*-nitrosourea induced rat mammary carcinogenesis. *Cancer Lett* 1996; **102**: 199–204.

57 Balasenthil S *et al*. Prevention of 4-nitroquinoline-1-oxide-induced rat tongue carcinogenesis by garlic. *Fitoterapia* 2001; **72**: 524–531.

58 Sparnins VL *et al*. Effects of organosulfur compounds from garlic and onions on benzo[*a*]pyrene-induced neoplasia and glutathione S-transferase activity in the mouse. *Carcinogenesis* 1988; **9**: 131–134.

59 Siegers C-P *et al*. The effects of garlic preparations against human tumor cell proliferation. *Phytomedicine* 1999; **6**: 7–11.

60 Nakagawa H *et al*. Growth inhibitory effects of diallyl disulphide on human breast cancer cell lines. *Carcinogenesis* 2001; **22**: 891–897.

61 Liu JZ *et al*. Inhibition of 7,12-dimethylbenz(a)anthracene induced mammary tumours and DNA adducts by garlic powder. *Carcinogenesis* 1992; **13**: 1847–1851.

62 Lin X-Y *et al*. Dietary garlic suppresses DNA adducts caused by *N*-nitroso compounds. *Carcinogenesis* 1994; **15**: 349–352.

63 Fujita K-I, Kamataki T. Screening of organosulfur compounds as inhibitors of human CYP2A6. *Drug Metab Disposition* 2001; **29**: 983–989.

64 Guyonnet D *et al*. Antimutagenic activity of organosulfur compounds from Allium is associated with phase II enzyme induction. *Mutat Res Genet Toxicol Environ Mutagen* 2001; **495**: 135–145.

65 Moon D-G *et al*. *Allium sativum* potentiates suicide gene therapy for murine transitional cell carcinoma. *Nutr Cancer* 2000; **38**: 98–105.

66 Hirao Y *et al*. Activation of immunoresponder cells by the protein fraction from aged garlic extract. *Phytother Res* 1987; **1**: 161–164.

67 Lamm DL, Riggs DR. Enhanced immunocompetence by garlic: role in bladder cancer and other malignancies. *J Nutr* 2001; **131**(Suppl.3): S1067–S1070.

68 Burger RA *et al*. Enhancement of *in vitro* human immune function by *Allium sativum* L. (garlic) fractions. *Int J Pharmacog* 1993; **31**: 169–174.

69 Kyo E *et al*. Immunomodulatory effects of aged garlic extract. *J Nutr* 2001; **131**(Suppl.3): S1075–S1079.

70 Ahsan M, Islam SN. Garlic: a broad spectrum antibacterial agent effective against common pathogenic bacteria. *Fitoterapia* 1996; **67**: 374–376.

71 Tsao S-M, Yin M-C. *In vitro* activity of garlic oil and four diallyl sulphides against antibiotic-resistant *Pseudomonas aeruginosa* and *Klebsiella pneumoniae*. *J Antimicrob Chemother* 2001; **47**: 665–670.

72 Tsao S-M, Yin M-C. *In vitro* antimicrobial activity of four diallyl sulphides occurring naturally in garlic and Chinese leek oils. *J Med Microbiol* 2001; **50**: 646–649.

73 Delaha ED, Garagusi VF. Inhibition of mycobacteria by garlic extract (*Allium sativum*). *Antimicrob Agents Chemother* 1985; **27**: 485–486.

74 Deshpande RG *et al*. Inhibition of *Mycobacterium avium* complex isolates from AIDS patients by garlic (*Allium sativum*). *J Antimicrob Chemother* 1993; **32**: 623–626.

75 Cellini L *et al*. Inhibition of *Helicobacter pylori* by garlic extract (*Allium sativum*). *FEMS Immunol Med Microbiol* 1996; **13**: 273–277.

76 Chung JG *et al*. Effects of garlic compounds diallyl sulfide and diallyl disulfide on arylamine N-acetyltransferase activity in strains of *Helicobacter pylori* from peptic ulcer patients. *Am J Chin Med* 1998; **26**: 353–364.

77 Feldberg RS *et al*. In vitro mechanism of inhibition of bacterial cell growth by allicin. *Antimicrob Agents Chemother* 1988; **32**: 1763–1768.

78 Adetumbi M *et al*. *Allium sativum* (garlic) inhibits lipid synthesis by *Candida albicans*. *Antimicrob Agents Chemother* 1986; **30**: 499–501.

79 Graham HD, Graham EJF. Inhibition of *Aspergillus parasiticus* growth and toxin production by garlic. *J Food Safety* 1987; **8**: 101–108.

80 Ankri S *et al*. Allicin from garlic strongly inhibits cysteine proteinases and cytopathic effects of *Entamoeba histolytica*. *Antimicrob Agents Chemother* 1997; **41**: 2286–2288.

81 Harris JC *et al*. The microaerophilic flagellate *Giardia intestinalis*: *Allium sativum* (garlic) is an effective antigiardial. *Microbiology* 2000; **146**: 3119–3127.

82 Hughes BG *et al*. Antiviral constituents from *Allium sativum*. *Planta Med* 1989; **55**: 114.

83 Tsai Y *et al*. Antiviral properties of garlic: *In vitro*

effects on influenza B, Herpes simplex and Coxsackie viruses. *Planta Med* 1985; **51**: 460–461.

84 Joshi DJ *et al*. Gastrointestinal actions of garlic oil. *Phytother Res* 1987; **1**: 140–141.

85 Hikino H *et al*. Antihepatotoxic actions of *Allium sativum* bulbs. *Planta Med* 1986; **52**: 163–168.

86 Nakagawa S *et al*. Prevention of liver damage by aged garlic extract and its components in mice. *Phytother Res* 1989; **3**: 50–53.

87 Sheen L-Y *et al*. Effect of diallyl sulfide and diallyl disulfide, the active principles of garlic, on the aflatoxin B_1-induced DNA damage in primary rat hepatocytes. *Toxicol Lett* 2001; **122**: 45–52.

88 Saxena KK *et al*. Effect of garlic pretreatment on isoprenaline-induced myocardial necrosis in albino rats. *Indian J Physiol Pharmacol* 1980; **24**: 233–236.

89 Senapati SK *et al*. Effect of garlic (*Allium sativum* L.) extract on tissue lead level in rats. *J Ethnopharmacol* 2001; **76**: 229–232.

90 Horie T *et al*. Alleviation by garlic of antitumor drug-induced damage to the intestine. *J Nutr* 2001; **131**(Suppl.3): S1071–S1074.

91 Nishiyama N *et al*. Ameliorative effect of S-allylcysteine, a major thioallyl constituent in aged garlic extract, on learning deficits in senescence-accelerated mice. *J Nutr* 2001; **131**(Suppl.3): S1093–S1095.

92 Brahmachari HD, Augusti KT. Orally effective hypoglycaemic agents from plants. *J Pharm Pharmacol* 1962; **14**: 254–255.

93 Dirsch VM, Vollmar AM. Ajoene, a natural product with non-steroidal anti-inflammatory drug (NSAID)-like properties?. *Biochem Pharmacol* 2001; **61**: 587–593.

94 Koch HP. Metabolismus und pharmakokinetik der Inhaltsstoffe des Knoblauchs: was Wissen wir darüber?. *Z Phytother* 1992; **13**: 83–90.

95 Jandke J, Spiteller G. Unusual conjugates in biological profiles originating from consumption of onions and garlic. *J Chromatog* 1987; **421**: 1–8.

96 De Rooij BM *et al*. Urinary excretion of *N*-acetyl-*S*-allyl-L-cysteine upon garlic consumption by human volunteers. *Arch Toxicol* 1996; **70**: 635–639.

97 Mennella JA, Beauchamp GK. Maternal diet alters the sensory qualities of human milk and the nursling's behavior. *Pediatrics* 1991; **88**: 737–744.

98 Mennella JA *et al* Garlic ingestion by pregnant women alters the odor of amniotic fluid. *Chem Senses* 1995; **20**: 207–209.

99 Bordia A *et al*. Effect of garlic (*Allium sativum*) on blood lipids, blood sugar, fibrinogen and fibrinolytic activity in patients with coronary artery disease. *Prostaglandins Leukot Essent Fatty Acids* 1998; **58**: 257–263.

100 Steiner M, Lin RS. Changes in platelet function and susceptibility of lipoproteins to oxidation associated with administration of aged garlic extract. *J Cardiovasc Pharmacol* 1998; **31**: 904–908.

101 Warrshafsky S *et al*. Effect of garlic on total serum cholesterol. A meta-analysis. *Ann Intern Med* 1993; **119**: 599–605.

102 Silagy C, Neil A. Garlic as a lipid lowering agent – a meta-analysis. *J R Coll Phys Lond* 1994; **28**: 2–8.

103 Neil HAW *et al*. Garlic powder in the treatment of moderate hyperlipidaemia: a controlled trial and meta-analysis. *J R Coll Phys Lond* 1996; **30**: 329–334.

104 Stevinson C *et al*. Garlic for treating hypercholesterolaemia. A meta-analysis of randomized clinical trials. *Ann Intern Med* 2000; **133**: 420–429.

105 Berthold HK *et al*. Effect of a garlic oil preparation on serum lipoproteins and cholesterol metabolism. A randomized controlled trial. *JAMA* 1998; **279**: 1900–1902.

106 Issacsohn JL *et al*. Garlic powder and plasma lipids and lipoproteins. A multicenter, randomized, placebo-controlled trial. *Arch Intern Med* 1998; **158**: 1189–1194.

107 Adler AJ, Holub BJ. Effect of garlic and fish-oil supplementation on serum lipid and lipoprotein concentrations in hypercholesterolaemic men. *Am J Clin Nutr* 1997; **65**: 445–450.

108 Gardner CD *et al*. The effect of a garlic preparation on plasma lipid levels in moderately hypercholesterolaemic adults. *Atherosclerosis* 2001; **154**: 213–220.

109 Lawson LD. Effect of garlic on serum lipids. *JAMA* 1998; **280**: 1568.

110 Ackermann RT *et al*. Garlic shows promise for improving some cardiovascular risk factors. *Arch Intern Med* 2001; **161**: 813–824.

111 Koscielny J *et al*. The anti-atherosclerotic effect of *Allium sativum*. *Atherosclerosis* 1999; **144**: 237–249.

112 Jepson RG *et al* Garlic for peripheral arterial occlusive disease (Cochrane review). In: *The Cochrane Library*, Issue 3, 2001. Oxford: Update Software.

113 Breithaupt-Grögler K *et al*. Protective effect of chronic garlic intake on elastic properties of aorta in the elderly. *Circulation* 1997; **96**: 2649–2655.

114 Ali M, Thomson M. Consumption of a garlic clove a day could be beneficial in preventing thrombosis. *Prostaglandins Leukot Essent Fatty Acids* 1995; **53**: 211–212.

115 Byrne DJ *et al*. A pilot study of garlic consumption shows no significant effect on markers of oxidation or sub-fraction composition of low-density lipoprotein including lipoprotein(a) after

allowance for non-compliance and the placebo effect. *Clin Chim Acta* 1999; **285**: 21–33.

116 Orekhov AN *et al.* Garlic powder tablets reduce atherogenicity of low density lipoprotein. A placebo-controlled double-blind study. *Nutr Metab Cardiovasc Dis* 1996; **6**: 21–31.

117 Grune T *et al.* Influence of *Allium sativum* on oxidative stress status – a clinical investigation. *Phytomedicine* 1996; **2**: 205–207.

118 Silagy CA, Neil HAW. A meta-analysis of the effect of garlic on blood pressure. *J Hypertens* 1994; **12**: 463–468.

119 Ernst E. Can *Allium* vegetables prevent cancer?. *Phytomedicine* 1997; **4**: 79–83.

120 You W-C *et al.* *Helicobacter pylori* infection, garlic intake and precancerous lesions in a Chinese population at low risk of gastric cancer. *Int J Epidemiol* 1998; **27**: 941–944.

121 Ledezma E *et al.* Efficacy of ajoene, an organosulphur compound from garlic, in the short-term therapy of tinea pedis. *Mycoses* 1996; **39**: 393–395.

122 Stjernberg L, Berglund J. Garlic as an insect repellant. *JAMA* 2000; **284**: 831.

123 Abrams GA, Fallon MB. Treatment of hepatopulmonary syndrome with *Allium sativum* L. (Garlic): a pilot trial. *J Clin Gastroenterol* 1998; **27**: 232–235.

124 Nakagawa S *et al.* Acute toxicity test of garlic extract. *J Toxicol Sci* 1984; **9**: 57–60.

125 Papageorgiou C *et al.* Allergic contact dermatitis to garlic (*Allium sativum* L.) Identification of the allergens: The role of mono-, di-, and trisulfides present in garlic. *Arch Dermatol Res* 1983; **275**: 229–234.

126 Lautier R, Wendt V. Contact allergy to Alliaceae/ case-report and literature survey. *Dermatosen* 1985; **33**: 213–215.

127 Asero R *et al.* A case of garlic allergy. *J Allergy Clin Immunol* 1998; **101**: 427–428.

128 Hallel-Halevy D *et al.* Multifaceted dermatitis caused by garlic. *J Eur Acad Dermatol Venereol* 1997; **9**: 185–187.

129 Farrell AM, Staughton RCD. Garlic burns mimicking herpes zoster. *Lancet* 1996; **347**: 1195.

130 Rafaat M, Leung AKC. Garlic burns. *Pediatr Dermatol* 2000; **17**: 475–476.

131 Sunter W. Warfarin and garlic. *Pharm J* 1991; **246**: 722.

132 Stockley IH. *Drug Interactions*, 5th edn. London: Pharmaceutical Press, 1999.

133 Ruffin J, Hunter SA. An evaluation of the side effects of garlic as an antihypertensive agent. *Cytobios* 1983; **37**: 85–89.

134 Sumiyoshi H *et al.* Chronic toxicity test of garlic extract in rats. *J Toxicol Sci* 1984; **9**: 61–75.

135 Yoshida S *et al.* Mutagenicity and cytotoxicity tests of garlic. *J Toxicol Sci* 1984; **9**: 77–86.

136 Abraham SK, Kesavan PC. Genotoxicity of garlic, turmeric and asafoetida in mice. *Mutat Res* 1984; **136**: 85–88.

137 Mennella JA, Beauchamp GK. The effects of repeated exposure to garlic-flavoured milk on the nursling's behavior. *Pediatr Res* 1993; **34**: 805–808.

Gentian

Species (Family)

Gentiana lutea L. (Gentianaceae)

Synonym(s)

Bitter Root, Gentiana, Yellow Gentian

Part(s) Used

Rhizome, root

Pharmacopoeial and Other Monographs

BHC 1992[G6]
BHP 1996[G9]
BP 2001[G15]
Complete German Commission E[G3]
ESCOP 1997[G52]
Martindale 32nd edition[G43]
PDR for Herbal Medicines 2nd edition[G36]
Ph Eur 2002[G28]

Legal Category (Licensed Products)

GSL[G37]

Constituents[G2,G6,G22,G41,G60,G62,G64]

Alkaloids Pyridine-type. Gentianine 0.6–0.8%, gentialutine.

Bitters Major component is secoiridoid glycoside gentiopicroside (also known as gentiamarin and gentiopicrin) 2%, with lesser amounts of amarogentin (0.01–0.04%) and swertiamarine.[1] Gentianose (a trisaccharide bitter principle). The glycosides amaropanin and amaroswerin are reported to be present in the related species *Gentiana pannonica*, *Gentiana punctata* and *Gentiana purpurea*, but are absent from *Gentiana lutea*.

Xanthones Gentisein, gentisin (gentianin), isogentisin and 1,3,7-trimethoxyxanthone.

Other constituents Carbohydrates (e.g. gentiobiose, sucrose and other common sugars), pectin, tannin (unspecified), triterpenes (e.g. β-amyrin, lupeol) and volatile oil (trace).

Food Use

Gentian (root, herbs and preparations) is listed by the Council of Europe as a natural source of food flavouring (category 4, with limits on xanthones) (*see* Appendix 23).[G17] In the USA, gentian is approved for food use.[G41]

Herbal Use[G2,G4,G6,G8,G32,G43,G52,G54,G56,G60,G64]

Gentian is stated to possess bitter, gastric stimulant, sialogogue and cholagogue properties. Traditionally, it has been used for anorexia, atonic dyspepsia, gastrointestinal atony, and specifically for dyspepsia with anorexia. The German Commission E approved use for digestive disorders such as loss of appetite, fullness and flatulence.[G3] Gentian is used in combination with angelica root and caraway fruit or with ginger and wormwood for loss of appetite and peptic discomfort.[G3]

Dosage

Dried rhizome/root 0.6–2 g or by infusion or decoction three times daily.[G6]

Tincture 1–4 mL (1 : 5 in 45% alcohol) three times daily.[G6]

Pharmacological Actions

In vitro and animal studies

The pharmacological activites of gentian root have been reviewed.[G52] A summary of this information is provided below.

Root extracts have antifungal activity, and are reported to stimulate phagocytic activity of human lymphocytes, indicating immunostimulant activity.[G52] Choleretic properties have been documented for gentian,[G41] and gentianine has been reported to possess anti-inflammatory activity.[G22] The bitter principles stimulate secretion of gastric juices and bile, thus aiding appetite and digestion. Elevation of gastric secretion by up to 30% has been reported following the administration of gentian tincture to dogs. An infusion given orally to sheep as a single daily dose (5 g) stimulated enzyme secretion in the small intestine. A root extract (12 mg/kg/day) applied by gavage to rats for three days elevated bronchosecretion. A standardised extract perfused into the stomachs of anaesthetised rats increased gastric secretion in a dose-dependent manner. Lower doses caused no changes in gastric pH, whereas higher doses increased pH from 4.25 to 4.85. A dose of 0.5 mL/kg did not affect the incidence of gastric ulceration in rats.

Clinical studies

In an open, uncontrolled study, a single dose of an alcoholic extract of gentian (equivalent to 0.2 g), given to 10 healthy volunteers, was reported to result in a stimulation of gastric juice secretion.[2] Gall-bladder emptying was increased and prolonged whilst protein and fat digestion was enhanced. Nineteen patients with inflammatory conditions of the gastrointestinal tract (colitis, Crohn's disease, nonspecific inflammation) and elevated secretory immunoglobulin A (IgA) concentrations and eight healthy individuals were treated with gentian tincture (3 × 20 drops/day) for eight days.[G52] IgA concentrations decreased in both groups.[G52]

Side-effects, Toxicity

Extracts of gentian are considered to be non-toxic, and are generally well-tolerated.[G52]

An acute oral LD_{50} value in mice was reported to be 25 mL/kg of extract (37% ethanol, bitterness value: 200 Swiss Pharmacopoeia units/g), and was the same as that of 37% ethanol. Rabbits treated with gentian extract (12.6 mg/day for three days) showed no toxic or abnormal concentration of serum parameters, with the exception of slightly higher erythrocyte concentrations in treated animals. Gentian may occasionally cause headache in some individuals.[G3] Mutagenic activity in the Ames test (*Salmonella typhimurium* TA100 with S9 mix) has been documented for gentian, with gentisin and isogentisin identified as mutagenic components.[3] Gentian root 100 g was reported to yield approximately 100 mg total mutagenic compounds, of which gentisin and isogentisin comprised approximately 76 mg.[3]

Contra-indications, Warnings

Gentian is stated to be contra-indicated in individuals with high blood pressure,[G60] although no rationale is given for this statement, and in individuals with hyperacidity, gastric or duodenal ulcers.[G52,G3].

Pregnancy and lactation Gentian is reputed to affect the menstrual cycle,[G22,G60] and it has been stated that gentian should not be used in pregnancy.[G60] In view of this and the documented mutagenic activity, gentian is best avoided in pregnancy and lactation.

Pharmaceutical Comment

The major constituents of pharmacological importance in gentian are the bitter principles; limited information is available on the other compounds present. The herbal uses of gentian are supported by the known properties of the bitter principles present in the root. Excessive doses should be avoided in view of the lack of toxicity data.

References

See also General References G2, G3, G6, G9, G12, G13, G15, G16, G22, G24, G25, G29, G31, G32, G36, G37, G41, G43, G52, G54, G56, G60, G62 and G64.

1　Verotta L. Isolation and HPLC determination of the active principles of *Rosmarinus officinalis* and *Gentiana lutea*. *Fitoterapia* 1985; **56**: 25–29.
2　Glatzel vonH, Hackenberg K. Röntgenologische untersuchungen der wirkungen von bittermitteln auf die verdauunogsorgane. *Planta Med* 1967; **15**: 223–232.
3　Morimoto I *et al.* Mutagenic activities of gentisin and isogentisin from Gentianae radix (Gentianaceae). *Mutat Res* 1983; **116**: 103–117.

Ginger

Species (Family)

Zingiber officinale Roscoe (Zingiberaceae)

Synonym(s)

Zingiber

Part(s) Used

Rhizome

Pharmacopoeial and Other Monographs

BHC 1992[G6]
BHP 1996[G9]
BP 2001[G15]
BPC 1973[G12]
ESCOP 1996[G52]
Martindale 32nd edition[G43]
Mills and Bone[G50]
PDR for Herbal Medicines 2nd edition[G36]
Ph Eur 2002[G28]
USP/NF19[G61]
WHO 1999 volume 1[G63]

Legal Category (Licensed Products)

GSL[G37]

Constituents[1,G2,G6,G37,G41,G64]

Carbohydrates Starch (major constituent, up to 50%).

Lipids 6–8%. Free fatty acids (e.g. palmitic acid, oleic acid, linoleic acid, caprylic acid, capric acid, lauric acid, myristic acid, pentadecanoic acid, heptadecanoic acid, stearic acid, linolenic acid, arachidic acid);[2] triglycerides, phosphatidic acid, lecithins; gingerglycolipids A, B and C.[3]

Oleo-resin Gingerol homologues (major, about 33%) including derivatives with a methyl side-chain,[4] shogaol homologues (dehydration products of gingerols), zingerone (degradation product of gingerols), 1-dehydrogingerdione,[5] 6-gingesulfonic acid[3] and volatile oils.

Volatile oils 1–3%. Complex, predominately hydrocarbons. β-Bisabolene and zingiberene (major); other sesquiterpenes include zingiberol, zingiberenol, *ar*-curcumene, β-sesquiphellandrene, β-sesquiphellandrol (*cis* and *trans*); numerous monoterpene hydrocarbons, alcohols and aldehydes (e.g. phellandrene, camphene, geraniol, neral, linalool, *d*-nerol).

Other constituents Amino acids (e.g. arginine, aspartic acid, cysteine, glycine, isoleucine, leucine, serine, threonine and valine), protein (about 9%), resins, diterpenes (galanolactone[6]), vitamins (especially nicotinic acid (niacin) and vitamin A), minerals.[2]

The material contains not less than 4.5% of alcohol (90%)-soluble extractive and not less than 10% of water-soluble extractive.[G15]

Food Use

Ginger is listed by the Council of Europe as a natural source of food flavouring (category N2). This category indicates that ginger can be added to foodstuffs in small quantities, with a possible limitation of an active principle (as yet unspecified) in the final product.[G16] It is used widely in foods as a spice. In the USA, ginger is listed as GRAS (Generally Recognised As Safe).[G41]

Herbal Use

Ginger is stated to possess carminative, diaphoretic and antispasmodic properties. Traditionally, it has been used for colic, flatulent dyspepsia, and specifically for flatulent intestinal colic.[7,G2,G6–G8,G32,G64] Modern interest in ginger is focused on its use in the prevention of nausea and vomiting, particularly motion (travel) sickness, as a digestive aid, and as an adjunctive treatment for inflammatory conditions, such as osteoarthritis and rheumatoid arthritis.

Dosage

Anti-emetic

Powdered rhizome Single dose of 1–2 g,[G6] 30 minutes before travel for prevention of motion sickness,[G52] or 0.5 g, two to four times daily.[G63]

Other uses

Powdered rhizome 0.25–1 g, three times daily.[G6]

Tincture 1.5–3 mL (1 : 5) three times daily,[G6] 1.7–5 mL daily.[G50]

Pharmacological Actions

Several pharmacological activities, including anti-emetic, antithrombotic, antimicrobial, anticancer, antioxidant and anti-inflammatory properties, have been documented for preparations of ginger in *in vitro* and/or animal studies. Also, ginger has been reported to have hypoglycaemic, hypo- and hypertensive, cardiac, prostaglandin and platelet aggregation inhibition, antihypercholesterolaemic, cholagogic and stomachic properties.

Clinical studies have focused mainly on the effects of ginger in the prevention of nausea and vomiting.

In vitro and animal studies

In vitro studies have demonstrated that constituents of ginger, such as 6-, 8- and 10-gingerols and gala-nolactone, have antiserotonergic activity.[6,8]

Anti-emetic activity and effects on gastrointestinal motility The older literature contains examples of studies documenting the antiemetic effects of ginger extract *in vivo* (e.g. dogs).[9] Oral administration of constituents of ginger (certain shogaols and gingerols at doses of 100 mg/kg body weight) inhibited emesis induced by oral administration of copper sulfate in leopard and ranid frogs.[10] Emetic latency was reported to be prolonged by over 150% by a trichloromethane extract of ginger at a dose of 1 g/kg body weight.

The anti-emetic activity of ginger extracts has also been assessed in dogs.[11] Acetone and ethanolic extracts of ginger, administered intragastrically at doses of 25, 50, 100 and 200 mg/kg, protected against cisplatin-induced emesis (3 mg/kg administered intravenously 30 minutes before ginger extract), compared with control. However, ginger extracts were less effective in preventing emesis than the 5-HT$_3$ receptor antagonist granisetron, and were ineffective against apomorphine-induced emesis.

Compared with control, an acetone extract of ginger at doses of 200 and 500 mg/kg administered orally reversed the delay in gastric emptying induced by intraperitoneal cisplatin 10 mg/kg in rats.[12] Ginger juice (2 and 4 mL/kg) had a similar effect. A 50% ethanolic extract of ginger also reversed the cisplatin-induced delay in gastric emptying, although only at a dose of 500 mg/kg. In mice, oral administration of an acetone extract of ginger (75 mg/kg), 6-shogaol (2.5 mg/kg) and 6-, 8- and 10-gingerol (5 mg/kg) enhanced the transportation of a charcoal meal, indicating enhancement of gastrointestinal motility.[13]

Anti-ulcer activity The effect of ginger (acetone extract) and zingiberene on hydrochloric acid/ethanol-induced gastric lesions in rats has been examined.[14] (6)-Gingerol and zingiberene, both 100 mg/kg body weight by mouth, significantly inhibited gastric lesions by 54.5% and 53.6%, respectively. The total extract inhibited lesions by 97.5% at 1 g/kg. Oral administration of both aqueous and methanol ginger extracts to rabbits has been reported to reduce gastric secretions (gastric juice volume, acid and pepsin output).[15] Both extracts were found to be comparable with cimetidine (50 mg/kg) with respect to gastric juice volume; the aqueous extract was comparable with cimetidine and superior to the methanol extract for pepsin output, and the methanol extract superior to both the aqueous extract and comparable to cimetidine for acid output. In rats, 6-gingerol, 6-shogaol and 6-gingesulfonic acid at doses of 150 mg/kg protected against hydrochloric acid/ethanol-induced gastric lesions, compared with control.[3] 6-Gingesulfonic acid 300 mg/kg provided almost 100% protection against gastric lesions in this model. Other studies in rats found that oral administration of an ethanolic extract of ginger (500 mg/kg) inhibited gastric lesions induced by ethanol (80%), hydrochloric acid (0.6 mol/L), sodium hydroxide (0.2 mol/L), and 25% sodium chloride, compared with control.[16] The same dose of extract protected against gastric mucosal damage induced by the non-steroidal anti-inflammatory drugs (NSAIDs) indometacin and aspirin in rats. In pylorus-ligated rats, oral administration of acetone and ethanol extracts of ginger inhibited gastric secretion.[17] These extracts, at doses of 62 mg/kg, also protected against the development of stress-induced lesions, although to a lesser extent than cimetidine.

Antiplatelet activity (6)-Gingerol, (6)- and (10)-dehydrogingerdione, (6)- and (10)-gingerdione have been reported to be potent inhibitors of prostaglandin biosynthesis (PG synthetase) *in vitro*, with the latter four compounds stated to be more potent than indometacin.[18] Dose-dependent inhibition of platelet aggregation, *in vitro*, induced by ADP, adrenaline, collagen and arachidonic acid has been described for an aqueous ginger extract.[19] Ginger was also found to reduce platelet synthesis of prostaglandin-endoperoxides, thromboxane and prostaglandins. A good correlation was reported between concentrations of the extract required to inhibit platelet aggregation and concentrations necessary to inhibit platelet thromboxane synthesis.[19]

Anti-atherosclerotic and antioxidant activity Ginger oleo-resin, by intragastric administration, has been reported to inhibit elevation in serum and hepatic cholesterol concentrations in rats by impairing cholesterol absorption.[20] Antihypercholesterolaemic activity has also been documented for dried ginger rhizome when given to both rats fed a cholesterol-rich diet and those with existing hypercholesterolaemia.[21] Fresh ginger juice was not found to have an effect on serum cholesterol concentrations within 4 hours of administration. In addition, serum cholesterol concentrations were not greatly increased within 4 hours of cholesterol administration.

An ethanol (50%) extract of ginger administered orally at a dose of 500 mg/kg to hyperlipidaemic rabbits led to a significant reduction in blood serum cholesterol concentrations, compared with those in control rabbits.[22] In a study in rabbits fed cholesterol for 10 weeks, administration of an ethanolic extract of ginger (200 mg/kg orally) decreased raised serum and tissue concentrations of cholesterol, serum triglycerides and serum lipoproteins.[23]

An ethanolic ginger extract, standardised to contain 40 mg/g gingerols, shogaols and zingerone, and 90 mg/g total polyphenols, was reported to inhibit low-density lipoprotein oxidation and to reduce the development of atherosclerosis in atherosclerotic mice, when compared with control.[24] In rats fed a high-fat diet for 10 weeks, an aqueous preparation of ginger powder administered orally at doses of 35 and 70 mg/kg demonstrated antioxidant activity, as measured by raised tissue concentrations of thiobarbituric acid reactive substances and hydroperoxides, and reduced activities of superoxide dismutase and catalase.[25]

The antioxidant activity of ginger constituents has been documented *in vitro*.[26]

Anti-inflammatory activity Constituents of ginger have been shown to have anti-inflammatory activity *in vitro*. In a study in intact human airway epithelial cells (A549 cells), 8-paradol and 8-shogaol inhibited cyclooxygenase 2 (COX-2) enzyme activity in a concentration-dependent manner (IC_{50} values ranged from 1 to 25 µmol/L).[27] In other studies, an acetone extract of ginger inhibited inflammation of the chorioallantoic membrane of fertilised hen's eggs in a concentration-dependent manner.[28] In another assay, the extract exhibited anti-inflammatory properties by inhibiting the release of nitric oxide in a concentration-dependent manner.[28] Ginger oil has demonstrated anti-inflammatory activity in a study in rats with severe chronic adjuvant arthritis induced by injection of 0.05 mL of a suspension of dead *Mycobacterium tuberculosis* bacilli.[29] Ginger oil 33 mg/kg administered orally for 26 days caused a significant suppression of paw and joint swelling, compared with control (no ginger oil).

Other studies documenting anti-inflammatory activity for ginger constituents have been summarised.[26]

Antimicrobial activity In vitro activity against rhinovirus IB has been reported for sesquiterpenes isolated from ginger rhizomes.[1] The most active compound was β-sesquiphellandrene (IC_{50} 0.44 µmol/L). *In vitro* anthelmintic activity against *Ascaridia galli* Schrank has been documented for the volatile oil of *Zingiber purpureum* Roxb.[30] Activity exceeding that of piperazine citrate was exhibited by the oxygenated compounds fractionated from the volatile oil.

Anticancer activity Extracts of ginger or constituents of ginger have been shown to have cancer chemopreventive and cytotoxic or cytostatic activity *in vitro* and *in vivo* (animals). Application of an ethanolic extract of fresh ginger in a mouse skin tumorigenesis model (SENCAR mice) resulted in significant inhibition of 12-O-tetradecanoylphorbol-13-acetate (TPA)-induced induction of epidermal ornithine decarboxylase, cyclooxygenase and lipoxygenase activities in a concentration-dependent manner.[31] Preapplication of ginger extract also inhibited TPA-induced epidermal oedema and hyperplasia. Application of ginger extract 30 minutes before application of two tumour inducers to the skin of SENCAR mice protected against skin tumour incidence, compared with control. In another mouse model, topical application of 6-gingerol or 6-paradol before application of tumour inducers attenuated skin papillomagenesis.[32] Other studies documenting the cancer chemopreventive potential of ginger and its constituents have been summarised.[26]

In vitro, incubation of 6-gingerol with human promyelocytic leukaemia (HL-60) cells resulted in inhibitory effects on cell viability and DNA synthesis.[33] Microscopic examination of the incubated cells provided evidence of the induction of apoptosis by 6-gingerol.

Other activities In rats, the anxiolytic effects of pretreatment with a combination preparation of standardised extracts of ginger and *Ginkgo biloba* administered intragastrically at doses between 0.5

and 100 mg/kg were assessed in the elevated plus-maze test.[34] The combination was found to have an anxiolytic effect at lower doses, but appeared to have an anxiogenic effect at higher doses.

A hypoglycaemic effect in both non-diabetic and alloxan-induced diabetic rabbits and rats has been documented for fresh ginger juice administered orally. The effect was stated to be significant in the diabetic animals.[35]

The pharmacological actions of (6)-shogaol and capsaicin have been compared.[36] Both compounds caused rapid hypotension followed by a marked pressor response, bradycardia, and apnoea in rats after intravenous administration. The pressor response was thought to be a centrally acting mechanism. Contractile responses in isolated guinea-pig trachea with both compounds, and positive inotropic and chronotropic responses in isolated rat atria with (6)-shogaol were thought to involve the release of an unknown active substance from nerve endings.[36] A potent, positive inotropic action on isolated guinea-pig atria has been documented and gingerols were identified as the cardiotonic principles.[37]

A cholagogic action in rats has been described for an acetone extract of ginger administered intra-duodenally.[38] (6)-Gingerol and (10)-gingerol were reported to be the active components, the former more potent with a significant increase in bile secretion still apparent 4 hours after administration.

Utero-activity has been described for a phenolic compound isolated from *Zingiber cassumunar* Roxb.[39] The compound was found to exhibit a dose-related relaxant effect on the non-pregnant rat uterus *in situ*; the uterine response from pregnant rats was stated to vary with the stage of pregnancy, the post-implantation period being the most sensitive. The compound was thought to act by a similar mechanism to that of papaverine.[39]

Clinical studies

Clinical trials of ginger have focused mainly on its effects on the prevention and treatment of nausea and vomiting of various causes. Other clinical studies have assessed the effects of ginger preparations on gastrointestinal motility and on platelet function, and in vertigo and inflammatory conditions, such as osteoarthritis. Several of these studies are described below.

Nausea and vomiting and effects on gastrointestinal motility Ginger has been reported to be effective as a prophylactic against seasickness.[40,41] Ingestion of powdered ginger root 1 g was found to significantly reduce the tendency to vomit and experience cold

sweating in 40 naval cadets, compared with 39 cadets who received placebo.[40] Powdered ginger root 1.88 g has been reported to be superior to dimenhydrinate 100 mg in preventing the gastrointestinal symptoms of motion sickness induced by a rotating chair.[41] However, a second study reported ginger (500 mg powdered, 1 g powdered/fresh) to be ineffective in the prevention of motion sickness induced by a rotating chair.[42] The study concluded hyoscine 600 µg and dexamphetamine 10 mg to be the most effective combination, with dimenhydrinate 50 mg as the over-the-counter motion sickness medication of choice.[42]

A systematic review of 6 randomised controlled trials of ginger preparations included three trials involving patients with post-operative nausea and vomiting, and three further trials in patients with seasickness (motion sickness), morning sickness (emesis of pregnancy) and cancer chemotherapy-induced nausea (one trial in each condition).[43] Two of the three studies assessing the effects of ginger in post-operative nausea and vomiting found that ginger was more effective than placebo and as effective as metoclopramide in reducing nausea. However, when the data from the three studies were pooled, the difference between the ginger and placebo groups was statistically non-significant.[43]

A randomised, double-blind, crossover trial involving women with nausea of pregnancy assessed the effects of capsules of powdered ginger root 250 mg, or placebo, administered orally four times daily for four days.[44] It was reported that symptom relief was significantly greater during treatment with ginger than with placebo, and that significantly more women stated a preference for ginger treatment than for placebo (as later disclosed). A more recent randomised, double-blind trial involving 70 women with nausea and vomiting of pregnancy assessed the effectiveness of capsules of powdered fresh ginger root 250 mg four times daily, or placebo, for four days.[45] At the end of the study, ginger recipients had significantly lower scores for nausea and fewer vomiting episodes than did the placebo group.

Studies involving healthy volunteers have investigated the effects of ginger on gastric emptying as a possible mechanism for the anti-emetic effects of ginger. A randomised, double-blind, placebo-controlled, crossover trial involving 16 volunteers assessed the effects of capsules containing powdered ginger 1 g for one week, followed by a one-week washout period before crossing over to the opposite arm of the study.[46] Gastric emptying was measured using a paracetamol absorption technique by comparing the effects of ginger administration on mean and peak plasma paracetamol concentrations. The results indicated that the rate of absorption of oral paracetamol was not affected by simultaneous ingestion of ginger. Another randomised, double-blind, placebo-controlled trial involving 12 healthy volunteers assessed the effects of ginger rhizome extract on fasting and postprandial gastroduodenal motility.[47] The results of this study indicated that oral administration of ginger improved gastroduodenal motility in both the fasting state and after a test meal.

A randomised, double-blind, placebo-controlled, crossover trial involving eight healthy volunteers tested the effects of powdered ginger root 1 g on experimentally induced vertigo.[48] One hour after ginger or placebo administration, participants' vestibular system was stimulated by water irrigation of the left ear. It was reported that ginger significantly reduced vertigo, when compared with placebo

Other effects In a randomised, double-blind, placebo-controlled, crossover trial involving 75 patients with osteoarthritis of the knee or hip, the effects of capsules of ginger extract 170 mg three times daily were compared with those of ibuprofen 400 mg three times daily, or placebo, for three weeks with a one-week washout period between each treatment period.[49] At the end of the study, data for the 56 evaluable participants indicated that there was no strong evidence of an effect for ginger extract over that of placebo on parameters of pain.

A reduction in joint pain and improvement in joint movement in seven rheumatoid arthritis sufferers has been documented for ginger, with a dual inhibition of cyclooxygenase and lipoxygenase pathways reported as a suggested mechanism of action.[50,51] Patients took either fresh ginger in amounts ranging from 5 to 50 g or powdered ginger 0.1–1.0 g daily.

A placebo-controlled study assessed the effects of two doses of ginger powder (4 g daily for three months, and 10 g as a single dose) on platelet aggregation and fibrinolytic activity in patients with coronary artery disease (CAD).[52] The results indicated that long-term administration of ginger powder did not affect ADP- and epinephrine (adrenaline)-induced platelet aggregation and had no effects on fibrinolytic activity or fibrinogen concentrations, compared with placebo administration. By contrast, administration of a single dose of ginger powder to 10 patients with CAD produced a significant reduction in platelet aggregation, compared with placebo administration ($n = 10$ patients with CAD).

In a study involving seven women, oral raw ginger 5 g reduced thromboxane B_2 concentrations in serum collected after clotting,[50] thus indicating a reduction in eicosanoid synthesis (associated with platelet aggregation).

Side-effects, Toxicity

None documented for ginger. Ginger oil is stated to be non-irritating and non-sensitising although dermatitis may be precipitated in hypersensitive individuals. Phototoxicity is not considered to be of significance.[53] Ginger oil is stated to be of low toxicity[G58] with acute LD_{50} values (rat, by mouth; rabbit, dermal) reported to exceed 5 g/kg.[53]

Mutagenic activity has been documented for an ethanolic ginger extract, gingerol and shogaol in *Salmonella typhimurium* strains TA100 and TA1535 in the presence of metabolic activation (S9 mix) but not in TA98 or TA1538 with or without S9 mix.[54] Zingerone was found to be non-mutagenic in all four strains with or without S9 mix, and was reported to suppress mutagenic activity of gingerol and shogaol. Ginger juice has been reported to exhibit antimutagenic activity, whereas mutagenic activity has been described for (6)-gingerol in the presence of known chemical mutagens.[55] It was suggested that certain mutagens may activate the mutagenic activity of (6)-gingerol so that it is not suppressed by antimutagenic components present in the juice.[55]

Contra-indications, Warnings

Ginger has been reported to possess both cardiotonic and antiplatelet activity *in vitro* and hypoglycaemic activity in *in vivo* studies. Excessive doses may therefore interfere with existing cardiac, antidiabetic or anticoagulant therapy. An oleo-resin component, (6)-shogaol has been reported to affect blood pressure (initially decrease then increase) *in vivo*.

Pregnancy and lactation Ginger is reputed to be an abortifacient[G30] and uteroactivity has been documented for a related species. Doses of ginger that greatly exceed the amounts used in foods should not be taken during pregnancy or lactation.

Pharmaceutical Comment

The chemistry of ginger is well documented with respect to the oleo-resin and volatile oil. Oleo-resin components are considered to be the main active principles in ginger and documented pharmacological actions generally support the traditional uses. In addition, a number of other pharmacological activities have been documented, including hypoglycaemic, antihypercholesterolaemic, anti-ulcer and inhibition of prostaglandin synthesis, all of which require further investigation. The use of ginger as a prophylactic remedy against motion sickness is contentious. It seems likely that ginger may act by a local action on the gastro-intestinal tract, rather than by a centrally mediated mechanism.

References

See also General References G2, G3, G5, G6, G9, G12, G15, G16, G18, G21, G29, G31, G32, G36, G41, G43, G50, G52, G58, G61, G63 and G64.

1 Denyer CV *et al*. Isolation of antirhinoviral sesquiterpenes from ginger (*Zingiber officinale*). *J Nat Prod* 1994; **57**: 658–662.
2 Lawrence BM, Reynolds RJ. Major tropical spices – ginger (*Zingiber officinale* Rosc.). *Perf Flav* 1984; **9**: 1–40.
3 Yoshikawa M *et al*. 6-Gingesulfonic acid, a new anti-ulcer principle, and gingerglycolipids A, B and C, three new monoacyldigalactosylglycerols from Zingiberis rhizoma originating in Taiwan. *Chem Pharm Bull* 1992; **40**: 2239–2241.
4 Chen C-C *et al*. Chromatographic analyses of gingerol compounds in ginger (*Zingiber officinale* Roscoe) extracted by liquid carbon dioxide. *J Chromatogr* 1986; **360**: 163–174.
5 Charles R *et al*. New gingerdione from the rhizomes of *Zingiber officinale*. *Fitoterapia* 2000; **71**: 716–718.
6 Huang Q *et al*. Anti-5-hydroxytryptamine3 effect of galanolactone, diterpenoid isolated from ginger. *Chem Pharm Bull* 1991; **39**: 397–399.
7 Langner E *et al*. Ginger: history and use. *Adv Ther* 1998; **15**: 25–44.
8 Yamahara J *et al*. Active components of ginger exhibiting anti-serotonergic action. *Phytother Res* 1989; **3**: 70–71.
9 Chang H-M, But PP-H, eds. *Pharmacology and Applications of Chinese Materia Medica*, vol 1. Singapore: World Scientific Publishing, 1986: 366–369.
10 Kawai T *et al*. Anti-emetic principles of *Magnolia obovata* bark and *Zingiber officinale* rhizome. *Planta Med* 1994; **60**: 17–20.
11 Sharma SS *et al*. Antiemetic activity of ginger (*Zingiber officinale*) against cisplatin-induced emesis in dogs. *J Ethnopharmacol* 1997; **57**: 93–96.
12 Sharma SS, Gupta YK. Reversal of cisplatin-induced delay in gastric emptying in rats by ginger (*Zingiber officinale*). *J Ethnopharmacol* 1998; **62**: 49–55.
13 Yamahara J *et al*. Gastrointestinal motility enhancing effect of ginger and its active constituents. *Chem Pharm Bull* 1990; **38**: 430–431.
14 Yamahara J *et al*. The anti-ulcer effect in rats of ginger constituents. *J Ethnopharmacol* 1988; **23**:

299–304.
15 Sakai K *et al*. Effect of extracts of Zingiberaceae herbs on gastric secretion in rabbits. *Chem Pharm Bull* 1989; **37**: 215–217.
16 Al-Yahya MA *et al*. Gastroprotective activity of ginger *Zingiber officinale* Rosc., in albino rats. *Am J Chin Med* 1998; **17**: 51–56.
17 Sertie JAA *et al*. Preventive anti-ulcer activity of the rhizome extract of *Zingiber officinale*. *Fitoterapia* 1992; **63**: 55–59.
18 Kiuchi F *et al*. Inhibitors of prostaglandin biosynthesis from ginger. *Chem Pharm Bull* 1982; **30**: 754–757.
19 Srivastava KC. Effects of aqueous extracts of onion, garlic and ginger on platelet aggregation and metabolism of arachidonic acid in the blood vascular system: in vitro study. *Prostaglandins Leukot Med* 1984; **13**: 227–235.
20 Gujral S *et al*. Effect of ginger (*Zingiber officinale* Roscoe) oleorosin on serum and hepatic cholesterol levels in cholesterol fed rats. *Nutr Rep Int* 1974; **17**: 183–189.
21 Giri J *et al*. Effect of ginger on serum cholesterol levels. *Indian J Nutr Diet* 1984; **21**: 433–436.
22 Sharma I *et al*. Hypolipidaemic and antiatherosclerotic effects of *Zingiber officinale* in cholesterol fed rabbits. *Phytother Res* 1996; **10**: 517–518.
23 Bhandari U *et al*. The protective action of ethanolic ginger (*Zingiber officinale*) extract in cholesterol fed rabbits. *J Ethnopharmacol* 1998; **61**: 167–171.
24 Fuhrman B *et al*. Ginger extract consumption reduces plasma cholesterol, inhibits LDL oxidation and attenates development of atherosclerosis in atherosclerotic, apolipoprotein E-deficient mice. *J Nutr* 2000; **130**: 1124–1131.
25 Jeyakumar SM *et al*. Antioxidant activity of ginger (*Zingiber officinale* Rosc) in rats fed a high fat diet. *Med Sci Res* 1999; **27**: 341–344.
26 Surh Y-J *et al*. Chemoprotective properties of some pungent ingredients present in red pepper and ginger. *Mutat Res* 1998; **402**: 259–267.
27 Tjendraputra E *et al*. Effect of ginger constituents and synthetic analogues on cyclooxygenase-2 enzyme in intact cells. *Bioorg Chem* 2001; **29**: 156–163.
28 Schuhbaum H *et al*. Anti-inflammatory activity of *Zingiber officinale* extracts. *Pharm Pharmacol Lett* 2000; **2**: 82–85.
29 Sharma JN *et al*. Suppressive effects of eugenol and ginger oil on arthritic rats. *Pharmacology* 1994; **49**: 314–318.
30 Taroeno *et al*. Anthelmintic activities of some hydrocarbons and oxygenated compounds in the essential oil of *Zingiber purpureum*. *Planta Med* 1989; **55**: 105.
31 Katiyar SK *et al*. Inhibition of tumor promotion in SENCAR mouse skin by ethanol extract of

Zingiber officinale rhizome. *Cancer Res* 1996; **56**: 1023–1030.

32 Surh Y-J *et al*. Anti-tumor-promoting activities of selected pungent phenolic substances in ginger. *J Environ Pathol Toxicol Oncol* 1999; **18**: 131–139.

33 Lee E, Surh Y-J. Induction of apoptosis in HL-60 cells by pungent vanilloids, [6]-gingerol and [6]-paradol. *Cancer Lett* 1998; **134**: 163–168.

34 Hasenohrl RU *et al*. Anxiolytic-like effect of combined extracts of *Zingiber officinale* and *Ginkgo biloba* in the elevated plus-maze. *Pharmacol Biochem Behav* 1996; **53**: 271–275.

35 Sharma M, Shukla S. Hypoglycaemic effect of ginger. *J Res Ind Med Yoga Homoeopath* 1977; **12**: 127–130.

36 Suekawa M *et al*. Pharmacological studies on ginger. V. Pharmacological comparison between (6)-shogaol and capsaicin. *Folia Pharmac Jpn* 1986; **88**: 339–347.

37 Shoji N *et al*. Cardiotonic principles of ginger (*Zingiber officinale* Roscoe). *J Pharm Sci* 1982; **71**: 1174–1175.

38 Yamahara J *et al*. Cholagogic effect of ginger and its active constituents. *J Ethnopharmacol* 1985; **13**: 217–225.

39 Kanjanapothi D *et al*. A uterine relaxant compound from *Zingiber cassumunar*. *Planta Med* 1987; **53**: 329–332.

40 Grontved A *et al*. Ginger root against seasickness. A controlled trial on the open sea. *Acta Otolaryngol* 1988; **105**: 45–49.

41 Mowrey DB, Clayson DE. Motion sickness, ginger, and psychophysics. *Lancet* 1982; **i**: 655–657.

42 Wood CD *et al*. Comparison of efficacy of ginger with various antimotion sickness drugs. *Clin Res Pract Drug Reg Affairs* 1988; **6**: 129–136.

43 Ernst E, Pittler MH. Efficacy of ginger for nausea and vomiting. A systematic review of randomised clinical trials. *Br J Anaesthesia* 2000; **84**: 367–371.

44 Fischer-Rasmussen W *et al*. Ginger treatment of hyperemesis gravidarum. *Eur J Obs Gyn Reprod Biol* 1990; **38**: 19–24.

45 Vutyavanich T *et al*. Ginger for nausea and vomiting in pregnancy: randomised, double-masked, placebo-controlled trial. *Obstet Gynecol* 2001; **97**: 577–582.

46 Phillips S *et al*. *Zingiber officinale* does not affect gastric emptying rate. A randomised, placebo-controlled, crossover trial. *Anaesthesia* 1993; **48**: 393–395.

47 Micklefield GH *et al*. Effects of ginger on gastroduodenal motility. *Int J Clin Pharmacol Ther* 1999; **37**: 341–346.

48 Grontved A, Hentzer E. Vertigo-reducing effect of ginger root. A controlled clinical study. *ORL J Otorhinolaryngol* 1986; **48**: 282–286.

49 Bliddal H *et al*. A randomized, placebo-controlled, cross-over study of ginger extracts and ibuprofen in osteoarthritis. *Osteoarthritis Cartilage* 2000; **8**: 9–12.

50 Srivastava KC. Effect of onion and ginger consumption on platelet thromboxane production in humans. *Prostaglandins Leukot Essent Fatty Acids* 1989; **35**: 183–185.

51 Srivastava K *et al*. Ginger and rheumatic disorders. *Med Hypoth* 1989; **29**: 25–28

52 Bordia A *et al*. Effect of ginger (*Zingiber officinale* Rosc.) and fenugreek (*Trigonella foenumgraecum* L.) on blood lipids, blood sugar and platelet aggregation in patients with coronary artery disease. *Prostaglandins Leukot Essent Fatty Acids* 1997; **56**: 379–384.

53 Opdyke DLJ. Ginger oil. *Food Cosmet Toxicol* 1974; **12**: 901–902.

54 Nagabhushan M *et al*. Mutagenicity of ginergol and shogaol and antimutagenicity of zingerone in salmonella/microsome assay. *Cancer Lett* 1987; **36**: 221–233.

55 Nakamura H, Yamamoto T. Mutagen and antimutagen in ginger, *Zingiber officinale*. *Mutat Res* 1982; **103**: 119–126.

Ginkgo

Species (Family)

Ginkgo biloba L. (Ginkgoaceae)

Synonym(s)

Fossil Tree, Kew Tree, Maidenhair Tree

Part(s) Used

Leaf

Pharmacopoeial and Other Monographs

BHP 1996[G9]
Complete German Commission E[G3]
Martindale 32nd edition[G43]
Mills and Bone[G50]
PDR for Herbal Medicines 2nd edition[G36]
Ph Eur 2002[G28]
WHO volume 1 1999[G63]

Legal Category (Licensed Products)

Ginkgo is not included in the GSL.[G37]

Constituents[1,2,G64]

Leaf

Amino acids 6-Hydroxykynurenic acid (2-carboxy-4-one-6-hydroxyquinoline), a metabolite of tryptophan.[3–5]

Flavonoids Dimeric flavones (e.g. amentoflavone, bilobetin, ginkgetin, isoginkgetin, sciadopitysin);[6] flavonols (e.g. quercetin, kaempferol) and their glycosides[3,7] and coumaroyl esters.

Proanthocyanidins

Terpenoids Sesquiterpenes (e.g. bilobalide), diterpenes (e.g. ginkgolides A, B, C, J, M, which are unique cage molecules,[8,9,G48] and triterpenes (e.g. sterols).

Other constituents Benzoic acid, allergenic ginkgolic acids, 2-hexenal, polyprenols (e.g. di-*trans*-poly-*cis*-octadecaprenol), sugars, waxes,[1] a peptide.[10]

Seeds

Alkaloids Ginkgotoxin (4-O-methylpyridoxine).[11]

Amino acids

Cyanogenetic glycosides Allergenic ginkgolic acids. Ginkbilobin.[12]

Standardised extracts of *G. biloba* leaves are standardised on the content of ginkgo flavonoid glycosides (22–27%; determined as quercetin, kaempferol and isorhamnetin), and terpene lactones (5–7%; comprising around 2.8–3.4% ginkgolides A, B and C, and 2.6–3.2% bilobalide, and less than 5 ppm ginkgolic acids).[G3,G56]

Food Use

Ginkgo biloba is not used in foods.

Herbal Use

Ginkgo has a long history of medicinal use, dating back to 2800BC. Traditional Chinese medicine used the seeds (kernel/nuts) for therapeutic purposes. The seed is used in China as an antitussive, expectorant and anti-asthmatic, and in bladder inflammation.[1,11,G50] In China, the leaves of *Ginkgo biloba* were also used in asthma and in cardiovascular disorders,[1] although the leaves have little history of traditional use in the West. Today, standardised concentrated extracts of *G. biloba* leaves are marketed in several European countries, and are used in cognitive deficiency, intermittent claudication (generally resulting from peripheral arterial occlusive disease), and vertigo and tinnitus of vascular origin (*see* Pharmacological Actions, Clinical studies).[G3,G32,G56,G63]

Dosage

Cognitive deficiency

Leaf extract 120–240 mg dry extract orally in two or three divided doses.[G3]

Peripheral arterial occlusive disease and vertigo/tinnitus

Leaf extract   120–160 mg dry extract orally in two or three divided doses.[G3]

Clinical trials of standardised extracts of G. biloba leaves (EGb 761, Willmar Schwabe GmbH and LI 1370, Lichtwer Pharma GmbH) in patients with cognitive deficiency have generally used oral doses ranging from 120 to 240 mg daily, usually for 8–12 weeks, although some studies have continued treatment for up to 24 or 52 weeks.[G56] Clinical trials in peripheral arterial occlusive disease used oral doses of 120–160 mg extract daily for 3–6 months.[G56]

Pharmacological Actions

In vitro and animal studies

There is a vast literature describing basic scientific research relating to the effects of ginkgo. Several pharmacological activities have been documented for ginkgo leaf extracts and/or their constituents. These include effects on behaviour, learning and memory, cardiovascular activities, effects on blood flow and antioxidant activity. The most important active principles of ginkgo extract include the ginkgo flavonoid glycosides and the terpene lactones.[1] Ginkgo has been described as having polyvalent action, i.e. the combined activity of several of its constituents is likely to be responsible for its effects.[13]

The pharmacological activities of ginkgo have been reviewed,[1,8,9,13–15] and other texts bring together several studies in specific areas, e.g. neuroprotective effects.[16] A summary of some of the literature on the *in vitro* and *in vivo* (animals) effects of ginkgo leaf is given below.

Effects on behaviour, learning and memory   The effects of a standardised extract of ginkgo leaf (EGb 761) on learning and memory, and on behaviour in relation to ageing and in recovery from brain injury, have been well studied.[13] Animal models (rats and mice) designed to test aspects of learning and memory (e.g. acquisition and retention) have documented improvements in animals treated with oral, intraperitoneal or subcutaneous EGb 761, compared with controls.[13] Studies involving rats reported improvements in acquisition and retention in older (24-month-old), but not younger (eight-month-old) rats. Other experiments involving rats of different ages have found that older rats (12- and 18-months old) showed improved performance in an eight-arm radial maze test following oral administration of EGb 761

30 or 60 mg/kg/day, whereas performance was stable among young rats (eight weeks old) following EGb 761 administration.[13] EGb 761 200 mg/kg administered orally to rats aged more than 26 months old led to significant improvements in aspects of cognitive behaviour.[17] *In vivo* studies have also shown that oral administration of EGb 761 (50 or 100 mg/kg/day for three weeks) to rats prevented the short-term memory-impairing effects of scopolamine administered intraperitoneally (0.125 mg/kg).[13]

The anxiolytic effects of a range of doses (0.01–10 mg/kg) of combination preparations containing different mixture ratios of standardised extracts of ginkgo leaf and ginger root have been tested in rats using the elevated plus-maze test.[18] Compared with controls, rats treated with the combination preparation (mixture ratio of ginger extract to ginkgo extract, 2.5 : 1; 1 mg/kg, intragastrically) spent increased amounts of time in the open arms of the maze, whereas the behaviour of rats treated with preparations of a mixture ratio of 1 : 1 and 1 : 2.5 did not change.

Several studies have reported that treatment with EGb 761, compared with control, aids recovery of function following brain injury, as demonstrated by behavioural tests in rats who had undergone bilateral frontal lobotomy or septohippocampal deafferentation, and in rat models of cortical hemiplegia.[13]

It has been suggested that the effects of EGb 761 in the experimental animal models described above may involve aspects of neuronal plasticity, e.g. neuronal regeneration.[13] Studies in rats have investigated, for example, the effects of EGb 761 administration on expression of neurotrophins and apolipoprotein E, and on behavioural recovery, following entorhinal cortex lesions, and on regeneration of primary olfactory neurons following olfactory bulbectomy. Research investigating the effects of EGb 761 on neuronal plasticity has been summarised.[1,13,19]

Cardiovascular and haemorheological activities   Studies investigating the molecular mechanisms that may contribute to the vasoregulatory (vasodilatation and vasoconstriction) effects of standardised ginkgo leaf extract (EGb 761) have been described.[13,20] *In vitro* experiments using isolated rabbit aorta suggested that possible mechanisms include effects on cyclic-GMP phosphodiesterase, prostaglandin I_2 and nitric oxide (NO). *Ex vivo* studies using isolated guinea-pig heart showed that EGb 761 led to a concentration-dependent increase in coronary blood flow. In studies involving isolated rat heart and in anaesthetised rabbits, EGb 761 administration has been reported to protect against myocardial ischaemia-reperfusion injury; the antioxidant and free-radical scavenging effects of EGb 761 (*see below*) may be important in this regard.[13] One study using isolated rat hearts suggested that the cardio-protective effects were due to the terpenoid constituents of EGb 761, and that the mechanism was independent of direct free radical-scavenging activity.[21] An *in vitro* study with endothelial cells suggested that the anti-ischaemic activity of EGb 761 may be due partly to the effects of the constituent bilobalide in protecting mitochondrial activity.[22]

The effects of ginkgo leaf extract have been studied in normal rats and those with ischaemic brain damage with middle cerebral artery occlusion.[23] Oral administration of ginkgo extract 100 mg/kg was reported to increase cerebral blood flow in normal rats, but the increase was less marked in rats with cerebral artery occlusion.

In vitro studies using human blood cells have documented effects of EGb 761 on several haemo-rheological parameters.[13] For example, *in vitro*, EGb 761 normalised changes in erythrocyte viscosity and in the viscoelastic properties of the erythrocyte membrane induced by standard metabolic challenge (pH 6.8; 380 mosmol/L) in six human blood donors. In other *in vitro* experiments, EGb 761 protected against hydrogen peroxide-induced damage in human erythrocytes. In studies using blood from patients with circulatory disorders, incubation with EGb 761 was reported to decrease erythrocyte aggregation. *In vitro* experiments using human neutrophils have found that EGb 761 at a concentration of 10 µmol/L inhibits release of hydrogen peroxide from these cells. The effects of EGb 761 on inhibition of human platelet aggregation elicited by substances such as thrombin and collagen have been documented.[13] A study using blood donated by healthy volunteers ($n = 35$) reported that a standardised extract of ginkgo leaf inhibited ADP- and collagen-induced platelet aggregation in platelet-rich plasma, gel-filtered platelets and in whole blood in a concentration-dependent manner.[24]

Platelet-activating factor antagonism Ginkgolides have been reported to competitively inhibit the binding of platelet-activating factor (PAF) to its membrane receptor.[8,9,25]

Ginkgolide B antagonises thrombus formation induced by PAF and, in guinea-pigs, it also induces a rapid curative thrombolysis. A protective effect is exerted by ginkgolides on PAF-induced broncho-constriction and airway hyperactivity in immuno-anaphylaxis and in antigen-induced bronchial provocation tests. Oral or intravenous injection of ginkgolide B antagonises cardiovascular impairments and bronchoconstriction induced by PAF. Ginkgolide B does not appear to interfere with cyclooxygenase, but at an earlier step involving PAF receptors and phospholipase activation. Eosinophil infiltration occurs in asthma and in allergic reactions, the number of eosinophils increasing during late phase. Since PAF is a potent activator of eosinophil function, it has been argued that ginkgolide B may interfere with the late-phase response.[25]

Pre-administration of ginkgolide B (1–5 mg/kg, intravenous) to rats has been reported to reduce PAF-induced decreases in diastolic and systolic arterial blood pressure in anaesthetised normotensive rats; this effect has also been reported in this animal model when ginkgolide B is administered shortly after PAF administration.[13]

Ginkgolide B has also been documented to have some beneficial effects in endotoxic shock; PAF is believed by some to be implicated in shock states. In anaesthetised guinea-pigs, intravenous administration of ginkgolide B (1 or 6 mg/kg) prior to injection of *Salmonella typhimurium* endotoxin reduced the initial rapid decrease in blood pressure, and intravenous administration of ginkgolide B during the prolonged phase of shock (1 hour after endotoxin administration) immediately and dose dependently reversed the decrease in blood pressure.[13] Other studies have found that ginkgolide B reduced arterial blood pressure in the secondary, but not the early, phase following administration of *Escherichia coli* endotoxin.[13]

Antioxidant activity The free radical-scavenging effects and antioxidant activity of EGb 761 *in vitro* are well documented.[13] EGb 761 scavenges several reactive oxygen species, including hydroxyl, super-oxide and peroxyl radicals.[13,26,27] In rat cerebellar neurons and cerebellar granule cells, ginkgo extract was reported to protect against oxidative stress induced by hydrogen peroxide, another reactive oxygen species.[28,29] In cultures of rat hippocampal cells, incubation with EGb 761 protected against cell death induced by β-amyloid, protected against toxicity induced by hydrogen peroxide, and blocked β-amyloid-induced events, such as accumulation of reactive oxygen species.[30] Bilobalide has also been documented to protect neurons against oxidative stress induced by reactive oxygen species *in vitro*.[31] Experiments in gerbils have suggested that the neuroprotective effects of gingko extract may be due to inhibition of nitric oxide formation.[32]

Other studies which have described neuroprotective effects of EGb 761 have suggested that antioxidant activity may be involved.[16] *In vitro*, a standardised ginkgo leaf extract was found to inhibit photo-induced formation of cholesterol oxides in a concentration-dependent manner.[33]

Antioxidant activity has been documented for EGb 761 *in vivo*. In rats, treatment with EGb 761 increased the concentrations of circulating and cellular polyunsaturated fatty acids, and reduced erythrocyte cell lysis induced by hydrogen peroxide.[34] Also in rats, oral administration of EGb 761 was reported to increase activity of the enzymes catalase and superoxide dismutase in the hippocampus, striatum and substantia nigrum.[35] Other data collected in this study suggested a decrease in lipid peroxidation in rat hippocampus in EGb 761-treated rats. In another study in rats, EGb 761 (200 mg/kg/day for four weeks) protected against carbon tetrachloride-induced (1.5 mL/kg) liver damage, as determined by malondialdehyde concentrations (a breakdown product of lipid peroxidation).[36]

Other activities   *In vivo* studies have suggested that EGb 761 may protect against chemically induced carcinogenesis. In mice, oral administration of EGb 761 (150 mg/kg daily for two weeks), compared with control, was reported to reduce tumour multiplicity; however, the inhibitory effect was not statistically significant.[37] It was also reported that EGb 761-treatment reduced the cardiotoxicity of doxorubicin.

EGb 761 and ginkgolide B have been shown to inhibit peripheral-type benzodiazepine receptor (PBR) expression and cell proliferation in the human breast cancer cell line MDA-231, which is known to be rich in PBR.[38] By contrast, the proliferation of MCF-7 breast cancer cells, which are low in PBR, was not affected.

In rats, oral administration of standardised ginkgo leaf extract 300 mg/kg was shown to ameliorate nephrotoxicity induced by administration of gentamicin 80 mg/kg.[39]

Aqueous extracts of dried ginkgo leaves have been reported to inhibit monoamine oxidases (MAO) A and B.[40] A study investigating the effects of bilobalide on gamma-aminobutyric acid (GABA) concentrations and on glutamic acid decarboxylase activity in mouse brain found that GABA concentrations and glutamic acid decarboxylase activity were significantly higher in animals treated orally with bilobalide 30 mg/kg daily for four days.[41] However, there were no differences between treated and control mice with regard to glutamate concentrations.

Several *in vivo* studies have documented adaptive effects for EGb 761.[20]

A peptide isolated from the leaves of *Ginkgo biloba* has been reported to have antifungal activity against several fungi, including *Pellicularia sasakii* and *Alternaria alternata*.[10]

Three long-chain phenols, anacardic acid, bilobol and cardanol, isolated from seeds of *G. biloba* are active against Sarcoma 180 ascites in mice.[42]

Clinical studies

Pharmacokinetics   Data on the pharmacokinetics of standardised extracts of ginkgo leaf have been summarised.[1,15,G18,G21] Mean bioavailabilities of ginkgolide A, ginkgolide B and bilobalide following oral administration of ginkgo extract 120 mg to fasting healthy volunteers were 80%, 88% and 79%, respectively. Food intake increased the time taken to reach peak concentration (suggesting slower absorption), but did not affect bioavailability.[1,G18] Peak concentrations of ginkgolides A and B and bilobalide observed in fasting volunteers ranged from 16.5 to 33.3 ng/mL, and from 11.5 to 21.1 ng/mL in volunteers who had consumed food.[1] Urinary excretion of ginkgolides A and B, and bilobalide, is around 70%, 50% and 30%, respectively, of the dose administered orally.[G18]

Therapeutic effects   Most clinical trials of ginkgo have explored its effects in the treatment of cognitive deficiency or cerebral insufficiency,[43,G56] a term used to describe a collection of symptoms thought to arise from an age-related reduction in cerebral blood flow. These symptoms include forgetfulness, poor concentration, poor perception, debilitation, dizziness, fatigue, sleep disturbances, listlessness, depressed mood, headache, mood swings, restlessness, tinnitus, anxiety, hearing loss and disorientation.[43,G56] Several studies have tested the effects of standardised ginkgo leaf extracts on cognitive function in patients with Alzheimer's disease[44] and/or multi-infarct dementia.[45] Both are conditions which share several symptoms (e.g. memory impairment) with cerebral insufficiency. Several other trials have explored the effects of ginkgo extracts on cognitive ability in individuals with no history of significant cognitive impairment. A few studies have explored the effects of ginkgo on tinnitus alone.[46]

Clinical research with ginkgo extracts has also focused on effects in improving pain-free walking distance in patients with intermittent claudication/peripheral arterial occlusive disease.[47,G56] Other studies have explored the effects of ginkgo in patients with chronic venous insufficiency, antidepressant-related sexual dysfunction, seasonal affective disorder (SAD), and symptoms of depression.

Almost all clinical trials of ginkgo have investigated the effects of the standardised ginkgo leaf extracts EGb 761 and LI 1370.

Cognitive deficiency, dementia in Alzheimer's disease, multi-infarct dementia A review of controlled clinical trials of ginkgo in patients with cerebral insufficiency identified 40 studies.[43] Generally, trials tested oral doses of standardised extracts of ginkgo leaf of 120 mg daily administered for at least four to six weeks. Most trials reported significant results or positive (but not statistically significant) trends in favour of ginkgo, compared with control. However, it was reported that most trials were of poor methodological quality; only eight studies were considered to be well-conducted. All of these eight studies reported statistically significant results for ginkgo, compared with placebo. Nevertheless, further randomised, double-blind, controlled trials involving larger numbers of patients were deemed necessary.[43] Details of 39 controlled studies of the ginkgo extracts EGb 761 and LI 1370 have been summarised.[G56] All but two[48,49] of these studies were conducted before new guidelines for testing the efficacy of nootropic drugs were developed.[G56] Details of the two studies that did meet the methodological criteria described in the guidelines are given below.

In a randomised, double-blind, placebo-controlled trial, after a four-week placebo run-in period, 216 patients with mild-to-moderate primary degenerative dementia of the Alzheimer type, or multi-infarct dementia, received standardised ginkgo leaf extract (EGb 761) 120 mg orally twice daily, or placebo, for 24 weeks.[48] At the end of the study, data for 156 patients were eligible for analysis. There were significantly more responders to treatment (defined as a response to at least two of the three primary outcome measures – a psychopathological assessment, an assessment of cognitive performance and a behavioural assessment of activities of daily life) in the ginkgo group, compared with the placebo group (28% versus 10% of ginkgo and placebo recipients, respectively; $p = 0.005$). The difference was also statistically significant in an intention-to-treat analysis (23% versus 10% of ginkgo and placebo recipients, respectively; $p = 0.005$).

A randomised, double-blind, placebo-controlled study involved 327 patients with mild-to-severe dementia related to Alzheimer's disease or multi-infarct dementia.[49] Participants received standardised ginkgo leaf extract (EGb 761) 40 mg orally three times daily ($n = 166$), or placebo ($n = 161$), for 52 weeks, and underwent a battery of assessments at 12, 26 and 52 weeks. The primary outcome measures were the Alzheimer's Disease Assessment Scale Cognitive Subscale (Adas-Cog), the Geriatric Evaluation by Relative's Rating Instrument (GERRI) and the Clinical Global Impression of Change (CGIC). In an intention-to-treat analysis ($n = 309$), ginkgo recipients scored significantly better than did placebo recipients on the Adas-Cog and the GERRI ($p = 0.04$ and $p = 0.004$, respectively). A slight worsening on the CGIC was observed for both groups. The average end-points for the intention-to-treat analysis were 38.6 and 34.6 weeks for the ginkgo and placebo groups, respectively.

A systematic review of randomised, double-blind, placebo-controlled trials assessing the effects of standardised ginkgo leaf extracts on cognitive function in patients with Alzheimer's disease, characterised according to recognised criteria, included four studies.[44] These involved oral administration of ginkgo extract 120 or 240 mg daily for 12–26 weeks, and involved a total of 212 patients each in the ginkgo and placebo groups. A meta-analysis of the results of the four studies indicated a modest effect for ginkgo, compared with placebo (difference of 3% on the Adas-Cog).

Another systematic review included nine randomised, double-blind, placebo-controlled trials of standardised ginkgo leaf extracts in patients with dementia of the Alzheimer type and/or multi-infarct dementia.[45] The review included two studies described above.[48,49] Studies generally involved the administration of oral doses of ginkgo extract 120 or 240 mg daily for 6–12 weeks, although two studies involved a 24-week[48] or 52-week[49] administration period. One study involved the administration of intravenous infusions of ginkgo extract 200 mg four times per week for four weeks. It was reported that, overall, the studies provided evidence to support the efficacy of standardised ginkgo leaf extracts in the symptomatic treatment of dementia. However, methodological limitations of several of the included studies (e.g. poorly defined inclusion and exclusion criteria and method of randomisation, treatment period less than six months, small sample sizes) were also emphasised. It was concluded that further studies are required to establish the benefits of ginkgo in dementia.[45]

In a randomised, double-blind, placebo-controlled study, 60 elderly volunteers with mild-to-moderate, age-related cognitive dysfunction received oral ginkgo extract (GB-8; no further details provided) 40 mg, 80 mg or placebo, three times daily for three months.[50] At the end of the study, for the 54 patients who completed, it was reported that memory function (as assessed by the Wechsler Memory Scale) improved significantly in the low-dose ginkgo group, compared with baseline values ($p = 0.016$), but that there was no significant improvement in the placebo or high-dose ginkgo groups, compared with baseline values. A significant decrease in diastolic blood pressure, compared with baseline values, was also reported for the low-dose ginkgo group ($p = 0.04$). This study, however, had methodological limitations (e.g. small sample size), and the report of the study did not include statistical analyses between groups.

A more methodologically rigorous randomised, double-blind, placebo-controlled trial involving patients with age-related impairment of memory and/or concentration assessed the effects of an alcohol/water extract of fresh leaves of ginkgo (drug extract ratio 1 : 4; total flavonoid glycosides 0.20 mg/mL, total ginkgolides 0.34 mg/mL).[51] Participants received undiluted ginkgo extract ($n = 77$), diluted ginkgo extract (1 : 1 with placebo) ($n = 82$), or placebo ($n = 82$), 40 drops (1.9 mL) three times daily for 24 weeks. At the end of the treatment period, a check for blinding indicated that participants were unable to identify the treatment they received. There were no statistically significant differences between the three groups in subjective perceptions of memory and concentration, and in the following objective measures: the Expended Mental Control Test (a measure of attention and concentration), and Rey test parts 1 and 2 (which measure short-term memory and learning curve, and long-term memory and recognition, respectively). However, a significant difference between groups was observed in the Benton test of visual retention-revised (a measure of short-term visual memory) – increases in baseline scores of 18, 26 and 11% were recorded for the high-dose ginkgo, low-dose ginkgo and placebo groups, respectively ($p = 0.0076$).[51]

In an open study, 18 elderly patients with 'possible or probable' Alzheimer's disease were randomised to receive a single oral dose of tacrine 40 mg or a standardised extract of ginkgo leaf (SeGb; no further details provided) 240 mg in two separate sessions within three- to seven-day intervals.[52] It was reported that both interventions induced pharmacological effects in the central nervous system (CNS), as assessed by quantitative pharmaco-electroencephalogram measurements. It should be noted that this was an uncontrolled study.

Cognitive enhancement in healthy volunteers Ginkgo has been tested for its cognitive enhancing effects in healthy (i.e. cognitively intact) individuals in addition to investigations into its effects in patients with cognitive deficiency.

In a double-blind, placebo-controlled, cross-over study, 20 healthy volunteers aged 19–24 years received a standardised extract of ginkgo leaf (GK501) at doses of 120 mg, 240 mg and 360 mg.[53] A battery of tests used to assess cognitive performance was carried out immediately before and at 1, 2.5, 4 and 6 hours after ginkgo administration. It was reported that with doses of ginkgo extract of 240 and 360 mg, there was a statistically significant improvement in 'speed of attention' (a measure of reaction time) from 2.5 hours up to 6 hours (the last measurement point) after ginkgo administration.

In a randomised, double-blind, placebo-controlled, crossover study, eight healthy female volunteers (mean age 32 years) were given a standardised extract of G. biloba leaf at doses of 120, 240 and 600 mg.[54] One hour after treatment, volunteers undertook a series of psychological tests. Memory was found to be significantly improved with G. biloba leaf 600 mg, compared with placebo.

A randomised, double-blind, placebo-controlled, crossover trial involving 31 volunteers aged 30–59 years tested the effects of a standardised extract of ginkgo leaf (LI 1370) 50 mg three times daily, 100 mg three times daily, 120 mg each morning, 240 mg each morning, and placebo, each taken for two days followed by a washout period of at least five days.[55] A battery of tests to assess memory and cognitive and psychomotor performance was carried out 30 minutes before ginkgo administration and then hourly for 12 hours. It was reported that there was a 'marginally significant' effect of treatment, compared with placebo, in a test assessing short-term memory, although the *p*-value given for this was greater than 0.05 ($p = 0.053$). Post-hoc analyses suggested that ginkgo extract 120 mg each morning was associated with better performance in this test than other doses of ginkgo extract (including ginkgo extract 50 mg three times daily) and placebo. There were no statistically significant effects of treatment on immediate and delayed word recall and choice reaction time.

Other studies have assessed the cognitive-enhancing effects of ginkgo extracts in older volunteers. In a randomised, double-blind, placebo-controlled trial, 48 cognitively intact individuals aged over 55 years received a standardised ginkgo leaf extract (EGb 761) 60 mg three times daily, or placebo, for six weeks.[56] A battery of neuropsychological tests was carried out before treatment and at the end of the study. Ginkgo extract recipients experienced a significant improvement in tests assessing speed of processing abilities, compared with placebo recipients ($p < 0.03$). However, no statistically significant differences between the ginkgo extract and placebo groups were evident for tests assessing memory.

In a questionnaire survey, the effects of administration of a standardised ginkgo leaf extract (LI 1370) 120 mg daily for four months on the activities of daily living were assessed in volunteers aged 32–97 years (mean (SD) 68.9 (8.4) years).[57] Volunteers were recruited via editorial in a magazine. Of 8557 initial respondents, 5028 were eligible for the survey. In total, 1000 volunteers (who were not currently using any ginkgo products) were said to be randomly allocated to receive ginkgo extract; all other respondents were allocated to the no-treatment control group, unless they had stated that they only wished to receive ginkgo. It was reported that ginkgo extract recipients achieved significantly better scores than the control group on a scale assessing ability to perform activities of daily living, self-assessment of ability to cope, and visual analogue scales for mood and sleep. However, for several reasons, the results of this study should be interpreted cautiously. For example, the study was carried out by post, therefore investigators did not meet participants at any time, the study was not truly randomised, the study was open, the control group did not receive placebo tablets, and there was no check on compliance.

Tinnitus and hearing loss Tinnitus and hearing loss are two of the symptoms of dementia.[G56] Several studies have assessed the effects of ginkgo on these conditions alone.

A systematic review of randomised, controlled trials of ginkgo extracts in tinnitus included five studies – four studies compared ginkgo extracts with placebo, and one study compared ginkgo extract with conventional drugs. Three trials tested the standardised ginkgo leaf extract EGb 761; full details of other extracts tested in the other studies are not given in the review. The review concluded that, overall, the studies identified provided evidence to support ginkgo extracts as a treatment for tinnitus, but that further investigation was required to fully establish the benefits. Typically, at least two of the studies had methodological flaws.[46]

A double-blind, controlled trial, published since the systematic review, tested the effects of a standardised ginkgo leaf extract (LI 1370) 50 mg, or placebo, three times daily for 12 weeks in 1121 individuals, aged 18–70 years, with tinnitus who were otherwise healthy.[58] Participants were recruited via advertisements placed in the UK national press and in a British Tinnitus Association's publication. The main outcome measure was participants' self-assessment of tinnitus (loudness and 'how troublesome') before, during and after treatment, carried out via postal questionnaires and telephone calls. Participants were paired where possible (489 pairs, i.e. 978 of 1121 participants were matched) and then randomly allocated to active or placebo. At the end of the study, the results indicated that ginkgo extract (LI 1370) 50 mg three times daily was 'no more effective than

placebo in treating tinnitus'.[58] The design of this study has been criticised. For example, participants did not have face-to-face contact with an investigator at any time during the study.[59]

In a randomised, controlled trial, 28 patients with untreated sudden loss of hearing received intravenous infusions of 6% hydroxyethyl starch (HES), or intravenous and oral ginkgo extract, for 10 days.[60] There were no statistically significant differences between the two groups in improvements in hearing. Further studies involving larger numbers of participants are required.[60]

Peripheral arterial occlusive disease/intermittent claudication The effects of standardised extracts of ginkgo have been investigated in patients with Fontaine stage II peripheral arterial occlusive disease. This condition is characterised by the onset of pain, as a result of oxygen deficit in the leg muscles, on walking distances greater than around 30–300 metres.[G56] The rationale for using ginkgo in this condition is for its effects in improving blood flow.

A meta-analysis of randomised, double-blind, placebo-controlled trials of ginkgo extract for the treatment of intermittent claudication included eight studies that assessed effects on walking distance.[61] The trials involved a total of 415 patients who received a standardised extract of ginkgo leaf at doses of 120 or 160 mg daily, or placebo, for 6, 12 (one trial each) or 24 weeks. The pooled results from all trials indicated a statistically significant increase in pain-free walking distance for ginkgo-treated patients, compared with placebo recipients (weighted mean difference (WMD): 34 metres; 95% confidence intervals (CI): 26–43 metres). A similar result was obtained when results for the six studies of good methodological quality were pooled (WMD: 37 metres; 95% CI: 26–47 metres). It is questionable whether the extent of these increases in pain-free walking distance is clinically relevant.[61]

Chronic venous insufficiency and venous ulcers A randomised, double-blind, placebo-controlled trial assessed the protective effects of a combination preparation (Ginkgor Forte) containing a standardised extract of ginkgo (2.3%), troxerutine (48.85%) and heptaminol (48.85%) against venous wall injury in 48 female patients with chronic venous insufficiency.[62] Ginkgor Forte 625 mg daily, or placebo, was given for four weeks. In total, 42 patients completed the study, but only 28 were included in the final analysis because of protocol violations. Circulating endothelial cell (CEC) count was used as a measure of injury to the vascular endothelium (CEC counts are raised in patients with chronic venous insufficiency.[62] After four weeks' treatment, CEC counts decreased significantly in both the treatment and placebo groups (by 14.5% and 8.4%, respectively), compared with baseline values ($p = 0.0021$ and $p = 0.0146$, respectively). The mean change in CEC count after four weeks' treatment was reported to be significantly greater for the treatment group, compared with the placebo group ($p = 0.039$).

In another double-blind trial, 213 patients with chronic venous or mixed ulcers located at the malleolus (rounded protuberance on ankle joint) received ginkgo extract 160 mg daily, or placebo, together with standard care (elastic stockings, local dressings and cleansing of ulcers) for 12 weeks.[1] At the end of the study, ginkgo extract recipients, compared with placebo recipients, showed a significant reduction in ulcer area.

Asthma, PAF antagonism Intradermal injections of PAF induce a biphasic inflammatory response similar to that observed in sensitised individuals subjected to moderate doses of allergen. A single dose of a mixture of ginkgolides has been reported to antagonise this response.[63] Oral administration of ginkgolides resulted in a reduction of eosinophil infiltration in atopic patients given intracutaneous injections of PAF.[63]

In a randomised, double-blind, crossover study, 80 and 120 mg capsules containing a standardised mixture of ginkgolides A, B and C (ratio of 40 : 40 : 20) were given as a single oral dose 2 hours before challenge by intradermal PAF/histamine. Both dose ranges inhibited flare which was maximal after 5 minutes. Within 15–30 minutes wheal volume was reduced, with the greatest effect being observed for the higher dose treatments. The protection was still present 8 hours after oral dosing.[8] Similar inhibition of PAF was observed for platelet aggregation with single oral doses of 80 and 120 mg extract which were given 2 hours before blood withdrawal. The ginkgolide mixture given orally also blocked PAF-induced airway hyper-responsiveness.

Antagonism of the effects of PAF by a standardised mixture of ginkgolides was assessed in a double-blind, placebo-controlled crossover study in six healthy subjects aged 25–35 years.[64] Wheal and flare responses to PAF examined 2 hours after ingestion of 80 mg and 120 mg of ginkgolide mixture were inhibited in a dose-related manner. Both doses significantly inhibited PAF-induced platelet aggregation in platelet-rich plasma.[64]

A randomised, double-blind, crossover study involved patients with atopic asthma who were challenged with their specific dust or pollen antigen.[8] After 6.5 hours, participants were subjected to a provocation test with acetylcholine so that the treatment of later stages of an asthma attack could be assessed. Mixed ginkgolide standardised extract, 40 mg three times daily, or placebo, were given during the three days before the test and a final single dose of 120 mg of extract was given 2 hours before the challenge. The results suggested that ginkgolides were effective in both the early phase and the late phase of airway hyperactivity.[8]

A study involving six patients with a history of exercise-induced asthma assessed the effects of a specific PAF antagonist (BN 52063, a standardised mixture of ginkgolides A, B and C, ratio of 40 : 40 : 20) on the response to isocapnic hyperventilation with dry cold air.[65] Participants were randomised to receive BN 52063 240 mg orally 2 hours before cold air challenge, 2.4 mg by metered dose inhaler 30 minutes before cold air challenge, or placebo. It was reported that oral BN 52063 did not reduce bronchoconstriction during challenge. A significant increase in airways resistance was observed after inhalation of BN 52063. In another study, six patients with a history of exercise-induced asthma received BN 52063 120 mg orally twice daily, 1 mg by spinhaler three times daily, or placebo, for three days, then, on the test day, 240 mg orally 3 hours before exercise challenge, 5 mg by spinhaler 1 hour before challenge, or placebo, respectively. With oral treatment, the prolonged reduction in peak expiratory flow was significantly attenuated ($p < 0.05$).[65]

Antidepressant-related sexual dysfunction Two open, uncontrolled studies have explored the effects of ginkgo extract in sexual dysfunction associated with treatment with antidepressant drugs.[66,67] One of these studies involved 63 men and women who were receiving treatment with selective serotonin reuptake inhibitors (SSRIs), venlafaxine, nefazodone, bupropion, phenelzine or protriptyline, and experiencing sexual dysfunction, including decreased libido, erectile difficulties, delayed or inhibited orgasm and/or ejaculatory failure.[66] All participants received ginkgo extract 40 or 60 mg twice daily, titrated up to a maximum of 120 mg twice daily (average daily dose 207 mg), for four weeks. It was reported that sexual dysfunction was relieved, as assessed by clinical interview and self-report, in 91% and 76% of female and male participants, respectively. An open, prospective pilot study involved 14 patients with sexual dysfunction (severe or complete loss of libido, with or without inability to achieve or maintain erection, failure or delay in ejaculation, anorgasmia) associated with current treatment with antidepressant drugs, mainly SSRIs, but also hypericum (St. John's wort) extract, amitriptyline and clomipramine.[67] Participants received a standardised extract of ginkgo 240 mg daily for six weeks. Assessment included an eight-item 'sexual stress' score, 'sleep problems' score, and the Hamilton Anxiety and Depression Scale scores. Among the 12 individuals who completed the study statistically significant improvements in scores were observed for anxiety at week 6 ($p < 0.05$) and sexual stress at weeks 3 and 6 ($p < 0.01$ for both), all compared with baseline values.

One of these studies[66] has been criticised for its methodological limitations and poor quality of the report.[68] Owing to their open, uncontrolled designs, neither study provides reliable evidence of the effects of gingko extract in antidepressant-related sexual dysfunction, as the observed effects cannot be reliably attributed to treatment with ginkgo.

Other conditions A Cochrane review of the effects of ginkgo extract in age-related macular degeneration identified one randomised, controlled trial involving 20 patients.[69] The study design did not include blinding of the assessment of outcome. The review concluded that the effects of ginkgo extract in preventing progression of age-related macular degeneration had not yet been adequately assessed.

In a randomised, double-blind, controlled trial, 27 patients with seasonal affective disorder (SAD) received standardised extract of ginkgo leaf (Bio-Biloba, containing flavone glycosides 24 mg and terpene lactones 6 mg) one tablet twice daily ($n = 15$), or placebo ($n = 12$), for 10 weeks or until development of depression requiring treatment.[70] All participants began the trial during October to December; assessments were carried out at baseline and on termination of study medication. Six of the 15 ginkgo recipients and two of the 12 placebo recipients terminated the study treatment because of emerging symptoms of SAD ('winter depression'). It was reported that this difference between groups was not statistically significant, according to Fisher's exact test. Also, there were no statistically significant differences between groups on the Montgomery–Asberg Depression Rating Scale, the ATYP scale (for symptoms of hypersomnia, hyperphagia and carbohydrate craving) and on self-assessed symptoms (energy, tiredness, appetite, carbohydrate craving, depressed mood). The results of this study cannot be considered definitive because of the small sample size of the study and other limitations.[70]

An open pilot study explored the effects of a standardised dried extract of ginkgo leaf (LI 1370) on cognitive performance in patients with major depression who were receiving trimipramine 200 mg daily.[71] Eight participants received trimipramine for six weeks, and ginkgo extract 120 mg twice daily from day 8 to day 35 of the study. The data for these individuals were compared with those for eight age- and sex-matched controls who received trimipramine only for six weeks. At the end of the study, there was a significantly higher response rate (determined by a reduction of 50% or more in baseline Hamilton Depression Rating Scale scores) among patients who received trimipramine only, compared with those who received trimipramine plus ginkgo extract ($p \leqslant 0.05$). However, duration of illness before enrolment in the study was reported to be significantly longer for ginkgo extract recipients than for controls ($p \leqslant 0.05$). It was claimed that the ginkgo extract group, compared with the control group (trimipramine only), had improved sleep efficiency and augmented non-REM (random eye movement) sleep, although p-values were not given. Furthermore, by contrast, sleep time was found to be significantly prolonged in participants receiving trimipramine only. The design of the study, together with conflicting results, do not allow any definitive conclusions regarding the effects on sleep of ginkgo extract in addition to trimipramine treatment.

A placebo-controlled trial involving 165 women with premenstrual syndrome explored the effects of standardised ginkgo leaf extract (EGb 761) 160 mg daily, or placebo, taken from day 16 of the menstrual cycle to day 5 of the following cycle, for two cycles.[72] Both groups experienced improvements in symptoms, compared with baseline values, although ginkgo recipients, compared with placebo recipients, were reported to experience significantly greater improvements in breast tenderness (as evaluated by the physician).

The effects of ginkgo extract have been explored in patients with schizophrenia. The rationale for this is based on the theory that excess free radical formation may occur in patients with schizophrenia, since superoxide dismutase (SOD) concentrations have been reported to be higher in certain tissues in such patients. (SOD is an enzyme that detoxifies superoxide radicals.) In a double-blind, placebo-controlled trial, 82 inpatients with chronic schizophrenia (illness for at least five years) were 'divided randomly' to receive haloperidol 0.25 mg/kg daily, with or without ginkgo extract 360 mg daily, for 12 weeks.[73] At the end of the study, mean SOD concentrations (expressed as ng/mL haemoglobin) were reported to be significantly lower, compared with baseline values, for ginkgo recipients (mean (SD): 815.8 (697.8) and 596.7 (148.3), respectively; $p = 0.021$). In participants who received haloperidol only, mean

(SD) SOD concentrations fell from 780.4 (605.4) at baseline to 617.6 (189.7) at the end of the study, although this decrease was reported to be statistically non-significant. A between-group comparison was not reported. Mean (SD) SOD concentrations in a group of 30 age- and sex-matched healthy volunteers were 515.8 (70.4).[73]

The effects of a preparation comprising *Ginkgo biloba* dimeric flavonoids in a 1:2 complex with phosphatidylcholine (GBDF-Phytosome) on the microcirculation of the skin have been investigated using various techniques including, infrared photo-pulse plethysmography, laser doppler flowmetry, high-performance contact thermography and computerised videothermography.[74] In a controlled study, small numbers of healthy individuals and volunteers with acrocyanosis or cellulitis were treated with 0.5 mL of a cream (oil-in-water emulsion) containing 3% GBDF-Phytosome or an oil-in-water emulsion of 2% phosphatidylcholine (control). Participants who received the GBDF-Phytosome preparation were reported to experience significant increases in capillary blood flow and skin temperature, compared with baseline values, whereas no significant changes were observed for the control group. No between-group comparisons were reported.[74] These preliminary findings suggest that the effects of this preparation on skin microcirculation may deserve further investigation.

A phase II (open, uncontrolled) study explored the effects of standardised ginkgo leaf extract (EGb 761) given in combination with 5-fluorouracil (5-FU) in 44 patients with advanced progressive colorectal cancer who had previously received 5-FU.[75] The rationale for including ginkgo extract in the regimen was based on its reputed ability to increase local blood flow. Thus, it was hypothesised that ginkgo extract might 'enhance local tumour blood flow and thus improve the distribution of 5-FU'. In the study, participants received ginkgo extract 350 mg in 250 mL saline intravenously over 30 minutes on days 1–6, and 5-FU 500 mg/m^2 in 250 mL saline intravenously over 30 minutes on days 2–6. The regimen was repeated every three weeks until recurrence of tumour progression. Data from 32 patients who had received at least two courses of treatment were eligible for analysis. Of these patients, 69% experienced progression of disease, 25% experienced no change, and 6.3% ($n = 2$) were in partial remission.[75]

Side-effects, Toxicity

The safety and toxicity of ginkgo have been reviewed.[G18,G21] Available data indicate that stan-dardised extracts of ginkgo leaf are well tolerated when used at recommended doses.[43,G21] Adverse effects are uncommon. A postmarketing surveillance study involving 10 815 patients who received a standardised extract (LI 1370) of ginkgo leaf reported that the frequency of adverse effects was 1.7%.[G56] Adverse effects reported with standardised extracts of ginkgo leaf are generally mild, and include nausea, headache, gastrointestinal upset and diarrhoea; allergic skin reactions occur rarely.[76,G21,G56]

A systematic review of nine randomised, double-blind, placebo-controlled trials of standardised ginkgo leaf extracts in patients with dementia of the Alzheimer type and/or multi-infarct dementia concluded that, overall, the frequency of adverse effects reported for ginkgo was not markedly different than that for placebo.[45] The largest trial included in this review involved 327 patients with mild-to-severe dementia related to Alzheimer's disease or multi-infarct dementia who received standardised ginkgo leaf extract (EGb 761) 40 mg orally three times daily ($n = 166$), or placebo ($n = 161$), for 52 weeks.[49] It was reported that there was no statistically significant differences between ginkgo and placebo in the number of participants reporting adverse events, or in the frequency and severity of adverse events. Of 188 adverse events reported during the study, 97 were reported by ginkgo recipients and 91 by placebo recipients. However, clinical trials generally only have the statistical power to detect common, acute adverse effects. Similar findings were reported in another systematic review/meta-analysis which included eight randomised, double-blind, placebo-controlled trials of ginkgo extract for the treatment of intermittent claudication, involving a total of 415 patients who received standardised extract of ginkgo leaf at doses of 120 or 160 mg daily, or placebo, for up to 24 weeks.[47] Five of the eight studies included reported (rarely) mild, transient adverse events occurring in ginkgo recipients; the remaining three studies, comprising almost 50% of the total number of patients, did not report any adverse events.

There are isolated reports of bleeding associated with ingestion of *Ginkgo biloba* extract. One report describes a 70-year-old man who experienced spontaneous bleeding from the iris into the anterior chamber of the eye one week after he began taking standardised ginkgo extract 80 mg daily.[77] A 61-year-old man who had taken ginkgo extract 120 mg or 160 mg daily for six months experienced a subarachnoid haemorrhage.[78] Another report describes a 33-year-old woman who began experiencing increasingly severe headaches, as well as double vision and nausea and vomiting, over several months.[79] During the course of investigations, it was revealed that she had been consuming standardised ginkgo extract 120 mg daily for two years. Her symptoms improved, although her headaches were not entirely relieved, after evacuation of bilateral subdural haematomas which were identified following an MRI scan. On stopping ginkgo extract, her prolonged bleeding time was reduced, and on follow-up she was symptom-free. A causal relationship between ginkgo ingestion and bleeding in these cases has not been definitively established.

There is a report of acute myoglobinuria in a 29-year-old man who was a regular weight-trainer and who had been taking a combination preparation containing extracts of ginkgo (200 mg), guarana (*Paullinia cupana*, 500 mg) and kava (*Piper methysticum*, 100 mg).[80] The man was admitted to an intensive care unit with severe muscle pain and blood creatine kinase and myoglobin concentrations of 100 500 IU/L (normal values: 0–195) and 10 000 ng/mL (normal values: 0–90), respectively. Signs and symptoms subsided within six weeks. The relevance, if any, of ginkgo ingestion to the man's condition, is unclear.

Contact or ingestion of the fruit pulp has produced severe allergic reactions including erythema, oedema, blisters and itching.[63] The seed contains the toxin 4-O-methylpyridoxine which is reported to be responsible for 'gin-nan' food poisoning in Japan and China.[11] The main symptoms are convulsion and loss of consciousness and lethality is estimated in about 27% of cases in Japan, infants being particularly vulnerable.

Contra-indications, Warnings

The fruit pulp has produced severe allergic reactions and should not be handled or ingested. The seed causes severe adverse effects when ingested.

Ginkgo extract should only be used with caution in patients taking anticoagulant or antiplatelet agents.

Pregnancy and lactation No studies appear to have been reported on the effects of *G. biloba* leaf extracts or ginkgolides in pregnant or lactating women. In view of the many pharmacological actions documented and the lack of toxicity data, use of ginkgo during pregnancy and lactation should be avoided.

Pharmaceutical Comment

There is a vast scientific literature describing the pharmacological effects of ginkgo leaf extracts and their constituents.[81] These data provide some supporting evidence for the modern clinical uses of standardised ginkgo leaf extracts.[1,2,8,13,14,16,19,20,76,82,83]

Also, standardised ginkgo leaf extracts are among the herbal preparations that have undergone most extensive clinical investigation. The effects of ginkgo extracts in dementia have been tested clinically mostly in trials involving patients with cognitive deficiency, Alzheimer's disease[44] and/or multi-infarct dementia. Some high-quality studies involving patients with dementia have reported significant beneficial effects for standardised ginkgo leaf extracts.[48,49] However, systematic reviews/meta-analysis of all relevant randomised, double-blind, placebo-controlled trials have reported modest effects for ginkgo extract, compared with placebo,[44] and have concluded that further high-quality studies are required to establish the benefits of ginkgo in dementia.[45] Small randomised, double-blind, placebo-controlled trials investigating the cognitive enhancing effects of ginkgo extracts in healthy volunteers have reported conflicting results. Further study is required to determine whether ginkgo extracts are of value in cognitively intact individuals. The effects of ginkgo extract in patients with tinnitus have not been definitively established by trials carried out to date. A meta-analysis of trials of standardised ginkgo leaf extract in peripheral arterial occlusive disease found that ginkgo significantly improved pain-free walking distance, although the clinical relevance of the extent of improvement is questionable.[47]

Generally, the intended uses of ginkgo are not suitable for self-medication.

References

See also General References G3, G5, G18, G21, G29, G31, G32, G36, G43, G50, G54, G56, G63 and G64.

1 Van Beek TA *et al*. Ginkgo biloba L. *Fitoterapia* 1998; **69**: 195–244.

2 Van Beek TA, ed. *Ginkgo. The Genus Ginkgoaceae*. Amsterdam: Harwood Academic Publishers, 1998.

3 Victoire C *et al*. Isolation of flavonoid glycosides from *Ginkgo biloba* leaves. *Planta Med* 1988; **54**: 245–247.

4 Schenne A, Holzl J. 6-Hydroxykynurensaure, die erste N- haltige Verbindung aus den Blattern von *Ginkgo biloba*. *Planta Med* 1986; **52**: 235–236.

5 Nasr C, *et al*. 2-Quinoline carboxylic acid-4,6-dihydroxy from *Ginkgo biloba*. Paper presented at the Phytochemical Society of Europe Symposium: Biologically Active Natural Products, Lausanne, 1986, p. 9.

6 Briancon-Scheid F *et al*. HPLC separation and quantitative determination of biflavones in leaves from *Ginkgo biloba*. *Planta Med* 1983; **49**: 204–220.

7 Vanhaelen M, Vanhaelen-Fastre R. Kaempferol-3-O-β-glucoside (astragalin) from *Ginkgo biloba*. *Fitoterapia* 1988; **59**: 511.

8 Braquet P. The ginkgolides: potent platelet-activating factor antagonists isolated from *Ginkgo biloba* L.: Chemistry, pharmacology and clinical applications. *Drugs of the Future* 1987; **12**: 643–699.

9 Anonymous. Extract of *Ginkgo biloba* (EGb 761). *Presse Med* 1986; **15**: 1438–1598.

10 Huang X *et al*. Characteristics and antifungal activity of a chitin binding protein from *Ginkgo biloba*. *FEBS* 2000; **478**: 123–126.

11 Wada K *et al*. Studies on the constitution of edible medicinal plants. 1. Isolation and identification of 4-O-methylpyridoxine, toxic principle from the seed of *Ginkgo biloba* L. *Chem Pharm Bull* 1988; **36**: 1779–1782.

12 Wang H, Ng TB. Ginkbilobin, a novel antifungal protein from *Ginkgo biloba* seeds with sequence similarity to embryo-abundant protein. *Biochem Biophys Res Commun* 2000; **279**: 407–411.

13 DeFeudis FV. *Ginkgo biloba. From Chemistry to Clinic*. Wiesbaden, Germany: Ullstein Medical, 1998.

14 Clostre F, De Feudis FV, eds. *Cardiovascular Effects of Ginkgo biloba Extract (EGb761). Advances in Ginkgo biloba Extract Research*, vol 3. Paris: Elsevier, 1994: 1–162.

15 Reuter HD. *Ginkgo biloba* – botany, constituents, pharmacology and clinical trials. *Br J Phytother* 1995/6; **4**: 3–20.

16 Christen Y, ed. *Ginkgo biloba Extract (EGb 761) as a Neuroprotective Agent: From Basic Studies to Clinical Trials. Advances in Ginkgo biloba Extract Research*, vol 8. Paris: Elsevier, 2001.

17 Winter JC. The effects of an extract of Ginkgo biloba, EGb 761, on cognitive behaviour and longevity in the rat. *Physiol Behav* 1998; **63**: 425–433.

18 Hasenöhrl RU *et al*. Dissociation between anxiolytic and hypomnestic effects for combined extracts of *Zingiber officinale* and *Ginkgo biloba*, as opposed to diazepam. *Pharmacol Biochem Behav* 1998; **59**: 527–535.

19 Christen Y *et al*., eds. *Effects of Ginkgo biloba Extract (EGb 761) on Neuronal Plasticity. Advances in Ginkgo biloba Extract Research*, vol 5. Paris: Elsevier, 1996.

20 Papadopoulos V *et al*. *Adaptive Effects of Ginkgo biloba Extract (EGb 761). Advances in Ginkgo biloba Extract Research*, vol 6. Paris: Elsevier, 1997.

21 Liebgott T *et al*. Complementary cardioprotective effects of flavonoid metabolites and terpenoid constituents of *Ginkgo biloba* extract (EGb 761) during ischemia and reperfusion. *Basic Res Cardiol* 2000; **95**: 368–377.

22 Janssens D *et al*. Protection by bilobalide of the ischaemia-induced alterations of the mitochondrial respiratory activity. *Fund Clin Pharmacol* 2000; **14**: 193–201.

23 Zhang WR *et al*. Protective effect of Ginkgo extract on rat brain with transient middle cerebral artery occlusion. *Neurol Res* 2000; **22**: 517–521.

24 Dutta-Roy AK *et al*. Inhibitory effect of *Ginkgo biloba* extract on human platelet aggregation. *Platelets* 1999; **10**: 298–305.

25 Hosford D, *et al*. Natural antagonists of platelet-activating factor. *Phytother Res* 1988; **2**: 1–17.

26 Maitra I *et al*. Peroxyl radical scavenging activity of *Ginkgo biloba* extract EGb 761. *Biochem Pharmacol* 1995; **49**: 1649–1655.

27 Lee S-L *et al*. Superoxide scavenging effect of *Ginkgo biloba* extract on serotonin-induced mitogenesis. *Biochem Pharmacol* 1998; **56**: 527–533.

28 Oyama Y *et al*. *Ginkgo biloba* extract protects brain neurons against oxidative stress induced by hydrogen peroxide. *Brain Res* 1996; **712**: 349–352.

29 Wei T *et al*. Hydrogen peroxide-induced oxidative damage and apoptosis in cerebellar granule cells: protection by *Ginkgo biloba* extract. *Pharmacol Res* 2000; **41**: 427–433.

30 Bastianetto S *et al*. The ginkgo biloba extract (EGb 761) protects hippocampal neurons against cell death induced by β-amyloid. *Eur J Neurosci* 2000; **12**: 1882–1890.

31 Zhou L-J, Zhu X-Z. Reactive oxygen species-induced apoptosis in PC12 cells and protective effect of bilobalide. *J Pharmacol Exp Ther* 2000; **293**: 982–988.

32 Calapai G *et al*. Neuroprotective effects of *Ginkgo biloba* extract in brain ischaemia are mediated by inhibition of nitric oxide synthesis. *Life Sci* 2000; **67**: 2673–2683.

33 Rasetti MF *et al*. Extracts of *Ginkgo biloba* L. leaves and *Vaccinium myrtillus* L. fruits prevent photo induced oxidation of low density lipoprotein cholesterol. *Phytomedicine* 1996/97; **3**: 335–338.

34 Drieu K *et al*. Effect of the extract of *Ginkgo biloba* (EGb 761) on the circulating and cellular profiles of polyunsaturated fatty acids: correlation with the anti-oxidant properties of the extract. *Prostaglandins Leukot Essent Fatty Acids* 2000; **63**: 293–300.

35 Bridi R *et al*. The antioxidant activity of standardized extract of *Ginkgo biloba* (EGb 761) in rats. *Phytother Res* 2001; **15**: 449–451.

36 Bahcecioglu IH *et al*. Protective effect of *Ginkgo biloba* extract on CCl_4-induced liver damage.

Hepatol Res 1999; **15**: 215–224.

37 Agha AM *et al*. Chemopreventive effect of *Ginkgo biloba* extract against benzo(a)pyrene-induced forestomach carcinogenesis in mice: amelioration of doxorubicin cardiotoxicity. *J Exp Clin Cancer Res* 2001; **20**: 39–50.

38 Papadopoulos V *et al*. Drug-induced inhibition of the peripheral-type benzodiazepine receptor expression and cell proliferation in human breast cancer cells. *Anticancer Res* 2000; **20**: 2835–2848.

39 Naidu MUR *et al*. *Ginkgo biloba* extract ameliorates gentamicin-induced nephrotoxicity in rats. *Phytomedicine* 2000; **7**: 191–197.

40 White HL *et al*. Extracts of *Ginkgo biloba* leaves inhibit monoamine oxidase. *Life Sci* 1996; **58**: 1315–1321.

41 Sasaki K *et al*. Effects of bilobalide on gamma-aminobutyric acid levels and glutamic acid decarboxylase in mouse brain. *Eur J Pharmacol* 1999; **367**: 165–173.

42 Itokawa H *et al*. Antitumour principles from *Ginkgo biloba* L. *Chem Pharm Bull* 1987; **35**: 3016–3020.

43 Kleijnen J, Knipschild P. *Ginkgo biloba* for cerebral insufficiency. *Br J Clin Pharmacol* 1992; **34**: 352–358.

44 Oken BS *et al*. The efficacy of *Ginkgo biloba* on cognitive function in Alzheimer disease. *Arch Neurol* 1998; **55**: 1409–1415.

45 Ernst E, Pittler MH. *Ginkgo biloba* for dementia. A systematic review of double-blind, placebo-controlled trials. *Clin Drug Invest* 1999; **17**: 301–308.

46 Ernst E, Stevinson C. *Ginkgo biloba* for tinnitus: a review. *Clin Otolaryngol* 1999; **24**: 164–167.

47 Pittler MH, Ernst E. *Ginkgo biloba* extract for the treatment of intermittent claudication: a meta-analysis of randomized trials. *Am J Med* 2000; **108**: 276–281.

48 Kanowski S *et al*. Proof of efficacy of the *Ginkgo biloba* special extract Egb 761 in outpatients suffering from mild to moderate primary degenerative dementia of the Alzheimer type or multi-infarct dementia. *Phytomedicine* 1997; **4**: 3–13.

49 Le Bars P *et al*. A placebo-controlled, double-blind, randomized trial of an extract of *Ginkgo biloba* for dementia. *JAMA* 1997; **278**: 1327–1332.

50 Winther K *et al*. Effects of *Ginkgo biloba* extract on cognitive function and blood pressure in elderly subjects. *Curr Ther Res* 1998; **59**: 881–888.

51 Brautigam MRH *et al*. Treatment of age-related memory complaints with *Ginkgo biloba* extract: a randomized double blind placebo-controlled study. *Phytomedicine* 1998; **5**: 425–434.

52 Itil TM *et al*. The pharmacological effects of *Ginkgo biloba*, a plant extract, on the brain of dementia patients in comparison with tacrine.

Psychopharmacol Bull 1998; **34**: 391–397.

53 Kennedy DO *et al*. The dose-dependent cognitive effects of acute administration of *Ginkgo biloba* to healthy young volunteers. *Psychopharmacology* 2000; **151**: 416–423.

54 Subhan Z, Hindmarsh I. The psychopharmacological effects of *Ginkgo biloba* extract in normal healthy volunteers. *Int J Clin Pharmacol Res* 1984; **4**: 89–93.

55 Rigney U *et al*. The effects of acute doses of standardized *Ginkgo biloba* extract on memory and psychomotor performance in volunteers. *Phytother Res* 1999; **13**: 408–415.

56 Mix JA, Crews WD. An examination of the efficacy of *Ginkgo biloba* extract EGb 761 on the neuropsychological functioning of cognitively intact older adults. *J Altern Complement Med* 2000; **6**: 219–229.

57 Cockle SM *et al*. The effects of *Ginkgo biloba* extract (LI 1370) supplementation on activities of daily living in free living older volunteers: a questionnaire survey. *Hum Psychopharmacol* 2000; **15**: 227–235.

58 Drew S, Davies E. Effectiveness of *Ginkgo biloba* in treating tinnitus: double blind, placebo controlled trial. *BMJ* 2001; **322**: 73–75.

59 Ernst E. Marketing studies and scientific research must be distinct. *BMJ* 2001; **322**: 1249.

60 Bukovics K *et al*. Vergleich von Ginkgo biloba und 6% HES 200/0,5 in der Behandlung des akuten Hörsturzes. *J Pharmakol Ther* 1999; **2**: 48–56.

61 Pittler MH, Ernst E. *Ginkgo biloba* extract for the treatment of intermittent claudication: a meta-analysis of randomised trials. *Am J Med* 2000; **108**: 276–281.

62 Janssens D *et al*. Increase in circulating endothelial cells in patients with primary chronic venous insufficiency: protective effect of Ginkor Fort in a randomized double-blind, placebo-controlled clinical trial. *J Cardiovasc Pharmacol* 1999; **33**: 7–11.

63 Pizzorno JE, Murray MT. *A Textbook of Natural Medicine*. Seattle, WA: John Bastyr College Publications, 1985 (looseleaf).

64 Chung KF. Effect of a ginkgolide mixture (BN 52063) in antagonising skin and platelet responses to platelet activating factor in man. *Lancet* 1987; **i**: 248–251.

65 Wilkens JH *et al*. Effects of a PAF-antagonist (BN 52063) on bronchoconstriction and platelet activation during exercise-induced asthma. *Br J Clin Pharmacol* 1990; **29**: 85–91.

66 Cohen AJ, Bartlik B. *Ginkgo biloba* for antidepressant-induced sexual dysfunction. *J Sex Marital Ther* 1998; **24**: 139–143.

67 Wheatley D. *Ginkgo biloba* in the treatment of sexual dysfunction due to antidepressant drugs. *Hum Psychopharmacol* 1999; **14**: 511–513.

68 Balon R. *Ginkgo biloba* for antidepressant-induced sexual dysfunction? *J Sex Marital Ther* 1999; **10**: 1–2.

69 Evans JR. *Ginkgo biloba* extract for age-related macular degeneration (Cochrane review). In: *The Cochrane Library*, Issue 3, 2001. Oxford: Update Software, 2001.

70 Lingjaerde O *et al*. Can winter depression be prevented by *Ginkgo biloba* extract? A placebo-controlled trial. *Acta Psychiatr Scand* 1999; **100**: 62–66.

71 Hemmeter U *et al*. Polysomnographic effects of adjuvant *Ginkgo biloba* therapy in patients with major depression medicated with trimipramine. *Pharmacopsychiatry* 2001; **34**: 50–59.

72 Tamborini A, Taurelle R. *Rev Fr Gynecol Obstet* 1993; **88**: 147. Cited by Bone K. Treatment of congestive symptoms of premenstrual syndrome with ginkgo. *Br J Phytother* 1995/96; **4**: 46.

73 Zhang XY *et al*. The effect of extract of *Ginkgo biloba* added to haloperidol on superoxide dismutase in inpatients with chronic schizophrenia. *J Clin Psychopharmacol* 2001; **21**: 85–88.

74 Bombardelli E *et al*. Activity of phospholipid-complex of *Ginkgo biloba* dimeric flavonoids on the skin microcirculation. *Fitoterapia* 1996; **67**: 265–273.

75 Hauns B *et al*. Phase II study of combined 5-fluorouracil/*Ginkgo biloba* extract (GBE 761 ONC) therapy in 5-fluorouracil pretreated patients with advanced colorectal cancer. *Phytother Res* 2001; **15**: 34–38.

76 DeFeudis FV. Safety of EGb 761-containing products. In: DeFeudis FV, ed. *Ginkgo biloba Extract (EGb 761). Pharmacological Activities and Clinical Applications*. Amsterdam: Elsevier, 1991.

77 Rosenblatt M, Mindel J. Spontaneous hyphema associated with ingestion of *Ginkgo biloba* extract. *N Engl J Med* 1997; **336**: 1108.

78 Vale S. Subarachnoid haemorrhage associated with *Ginkgo biloba*. *Lancet* 1998; **352**: 36.

79 Rowin J, Lewis SL. Spontaneous bilateral subdural hematomas associated with chronic *Ginkgo biloba* ingestion. *Neurology* 1996; **46**: 1775–1776.

80 Donadio V *et al*. Myoglobinuria after ingestion of extracts of guarana, *Ginkgo biloba* and kava. *Neurol Sci* 2000; **21**: 124.

81 Houghton PJ. Ginkgo. *Pharm J* 1994; **253**: 122–123.

82 Braquet P, ed. *Ginkgolides – Chemistry, Biology, Pharmacology and Clinical Perspectives*, vol 1. Barcelona: JR Prous, 1988.

83 Braquet P, ed. *Ginkgolides – Chemistry, Biology, Pharmacology and Clinical Perspectives*, vol 2. Barcelona: JR Prous, 1989.

Ginseng, Eleutherococcus

Species (Family)

Eleutherococcus senticosus (Rupr. & Maxim.) Maxim. (Araliaceae)

Synonym(s)

Acanthopanax senticosus, Devil's Shrub, Eleuthero, *Hedera senticosa*, Siberian Ginseng, Touch-Me-Not, Wild Pepper

Part(s) Used

Root

Pharmacopoeial and Other Monographs

BHC 1992[G6]
BHP 1996[G9]
BP 2001[G15]
Complete German Commission E[G3]
Martindale 32nd edition[G43]
Mills and Bone[G50]
PDR for Herbal Medicines 2nd edition[G36]
Ph Eur 2002[G28]

Legal Category (Licensed Products)

Eleutherococcus ginseng is not included in the GSL.[G37]

Constituents[1,2,G6]

Eleutherosides A–M Heterogeneous group of compounds including sterol(A), phenylpropanoid(B), coumarin (B1, B3), monosaccharide(C), and lignan(B₄,D,E) structural types; many present as glycosides. Characterised eleutherosides include daucosterol(A), syringin(B), isofraxidin glucoside(B₁), (−)-sesamin(B₄), methyl-α-D-galactoside(C), (−)-syringaresinol glucoside(D), acanthoside D(E) and hedera-saponin B(M).

Carbohydrates Polysaccharides (glycans); some have been referred to as eleutherans.[3] Galactose, glucose, maltose, sucrose.

Some of the additional documented constituents represent aglycones of the eleutherosides, namely β-sitosterol, isofraxidin, (−)-syringaresinol and sinapyl alcohol.

Phenylpropanoids Caffeic acid and ester, coniferyl aldehyde.

Terpenoids Oleanolic acid.

Volatile oils 0.8%. Individual components not documented.

Food Use

Eleutherococcus ginseng is not used in foods.

Herbal Use

Eleutherococcus ginseng does not have a traditional herbal use in the UK, although it has been used for many years in the former Soviet Union. Like Panax ginseng, Eleutherococcus ginseng is claimed to be an adaptogen in that it increases the body's resistance to stress and builds up general vitality.[G6,G8,G49]

Dosage

Dry root 0.6–3 g daily for up to one month has been recommended.[G6,G49] Russian studies in healthy human subjects have involved the administration of an ethanolic extract in doses ranging from 2 to 16 mL one to three times daily, for up to 60 consecutive days.

Doses in non-healthy individuals ranged from 0.5 to 6.0 mL one to three times daily for up to 35 days. In both groups, multiple dosing regimens were separated by an extract-free period of two to three weeks.[1]

Pharmacological Actions

The adaptogenic properties of Eleutherococcus ginseng have been extensively investigated in the countries of the former USSR. Pharmacological studies on extracts of Eleutherococcus ginseng started in the 1950s and have been primarily reported by two groups of Russian scientists. In 1962, a 33% ethanolic extract of *Eleutherococcus senticosus* was approved for human use by the Pharmacological Committee of USSR Ministry of Health, and in 1976 it was estimated that some three million people were regularly using this extract.[1]

A review by Farnsworth *et al.*[1] describes the chemistry and toxicity of Eleutherococcus ginseng and documents results of *in vitro*, *in vivo* and human studies involving the oral administration of an ethanolic extract.

The majority of literature on Eleutherococcus ginseng has been published in the Russian language and therefore great difficulty is encountered in obtaining translations.[1] This monograph will draw mainly on data included in the Farnsworth review as well as on more recent papers that have been published in English. When used in this monograph , 'ginseng' will refer to Eleutherococcus ginseng unless indicated otherwise.

In vitro and animal studies

Hypo/hyperglycaemic activity Hypo/hyperglycaemic activity has been documented in both normal animals and in those with induced hyperglycaemia (rabbit, mouse), but with little effect on alloxaninduced hyperglycaemia (rat).[1,4] Hypoglycaemic activity (mice, intraperitoneal injection) of an aqueous ginseng extract has been attributed to polysaccharide components termed eleutherans A–G.[5]

Central nervous system effects Sedative actions (rat, mouse), CNS-stimulant effects (intravenous/subcutaneous injection, rabbit), and a decrease/increase in barbiturate sleeping time has been reported.[1,6]

Immunostimulant, antitoxic actions Increased resistance to induced listeriosis infection (mouse, rabbit) with prophylactic ginseng administration and reduced resistance with simultaneous administration, stimulation of specific antiviral immunity (guinea-pig, mouse), regulation of complement titre and lysozyme activity post immunisation have been documented.[1] In addition, protection against cardiac glycoside (intravenous injection, frog), diethylglycolic acid (mouse) and alloxan (rat) toxicity has also been described.[1] Immune stimulant effects have been reported for polysaccharide components, together with an ability to lessen thioacetamide, phytohaemagglutinin and X-ray toxicity, and to exhibit antitumour effects.[5] Immunostimulant activity *in vitro* (using granulocyte, carbon clearance and lymphocyte-transformation tests) has been documented for high molecular weight polysaccharide components.[7,8]

Effects on overall performance A beneficial action on parameters indicative of stress (rat) and on overall work capacity (mouse) has been reported,[1] although a lack of adaptogenic response has also been reported in mice receiving various ginseng infusions (Siberian, Korean and American).[9,10] In one study, mice receiving a commercial concentrated extract of eleutherococcus ginseng were noted to exhibit significantly more aggressive behaviour.[9] Ginseng is claimed to result in a more economical utilisation of glycogen and high-energy phosphorus compounds, and in a more intense metabolism of lactic and pyruvic acids during stress.[1] It has been claimed that the adaptogenic effect of ginseng involves regulation of energy, nucleic acid, and protein metabolism in tissues.[1]

Steroidal activity Gonadotrophic activity in immature male mice (intraperitoneal injection), oestrogenic activity in immature female mice, and an anabolic effect in immature rats (intraperitoneal injection) has been reported.[1] *In vitro* studies have reported that ginseng extracts bind to progestin, mineralocorticoid, glucocorticoid and oestrogen receptors.[1]

Cardiovascular activity 3,4-Dihydroxybenzoic acid (DBA) has been identified as an anti-aggregatory component in eleutherococcus ginseng.[3] Compared with aspirin, activity of DBA was comparable versus collagen- and ADP-induced platelet aggregation, but less potent versus arachidonic acid-induced platelet aggregation.[3] Anti-oedema and anti-inflammatory actions (intravenous injection, mouse), have also been described.[1]

Effect on reproductive capacity Ginseng has been reported to improve the reproductive capacity of bulls and cows, and to have no adverse effects on the various blood parameters (haemoglobin, total plasma protein, albumin and globulin, protein coefficient) measured.[1]

Other actions documented for ginseng include the stimulation of liver regeneration in partially hepatectomised mice,[1] an increase in catecholamine concentrations in the brain, adrenal gland and urine,[1] a variable effect on induced hypothermia (rabbit, rat, mouse),[1] and *in vitro* inhibition (66%) of hexobarbitone metabolism.[6]

Clinical studies

In Russia, ginseng extract has been administered orally to more than 4300 human subjects in studies involving either healthy or non-healthy individuals.[1]

Administration to healthy subjects These studies were designed to investigate the adaptogenic effects of ginseng and measured parameters such as the ability of humans to withstand adverse conditions (heat, noise, motion, workload increase, exercise, decompression), improvement in auditory disturbances, quality of work under stress conditions and in athletic performance, and increase in mental alertness and work output.[1] The studies involved more than 2100 subjects and included both male and female subjects ranging in age from 19 to 72 years. Doses ranged from 2 to 16 mL of an ethanolic extract (33%), administered orally one to three times daily, for periods of up to 60 consecutive days. Multiple dosing regimens usually involved a two- to three-week interval between courses.[1] For many of the studies, it is unclear whether ginseng had a beneficial effect. However, ginseng was found to exert favourable effects in a number of situations including ability to perform physical labour, quality of proofreading, adaptation to a high-temperature environment, speed and quality of work by radiotelegraphers in noisy conditions, resistance to hypoxaemia and physical burdens in skiers, ability to withstand conditions designed to induce motion sickness, capillary resistance, haematological parameters in blood donors, and number of days lost to sickness amongst factory workers. Ginseng was also reported to increase excretion of vitamins B_1, B_2 and C given concurrently with ginseng. On its own, ginseng did not affect the excretion of water-soluble vitamins.

Administration to non-healthy subjects These studies involved more than 2200 subjects with various ailments and included both males and females ranging in age from 19 to 60 years. Ginseng doses ranging from 0.5 to 6 mL were administered orally between one to three times daily for up to 35 days, with as many as eight courses employed. Multiple dosing regimens involved a two- to three-week ginseng-free interval in between courses.[1] A favourable effect was noted in atherosclerosis (although treatment was stated to be less effective in patients with high blood pressure), acute pyelonephritis, various forms of diabetes mellitus (although no marked effect was noted in another study), hypertension and hypotension (tendency to normalisation), acute craniocerebral trauma, various types of neuroses, rheumatic heart disease (reduced blood coagulation properties), chronic bronchitis, and in children with abating forms of pulmonary tuberculosis.[1] An increase in the working capacity of six males, in a single blind crossover study using placebo and no treatment as comparators, has been reported for a 33% ethanolic ginseng extract.[11] The observed increase in working capacity was partially attributed to an improvement in bodily oxygen metabolism, reflected by the increase in all four measured parameters (oxygen

uptake, oxygen pulse, total work and exhaustion time).[12]

Immunostimulant activity A strong immunomodulatory effect has been documented for an ethanolic extract of ginseng, in a placebo-controlled double-blind study using healthy volunteers.[13] A significant increase in the total lymphocyte count, especially in the T lymphocyte cells, was noted in the ginseng-treated group who received a daily dose of 30–40 mL extract (eleutheroside B 0.2% w/v). Specificity of action on the lymphocytes was confirmed by the fact that neither granulocyte or monocyte levels were significantly altered.[13]

Side-effects, Toxicity

No side-effects were documented from Russian studies involving more than 2100 healthy subjects.[1] Studies involving patients with various ailments have reported a few side-effects: insomnia, shifts in heart rhythm, tachycardia, extrasystole and hypertonia in some atherosclerotic patients; headaches, pericardial pain, palpitations, and elevated blood pressure in 2 of 55 patients (at high dose level) with rheumatic heart disease; insomnia, irritability, melancholy and anxiety in hypochondriac patients receiving higher doses of extract; hypersensitivity reaction (symptoms unspecified) in stressed individuals.[1] Hypertension and mastalgia have been documented as side-effects of ginseng (species unknown).[11]

Results of various animal toxicity studies have indicated ginseng to be non-toxic.[1] Many species have been exposed to extracts including mice, rats, rabbits, dogs, minks, deer, lambs, and piglets.[1] Documented acute oral LD_{50} values for various preparations include: 23 mL/kg and 14.5 g/kg (mice), and greater than 20 mL/kg (dogs) for a 33% ethanolic extract[1,4]; 31 g/kg (mice) for the powdered root; greater than 3 g/kg (mice) for an aqueous aqueous (equivalent to 25 g dried roots/kg).[4] No deaths occurred in mice administered single 3 g/kg doses of a freeze-dried aqueous extract.[12] Symptoms observed in dogs receiving 7.1 mL/kg doses of the ethanolic extract (sedation, ataxia, loss of righting reflex, hypopnoea, tremors, increased salivation and vomiting) were attributed to the ethanol content of the extract.[1] A chronic toxicity study reported no toxic manifestations or deaths in rats fed 5 mL/kg ethanolic extract for 320 days.[1]

Teratogenicity studies in male and female rats, pregnant minks, rabbits and lambs have reported no abnormalities in the offspring and no adverse effects in the animals administered the extracts. Premature death in parent female rabbits fed 13.5 mL/kg ethanolic extract daily was attributed to ethanol intoxication.[1]

Mutagenicity studies using *Salmonella typhimurium* TA100 and TA98, and the micronucleus test in mice have reported no activity for ginseng.[14] Differences in various serum biochemical parameters have been reported between test (ginseng) and control groups.[14] Parameters affected included alkaline phosphatase and gamma-glutamyl transferase enzymes (increased), serum triglycerides (decreased), and creatinine and blood urea nitrogen (increased).[14] No pathological changes were found in rats receiving a ginseng extract.[14]

Contra-indications, Warnings

It has been stated that ginseng should be avoided by individuals who are highly energetic, nervous, tense, hysteric, manic or schizophrenic, and that it should not be taken with stimulants, including coffee, antipsychotic drugs or during treatment with hormones.[11] In view of documented pharmacological actions, ginseng may interfere with a number of therapies including cardiac, anticoagulant, hypoglycaemic and hypo/hypertensive. Ginseng is stated to be unsuitable for individuals with high blood pressure (180/90 mmHg or greater)[1] and has been advised to be avoided by premenopausal women.[11]

Russian recommendations advise that healthy people under the age of 40 should not use ginseng and that middle-aged people can be treated with small doses of ginseng on a daily basis.[11] Individuals considered suitable to use ginseng are recommended to abstain from alcoholic beverages, sexual activity, bitter substances and spicy foods.[11]

In general, long-term use of ginseng is not recommended and one author has documented that the main side-effect of prolonged use manifests as an inflamed nerve, frequently the sciatic, which then causes muscle spasm in the affected area.[11] Human studies involving long-term administration of ginseng have involved ginseng-free periods of 2–3 weeks every 30–60 days.

Pregnancy and lactation Teratogenicity studies in various animal species have not reported any teratogenic effects for ginseng. However, in view of the many pharmacological actions documented for ginseng, and the general recommendation that it should not be used by premenopausal women, the use of ginseng during both pregnancy and lactation should be avoided. It is unknown whether the pharmacologically active constituents in ginseng are secreted in the breast milk.

Pharmaceutical Comment

Phytochemical studies have revealed that there is no one constituent type that is characteristic of Eleutherococcus ginseng. Studies have shown that components thought to represent the main active constituents ('eleutherosides') consist of a heterogeneous mixture of common plant constituents. Since the 1950s, many studies (animal and human) have been carried out in Russia, and more recently in Western countries, to investigate the reputed adaptogen properties of Eleutherococcus ginseng. An adaptogen is a substance that is defined as having three characteristics, namely lack of toxicity, non-specific action, and a normalising action.[1] Results of numerous studies in animals and humans seem to support these three criteria for Eleutherococcus ginseng, although pharmacological explanations for the observed actions are less well understood.[1] As with Panax ginseng, Eleutherococcus ginseng has been shown to possess a wide range of pharmacological activities. Consequently, it should be used with appropriate regard to traditional guidelines that have been drawn up in China and Russia.

References

See also General References G3, G5, G6, G8, G9, G15, G28, G31, G32, G36, G37, G43, G49, G50 and G56.

1 Farnsworth NR *et al*. Siberian ginseng (*Eleutherococcus senticosus*): Current status as an adaptogen. In: Wagner H *et al*., eds. *Economics and Medicinal Plant Research*, vol 1, London: Academic Press, 1985: 155–209.

2 Phillipson JD, Anderson LA. Ginseng – quality, safety and efficacy? *Pharm J* 1984; **232**: 161–165.

3 Yun-Choi HS *et al*. Potential inhibitors of platelet aggregation from plant sources, III. *J Nat Prod* 1987; **50**: 1059–1064.

4 Medon PJ *et al*. Hypoglycaemic effect and toxicity of *Eleutherococcus senticosus* following acute and chronic administration in mice. *Acta Pharmacol Sin* 1981; **2**: 281–285.

5 Hikino H *et al*. Isolation and hypoglycaemic activity of eleutherans A, B, C, D, E, F, and G: Glycans of *Eleutherococcus senticosus* roots. *J Nat Prod* 1986; **49**: 293–297.

6 Medon PJ *et al*. Effects of *Eleutherococcus*

senticosus extracts on hexobarbital metabolism *in vivo* and *in vitro*. *J Ethnopharmacol* 1984; **10**: 235–241.

7   Wagner H *et al*. Immunstimulierend wirkende Polysaccharide (heteroglykane) aus höheren Pflanzen. *Arzneimittelforschung* 1985; **35**: 1069.

8   Wagner H. Immunostimulants from medicinal plants. In: Chang HM *et al*., eds. *Advances in Chinese Medicinal Materials Research*. Singapore: World Scientific, 1985: 159.

9   Lewis WH *et al*. No adaptogen response of mice to ginseng and *Eleutherococcus* infusions. *J Ethnopharmacol* 1983; **8**: 209–214.

10 Martinez B, Staba EJ. The physiological effects of *Aralia*, *Panax* and *Eleutherococcus* on exercised rats. *Jpn J Pharmacol* 1984; **35**: 79–85.

11 Baldwin CA *et al*. What pharmacists should know about ginseng. *Pharm J* 1986; **237**: 583.

12 Asano K *et al*. Effect of *Eleutherococcus senticosus* extract on human physical working capacity. *Planta Med* 1986; **52**: 175.

13 Bohn B *et al*. Flow-cytometric studies with *Eleutherococcus senticosus* extract as an immunomodulatory agent. *Arzneimittelforschung* 1987; **37**: 1193–1196.

14 Hirosue T *et al*. Mutagenicity and subacute toxicity of *Acanthopanax senticosus* extracts in rats. *J Food Hyg Soc Jpn* 1986; **27**: 380–386.

Ginseng, Panax

Species (Family)

Various *Panax* species (Araliaceae) including:
(i) *Panax ginseng* Meyer
(ii) *Panax quinquefolius* L.
(iii) *Panax notoginseng* (Burkh.) Hoo & Tseng

Synonym(s)

(i) Asiatic Ginseng, Chinese Ginseng, Japanese Ginseng, Jintsam, Korean Ginseng, Ninjin, Oriental Ginseng, *Panax pseudoginseng Wall.*, *Panax schinseng* Nees, Schinsent
(ii) American Ginseng, Sanchi Ginseng and Tienchi Ginseng
(iii) American Ginseng, Five-Fingers, Sang and Western Ginseng

Part(s) Used

Root. White ginseng represents the peeled and sun-dried root whilst red ginseng is unpeeled, steamed and dried.

Pharmacopoeial and Other Monographs

BHC 1992[G6]
BHP 1996[G9]
BP 2001[G15]
Complete German Commission E[G3]
Martindale 32nd edition[G43]
Mills and Bone[G50]
PDR for Herbal Medicines 2nd edition[G36]
Ph Eur 2002[G28]
USP24/NF19[G61]

Legal Category (Licensed Products)

GSL[G37]

Constituents[G2,G6,G41,G64]

Terpenoids Complex mixture of compounds (ginpanaxosides) involves three aglycone structural types – two tetracyclic dammarane-type sapogenins (protopanaxadiol and protopanaxatriol) and a pentacyclic triterpene oleanolic acid-type. Different naming conventions have been used for these compounds. In Japan, they are known as ginsenosides and are represented by R_x where 'x' indicates a particular saponin. For example, R_a, R_{b-1}, R_c, R_d, R_{g-1}. In Russia, the saponins are referred to as panaxosides and are represented as panaxoside X where 'X' can be A–F. The suffixes in the two systems are not equivalent and thus panaxoside A does not equal R_a but R_{g-1}.[1]

The saponin content varies between different *Panax* species. For example, in *P. ginseng* the major ginsenosides are R_{b-1}, R_c and R_{g-1} whereas in *P. quinquefolis* R_{b-1} is the only major ginsenoside.[1]

Other constituents Volatile oil (trace) mainly consisting of sesquiterpenes including panacene, limonene, terpineol, eucalyptol, α-phellandrene and citral,[2] sesquiterpene alcohols including the pana-sinsanols A and B, and ginsenol,[3,4] polyacetylenes,[5,6] sterols, polysaccharides (mainly pectins and glucans),[7] starch (8–32%), β-amylase,[8] free sugars, vitamins (B_1, B_2, B_{12}, panthotenic acid, biotin), choline (0.1–0.2%), fats, minerals.

The sesquiterpene alcohols are stated to be characteristic components of *Panax ginseng* in that they are absent from the volatile oils of other *Panax* species.[4]

Food Use

Ginseng is listed by the Council of Europe as a natural source of food flavouring (category N2). This category indicates that ginseng can be added to foodstuffs in small quantities, with a possible limitation of an active principle (as yet unspecified) in the final product.[G16]

Herbal Use

Ginseng is stated to possess thymoleptic, sedative, demulcent and stomachic properties, and is reputed to be an aphrodisiac. Traditionally, it has been used for neurasthenia, neuralgia, insomnia, hypotonia, and specifically for depressive states associated with sexual inadequacy.[G2,G6,G8,G64]

Ginseng has been used traditionally in Chinese medicine for many thousands of years as a stimulant, tonic, diuretic and stomachic.[9] Traditionally, ginseng use has been divided into two categories: short-term – to improve stamina, concentration, healing process, stress resistance, vigilance and work efficiency in healthy individuals, and long-term – to improve well-being in debilitated and degenerative conditions especially those associated with old age.

Dosage

Traditionally, dosage recommendations differ between the short-term use in healthy individuals and the long-term use in elderly or debilitated persons.

Short-term (for the young and healthy) 0.5–1.0 g root daily, as two divided doses, for a course generally lasting 15–20 days and with a root-free period of approximately two weeks between consecutive courses. Doses are recommended to be taken in the morning, 2 hours before a meal, and in the evening, not less than 2 hours after a meal.[9]

Long-term (for the old and sick) 0.4–0.8 g root daily. Doses may be taken continuously.[1]

Pharmacological Actions

In the 1950s, early studies on ginseng reported its ability to improve both physical endurance and mental ability in animals and humans.[10] In addition, the 'tonic' properties of ginseng were confirmed by the observation that doses taken for a prolonged period of time increased the overall well-being of an individual, measured by various parameters such as appetite, sleep and absence of moodiness, resulting in an increased work efficiency. Furthermore, these effects were felt for some time after cessation of ginseng treatment.[10] In addition, gonadotrophic activity, slight anti-inflammatory activity and an effect on carbohydrate metabolism were noted.[10] Since then, numerous studies have investigated the complex pharmacology of ginseng in both animals and humans. The saponin glycosides (ginsenosides/ panaxosides) are generally recognised as the main active constituents in ginseng, although pharmacological activities have also been associated with non-saponin components.

The following sections on animal and human studies are intended to give an indication of the type of research that has been published for ginseng rather than to provide a comprehensive bibliography of ginseng research papers.

In vitro and animal studies

Corticosteroid-like activity Many of the activities exhibited by Panax ginseng have been compared to corticosteroid-like actions and results of endocrinological studies have suggested that the ginsenosides may primarily augment adrenal steroidogenesis via

an indirect action on the pituitary gland.[11] Ginsenosides have increased adrenal cAMP in intact but not in hypophysectomised rats and dexamethasone, a synthetic glucocorticoid that provides positive feedback at the level of the pituitary gland, has blocked the effect of ginsenosides on pituitary corticotrophin and adrenal corticosterone secretion.[11] Hormones produced by the pituitary and adrenal glands are known to play a significant role in the adaptation capabilities of the body.[12] Working capacity is one of the indices used to measure adaptation ability and ginseng has been shown to increase the working capacity of rats following single (132%) and seven-day (179%) administration (intraperitoneal). Furthermore, seven-day administration of ginseng decreased the reduction seen in working capacity when the pituitary–adrenocortical system is blocked by prior administration of hydrocortisone.[12]

Hypoglycaemic activity Hypoglycaemic activity has been documented for ginseng and attributed to both saponin and polysaccharide constituents. *In vitro* studies using isolated rat pancreatic islets have shown that ginsenosides promote an insulin release which is independent of extracellular calcium and which utilises a different mechanism to that of glucose.[13] In addition, *in vivo* studies in rats have reported that a ginseng extract increases the number of insulin receptors in bone marrow and reduces the number of glucocorticoid receptors in rat brain homogenate.[14] Both of these actions are thought to contribute to the antidiabetic action of ginseng, in view of the known diabetogenic action of adrenal corticoids and the knowledge that the number of insulin receptors generally decreases with ageing.[14]

Hypoglycaemic activity observed in both normal and alloxan-induced hyperglycaemic mice administered ginseng (intraperitoneal) has also been attributed to non-saponin but uncharacterised principles[15–18] and to glycan (polysaccharide) components, Panaxans A–E and Q–U.[19–23] Glycans isolated from Korean ginseng or Chinese ginseng (A–E) were found to possess stronger hypoglycaemic activity than those isolated from Japanese ginseng (Q–U).[23] Proposed mechanisms of action have included elevated plasma insulin concentration due to an increase of insulin secretion from pancreatic islets, and enhancement of insulin sensitivity.[21] However, these mechanisms do not explain the total hypoglycaemic activity that has been exhibited by the polysaccharides and further mechanisms are under investigation.[21]

The effect of panaxans A and B on the activities of key enzymes participating in carbohydrate metabolism has been studied.[18] DPG-3-2, a non-saponin component isolated from ginseng, has been shown to stimulate insulin biosynthesis in pancreatic preparations from various hyperglycaemic (but not normoglycaemic) animals; ginsenosides Rb_1 and Rg_1 were found to decrease islet insulin concentrations to an undetectable level.[16]

Cardiovascular activity Individual saponins have been reported to have different actions on cardiac haemodynamics.[24] For instance R_g, R_{g-1} and total flower saponins have increased cardiac performance whilst R_b and total leaf saponins have decreased it; calcium antagonist activity has been reported for R_b but not for R_g; R_b but not R_g has produced a protective effect on experimental myocardial infarction in rabbits.[24] Negative chronotropic and inotropic effects *in vitro* have been observed for ginseng saponins and a mechanism of action similar to that of verapamil has been suggested.[25] *In vitro* studies on the isolated rabbit heart have reported an increase in coronary blood flow together with a positive inotropic effect.[26] Anti-arrhythmic action on aconitine and barium chloride (rat) and adrenaline (rabbit)-induced arrhythmias, and prolongation of RR, PR and QT_c intervals (rat), have been documented for saponins R_{c-1} and R_{d-1}. The mode of action was thought to be similar to that of amiodarone.[27] Ginsenosides (i.p.) have been reported to protect mice against metabolic disturbances and myocardial damage associated with conditions of severe anoxia.[28]

Ginseng has produced a marked hypotensive response together with bradycardia following intravenous administration to rats. The dose-related effect was blocked by many antagonists suggesting multi-site activity.[26] Higher doses of ginseng were found to cause vasoconstriction rather than vasodilation in renal, mesenteric and femoral arteries.[26]

The total ginseng saponin fraction has been reported to be devoid of haemolytic activity. However, individual ginsenosides have been found to exhibit either haemolytic or protective activities. Protective ginsenosides include R_c, R_{b-2} and R_e, whereas haemolytic saponins have included R_g, R_h and R_f.[29] The number and position of sugars attached to the sapogenin moiety was thought to determine activity.[29] Haemostatic activity has also been documented for ginseng.[30]

Oral administration of ginseng to rats fed a high cholesterol diet reduced serum cholesterol and triglycerides, increased high-density lipoprotein (HDL) cholesterol, decreased platelet adhesiveness, and decreased fatty changes to the liver.[31] Ginseng has also been reported to reduce blood coagulation and enhance fibrinolysis.[32] Panaxynol and the ginsenosides R_o, R_{g-1} and R_{g-2} have been documented as the main antiplatelet components in ginseng inhibiting aggregation, release reaction and thromboxane formation *in vitro*.[32] Anti-inflammatory activity and inhibition of thromboxane B_2 have previously been described for panaxynol.[32] Anticomplementary activity *in vitro* (human serum) has been documented for ginseng polysaccharides with highest activity observed in strongly acidic polysaccharide fractions.[7]

Effects on neurotransmitters Studies in rats have shown that a standardised ginseng extract (G115) inhibits the development of morphine tolerance and physical dependence, of a decrease in hepatic glutathione concentrations, and of dopamine receptor sensitivity without antagonising morphine analgesia, as previously documented for the individual saponins.[33] The inhibition of tolerance was thought to be associated with a reduction in morphinone production, a toxic metabolite which irreversibly blocks the opiate receptor sites, and with the activation of morphinone–glutathione conjugation, a detoxication process. The mechanism of inhibition of physical dependence was unclear but thought to be associated with changed ratios of adrenaline, noradrenaline, dopamine and serotonin in the brain.[33]

A total ginsenoside fraction has been reported to inhibit the uptake of various neurotransmitters into rat brain synaptosomes in descending order of gamma-aminobutyrate and noradrenaline, dopamine, glutamate and serotonin.[34–36] The fraction containing ginsenoside R_d was most effective. Uptake of metabolic substrates 2-deoxy-D-glucose and leucine was only slightly affected and therefore it was proposed that the ginseng extracts were acting centrally rather than locally as surface active agents.

Studies in rats have indicated that the increase in dopaminergic receptors in the brain observed under conditions of stress is prevented by pretreatment with ginseng.[37]

Hepatoprotective activity Antioxidant and detoxifying activities have been documented for ginseng.[38] Protection against carbon tetrachloride- and galactosamine-induced hepatotoxicity has been observed in cultured rat hepatocytes for specific ginsenosides (oleanolic acid and dammarane series).[38,39] However, at higher doses certain ginsenosides from both series were found to exhibit simultaneous cytotoxic activity.[36]

Cytotoxic and antitumour activity Cytotoxic activity (ED_{50} 0.5 µg/mL) versus L1210 has been documented for polyacetylenes isolated from the root.[5,6,40] The antitumour effect of ginseng polysaccharides in tumour-bearing mice has been associated with an immunological mechanism of action.[41] Ginseng polysaccharides have been reported to increase the lifespan of tumour-bearing mice and to inhibit the growth of tumour cells *in vivo*, although cytocidal action was not seen *in vitro*.[41] Antitumour activity *in vitro* versus several tumour cell lines has been documented for a polyacetylene, panaxytriol.[42,]

Antiviral activity Antiviral activity (versus Semliki forest virus; 34–40% protection) has been documented for ginseng extract (G115,, Pharmaton) administered orally to rats.[37] The ginseng extract also enhanced the level of protection afforded by 6-MFA,[43] an interferon-inducing agent of fungal origin.[43] Ginseng has been found to induce *in vitro* and *in vivo* production of interferon and to augment the natural killer and antibody dependent cytotoxic activities in human peripheral lymphocytes.[43,44] In addition, ginseng enhances the antibody-forming cell response to sheep red blood cells in mice and stimulates cell mediated immunity both *in vitro* and *in vivo*.[43,44] In view of these observations, it has been proposed that the antiviral activity of ginseng may be immunologically mediated.[43,44]

Clinical studies

Improvements in serum total cholesterol, HDL cholesterol, triglycerides, non-essential fatty acids and lipoperoxides have been observed in 67 hyperlipidaemic patients administered 2.7 g/day red ginseng.[27] The addition of ginseng (3 g/65 kg body weight) to alcohol consumption (72 g/65 kg body weight of 25% ethanol) has been reported to enhance blood alcohol clearance by 32–51%.[45]

A preparation containing ginseng extract with multivitamins and trace elements has been shown to modify some indices of metabolic and liver function in elderly patients with chronic hepatotoxicity induced by alcohol and drugs.[46] Patients who received ginseng exhibited an increase in bromo-sulphthalein excretion (which is related to hepatic detoxification) and improved serum zinc concentrations.[46]

A favourable effect on various tests of psychomotor performance (attention, processing, integrated sensory motor function and auditory reaction time) in healthy individuals receiving a ginseng extract (200 mg daily for 12 weeks) has been documented in a double-blind placebo-controlled study.[47] No difference was observed between ginseng and placebo groups in tests of pure motor function, recognition and visual reaction time.[47]

Ginseng has been reported to improve the overall control of status asthmaticus when added to conventional steroid, bronchodilator and antibiotic therapies.[48]

Ginseng has been shown to reduce blood sugar concentrations in both diabetics and non-diabetics,[1] such that in one study insulin therapy was no longer required in a proportion of the patients investigated.[1]

Ginseng has also been reported to normalise both high and low blood pressure states.[1]

Ginseng has been found to affect concentrations of corticosteroids such as adrenocorticotrophic hormone (ACTH) and cortisol and noradrenaline.[1]

Ginseng has been reported to successfully treat cases of diabetic polyneuropathy, reactive depression, psychogenic impotence, enuresis and various child psychiatric disorders.[49]

Side-effects, Toxicity

In Japan, ginseng (panax) has been given to more than 500 individuals over the course of two studies with no side-effects experienced.[1] However, suspected adverse events associated with ginseng treatment have been documented although it is often difficult to assess individual cases due to a lack of information concerning dose, duration of treatment, species of ginseng used, and concurrent medication.[1] Nevertheless, symptoms documented include hypertension[1] (ginseng species unspecified), diarrhoea,[1] insomnia[1] (as a result of over stimulation), mastalgia,[1] skin eruptions[1] and vaginal bleeding[1]. A case of vaginal bleeding in a postmenopausal woman has been associated with the use of a ginseng face cream.[50] In 1979, two studies referred to a ginseng abuse syndrome (GAS) which emphasised that most side-effects documented for ginseng were associated with the ingestion of large doses of ginseng together with other psychomotor stimulants, including tea and coffee.[1] GAS was defined as diarrhoea, hypertension, nervousness, skin eruptions and sleeplessness. Other symptoms occasionally observed included amenorrhoea, decreased appetite, depression, euphoria, hypotension and oedema. However, these two studies have been widely criticised over the variety of ginseng and other preparations used, and over the lack of authentication of the ginseng species ingested.[1] Elsewhere, symptoms of overdose have been described as those exhibited by individuals allergic to ginseng, namely palpitations, insomnia and pruritus, together with heart pain, decrease in sexual potency, vomiting, haemorrhagic diathesis, headache and epistaxis; ingestion of very large doses have even been reported to be fatal.[9]

Two cases of a suspected interaction between ginseng and phenelzine have been documented.[51] Symptoms of headache and tremulousness in one 64-year-old woman and of manic-like symptoms in a 42-year-old woman were described.[51]

Results documented for toxicity studies carried out in a number of animal species using standardised extracts (SE) indicate ginseng to be of low toxicity.[52–56]

Acute toxicity   Single doses of up to 2 g SE have been administered to mice and rats with no toxic effects observed.[55] LD_{50} values (p.o.) in mice and rats have been estimated at 2 g/kg and greater than 5 g/kg.[52] In addition, LD_{50} values (i.p., mice) have been estimated for individual ginsenosides as 305 mg/kg (R_{b-2}), 324 mg/kg (R_d), 405 mg/kg (R_e), 410 mg/kg (R_c), 1110 mg/kg (R_{b-1}), 1250 mg/kg (R_{g-1}), and 1340 mg/kg (R_f); an LD_{50} (i.v., mice) of 3806 mg/kg has been estimated for the saponins R_{c-1} and R_{d-1}.[52]

Subacute toxicity   Doses of approximately 720 mg of a ginseng extract (G115) have been administered orally to rats for 20 days with no side-effects documented.[56]

Chronic toxicity   Daily doses of up to 15 mg G115/kg body weight have been administered orally to dogs for 90 days with no toxic effects documented. An initial increase in excitability which disappeared after two to three weeks was the only observation reported in rats fed 200 mg G115/kg body weight for 25 weeks.[55]

P. quinquefolis has been reported to be devoid of mutagenic potential when investigated versus *Salmonella typhimurium* strain TM677.[57]

Contra-indications, Warnings

Ginseng may potentiate the action of monoamine oxidase inhibitors (MAOIs) (inhibits uptake of various neurotransmitter substances)[34] and two cases of suspected ginseng interaction with phenelzine have been documented.[51] The use of ginseng has been contraindicated during acute illness, any form of haemorrhage and during the acute period of coronary thrombosis[1]. It has been recommended that ginseng should be avoided by individuals who are highly energetic, nervous, tense, hysteric, manic or schizophrenic, and that it should not be taken with stimulants, including coffee, antipsychotic drugs or during treatment with hormones.[1,G49]

In view of documented pharmacological actions and side-effects, ginseng should also be used with caution in the following circumstances: cardiac disorders, diabetes, hyper- and hypotensive disorders, and with all steroid therapy. Women may experience oestrogenic side-effects.

In Russia, it is recommended that healthy people under the age of 40 should not use ginseng and that middle-aged people can be treated with small doses of ginseng on a daily basis. In general, long-term use of ginseng is not recommended and one author has documented that the main side-effect of prolonged use manifests as an inflamed nerve, frequently the sciatic, which then causes muscle spasm in the affected area.[1] In Russia, those individuals considered suitable to use ginseng are recommended to abstain from alcoholic beverages, sexual activity, bitter substances and spicy foods[9] Patients allergic to ginseng may exhibit symptoms of palpitation, insomnia, and pruritus.[9]

Pregnancy and lactation   No fetal abnormalities have been observed in rats and rabbits administered a standardised extract (40 mg/kg, p.o.) from day 1 to day 15 of pregnancy.[55] Ginseng has also been fed to two successive generations of rats in doses of up to 15 mg G115/kg body weight/day (equivalent to approximately 2700 mg ginseng extract) with no teratogenic effects observed.[52] However, the safety of ginseng during pregnancy has not been established in humans and therefore its use should be avoided. Similarly, there are no published data concerning the secretion of pharmacologically active constituents from ginseng into the breast milk and use of ginseng during lactation is therefore best avoided.

Pharmaceutical Comment

Phytochemical studies on panax ginseng are well documented and have initially concentrated on the saponin components (ginsenosides) which are generally considered to be the main active constituents. More recently, pharmacological actions documented for the non-saponin components, principally polysaccharides, have stimulated research into identifying non-saponin active constituents. Many of the pharmacological actions documented for ginseng directly oppose one another and this has been attributed to the actions of the individual ginsenosides. For example, ginsenoside R_{b1} exhibits CNS-depressant, hypotensive and tranquillising actions whilst ginsenoside R_{g1} exhibits CNS-stimulant, hypertensive and anti-fatigue actions. These opposing actions are thought to explain the 'adaptogenic' reputation of ginseng, that is the ability to increase the overall resistance of the body to stress and to balance bodily functions.

In summary, ginseng has been shown to possess a wide range of pharmacological activities and it should consequently be used with appropriate regard to the traditional guidelines drawn up in China, Japan and Russia, to the health of the individual and to any concomitant therapies. When used appropriately, ginseng appears to be relatively non-toxic and most documented side-effects are associated with inappropriate use when compared with traditional warnings and guidelines.

References

See also General References G2, G3, G5, G6, G8, G9, G16, G18, G28, G29, G31, G32, G36, G37, G41, G43, G46, G49, G50, G56, G61 and G64.

1 Baldwin CA *et al*. What pharmacists should know about ginseng. *Pharm J* 1986; **237**: 583–586.
2 Chung BS. Studies on the components of Korean ginseng (II) On the composition of ginseng essential oils. *Kor J Pharmacog* 1976; **7**: 41–44.
3 Iwabuchi H *et al*. Studies on the sesquiterpenoids of *Panax ginseng* C.A. Meyer III. *Chem Pharm Bull* 1989; **37**: 509–510.
4 Iwabuchi H *et al*. Studies on the sesquiterpenoids of *Panax ginseng* C.A. Meyer II. Isolation and structure determination of ginsenol, a novel sesquiterpene alcohol. *Chem Pharm Bull* 1988; **36**: 2447–2451.
5 Ahn B-Z *et al*. Acetylpanaxydol and panaxydolchlorohydrin, two new poly-ynes from Korean ginseng with cytotoxic activity against L1210 cells. *Arch Pharm (Weinheim)* 1989; **322**: 223–226.
6 Fujimoto Y, Satoh M. A new cytotoxic chlorine-containing polyacetylene from the callus of *Panax ginseng. Chem Pharm Bull* 1988; **36**: 4206–4208.
7 Gao Q-P *et al*. Chemical properties and anti-complementary activities of polysaccharide fractions from roots and leaves of *Panax ginseng. Planta Med* 1989; **55**: 9–12.
8 Yamasaki K *et al*. Purification and characterization of β-amylase from ginseng. *Chem Pharm Bull* 1989; **37**: 973–978.
9 Baranov AI. Medicinal uses of ginseng and related plants in the Soviet Union: recent trends in the Soviet literature. *J Ethnopharmacol* 1982; **6**: 339–353.
10 Brekhman II. *Panax* ginseng-1. *Med Sci Service* 1967; **4**: 17–26.
11 Li TB *et al*. Effects of ginsenosides, lectins and *Momordica charantia* insulin-like peptide on corticosterone production by isolated rat adrenal cells. *J Ethnopharmacol* 1987; **21**: 21–29.
12 Filaretov AA *et al*. Role of pituitary-adrenocortical system in body adaptation abilities. *Exp Clin Endocrinol* 1988; **92**: 129–136.
13 Guodong L, Zhongqi L. Effects of ginseng saponins on insulin release from isolated pancreatic

islets of rats. *Chin J Integr Trad Western Med* 1987; **7**: 326.
14 Yushu H, Yuzhen C. The effect of *Panax ginseng* extract (GS) on insulin and corticosteroid receptors. *J Trad Chin Med* 1988; **8**: 293–295.
15 Kimura M *et al*. Pharmacological sequential trials for the fractionation of components with hypoglycemic activity in alloxan diabetic mice from *Ginseng radix. J Pharm Dyn* 1981; **4**: 402–409.
16 Waki I *et al*. Effects of a hypoglycemic component of *Ginseng radix* on insulin biosynthesis in normal and diabetic animals. *J Pharm Dyn* 1982; **5**: 547–554.
17 Avakian EV *et al*. Effect of *Panax ginseng* extract on energy metabolism during exercise in rats. *Planta Med* 1984; **50**: 151–154.
18 Suzuki Y, Hikino H. Mechanisms of hypoglycemic activity of panaxans A and B, glycans of *Panax ginseng* roots: effects on the key enzymes of glucose metabolism in the liver of mice. *Phytother Res* 1989; **3**: 15–19.
19 Oshima Y *et al*. Isolation and hypoglycemic activity of quinquefolans A, B, and C, glycans of *Panax quinquefolium* roots. *J Nat Prod* 1987; **50**: 188–190.
20 Konno C, Hikino H. Isolation and hypoglycemic activity of panaxans M, N, O and P, glycans of *Panax ginseng* roots. *Int J Crude Drug Res* 1987; **25**: 53–56.
21 Suzuki Y, Hikino H. Mechanisms of hypoglycemic activity of panaxans A and B, glycans of *Panax ginseng* roots: effects of plasma level, secretion, sensitivity and binding of insulin in mice. *Phytother Res* 1989; **3**: 20–24.
22 Konno C *et al*. Isolation and hypoglycaemic activity of panaxans A, B, C, D and E, glycans of *Panax ginseng* roots. *Planta Med* 1984; **50**: 434–436.
23 Konno C *et al*. Isolation and hypoglycaemic activity of panaxans Q, R, S, T and U, glycans of *Panax ginseng* roots. *J Ethnopharmacol* 1985; **14**: 69–74.
24 Manren R *et al*. Calcium antagonistic action of saponins from *Panax notoginseng* (sanqi-ginseng). *J Trad Chin Med* 1987; **7**: 127–130.
25 Wu J-X, Chen J-X. Negative chronotropic and inotropic effects of *Panax saponins. Acta Pharmacol Sin* 1988; **9**: 409–412.
26 Lei X-L *et al*. Cardiovascular pharmacology of *Panax notoginseng* (Burk) F.H. Chen and *Salvia militiorrhiza. Am J Chin Med* 1986; **14**: 145–152.
27 Li XJ, Zhang BH. Studies on the antiarrhythmic effects of panaxatriol saponins (PTS) isolated from *Panax notoginseng. Acta Pharm Sin* 1988; **23**: 168–173.
28 Yunxiang F, Xiu C. Effects of ginenosides on myocardial lactic acid, cyclic nucleotides and

ultrastructural myocardial changes of anoxia on mice. *Chin J Integr Trad Western Med* 1987; **7**: 326.

29 Namba T *et al*. Fundamental studies on the evaluation of the crude drugs. (I). Hemolytic and its protective activity of ginseng saponins. *Planta Med* 1974; **28**: 28–38.

30 Kosuge T *et al*. Studies on antihemorrhagic principles in the crude drugs for hemostatics. I. On hemostatic activities of the crude drugs for hemostatics. *Yakugaku Zasshi [J Pharm Soc Jpn]* 1981; **101**: 501–503.

31 Yamamoto M, Kumagai M. Anti-atherogenic action of *Panax ginseng* in rats and in patients with hyperlipidemia. *Planta Med* 1982; **45**: 149–166.

32 Kuo S-C *et al*. Antiplatelet components in *Panax ginseng*. *Planta Med* 1990; **56**: 164–167.

33 Kim H-S *et al*. Antinarcotic effects of the standardized ginseng extract G115 on morphine. *Planta Med* 1990; **56**: 158–163

34 Tsang D *et al*. Ginseng saponins: Influence on neurotransmitter uptake in rat brain synaptosomes. *Planta Med* 1985; **51**: 221–224.

35 Kobayashi S *et al*. Inhibitory actions of phospholipase A_2 and saponins including ginsenoside Rb_1 and glycyrrhizin on the formation of nicotinic acetylcholine receptor clusters on cultured mouse myotubes. *Phytother Res* 1990; **4**: 106–111.

36 Tsang D *et al*. Ginenoside modulates K^+ stimulated noradrenaline release from rat cerebral cortex slices. *Planta Med* 1986; **52**: 266–268.

37 Saksena AK *et al*. Effect of *Withania somnifera* and *Panax ginseng* on dopaminergic receptors in rat brain during stress. *Planta Med* 1989; **55**: 95.

38 Nakagawa S *et al*. Cytoprotective activity of components of garlic, ginseng and ciuwjia on hepatocyte injury induced by carbon tetrachloride *in vitro*. *Hiroshima J Med Sci* 1985; **34**: 303–309.

39 Hikino H *et al*. Antihepatotoxic actions of ginsenosides from *Panax ginseng* roots. *Planta Med* 1985; **51**: 62–64.

40 Ahn B-Z, Kim SI. Heptadeca-1,8t-dien-4,6-diin-3,10-diol, ein weiteres, gegen L1210 – Zellen cytotoxisches Wirkprinzip aus der Koreanischen Ginsengwurzel. *Planta Med* 1988; **54**: 183.

41 Qian B-C *et al*. Effects of ginseng polysaccharides on tumor and immunological function in tumor-bearing mice. *Acta Pharmacol Sin* 1987; **8**: 277–288.

42 Matsunaga H *et al*. Studies on the panaxytriol of *Panax ginseng* C.A. Meyer. Isolation, determina-tion and antitumor activity. *Chem Pharm Bull* 1989; **37**: 1279–1281.

43 Singh VK *et al*. Combined treatment of mice with *Panax ginseng* extract and interferon inducer. *Planta Med* 1983; **47**: 235–236.

44 Singh VK *et al*. Immunomodulatory activity of *Panax ginseng* extract. *Planta Med* 1984; **50**: 462–465.

45 Lee FC *et al*. Effects of *Panax ginseng* on blood alcohol clearance in man. *Clin Exp Pharmac Physiol* 1987; **14**: 543–546.

46 Zuin M *et al*. Effects of a preparation containing a standardized ginseng extract combined with trace elements and multivitamins against hepatotoxin-induced chronic liver disease in the elderly. *J Int Med Res* 1987; **15**: 276–281.

47 D'Angelo L *et al*. A double-blind, placebo-controlled clinical study on the effect of a standardized ginseng extract on psychomotor performance in healthy volunteers. *J Ethnopharmacol* 1986; **16**: 15–22.

48 Peigen X, Keji C. Recent advances in clinical studies of Chinese medicinal herbs. 2. Clinical trials of Chinese herbs in a number of chronic conditions. *Phytother Res* 1988; **2**: 55–60.

49 Chong SKF, Oberholzer VG. Ginseng – is there a use in clinical medicine? *Postgrad Med J* 1988; **64**: 841–846.

50 Hopkins MP *et al*. Ginseng face cream and unexplained vaginal bleeding. *Am J Obstet Gynecol* 1988; **159**: 1121–1122.

51 Jones BD *et al*. Interaction of ginseng with phenelzine. *J Clin Psychopharmacol* 1987; **7**: 201–202.

52 Berté F. Toxicological investigation of the standardized ginseng extract G115 after unique administration [LD_{50}]. Manufacturer's data, on file. 1982, pp. 1–12.

53 Hess FG *et al*. Reproduction study in rats of ginseng extract G115. *Food Chem Toxicol* 1982; **20**: 189–192.

54 Hess FG *et al*. Effects of subchronic feeding of ginseng extract G115 in beagle dogs. *Food Chem Toxicol* 1983; **21**: 95–97.

55 Trabucchi E. Toxicological and pharmacological investigation of Geriatric Pharmaton. Manufacturer's data on file. 1971, pp. 1–22.

56 Savel J. Toxicological report on Geriatric Pharmaton. Manufacturer's data on file. 1971, pp. 1–31.

57 Chang YS *et al*. Evaluation of the mutagenic potential of American ginseng (*Panax quinquefolius*). *Planta Med* 1986; **52**: 338.

Golden Seal

Species (Family)

Hydrastis canadensis L. (Ranunculaceae)

Synonym(s)

Yellow Root

Yellow root also refers to *Xanthorhiza simplicissima* Marsh, which is also a member of the Ranunculaceae family and contains berberine as the major alkaloid constituent.

Part(s) Used

Rhizome, root

Pharmacopoeial and Other Monographs

BHC 1992[G6]
BHP 1996[G9]
Martindale 32nd edition[G43]
Mills and Bone (Hydrastis root)[G50]
PDR for Herbal Medicines 2nd edition[G36]

Legal Category (Licensed Products)

GSL[G37]

Constituents[G6,G22,G40,G41,G62,G64]

Alkaloids Isoquinoline-type. 2.5–6.0%. Hydrastine (major, 1.5–4.0%), berberine (0.5–6.0%), berberastine (2–3%), and canadine (1%), with lesser amounts of related alkaloids including candaline and canadaline.[1–3]

Other constituents Chlorogenic acid, carbohydrates, fatty acids (75% saturated, 25% unsaturated), volatile oil (trace), resin, meconin (meconinic acid lactone).

Food Use

Golden seal is not used in foods, although it is reported to be used in herbal teas.[G41] The concentration of berberine permitted in foods is limited to 0.1 mg/kg, and 10 mg/kg in alcoholic beverages.[G16]

Herbal Use

Golden seal is stated to be a stimulant to involuntary muscle, and to possess stomachic, oxytocic, anti-haemorrhagic and laxative properties. Traditionally it has been used for digestive disorders, gastritis, peptic ulceration, colitis, anorexia, upper respiratory catarrh, menorrhagia, post-partum haemorrhage, dysmenorrhoea, topically for eczema, pruritus, otorrhoea, catarrhal deafness and tinnitus, conjunctivitis, and specifically for atonic dyspepsia with hepatic symptoms.[G6,G7,G8]

Dosage

Dried rhizome 0.5–1.0 g or by decoction three times daily.[G6,G7]

Liquid Extract of Hydrastis (BPC 1949) 0.3–1.0 mL.

Tincture of Hydrastis (BPC 1949) 2–4 mL.

Pharmacological Actions

The pharmacological activity of golden seal is attributed to the isoquinoline alkaloid constituents, primarily hydrastine and berberine,[3,4] which are reported to have similar properties.[G41] Antibiotic, immunostimulant, anticonvulsant, sedative, hypotensive, uterotonic, choleretic and carminative activities have been described for berberine.[3]

In vitro and animal studies

Limited work has been documented for golden seal, although the pharmacology of berberine and hydrastine is well studied.

The total alkaloid fraction of golden seal has been reported to exhibit anticonvulsant activity in smooth muscle preparations (e.g. mouse intestine, uterus).[5] However, *in vitro*, canadine is reported to exhibit uterine stimulation in guinea-pig and rabbit tissues.[4] Berberine, canadine and hydrastine are all stated to exhibit utero-activity.[G30]

Berberine and hydrastine have produced a hypotensive effect in laboratory animals following intravenous administration.[6,7,G41] High doses of hydrastine are documented to produce an increase in blood pressure.[7] *In vitro*, berberine has been reported to decrease the anticoagulant action of heparin in canine and human blood.[7]

Berberine is reported to exert a stimulant action on the heart and to increase coronary blood flow, although higher doses are stated to inhibit cardiac activity.[7]

Antimuscarinic and antihistamine actions have been documented for berberine.[7]

In rats, berberine has exhibited antipyretic activity three times as effective as aspirin.[3]

Berberine potentiated barbiturate sleeping time, but did not exhibit any analgesic or tranquillising effects.[7]

A broad spectrum of antimicrobial activity against bacteria, fungi, and protozoa has been reported for berberine. Sensitive organisms include *Staphylococcus* spp., *Streptococcus* spp., *Chlamydia aureus*, *Corynebacterium diphtheriae*, *Salmonella typhi*, *Diplococcus pneumoniae*, *Pseudomonas aeruginosa*, *Shigella dysenteriae*, *Trichomonas vaginalis*, *Neisseria gonorrhoeae*, *Neisseria meningitidis*, *Treponema pallidum*, *Giardia lamblia* and *Leishmania donovani*.[3] Berberine is reported to be effective against diarrhoeas caused by enterotoxins such as *Vibrio cholerae* and *Escherichia coli*.[7] *In vivo* and *in vitro* studies in hamsters and rats have reported significant activity for berberine against *Entamoeba histolytica*.[3]

Anticancer activity has been reported for berberine in B1, KB and PS tumour systems.[G22] In addition, berberine sulfate was found to inhibit the action of teleocidin, a known tumour promoter, on the formation of mouse skin tumours initiated with 7,12-dimethylbenz[*a*]anthracene.[5]

Clinical studies

None documented for golden seal. Berberine is stated to have shown significant success in the treatment of acute diarrhoea in several clinical studies.[3] It has been found effective against diarrhoeas caused by *Escherichia coli*, *Shigella dysenteriae*, *Salmonella paratyphi* B, *Klebsiella*, *Giardia lamblia* and *Vibrio cholerae*.[3] Berberine has been used to treat trachoma, an infectious ocular disease caused by *Chlamydia trachomatis*, which is a major cause of blindness and impaired vision in developing countries.[3]

Clinical studies have shown berberine to stimulate bile and bilirubin secretion and to improve symptoms of chronic cholecystitis, and to correct raised levels of tyramine in patients with liver cirrhosis.[3]

Side-effects, Toxicity

Berberine and berberine-containing plants are considered to be non-toxic.[3] However, the alkaloid constituents are potentially toxic and symptoms of golden seal poisoning include stomach upset, nervous symptoms and depression; large quantities may even be fatal.[8] High doses of hydrastine are reported to cause exaggerated reflexes, convulsions, paralysis and death from respiratory failure.[4] The root may cause contact ulceration of mucosal surfaces.

Contra-indications, Warnings

Golden seal is contra-indicated in individuals with raised blood pressure.[G7,G22,G49] Prolonged use of golden seal may decrease vitamin B absorption.[G22] Coagulant activity opposing the action of heparin, and cardiac stimulant activity have been documented for berberine. The use of golden seal as a douche should be avoided because of the potential ulcerative side-effects.[G22] The alkaloid constituents of golden seal are potentially toxic and excessive use should be avoided.

Pregnancy and lactation Golden seal is contra-indicated for use during pregnancy.[3,G7,G49] Berberine, canadine, hydrastine and hydrastinine have all been reported to produce uterine stimulant activity.[G30] It is not known whether the alkaloids are excreted in breast milk. The use of golden seal during lactation should be avoided.

Pharmaceutical Comment

Golden seal is characterised by the isoquinoline alkaloid constituents. These compounds, primarily hydrastine and berberine, represent the main active components of golden seal. Numerous activities have been documented many of which support the traditional herbal uses of the root. However, in view of the pharmacological properties of the alkaloid constituents, excessive use of golden seal should be avoided.

References

See also General References G5, G6, G9, G10, G16, G22, G30, G31, G32, G36, G37, G40, G41, G43, G48, G50, G62 and G64.

1 Gleye J *et al*. La canadaline: nouvel alcaloide d'*Hydrastis canadensis*. *Phytochemistry* 1974; **13**: 675–676.
2 El-Masry S *et al*. Colorimetric and spectrophotometric determination of *Hydrastis* alkaloids in pharmaceutical preparations. *J Pharm Sci* 1980; **69**: 597–598.
3 Pizzorno JE, Murray MT. *Hydrastis canadensis*, *Berberis vulgaris*, *Berberis aquitolium* and other berberine containing plants. In: *Textbook of Natural Medicine*. Seattle: John Bastyr College Publications, 1985 (looseleaf).
4 Genest K, Hughes DW. Natural products in

Canadian pharmaceuticals iv. *Hydrastis canadensis. Can J Pharm Sci* 1969; **4**: 41–45.

5   Nishino H *et al.* Berberine sulphate inhibits tumour-promoting activity of teleocidin in two-stage carcinogenesis on mouse skin. *Oncology* 1986; **43**: 131–134.

6   Wisniewski W, Gorta T. Effect of temperature on the oxidation of hydrastine to hydrastinine in liquid extracts and rhizomes of *Hydrastis cana-densis* in the presence of air and steam. *Acta Pol Pharm* 1969; **26**: 313–317.

7   Preininger V. The pharmacology and toxicology of the Papaveraceae alkaloids. In: Manske RHF, Holmes HL, eds. *The Alkaloids*, vol 15. New York: Academic Press, 1975: 239.

8   Hardin JW, Arena JM. *Human Poisoning from Native and Cultivated Plants*, 2nd edn. Durham, North Carolina: Duke University Press, 1974.

Gravel Root

Species (Family)

Eupatorium purpureum L. (Asteraceae/Compositae)

Synonym(s)

Joe-Pye Weed, Kydney Root, Purple Boneset, Queen of the Meadow

Part(s) Used

Rhizome, root

Pharmacopoeial and Other Monographs

BHP 1983[G7]

Legal Category (Licensed Products)

GSL[G37]

Constituents[G20,G40,G42,G48,G49,G64]

Little information is available on the chemistry of gravel root. It is stated to contain euparin (a benzofuran compound), eupatorin (a flavonoid), resin and volatile oil.

Other plant parts The herb is reported to contain echinatine, an unsaturated pyrrolizidine alkaloid.[1]

Food Use

Gravel root is not used in foods.

Herbal Use

Gravel root is stated to possess antilithic, diuretic and antirheumatic properties. Traditionally, it has been used for urinary calculus, cystitis, dysuria, urethritis, prostatitis, rheumatism, gout, and specifically for renal or vesicular calculi.[G7,G64]

Dosage

Dried rhizome/root 2–4 g or by decoction three times daily.[G7]

Liquid extract 2–4 mL (1 : 1 in 25% alcohol) three times daily.[G7]

Tincture 1–2 mL (1 : 5 in 40% alcohol) three times daily.[G7]

Pharmacological Actions

None documented.

Side-effects, Toxicity[G20]

None documented for gravel root although pyrrolizidine alkaloids are constituents of many species of *Eupatorium*.[1,G20] Pyrrolizidine alkaloids with an unsaturated pyrrolizidine nucleus are reported to be hepatotoxic in both animals and humans (*see* Comfrey). An unsaturated pyrrolizidine alkaloid, echinatine, has been reported for the aerial parts of gravel root.

Contra-indications, Warnings

None documented.

Pregnancy and lactation The safety of gravel root has not been established. In view of the lack of phytochemical, pharmacological and toxicological information the use of gravel root during pregnancy and lactation should be avoided.

Pharmaceutical Comment

The chemistry of gravel root is poorly studied and no scientific evidence was located to justify the herbal uses. Excessive use of gravel root should be avoided.

References

See also General References G7, G20, G31, G37, G40, G42, G48, G49 and G64.

1 *Pyrrolizidine Alkaloids. Environmental Health Criteria 80*. Geneva: WHO, 1988.

Ground Ivy

Species (Family)

Nepeta hederacea (L.) Trev. (Labiatae)

Synonym(s)

Glechoma hederacea L.

Part(s) Used

Herb

Pharmacopoeial and Other Monographs

BHC 1992[G6]
BHP 1996[G9]
PDR for Herbal Medicines 2nd edition[G36]

Legal Category (Licensed Products)

GSL[G37]

Constituents[G6,G22,G48,G64]

Amino acids Asparagic acid, glutamic acid, proline, tyrosine and valine.

Flavonoids Flavonol glycosides (e.g. hyperoside, isoquercitrin, rutin) and flavone glycosides (e.g. luteolin diglucoside, cosmosyin).[1]

Steroids β-Sitosterol.

Terpenoids Oleanolic acid, α-ursolic acid, β-ursolic acid.[2]

Volatile oils 0.03–0.06%. Various terpenoid components including *p*-cymene, linalool, limonene, menthone, α-pinene, β-pinene, pinocamphone, pulegone and terpineol; glechomafuran (a sesquiterpene).[3]

Other constituents Palmitic acid, rosmarinic acid, succinic acid, bitter principle (glechomin), choline, gum, diterpene lactone (marrubiin), saponin, tannin and wax.

Food Use

Ground ivy is listed by the Council of Europe as a natural source of food flavouring (category N3). This category indicates that ground ivy can be added to foodstuffs in the traditionally accepted manner, although there is insufficient information available for an adequate assessment of potential toxicity.[G16]

Herbal Use

Ground ivy is stated to possess mild expectorant, anticatarrhal, astringent, vulnerary, diuretic and stomachic properties. Traditionally, it has been used for bronchitis, tinnitus, diarrhoea, haemorrhoids, cystitis, gastritis, and specifically for chronic bronchial catarrh.[G6,G7,G8,G49,G64]

Dosage

Dried herb 2–4 g or by infusion three times daily.[G6,G7]

Liquid extract 2–4 mL (1 : 1 in 25% alcohol) three times daily.[G6,G7]

Pharmacological Actions

In vitro and animal studies

In vivo anti-inflammatory activity has been reported for an ethanolic extract of ground ivy, which was stated to exhibit a moderate inhibition (27%) of carrageenan-induced rat paw oedema.[4]

Ursolic acid analogues, 2α- and 2β-hydroxyursolic acid, have been documented to provide significant ulcer-protective activity in mice.[5]

The astringent activity documented for ground ivy has been attributed to rosmarinic acid, a polyphenolic acid.[6]

Glechomin and marrubiin are stated to be bitter principles, and α-terpineol is known to be an antiseptic component of volatile oils.[G48,G49]

Anti-inflammatory and astringent properties are generally associated with flavonoids and tannins, respectively. Anti-inflammatory properties have been documented for rosmarinic acid (*see* Rosemary).

In vitro antiviral activity against the Epstein–Barr virus has been documented for ursolic acid.[7] Both oleanolic and ursolic acids were found to inhibit tumour production by TPA in mouse skin, with activity comparable to that of retinoic acid, a known tumour-promoter inhibitor.[7]

Significant cytotoxic activity has also been reported for ursolic acid in lymphocytic leukaemia (P-388, L-1210) and human lung carcinoma (A-549), and marginal activity in KB cells, human colon (HCT-8), and mammary (MCF-7) tumour cells.[8]

Side-effects, Toxicity

Poisoning in cattle and horses has been documented in Eastern Europe.[9] Symptoms include accelerated weak pulse, difficulty in breathing, conjunctival haemorrhage, elevated temperature, dizziness, spleen enlargement, dilation of the caecum, and gastroenteritis revealed at post-mortem. Antitumour and cytotoxic activities have been reported for olea-nolic and ursolic acids (see In vitro and animal studies).

Ground ivy volatile oil contains many terpenoids and terpene-rich volatile oils are irritant to the gastrointestinal tract and kidneys. Pulegone is an irritant, hepatotoxic, and abortifacient principle of the volatile oil of pennyroyal. However, in comparison with pennyroyal the overall yield of volatile oil is much less (0.03–0.06% in ground ivy and 1–2% in pennyroyal).

Contra-indications, Warnings

Ground ivy is contra-indicated in epilepsy [G7] although no rationale for this statement has been found. Excessive doses may be irritant to the gastrointestinal mucosa and should be avoided by individuals with existing renal disease.

Pregnancy and lactation The safety of ground ivy has not been established. In view of the lack of toxicity data and the possible irritant and abortifacient action of the volatile oil, the use of ground ivy during pregnancy and lactation should be avoided.

Pharmaceutical Comment

The chemistry of ground ivy is well studied. Documented pharmacological activities support some of the herbal uses, although no references to human studies were located. In view of the lack of toxicity data and the reported cytotoxic activity of ursolic acid, excessive use of ground ivy should be avoided.

References

See also General References G6, G9, G16, G22, G31, G36, G37, G48, G49 and G64.

1 Zieba J. Isolation and identification of flavonoids from *Glechoma hederacea*. *Pol J Pharmacol Pharm* 1973; **25**: 593–597.
2 Zieba J. Isolation and identification of nonheteroside triterpenoids from *Glechoma hederacea*. *Pol J Pharmacol Pharm* 1973; **25**: 587–592.
3 Stahl E, Datta SN. New sesquiterpenoids of the ground ivy (*Glechoma hederacea*). *Justus Liebigs Ann Chem* 1972; **757**: 23–32.
4 Mascolo N *et al*. Biological screening of Italian medicinal plants for anti-inflammatory activity. *Phytother Res* 1987; **1**: 28–31.
5 Okuyama E *et al* IIsolation and identification of ursolic acid-related compounds as the principles of *Glechoma hederacea* having an antiulcerogenic activity. *Shoyakugaku Zasshi* 1983; **37**: 52–55.
6 Okuda T *et al*. The components of tannic activities in Labiatae plants. I. Rosmarinic acid from Labiatae plants in Japan. *Yakugaku Zasshi* 1986; **106**: 1108–1111.
7 Tokuda H *et al*. Inhibitory effects of ursolic and oleanolic acid on skin tumor promotion by 12-O-tetradecanoylphorbol-13-acetate. *Cancer Lett* 1986; **33**: 279–285.
8 Lee K-H *et al*. The cytotoxic principles of *Prunella vulgaris*, *Psychotria serpens*, and *Hyptis capitata*: Ursolic acid and related derivatives. *Planta Med* 1988; **54**: 308.
9 MAFF. *Poisonous Plants in Britain*. London: HMSO, 1984: 139.

Guaiacum

Species (Family)

(i) *Guaiacum officinale* L. (Zygophyllaceae)
(ii) *Guaiacum sanctum* L.

Synonym(s)

Guaiac, Guajacum, Lignum Vitae

Part(s) Used

Resin obtained from the heartwood

Pharmacopoeial and Other Monographs

BHC 1992[G6]
BHP 1996[G9]
Complete German Commission E[G3]
Martindale 32nd edition[G43]
PDR for Herbal Medicines 2nd edition[G36]

Legal Category (Licensed Products)

GSL[G37]

Constituents[G6,G48,G64]

Resins 15–20%. Guaiaretic acid, dehydroguaiaretic acid, guaiacin, isoguaiacin, α-guaiaconic acid (lignans), furoguaiacin and its monomethyl ether, furoguaiacidin, tetrahydrofuroguaiacin-A and tetrahydrofuroguaiacin-B (furano-lignans), furoguaiaoxidin (enedione lignan).[1-4]

Steroids β-Sitosterol.

Terpenoids Saponins, oleanolic acid.[5,6]

Food Use

Guaiacum is listed by the Council of Europe as a natural source of food flavouring (category N2). This category indicates that guaiacum can be added to foodstuffs in small quantities, with a possible limitation of an active principle (as yet unspecified) in the final product.[G16]

Herbal Use

Guaiacum is stated to possess antirheumatic, anti-inflammatory, diuretic, mild laxative and diaphoretic properties. Traditionally, it has been used for sub-acute rheumatism, prophylaxis against gout, and specifically for chronic rheumatism and rheumatoid arthritis.[G6,G7,G8,G64]

Dosage

Dried wood 1–2 g or by decoction three times daily.[G6,G7]

Liquid extract 1–2 mL (1:1 in 80% alcohol) three times daily.[G6,G7]

Tincture of Guaiacum (BPC 1934) 2–4 mL.

Pharmacological Actions

In vitro and animal studies

None documented. Antimicrobial properties are associated with lignans and much has been documented for nordihydroguaiaretic acid, the principal lignan constituent in chaparral (*see* Chaparral).

Side-effects, Toxicity

Guaiacum resin has been reported to cause contact dermatitis.[G51] The resin is documented to be of low toxicity; the oral LD_{50} in rats is greater than 5 g/kg body weight.[G48]

Contra-indications, Warnings

It is recommended that guaiacum is avoided by individuals with hypersensitive, allergic or acute inflammatory conditions.[G49]

Pregnancy and lactation The safety of guaiacum during pregnancy has not been established. In view of this, and the overall lack of pharmacological and toxicological data, the use of guaiacum during pregnancy and lactation should be avoided.

Pharmaceutical Comment

Guaiacum is characterised by the resin fraction of the heartwood and much has been documented on the constituents (principally lignans) of the resin, although little is known regarding other constituents. No scientific information was found to justify the herbal use of guaiacum as an antirheumatic or anti-inflammatory agent. In view of the lack of toxicity data, excessive use of guaiacum should be avoided.

References

See also General References G3, G6, G9, G16, G29, G36, G37, G43, G48, G49, G51 and G64.

1 King FE, Wilson JG. The chemistry of extractives from hardwoods. Part XXXVI. The lignans of *Guaiacum officinale* L. *J Chem Soc* 1964; 4011–4024.
2 Kratochvil JF *et al*. Isolation and characterization of α-guaiaconic acid and the nature of guaiacum blue. *Phytochemistry* 1971; **10**: 2529–3251.
3 Majumder PL, Bhattacharyya M. Structure of furoguaiacidin: a new furanoid lignan of the heartwood of *Guaiacum officinale* L. *Chem Ind* 1974; 77–78.
4 Majumder P, Bhattacharyya M. Furoguaiaoxidin – a new enedione lignan of *Guaiacum officinale*: a novel method of sequential introduction of alkoxy functions in the 3- and 4-methyl groups of 2,5-diaryl-3,4-dimethylfurans. *JCS Chem Commun* 1975; 702–703.
5 Ahmad VU *et al*. Officigenin, a new sapogenin of *Guaiacum officinale*. *J Nat Prod* 1984; **47**: 977–982.
6 Ahmad VU *et al*. Guaianin, a new saponin from *Guaiacum officinale*. *J Nat Prod* 1986; **49**: 784–786.

Hawthorn

Species (Family)

(i) *Crataegus laevigata* (Pois) DC. (Rosaceae)
(ii) *Crataegus monogyna* Jacq.

Synonym(s)

Whitethorn

Part(s) Used

Fruit

Pharmacopoeial and Other Monographs

American Herbal Pharmacopoeia[G1]
BHP 1996[G9]
BP 2001[G15]
Complete German Commission E[G3]
ESCOP 1999[G52]
Martindale 32nd edition[G43]
Mills and Bone[G50]
PDR for Herbal Medicines 2nd edition[G36]
Ph Eur 2002[G28]

Legal Category (Licensed Products)

Hawthorn is not included in the GSL.[G37]

Constituents[G1,G2,G22,G62,G64]

Amines Phenylethylamine, O-methoxyphenethylamine and tyramine.[1]

Flavonoids Flavonol (e.g. kaempferol, quercetin) and flavone (e.g. apigenin, luteolin) derivatives, rutin, hyperoside, vitexin glycosides, orientin glycosides[2–5] and procyanidins.[6,7]

Tannins Pharmacopoeial standard not less than 1.0% procyanidins, condensed (proanthocyanidins).

Other constituents Cyanogenetic glycosides and saponins.

Food Use

Hawthorn is not commonly used in foods. It is listed by the Council of Europe as a natural source of food flavouring (category N2). This category indicates that hawthorn can be added to foodstuffs in small quantities, with a possible limitation of an active principle (as yet unspecified) in the final product.[G16]

Herbal Use[G2,G3,G7,G43,G52]

Hawthorn is stated to possess cardiotonic, coronary vasodilator and hypotensive properties. Traditionally, it has been used for cardiac failure, myocardial weakness, paroxysmal tachycardia, hypertension, arteriosclerosis and Buerger's disease. The German Commission E did not approve therapeutic use.[G3]

Dosage

Dried fruit 0.3–1.0 g or by infusion three times daily.[G7]

Liquid extract 0.5–1.0 mL (1:1 in 25% alcohol) three times daily.[G7]

Tincture 1–2 mL (1:5 in 45% alcohol) three times daily.[G7]

Pharmacological Actions

In vitro and animal studies

Cardiovascular activity has been documented for hawthorn and attributed to the flavonoid components, in particular the procyanidins. Hawthorn extracts have been documented to increase coronary blood flow both *in vitro* (in the guinea-pig heart) and *in vivo* (in the cat, dog and rabbit), reduce blood pressure *in vivo* (in the cat, dog, rabbit and rat), increase (head, skeletal muscle and kidney) and reduce (skin, gastrointestinal tract) peripheral blood flow *in vivo* (in the dog) and reduce peripheral resistance *in vivo* (in the dog).[6,8–13] The hypotensive activity of hawthorn has been attributed to a vasodilation action rather than via adrenergic, muscarinic or histaminergic receptors.[12] Beta-adrenoceptor blocking activity (versus adrenaline-induced tachycardia) has been exhibited *in vivo* in the dog and *in vitro* in the frog heart using flower, leaf and fruit extracts standardised on their procyanidin content.[6] The authors reported a direct relationship between the concentration of procyanidin and observed actions.

Negative chronotropic and positive inotropic actions have been observed *in vitro* using the guinea-pig heart and attributed to flavonoid and proanthocyanidin fractions.[14] A positive inotropic effect has also been exhibited by amine constituents *in vitro* using guinea-pig papillary muscle.[1]

Hawthorn extracts have also been reported to lack any effect on the heart rate and muscle contractility in studies that have observed an effect on blood pressure in the dog and rat.[11,12] Hawthorn extracts have exhibited some prophylactic anti-arrhythmic activity in rabbits administered intravenous aconitine.[15] Extracts infused after aconitine did not affect the induced arrhythmias. *In vitro*, vitexin rhamnoside has been reported to have no effect on the action of ouabain and aconitine.[15] A crude extract of *Crataegus pinnatifidia* Bge. var *major* N.E.Br. and the flavonoid vitexin rhamnoside have been reported to exert a protective action on experimental ischaemic myocardium in anaesthetised dogs.[16] The extracts were observed to decrease left ventricular work, decrease the consumption of oxygen index, and increase coronary sinus blood oxygen concentrations, resulting in a decrease in oxygen consumption and balance of oxygen metabolism. In contrast to other studies, an increase in coronary blood flow was not observed. The authors attributed these opposing results to the variation in concentrations of active constituents between the different plant parts. *In vitro*, vitexin rhamnoside has been reported to exert a protective action towards cardiac cells deprived of oxygen and glucose.[17]

A mild CNS-depressant effect has been documented in mice that received oral administration of hawthorn flower extracts.[18] An increase in barbiturate sleeping time and a decrease in spontaneous basal motility were the most noticeable effects.

Free radicals have been linked with the ageing process. When fed to mice, a hawthorn fruit (*C. pinnatifidia*) extract has been reported to enhance the action of superoxide dismutase (SOD), which promotes the scavenging of free radicals.[19] An inhibition of lipid peroxidation, which can be caused by highly reactive free radicals was also documented.[19] The pharmacological actions of leaf with flowers include increase in cardiac contractility, increase in coronary blood flow and myocardial circulation, protection from ischaemic damage and decrease of peripheral vascular resistance.[G52]

Clinical studies

The effects of a commercial preparation containing 30 mg hawthorn extract standardised to 1 mg procyanidins were assessed in a double-blind, placebo-controlled study involving 80 patients.[20] Hawthorn extract was reported to exhibit greater overall improvement of cardiac function and of subjective symptoms, such as dyspnoea and palpitations, compared with placebo. Improvements in ECG recordings were not found to differ between the two groups.

A commercial product containing hawthorn, valerian, camphor and cereus was given to 2243 patients with functional cardiovascular disorders and/or hypotension or meteorosensitivity in an open multicentre study.[21] An improvement in 84% of treated individuals was reported.

In a randomised, double-blind, controlled trial involving 60 patients with stable angina, a commercial hawthorn preparation (60 mg three times daily) was reported to increase coronary perfusion and to economise myocardial oxygen consumption.[22]

A commercial hawthorn/passionflower extract (standardised on flavone and proanthocyanidin content) 6 mL daily for 42 days has been assessed in a randomised, double-blind, placebo-controlled trial involving 40 patients with chronic heart failure.[23] Significant improvements were noted for the active group, compared with placebo, in exercise capacity, heart rate at rest, diastolic blood pressure at rest, and concentrations of total plasma cholesterol and low-density lipids. Non-significant improvements were noted in the active group for maximum exercise capacity, breathlessness, and physical performance. The authors commented that a higher dose of the extract administered over a longer period was necessary for further investigation of the observed improvements.[23] Clinical studies with standardised extracts of leaf with flowers have demonstrated beneficial effects in patients with cardiac insufficiency.[G52]

Side-effects, Toxicity

Nausea[20] and fatigue, sweating and rash on the hands[23] have been reported as side-effects in clinical trials using commercial preparations of hawthorn.[20]

General symptoms of acute toxicity observed in a number of animal models (e.g. guinea-pig, frog, tortoise, cat, rabbit, rat) have been documented as bradycardia and respiratory depression leading to cardiac arrest and respiratory paralysis.[8–10] Acute toxicity (LD_{50}) of isolated constituents (mainly flavonoids) has been documented as 50–2600 mg/kg (by intravenous injection) and 6 g/kg (by mouth) in various animal preparations.[8–10] The documented acute toxicity of commercial hawthorn preparations has also been reviewed.[8–10]

Contra-indications, Warnings

Hawthorn has been reported to exhibit many cardiovascular activities and as such may affect the existing therapy of patients with various cardiovascular disorders such as hypertension, hypotension and cardiac disorders. These patient groups are likely to be most susceptible to the pharmacological actions of hawthorn.

Pregnancy and lactation   In *vivo* and in *vitro* uteroactivity (reduction in tone and motility) has been documented for hawthorn extracts.[8–10] In view of the pharmacological activities described for hawthorn, it should not be taken during pregnancy and lactation.

Pharmaceutical Comment

Hawthorn is characterised by its phenolic constituents, in particular the flavonoid components to which many of the pharmacological properties associated with hawthorn have been attributed. Pharmacological actions documented in both animal and human studies support the traditional actions of hawthorn and include cardioactive, hypotensive and coronary vasodilator.[24] Separate monographs for the fruit (berries) and leaf with flowers appear in the British Pharmacopoeia and European Pharmacopoeia.[G15,G28] The German Commission E did not approve the use of fruit for therapeutic purposes on the grounds of insufficient evidence. There is some evidence from clinical trials to support the use of the standardised extracts of leaf with flower for cardiac insufficiency. In view of the nature of the actions documented for hawthorn, it is not suitable for self-medication.

References

See also General References G1, G2, G3, G9, G15, G16, G18, G22, G28, G31, G32, G36, G43, G50, G52, G56, G62 and G64.

1 Wagner H, Grevel J. Cardioactive drugs IV. Cardiotonic amines from *Crataegus oxyacantha*. *Plant Med* 1982; **45**: 99–101.
2 Nikolov N *et al.* New flavonoid glycosides from *Crataegus monogyna* and *Crataegus pentagyna*. *Planta Med* 1982; **44**: 50–53.
3 Ficarra P *et al.* High-performance liquid chromatography of flavonoids in *Crataegus oxyacantha* L. *Il Farmaco Ed Pr* 1984; **39**: 148–157.
4 Ficcara P *et al.* Analysis of 2-phenyl-chromon derivatives and chlorogenic acid. II – High-performance thin layer chromatography and high-performance liquid chromatography in flowers, leaves and buds extractives of *Crataegus oxyacantha* L. *Il Farmaco Ed Pr* 1984; **39**: 342–354.
5 Pietta P *et al.* Isocratic liquid chormatographic method for the simultaneous determination of *Passiflora incarnata* L. and *Crataegus monogyna* flavonoids in drugs. *J Chromatogr* 1986; **357**: 233–238.
6 Rácz-Kotilla E *et al.* Hypotensive and beta-blocking effect of procyanidins of *Crataegus monogyna*. *Planta Med* 1980; **39**: 239.
7 Vanhaelen M, Vanhaelen-Fastre R. TLC-densitometric determination of 2,3-*cis*-procyanidin monomer and oligo-mers from hawthorn (*Crataegus laevigata* and *C. monogyna*). *J Pharm Biomed Anal* 1989; **7**: 1871–1875.
8 Ammon HPT, Händel M. Crataegus, toxicology and pharmacology. Part I: Toxicity. *Planta Med* 1981; **43**: 105–120.
9 Ammon HPT, Händel M. Crataegus, toxicology and pharmacology. Part II: Pharmacodynamics. *Planta Med* 1981; **43**: 209–239.
10 Ammon HPT, Händel M. Crataegus, toxicology and pharmacology. Part III: Pharmacodynamics and pharmacokinetics. *Planta Med* 1981; **43**: 313–322.
11 Lièvre M *et al.* Assessment in the anesthetized dog of the cardiovascular effects of a pure extract (hyperoside) from hawthorn. *Ann Pharm Fr* 1985; **43**: 471–477.
12 Abdul-Ghani A-S *et al.* Hypotensive effect of *Crateagus oxyacantha*. *Int J Crude Drug Res* 1987; **25**: 216–220.
13 Petkov V. Plants with hypotensive, antiatheromatous and coronarodilatating action. *Am J Chin Med* 1979; **7**: 197–236.
14 Leukel A *et al.* Studies on the activity of *Crataegus* compounds upon the isolated guinea pig heart. *Planta Med* 1986; **52**: 65.
15 Thompson EB *et al.* Preliminary study of potential antiarrhythmic effects of *Crataegus monogyna*. *J Pharm Sci* 1974; **63**: 1936–1937.
16 Lianda L *et al.* Studies on hawthorn and its active principle. I. Effect on myocardial ischemia and hemodynamics in dogs. *J Trad Chin Med* 1984; **4**: 283–288.
17 Lianda L *et al.* Studies on hawthorn and its active principle. II. Effects on cultured rat heart cells deprived of oxygen and glucose. *J Trad Chin Med* 1984; **4**: 289–292.
18 Della Loggia R *et al.* Depressive effect of *Crataegus oxyacantha* L. on central nervous system in mice. *Sci Pharm* 1983; **51**: 319–324.
19 Dai Y-R *et al.* Effect of extracts of some medicinal plants on superoxide dismutase activity in mice. *Planta Med* 1987; **53**: 309–310.

20 Iwamoto M *et al*. Klinische Wirkung von Crataegutt bei Herzerkrankungen ischämischer und/oder hypertensiver Genese. *Planta Med* 1981; **42**: 1–16.

21 Busanny-Caspari E *et al*. Indikationen Herzbeschwerden, Hypotonie und Wetterfühligkeit. *Therapiewoche* 1986; **36**: 2545– 2550.

22 Hanak Th, Brückel M-H. Behhandlung von leichten stabilen Formen der Angina pectoris mit Crataegutt novo. *Therapiewoche* 1983; **33**; 4331– 4333.

23 von Eiff M *et al*. Hawthorn/Passionflower extract and improvement in physical exercise capacity of patients with dyspnoea Class II of the NYHM functional classification. *Acta Ther* 1994; **20**: 47– 66.

24 Hobbs C, Foster S. Hawthorn – a literature review. *Herbalgram* 1990; **22**: 19–33.

Holy Thistle

Species (Family)

Cnicus benedictus L. (Asteraceae/Compositae)

Synonym(s)

Blessed Thistle, Carbenia Benedicta, Carduus Benedictus, Cnicus

Part(s) Used

Herb

Pharmacopoeial and Other Monographs

BHC 1992[G6]
BHP 1996[G9]
Complete German Commission E[G3]
Martindale 32nd edition[G43]
PDR for Herbal Medicines 2nd edition[G36]

Legal Category (Licensed Products)

GSL[G37]

Constituents[G2,G6,G30,G40,G62,G64]

Lignans Arctigenin, nortracheloside, 2-acetyl nortracheloside and trachelogenin.[1]

Polyenes Several polyacetylenes.[2]

Steroids Phytosterols (e.g. *n*-nonacosan, sitosterol, sitosteryl glycoside, stigmasterol).[3]

Tannins Type unspecified (8%).

Terpenoids Sesquiterpenes including cnicin 0.2–0.7%,[4] yielding salonitenolide as aglycone,[5] and artemisiifolin. Shoot and flowering head are reported to be devoid of cnicin.[4] Triterpenoids including α-amyrenone, α-amyrin acetate, α-amyrine, multiflorenol, multiflorenol acetate and oleanolic acid.[3]

Volatile oils Many components, mainly hydrocarbons.[6]

Other constituents Lithospermic acid, mucilage, nicotinic acid and nicotinamide complex, resin.

Food Use

Holy thistle is listed by the Council of Europe as natural source of food flavouring (category N2). This category indicates that holy thistle can be added to foodstuffs in small quantities, with a possible limitation of an active principle (as yet unspecified) in the final product.[G16] In the USA, holy thistle is permitted for use in alcoholic beverages.[G65]

Herbal Use[G2,G6,G7,G8,G64]

Holy thistle is stated to possess bitter stomachic, antidiarrhoeal, antihaemorrhagic, febrifuge, expectorant, antibiotic, bacteriostatic, vulnerary and antiseptic properties. Traditionally, it has been used for anorexia, flatulent dyspepsia, bronchial catarrh, topically for gangrenous and indolent ulcers, and specifically for atonic dyspepsia, and enteropathy with flatulent colic.

Dosage

Dried flowering tops 1.5–3.0 g or by infusion three times daily.[G6,G7]

Liquid extract 1.5–3.0 mL (1:1 in 25% alcohol) three times daily.[G6,G7]

Pharmacological Actions

In vitro and animal studies

Antibacterial activity has been reported for an aqueous extract of the herb, for cnicin, and for the volatile oil.[6–9] Activity has been documented against *Bacillus subtilis*, *Brucella abortus*, *Brucella bronchoseptica*, *Escherichia coli*, *Proteus* species, *Pseudomonas aeruginosa*, *Staphylococcus aureus* and *Streptococcus faecalis*. The antimicrobial activity of holy thistle has been attributed to cnicin and to the polyacetylene constituents.[9]

Cnicin has exhibited *in vivo* anti-inflammatory activity (carrageenan-induced rat-paw oedema test) virtually equipotent to indomethacin.[004,] Antitumour activity has been documented in mice against sarcoma 180 for the whole herb,[8] and against lymphoid leukaemia for cnicin;[8] cnicin has also been reported to exhibit *in vitro* activity against KB cells.[8] An α-methylene-γ-lactone moiety is thought to be necessary for the antibacterial and antitumour activities of cnicin.[8]

Lithospermic acid is thought to be responsible for the antigonadotrophic activity documented for holy thistle.[G30] The sesquiterpene lactone constituents are stated to be bitter principles.[G62]

Tannins are generally known to possess astringent properties.

Side-effects, Toxicity

None documented for holy thistle. The toxicity of cnicin has been studied in mice: the acute oral LD_{50} was stated to be 1.6–3.2 mmol/kg body weight and intraperitoneal administration was reported to cause irritation of tissue. In the writhing test, cnicin was found to cause abdominal pain with an ED_{50} estimated as 6.2 mmol/kg.[4]

Antitumour activity has been documented for the whole herb and for cnicin (*see In vitro* and animal studies).

Contra-indications, Warnings

None documented for holy thistle. Plants containing sesquiterpene lactones with an α-methylene-γ-lactone moiety are generally considered to be allergenic, although no documented hypersensitivity reactions to holy thistle were located. Holy thistle may cause an allergic reaction in individuals with a known hypersensitivity to other members of the Compositae (e.g. chamomile, ragwort, tansy).

Pregnancy and lactation The safety of holy thistle has not been established. In view of the lack of toxicity data, excessive use of holy thistle during pregnancy and lactation should be avoided.

Pharmaceutical Comment

The chemistry of holy thistle is well documented and the available pharmacological data support most of the stated herbal uses, although no references to human studies were located. In view of the lack of toxicity data, excessive use of holy thistle should be avoided.

References

See also General References G2, G3, G6, G9, G16, G30, G31, G36, G37, G40, G43, G56, G62 and G64.

1 Vanhaelen M, Vanhaelen-Fastré R. Lactonic lignans from *Cnicus benedictus*. *Phytochemistry* 1975; **14**: 2709.
2 Vanhaelen-Fastré R. Constituents polyacétyleniques de *Cnicus benedictus* L. *Planta Med* 1974; **25**: 47–59.
3 Ulubelen A, Berkan T. Triterpenic and steroidal compounds of *Cnicus benedictus*. *Planta Med* 1977; **31**: 375–377.
4 Schneider G, Lachner I. A contribution to analytics and pharmacology of Cnicin. *Planta Med* 1987; **53**: 247–251.
5 Vanhaelen-Fastré R, Vanhaelen M. Presence of saloniténolide in *Cnicus benedictus*. *Planta Med* 1974; **26**: 375–379.
6 Vanhaelen-Fastré R. Constitution and antibiotical properties of the essential oil of *Cnicus benedictus*. *Planta Med* 1973; **24**: 165–175.
7 Cobb E. Antineoplastic agent from *Cnicus benedictus*. British Patent 1,335,181 (Cl.A61k) 24 Oct 1973, Appl.54,800/69 (via *Chemical Abstracts* 1975; **83**: 48189j).
8 Vanhaelen-Fastré R. Antibiotic and cytotoxic activities of cnicin isolated from *Cnicus benedictus*. *J Pharm Belg* 1972; **27**: 683–688.
9 Vanhaelen-Fastré R. *Cnicus benedictus*: Separation of antimicrobial constituents. *Plant Med Phytother* 1968; **2**: 294–299.

Hops

Species (Family)

Humulus lupulus L. (Cannabinaceae/Moraceae)

Synonym(s)

Humulus, Lupulus

Part(s) Used

Strobile

Pharmacopoeial and Other Monographs

BHC 1992[G6]
BHP 1996[G9]
BP 2001[G15]
Complete German Commission E[G3]
ESCOP 1997[G52]
Martindale 32nd edition[G43]
PDR for Herbal Medicines 2nd edition[G36]
Ph Eur 2002[G28]

Legal Category (Licensed Products)

GSL[G37]

Constituents[G2,G6,G22,G41,G48,G49,G52,G64]

Flavonoids Astragalin, kaempferol, quercetin, quercitrin and rutin.

Chalcones Isoxanthohumol, xanthohumol, 6-isopentenylnaringenin, 3′-(isoprenyl)-2′,4-dihydroxy-4′,6′-dimethoxychalcone, 2′,6′-dimethoxy-4,4′-dihydroxychalcone.[1]

Oleo-resin 15–30%. Bitter principles (acylphloroglucides) in a soft and hard resin. The lipophilic soft resin consists mainly of α-acids (e.g. humulone, cohumulone, adhumulone, prehumulone, posthumulone), β-acids (e.g. lupulone, colupulone, adlupulone), and their oxidative degradation products including 2-methyl-3-buten-2-ol[2,3,G52] The hard resin contains a hydrophilic δ-resin and χ-resin.

Tannins 2–4%. Condensed; gallocatechin identified.[4]

Volatile oils 0.3–1.0%. More than 100 terpenoid components identified; primarily (at least 90%) β-caryophyllene, farnesene and humulene (sesquiter-monoterpene).

Other constituents Amino acids, phenolic acids, gamma-linoleic acids, lipids and oestrogenic substances (disputed).[5]

It has been stated that only low amounts of 2-methyl-3-buten- 2-ol, the sedative principle identified in hops, are present in sedative tablets containing hops.[2] However, it is thought that 2-methyl-3-buten-2-ol is formed *in vivo* by metabolism of the α-bitter acids and, therefore, the low amount of 2-methyl-3-buten-2-ol in a preparation may not indicate low sedative activity.[6] Interestingly, relatively high concentrations of 2-methyl-3-buten-2-ol were found in bath preparations, suggesting that high concentrations of 2-methyl-3-buten-2-ol may be achieved in both tea and bath products containing hops.[2]

Food Use

Hops are listed by the Council of Europe as a natural source of food flavouring (category N2). This category indicates that hops can be added to foodstuffs in small quantities, with a possible limitation of an active principle (as yet unspecified) in the final product.[G16] In the USA, hops is listed as GRAS (Generally Recognised As Safe).[G65]

Herbal Use[G2,G4,G6,G7,G8,G32,G43,G52,G54,G56,G64]

Hops are stated to possess sedative, hypnotic and topical bactericidal properties. Traditionally, they have been used for neuralgia, insomnia, excitability, priapism, mucous colitis, topically for crural ulcers, and specifically for restlessness associated with nervous tension headache and/or indigestion. The German Commission E approved use for mood disturbances such as restlessness and anxiety as well as sleep disturbances.[G3] Hops are used in combination with valerian root for nervous sleeping disorders and conditions of unrest.[G3]

Dosage

Dried strobile 0.5–1.0 g or by infusion; 1–2 g as a hypnotic.

Liquid extract 0.5–2.0 mL (1 : 1 in 45% alcohol).

Tincture 1–2 mL (1 : 5 in 60% alcohol).

Pharmacological Actions

In vitro and animal studies

Antibacterial activity, mainly against Gram-positive bacteria, has been documented for hops, and attributed to the humulone and lupulone constituents.[7] The activity of the bitter acids against Gram-positive bacteria is thought to involve primary membrane leakage. Resistance of Gram-negative bacteria to the resin acids is attributed to the presence of a phospholipid-containing outer membrane, as lupulone and humulone are inactivated by serum phospholipids.[7] Structure–activity studies have indicated the requirement of a hydrophobic molecule and a six-membered central ring for such activity.[8]

The humulones and lupulones are thought to possess little activity towards fungi or yeasts. However, antifungal activity has been documented for the bitter acids towards *Trichophyton*, *Candida*, *Fusarium* and *Mucor* species.[9] Flavonone constituents have also been documented to possess antifungal activity towards *Trichophyton* and *Mucor* species, and antibacterial activity towards *Staphylococcus aureus*.[10]

Antispasmodic activity has been documented for an alcoholic hop extract on various isolated smooth muscle preparations.[11] Hops have been reported to exhibit hypnotic and sedative properties.[G41] 2-Methyl-3-buten-2-ol, a bitter acid degradation product, has been identified as a sedative principle in hops.[2,3] 2-Methyl-3-buten-2-ol has been shown to possess narcotic properties in mice and motility depressant activity in rats, with the latter not attributable to a muscle-relaxant effect.[12] It has also been suggested that isovaleric acid residues present in hops may contribute towards the sedative action. In mice, hops extract administered intraperitoneally (100, 250, 500 mg/kg) 30 minutes prior to a series of behavioural tests, resulted in a dose-dependent suppression of spontaneous locomotor at doses of 250 mg/kg for up to one hour.[13] The time for mice to be able to remain on a rota rod was decreased by 59 and 65% at doses of 250 mg/kg and 500 mg/kg, respectively. The time of onset of convulsions and survival time after administration of pentylenetetrazole (100 mg/kg) was significantly lengthened. Hops extract (35 mg/kg, intraperitoneal administration) produced a dose-dependent increase in sleeping time in mice treated with pentobarbitol. An antinociceptive effect was noted by increased latency of licking forepaws in hotplate tests and hypothermic activity observed from a time-dependent fall of rectal temperature at a dose of 500 mg/kg.[13]

Hops have previously been reported to possess oestrogenic constituents.[5] However, when a number of purified components, including the volatile oil and the bitter acids, were examined using the uterine weight assay in immature female mice, no oestrogenic activity was found.[5]

Clinical studies

Clinical studies have generally assessed hops given in combination with one or more additional herbs. For example, hops has been reported to improve sleep disturbances when given in combination with valerian.[14]

Hops, in combination with chicory and peppermint, has been documented to relieve pain in patients with chronic cholecystitis (calculus and non-calculous).[15] A herbal product containing a mixture of plant extracts, including hops and uva-ursi, and alpha-tocopherol acetate was reported to improve irritable bladder and urinary incontinence.[16]

Side-effects, Toxicity

Respiratory allergy caused by the handling of hop cones have been documented;[17] a subsequent patch test using dried, crushed flowerheads proved negative. Positive patch test reactions have been documented for fresh hop oil, humulone, and lupulone. Myrcene, present in the fresh oil but readily oxidised, was concluded to be the sensitising agent in the hop oil.[G51] Contact dermatitis to hops has long been recognised[G51] and is attributed to the pollen.[G41] Small doses of hops are stated to be non-toxic.[G42] Large doses administered to animals by injection have resulted in a soporific effect followed by death, with chronic administration resulting in weight loss before death.[G39]

Contra-indications, Warnings

It has been stated that hops should not be taken by individuals suffering from depressive illness, as the sedative effect may accentuate symptoms.[G45,G49] The sedative action may potentiate the effects of existing sedative therapy and alcohol. Allergic reactions have been reported for hops, although only following external contact with the herb and oil. Reports of oestrogenic activity are inconclusive.[G52] It is claimed that hops are not oestrogenic,[G56] but hop flower is said to have oestrogenic-binding activity and physiological oestrogenic effects.[18] Concern has been expressed that herbs with oestrogenic effects, including hops, may stimulate breast cancer growth and oppose action of competative oestrogen receptor antagonists such as tamoxifen.[18]

Pregnancy and lactation *In vitro* antispasmodic activity on the uterus has been documented. In view of this and the lack of toxicity data, the excessive use of hops during pregnancy and lactation should be avoided.

Pharmaceutical Comment

The chemistry of hops is well documented and is characterised by the bitter acid components of the oleo-resin. Documented pharmacological activities justify the herbal uses, although excessive use should be avoided in view of the limited toxicity data.

References

See also General References G2, G3, G5, G6, G9, G11, G15, G16, G22, G28, G29, G31, G32, G36, G37, G39, G41, G42, G43, G48, G49, G51, G52, G54, G56 and G64.

1 Song-San S *et al*. Chalcones from *Humulus lupulus*. *Phytochemistry* 1989; **28**: 1776–1777.
2 Hänsel R *et al*. The sedative-hypnotic principle of hops. 3. Communication: Contents of 2-methyl-3-butene-2-ol in hops and hop preparations. *Planta Med* 1982; **45**: 224–228.
3 Wohlfart R *et al*. Detection of sedative–hypnotic hop constituents, V: Degradation of humulones and lupulones to 2-methyl-3-buten-2-ol, a hop constituent possessing sedative-hypnotic activity. *Arch Pharm (Weinheim)* 1982; **315**: 132–137.
4 Gorissen H *et al*. Separation and identification of (+)-gallocatechin in hops. *Arch Int Physiol Biochem* 1968; **76**: 932–934.
5 Fenselau C, Talalay P. Is oestrogenic activity present in hops? *Food Cosmet Toxicol* 1973; **11**: 597–603.
6 Hänsel R, Wohlfart R. Narcotic action of 2-methyl-3-butene-2-ol contained in the exhalation of hops. *Z Naturforsch* 1980; **35**: 1096–1097.
7 Teuber M, Schmalreck AF. Membrane leakage in *Bacillus subtilis* 168 induced by the hop constituents lupulone, humulone, isohumulone and humulinic acid. *Arch Mikrobiol* 1973; **94**: 159–171.
8 Schmalreck AF *et al*. Structural features determining the antibiotic potencies of natural and synthetic hop bitter resins, their precursors and derivatives. *Can J Microbiol* 1975; **21**: 205–212.
9 Mizobuchi S, Sato Y. Antifungal activities of hop bitter resins and related compounds. *Agric Biol Chem* 1985; **49**: 399–405.
10 Mizobuchi S, Sato Y. A new flavanone with antifungal activity isolated from hops. *Agric Biol Chem* 1984; **48**: 2771–2775.
11 Caujolle F *et al*. Spasmolytic action of hop (*Humulus lupulus*). *Agressologie* 1969; **10**: 405–10.
12 Wohlfart R *et al*. The sedative-hypnotic principle of hops. 4. Communication: Pharmacology of 2-methyl-3-buten-2-ol. *Planta Med* 1983; **48**: 120–123.
13 Lee KM *et al*. Effects of *Humulus lupulus* extract on the central nervous system in mice. *Planta Med* 1993; **59**: A691.
14 Müller-Limmroth W, Ehrenstein W. Untersuchungen über die Wirkung von Seda- Kneipp auf den Schlaf schlafgestörter Menschen. *Med Klin* 1977; **72**: 1119–1125.
15 Chakarski I *et al*. Clinical study of a herb combination consisting of *Humulus lupulus*, *Cichorium intybus*, *Mentha piperita* in patients with chronic calculous and non-calculous cholecystitis. *Probl Vatr Med* 1982; **10**: 65–69.
16 Lenau H *et al*. Wirksamkeit und Verträglichkeit von Cysto Fink bei Patienten mit Reizblase und/oder Harninkontinenz. *Therapiewoche* 1984; **34**: 6054.
17 Newmark FM. Hops allergy and terpene sensitivity: An occupational disease. *Ann Allergy* 1978; **41**: 311–312.
18 Stockley IH. *Drug Interactions*, 5th edn. London: Pharmaceutical Press, 1999.

Horehound, Black

Species (Family)

Ballota nigra L. (Labiatae)

Synonym(s)

Ballota

Part(s) Used

Herb

Pharmacopoeial and Other Monographs

BHP 1996[G9]
PDR for Herbal Medicines 2nd edition[G36]

Legal Category (Licensed Products)

Black horehound is not included in the GSL.[G37]

Constituents[G49,G64]

Limited chemical information is available for black horehound. Documented constituents include diterpenes (e.g. ballotenol, ballotinone, preleosibirin),[1–3] flavonoids, and volatile oil.

Food Use

Black horehound is listed by the Council of Europe as a natural source of food flavouring (category N3). This category indicates that black horehound can be added to foodstuffs in the traditionally accepted manner, although insufficient information is available for an adequate assessment of potential toxicity.[G16]

Herbal Use

Black horehound is stated to possess anti-emetic, sedative and mild astringent properties. Traditionally, it has been used for nausea, vomiting, nervous dyspepsia, and specifically for vomiting of central origin.[G7,G64]

Dosage

Dried herb 2–4 g or by infusion three times daily.[G7]

Liquid extract 1–3 mL (1 : 1 in 25% alcohol) three times daily.[G7]

Tincture 1–2 mL (1 : 10 in 45% alcohol) three times daily.[G7]

Pharmacological Actions

None documented.

Side-effects, Toxicity

None documented.

Contra-indications, Warnings

None documented.

Pregnancy and lactation Black horehound is reputed to affect the menstrual cycle.[G30] In view of the lack of phytochemical, pharmacological and toxicity data, the use of black horehound during pregnancy and lactation should be avoided.

Pharmaceutical Comment

Limited phytochemical or pharmacological information is available for black horehound to justify its use as a herbal remedy. In view of the lack of toxicity data, excessive use should be avoided.

References

See also General References G9, G16, G30, G36, G37, G49 and G64.

1 Bruno M *et al*. Preleosibirin, a prefuranic labdane diterpene from *Ballota nigra* subsp. *foetida*. *Phytochemistry* 1986; **25**: 538–539.
2 Savona G *et al*. Structure of ballotinone, a diterpenoid from *Ballota nigra*. *J Chem Soc Perkin Trans 1* 1976; 1607–1609.
3 Savona G *et al*. The structure of ballotenol, a new diterpenoid from *Ballota nigra*. *J Chem Soc Perkin Trans 1* 1977; 497–499.

Horehound, White

Species (Family)

Marrubium vulgare L. (Labiatae)

Synonym(s)

Common Hoarhound, Hoarhound, Horehound, Marrubium

Part(s) Used

Flower, leaf

Pharmacopoeial and Other Monographs

BHC 1992[G6]
BHP 1996[G9]
Complete German Commission E[G3]
Martindale 32nd edition[G43]
PDR for Herbal Medicines 2nd edition[G36]

Legal Category (Licensed Products)

GSL[G37]

Constituents[G2,G6,G41,G62,G64]

Alkaloids Pyrrolidine-type. Betonicine 0.3%, the *cis*-isomer turicine.

Flavonoids Apigenin, luteolin, quercetin, and their glycosides.[1]

Terpenoids Diterpenes including marrubiin 0.3–1.0%, a lactone, as the main component with lesser amounts of various alcohols (e.g. marrubenol, marrubiol, peregrinol and vulgarol). Marrubiin has also been stated to be an artefact formed from a precursor, premarrubiin, during extraction.[2]

Volatile oils Trace. Bisabolol, camphene, *p*-cymene, limonene, β-pinene, sabinene and others,[2] a sesquiterpene (unspecified).

Other constituents Choline, saponin (unspecified), β-sitosterol (a phytosterol), waxes (C_{26}-C_{34} alkanes).

Food Use

White horehound is listed by the Council of Europe as a natural source of food flavouring (category N2). This category indicates that white horehound can be added to foodstuffs in small quantities, with a possible limitation of an active principle (as yet unspecified) in the final product.[G16] In the USA, white horehound is listed as GRAS (Generally Recognised As Safe).[G65]

Herbal Use

White horehound is stated to possess expectorant and antispasmodic properties. Traditionally, it has been used for acute or chronic bronchitis, whooping cough, and specifically for bronchitis with non-productive cough.[G2,G6,G7,G8,G64]

Dosage

Dried herb 1–2 g or by infusion three times daily.[G6,G7]

Liquid extract 2–4 mL (1:1 in 20% alcohol) three times daily.[G6,G7]

Pharmacological Actions

In vitro and animal studies

Aqueous extracts have been reported to exhibit an antagonistic effect towards hydroxytryptamine *in vivo* in mice, and *in vitro* in guinea-pig ileum and rat uterus tissue.[3] Expectorant and vasodilatory properties have been documented for the volatile oil.[4] However, the main active expectorant principle in white horehound is reported to be marrubiin, which is stated to stimulate secretions of the bronchial mucosa.[G60,] Marrubiin has also been stated to be cardioactive, possessing anti-arrhythmic properties, although higher doses are reported to cause arrhythmias.[G60] Marrubin acid (obtained from the saponification of marrubiin) has been documented to stimulate bile secretion in rats, whereas marrubiin was found to be inactive.[5] White horehound is stated to possess bitter properties (BI 65 000 com-

294

pared to gentian BI 10 000–30 000) with marrubiin as the main active component.[G62]

Large doses of white horehound are purgative.[G10,G60] The volatile oil has antischistosomal activity.[6]

Side-effects, Toxicity

The plant juice of white horehound is stated to contain an irritant principle, which can cause contact dermatitis.[G51] No documented toxicity studies were located for the whole plant, although an LD_{50} (rat, by mouth) value for marrubin acid is reported as 370 mg/kg body weight.[5] The volatile oil is documented to be highly toxic to the flukes *Schistosoma mansoni* and *Schistosoma haematobium*.[6]

Contra-indications, Warnings

None documented. Cardioactive properties and an antagonism of 5-hydroxytryptamine have been documented in animals.

Pregnancy and lactation White horehound is reputed to be an abortifacient and to affect the menstrual cycle.[G30] Uterine stimulant activity in animals has been documented.[G30] In view of this and the lack of safety data, the use of white horehound during pregnancy should be avoided. Excessive use during lactation should be avoided.

Pharmaceutical Comment

The chemistry of white horehound is well documented. Limited pharmacological information is available, although expectorant properties have been reported which support some of the herbal uses. In view of the lack of toxicity data and suggested cardioactive properties, white horehound should not be taken in excessive doses.

References

See also General References G2, G3, G6, G9, G10, G16, G30, G31, G32, G36, G37, G41, G43, G48, G51, G60, G62 and G64.

1   Kowalewski Z, Matlawska I. Flavonoid compounds in the herb of *Marrubium vulgare* L. *Herba Pol* 1978; **24**: 183–186.
2   Henderson MS, McCrindle R. Premarrubiin. A diterpernoid from *Marrubium vulgare* L. *J Chem Soc* 1969; (C): 2014.
3   Cahen R. Pharmacologic spectrum of *Marrubium vulgare*. *C R Soc Biol* 1970; **164**: 1467–1472.
4   Karryev MO *et al.* Some therapeutic properties and phytochemistry of common horehound. *Izv Akad Nauk Turkm SSR Ser Biol Nauk* 1976; **3**: 86–88.
5   Krejcí I, Zadina R. Die Gallentreibende Wirkung von Marrubiin und Marrabinsäure. *Planta Med*; 1959; **7**: 1–7.
6   Saleh MM, Glombitza KW. Volatile oil of *Marrubium vulgare* and its anti-schistosomal activity. *Planta Med* 1989; **55**: 105.

Horse-chestnut

Species (Family)

Aesculus hippocastanum L. (Hippocastanaceae)

Synonym(s)

Aesculus

Part(s) Used

Seed

Pharmacopoeial and Other Monographs

BHP 1996[G9]
ESCOP 1999[G52]
Martindale 32nd edition[G43]
Mills and Bone[G50]
PDR for Herbal Medicines 2nd edition[G36]

Legal Category (Licensed Products)

GSL (for external use only)[G37]

Constituents[G22,G48,G52,G59,G62,G64]

Coumarins Aesculetin, fraxin (fraxetin glucoside), scopolin (scopoletin glucoside).

Flavonoids Flavonol (kaempferol, quercetin) glycosides including astragalin, isoquercetrin, rutin; leucocyanidin (quercetin derivative).

Saponins French pharmacopoeial standard, not less than 3% aescin. A mixture of saponins collectively referred to as 'aescin' (3–10%); α- and β-escin as major glycosides.

Tannins Type unspecified but likely to be condensed in view of the epicatechin content (formed during hydrolysis of condensed tannins).

Other constituents Allantoin, amino acids (adenine, adenosine, guanine), choline, citric acid, phytosterol.

Food Use

Horse-chestnut is not used in foods.

Herbal Use[G4,G49,G52]

Traditionally, horse-chestnut has been used for the treatment of varicose veins, haemorrhoids, phlebitis, diarrhoea, fever and enlargement of the prostate gland. The German Commission E approved use for treatment of chronic venous insufficiency in the legs.[G3]

Dosage

Fruit 0.2–1.0 g three times daily.[G49]

Preparations Extracts equivalent to 50–150 mg triterpenes calculated as aescin.[G52]

Pharmacological Actions

Documented studies have concentrated on the actions of the saponins, in particular, aescin.

In vitro and animal studies

Anti-inflammatory and anti-oedema effects Anti-inflammatory activity in rats has been documented for both a fruit extract and the saponin fraction.[1–4] Anti-inflammatory activity in the rat has been reported to be greater for a total horse-chestnut extract compared to aescin. In addition, an extract excluding aescin also exhibited activity, suggesting that horse-chestnut contains anti-inflammatory agents other than aescin.[5] No difference in activity was noted when the horse-chestnut extracts were administered prior to and after dextran (inflammatory agent). It has been proposed that aescin affects the initial phase of inflammation by exerting a 'sealing' effect on capillaries and by reducing the number and/or diameter of capillary pores.[3]

Effects on venous tone Horse-chestnut extract (16% aescin, 0.2 mg/mL) and also aescin (0.1 mg/mL) induced contractions in isolated bovine and human veins.[G52] Concentration-dependent contractions of isolated canine veins were observed with a horse-chestnut extract (16% aescin, 5×10^{-4} mg/mL).[G52] A standardised extract (16% aescin, 50 mg, given intravenously) increased femoral venous pressure in anaesthetised dogs, and decreased cutaneous capillary hyperpermeability in rats (200 mg/kg, given orally).[G52]

In addition, the saponin fraction has been reported to exhibit analgesic and antigranulation activities in rats,[3] to reduce capillary permeability,[6] and to produce an initial hypotension followed by a longer lasting hypertension in anaesthetised animals.[4] Prostaglandin production by venous tissue is thought to be involved in the regulation of vascular reactivity.[7] Prostaglandins of the E series are known to cause relaxation of venous tissues whereas those of the F_α series produce contraction. Increased venous tone induced by aescin *in vitro* was found to be associated with an increased $PGF_{2\alpha}$ synthesis in the venous tissue.

Other activities   *In vitro*, aescin has been documented to inhibit hyaluronidase activity (IC_{50} 150 μmol/L).[G52]

A saponin fraction of horse-chestnut has been reported to contract isolated rabbit ileum.[3]

Antiviral activity *in vitro* against influenza virus (A_2/Japan 305) has been described for aescin.[8]

Metabolism studies of aescin in the rat have concluded that aescin toxicity is reduced by hepatic metabolism.[9]

Flavonoids and tannins are generally recognised as having anti-inflammatory and astringent properties, respectively.

Clinical studies

Chronic venous insufficiency   Several studies have assessed the effects of horse-chestnut seed extract in patients with chronic venous insufficiency, a common condition which causes oedema of the lower leg.

A systematic review of randomised, double-blind, controlled trials of horse-chestnut seed extract in chronic venous insufficiency included 13 studies (eight placebo-controlled trials and five studies comparing horse-chestnut seed extract with reference medication or compression therapy).[10] Generally, trials involved the administration of horse-chestnut seed extract 100 or 150 mg daily for 3–12 weeks. The results of all the placebo-controlled studies indicated that horse-chestnut seed extract was superior. Four comparative studies indicated that horse-chestnut seed extract was as effective as O-(β-hydroxyethyl)-rutosides in relieving symptoms of chronic venous insufficiency; one study suggested that horse-chestnut seed extract was as effective as compression therapy. It was concluded that horse-chestnut seed extract is effective as a symptomatic, short-term treatment for chronic venous insufficiency, but that further well-designed clinical trials are required to confirm this.[10]

Other effects   Glycosaminoglycan hydrolyses are enzymes involved in the breakdown of substances (proteoglycans) that determine capillary rigidity and pore size (thus influencing the passage of macromolecules into the surrounding tissue). Proteoglycans also interact with collagen, stabilising the fibres and regulating their correct biosynthesis.[11] The activity of these enzymes was found to be raised in patients with varicosis, compared with healthy patients. In a study involving 15 patients with varicosis treated with horse-chestnut extract (900 mg daily) for 12 days, the activity of these enzymes was significantly reduced.[11] It was proposed that horse-chestnut may act at the site of enzyme release, exerting a stabilising effect on the lysosomal membrane.[11]

In a randomised, double-blind, placebo-controlled study involving 70 healthy individuals with haematomas, a topical gel (2% aescin) reduced sensitivity to pressure on affected areas.[G52]

The cosmetic applications of horse-chestnut have been reviewed;[12] these effects are attributed to properties associated with the saponin constituents.

Side-effects, Toxicity

Two incidences of toxic nephropathy have been reported and were stated as probably secondary to the ingestion of high doses of aescin.[13] In Japan, where horse-chestnut has been used as an anti-inflammatory drug after surgery or trauma, hepatic injury has been described in a male patient who received an intramuscular injection of a proprietary product containing horse-chestnut.[14] Liver function tests showed a mild abnormality and a diagnosis of giant cell tumour of bone (grade 2) by bone biopsy was made. Other side-effects stated to have been reported for the product include shock, spasm, mild nausea, vomiting and urticaria.[14]

The effect of aescin, both free and albumin-bound, on renal tubular transport processes has been studied in the isolated, artificially perfused frog kidney.[15] Aescin was found to primarily affect tubular, rather than glomerular, epithelium and it was noted that binding to plasma protein (approximately 50%) protects against this nephrotoxicity. Aescin was thought to be neither secreted nor reabsorbed in the tubules, and the concentration of unbound aescin filtered through the kidney (13%) was considered to be too low to have toxic effects. The authors commented that the symptoms of acute renal failure in humans are caused primarily by interference with glomeruli and in view of this, the nephrotoxic potential of aescin is probably only relevant when the kidneys are already damaged and also if the aescin is displaced from its binding to plasma protein.[15]

A proprietary product containing horse-chestnut (together with phenopyrazone and cardiac glycoside-containing plant extracts) has been associated with the development of a drug-induced auto-immune disease called 'pseudolupus syndrome' in Germany and Switzerland.[16,17] The individual component in the product responsible for the syndrome was not established.

It has been noted that death occurs rapidly in animals given large doses of aescin, due to massive haemolysis. Death is more prolonged in animals given smaller doses of aescin.[4]

LD_{50} values for aescin have been estimated in mice, rats and guinea-pigs and range from 134 to 720 mg/kg (by mouth) and from 1.4 to 15.2 mg/kg (intravenous injection).[G49] The total saponin fraction has been reported to be less toxic in mice (intraperitoneal injection) compared to the isolated aescin mixture (LD_{50} 46.5 mg/kg and 9.5 mg/kg, respectively).[3] The haemolytic index of horse-chestnut is documented as being 6000, compared with 9500 to 12 500 for aescin.[G62] Daily doses in rats (100 mg/kg, orally) of a standardised extract of horse-chestnut (16% aescin) did not produce teratogenic effects, and the extract was negative in the Ames test with *Salmonella typhimurium* TA98 without actuation.[G52]

Contra-indications, Warnings

Horse-chestnut may be irritant to the gastrointestinal tract due to the saponin constituents. Saponins are generally recognised to possess haemolytic properties, but are not usually absorbed from the gastrointestinal tract following oral administration. Horse-chestnut may interfere with anticoagulant/coagulant therapy (coumarin constituents). Aescin, the main saponin component in horse-chestnut, binds to plasma protein and may affect the binding of other drugs. Horse-chestnut should be avoided by patients with existing renal or hepatic impairment.

Pregnancy and lactation   The safety of horse-chestnut during pregnancy and lactation has not been established. In view of the pharmacologically active constituents present in horse-chestnut, use during pregnancy and lactation is best avoided.

Pharmaceutical Comment

Horse-chestnut is traditionally characterised by its saponin components, in particular aescin which represents a mixture of compounds. However, horse-chestnut also contains other pharmacologically active constituents including coumarins and flavonoids. The traditional use of horse-chestnut in peripheral vascular disorders has largely been substantiated by studies in animals and humans, in which anti-inflammatory and capillary stabilising effects have been observed. There is evidence from randomised, double-blind, controlled clinical trials to support the use of horse-chestnut seed extract in the treatment of symptoms of chronic venous insufficiency.

Many of the documented activities can probably be attributed to the saponin and flavonoid constituents in horse-chestnut.

References

See also General References G2, G9, G16, G22, G31, G36, G37, G43, G48, G49, G50, G52, G56, G59, G62 and G64.

1   Farnsworth NR, Cordell GA. A review of some biologically active compounds isolated from plants as reported in the 1974–75 literature. *Lloydia* 1976; **39**: 420–455.

2   Benoit PS *et al.* Biological and phytochemical evaluation of plants. XIV. Antiinflammatory evaluation of 163 species of plants. *Lloydia* 1976; **39**: 160–171.

3   Cebo B *et al.* Pharmacological properties of saponin fractions from Polish crude drugs: *Saponaria officinalis*, *Primula officinalis*, and *Aesculus hippocastanum*. *Herba Pol* 1976; **22**: 154–162.

4   Vogel G *et al.* Untersuchungen zum Mechanismus der therapeutischen und toxischen Wirkung des Rosskastanien-saponins aescin. *Arzneimittelforschung* 1970; **20**: 699–705.

5   Tsutsumi S, Ishizuka S. Anti-inflammatory effects of the extract *Aesculus hippocastanum* and seed. *Shikwa-Gakutto* 1967; **67**: 1324–1328.

6   De Pascale V *et al.* Effect of an escin-cyclonamine mixture on capillary permeability. *Boll Chim Farm* 1974; **113**: 600–614.

7   Longiave D *et al.* The mode of action of aescin on isolated veins: Relationship with $PGF_2\alpha$. *Pharmacol Res Commun* 1978; **10**: 145–153.

8   Rao SG, Cochran KW. Antiviral activity of triterpenoid saponins containing acylated β-amyrin aglycones. *J Pharm Sci* 1974; **63**: 471.

9   Rothkopf M. Effects of age, sex and phenobarbital pretreatment on the acute toxicity of the horse chestnut saponin aescin in rats. *Naunyn-Schmiedarchpharm* 1977; **297**(Suppl.): R18.

10 Pittler MH, Ernst E. Horse-chestnut seed extract for chronic venous insufficiency. A criteria-based systematic review. *Arch Dermatol* 1998; **134**: 1356–1360.

11 Kreysel HW *et al*. A possible role of lysosomal enzymes in the pathogenesis of varicosis and the reduction in their serum activity by Venostasin^R. *Vasa* 1983; **12**: 377– 382.

12 Proserpio G *et al*. Cosmetic uses of horse-chestnut (*Aesculum hippocastanum*) extracts, of escin and of the cholesterol/escin complex. *Fitoterapia* 1980; **51**: 113–128.

13 Grasso A, Corvaglia E. Two cases of suspected toxic tubulonephrosis due to escine. *Gazz Med Ital* 1976; **135**: 581–584.

14 Takegoshi K *et al*. A case of Venoplant^R-induced hepatic injury. *Gastroenterol Japonica* 1986; **21**: 62–65.

15 Rothkopf M *et al*. Animal experiments on the question of the renal toleration of the horse chestnut saponin aescin. *Arzneimittelforschung* 1977; **27**: 598–605.

16 Grob P *et al*. Drug-induced pseudolupus. *Lancet* 1975; **ii**: 144–148.

17 Russell AS. Drug-induced autoimmune disease. *Clin Immunol Allergy* 1981; **1**: 57–76.

Horseradish

Species (Family)

Radicula armoracia (L.) Robinson (Brassicaceae/Cruciferae)

Synonym(s)

Armoracia lopathifolia Gilib., *A. rusticana* (Gaertn.) Mey & Scherb., *Cochlearia armoracia* L., *Nasturtium armoracia* Fries, *Roripa armoracia* Hitch.

Part(s) Used

Root

Pharmacopoeial and Other Monographs

Complete German Commission E[G3]
PDR for Herbal Medicines 2nd edition[G36]

Legal Category (Licensed Products)

GSL[G37]

Constituents[G40,G48,G49,G57,G58,G62,G64]

Coumarins Aesculetin, scopoletin.[1]

Phenols Caffeic acid derivatives and lesser amounts of hydroxycinnamic acid derivatives. Concentrations of acids are reported to be much lower in the root than in the leaf.[1]

Volatile oils Glucosinolates (mustard oil glycosides) gluconasturtiin and sinigrin (*S*-glucosides), yielding phenylethylisothiocyanate and allylisothiocyanate after hydrolysis. Isothiocyanate content estimated as 12.2–20.4 mg/g freeze dried root.[2,3] Other isothiocyanate types include isopropyl, 3-butenyl, 4-pentenyl, phenyl, 3-methylthiopropyl and benzyl derivatives.[4]

Other constituents Ascorbic acid, asparagin, peroxidase enzymes, resin, starch and sugar.

Other plant parts Kaempferol and quercetin have been documented for the leaf.

Food Use

Horseradish is listed by the Council of Europe as a natural source of food flavouring (category N2). This category indicates that horseradish can be added to foodstuffs in small quantities, with a possible limitation of an active principle (as yet unspecified) in the final product.[G16] In the USA, horseradish is listed as GRAS (Generally Recognised As Safe).[G57] Horseradish is commonly used as a food flavouring.

Herbal Use

Horseradish is stated to possess antiseptic, circulatory and digestive stimulant, diuretic and vulnerary properties.[G42,G49,G64] Traditionally, it has been used for pulmonary and urinary infection, urinary stones, oedematous conditions, and externally for application to inflamed joints or tissues.[G49]

Dosage

Root (fresh) 2–4 g before meals.[G49]

Pharmacological Actions

In vitro and animal studies

A marked hypotensive effect in cats has been documented for horseradish peroxidase, following intravenous administration.[5] The effect was completely blocked by aspirin and indomethacin, but was not affected by antihistamines. It was concluded that horseradish peroxidase acts by stimulating the synthesis of arachidonic acid metabolites.

Side-effects, Toxicity

Isothiocyanates are reported to have irritant effects on the skin and also to be allergenic.[G51,G58] Animal poisoning has been documented for horseradish. Symptoms described include inflammation of the stomach or rumen, and excitement followed by collapse.[G33]

Contra-indications, Warnings

It is stated that horseradish may depress thyroid function, and should be avoided by individuals with hypothyroidism or by those receiving thyroxine.[G42,G49] No rationale for this statement is included except that this action is common to all members of the cabbage and mustard family.

Pregnancy and lactation Allylisothiocyanate is extremely toxic and a violent irritant to mucous membranes.[G58] Its use should be avoided during pregnancy and lactation.

Pharmaceutical Comment

The chemistry of horseradish is well established and it is recognised as one of the richest plant sources of peroxidase enzymes.[G48] Little pharmacological information was located, although the isothiocyanates and peroxidases probably account for the reputed circulatory stimulant and wound-healing actions, respectively. The oil is one of the most hazardous of all essential oils and it is not recommended for either external or internal use.[G58] Horseradish should not be ingested in amounts exceeding those used in foods.

References

See also General References G3, G10, G16, G31, G36, G40, G42, G48, G49, G51, G57, G58, G62 and G64.

1 Stoehr H, Herrman K. Phenolic acids of vegetables. III. Hydroxycinnamic acids and hydroxybenzoic acids of root vegetables. *Z Lebensm-Unters Forsch* 1975: **159**: 219–224.
2 Hansen H. Content of glucosinolates in horseradish (*Armoracia rusticana*). *Tidsskr Planteavl* 1974; **73**: 408–410.
3 Kojima M. Volatile components of *Wasabia japonica*. II. Volatile components other than isothiocyanates. *Hakko Kogaku Zasshi* 1971; **49**: 650–653.
4 Kojima M *et al.* Studies on the volatile components of *Wasabia japonica*, *Brassica juncea*, and *Cocholearia armoracia* by gas chromatography-mass spectrometry. *Yakugaku Zasshi* 1973; **93**: 453–459.
5 Sjaastad OV *et al.* Hypotensive effects in cats caused by horseradish peroxidase mediated by metabolites of arachidonic acid. *J Histochem Cytochem* 1984; **32**: 1328–1330.

Hydrangea

Species (Family)

Hydrangea arborescens L. (Saxifragaceae)

Synonym(s)

Mountain Hydrangea, Seven Barks, Smooth Hydrangea, Wild Hydrangea

Part(s) Used

Rhizome, Root

Pharmacopoeial and Other Monographs

BHP 1996[G9]
PDR for Herbal Medicines 2nd edition[G36]

Legal Category (Licensed Products)

GSL[G37]

Constituents[G22,G40,G41,G48,G64]

Limited information is available on the chemistry of hydrangea. It is stated to contain carbohydrates (e.g. gum, starch, sugars), flavonoids (e.g. kaempferol, quercetin, rutin), resin, saponins, hydrangin and hydrangenol, a stilbenoid,[1] and to be free from tannins.

Food Use

Hydrangea is not used in foods. In the USA, hydrangea is listed as a 'Herb of Undefined Safety'.[G22]

Herbal Use

Hydrangea is stated to possess diuretic and antilithic properties. Traditionally, it has been used for cystitis, urethritis, urinary calculi, prostatitis, enlarged prostate gland, and specifically for urinary calculi with gravel and cystitis.[G7,G64]

Dosage

Dried rhizome/root 2–4 g or by decoction three times daily.[G7]

Liquid extract 2–4 mL (1 : 1 in 25% alcohol) three times daily.[G7]

Tincture 2–10 mL (1 : 5 in 45% alcohol) three times daily.[G7]

Pharmacological Actions

In vitro and animal studies

None documented for hydrangea. Synthesised hydrangenol derivatives have been reported to possess anti-allergic properties, exhibiting a strong inhibitory action towards hyaluronidase activity and histamine release.[2]

Side-effects, Toxicity

Hydrangea has been reported to cause contact dermatitis,[G51] and it is stated that hydrangin may cause gastroenteritis.[G22] Symptoms of overdose are described as vertigo and a feeling of tightness in the chest.[G22] An extract has been reported to be non-toxic in animals.[G64]

Contra-indications, Warnings

None documented.

Pregnancy and lactation The safety of hydrangea has not been established. In view of the lack of phytochemical, pharmacological and toxicity data, the use of hydrangea during pregnancy and lactation should be avoided.

Pharmaceutical Comment

Limited information is available on the chemistry of hydrangea, although related species have been investigated more thoroughly.[G41] No scientific evidence was located to justify the herbal uses. In view of the lack of toxicity data, excessive use of hydrangea should be avoided.

References

See also General References G7, G9, G22, G32, G36, G37, G40, G41, G48, G51 and G64.

1 Harborne JB, Baxter H. *Phytochemical Dictionary*. London: Taylor and Francis, 1993.
2 Kakegawa H *et al.* Inhibitory effects of hydrangeol derivatives on the activation of hyaluronidase and their anti-allergic activities. *Planta Med* 1988; 54: 385–389.

Hydrocotyle

Species (Family)

Centella asiatica (L.) Urban (Umbelliferae)

Synonym(s)

Centella, Gotu Kola, *Hydrocotyle asiatica*, Indian Pennywort, Indian Water Navelwort

Part(s) Used

Herb

Pharmacopoeial and Other Monographs

BHP 1983[G7]
Martindale 32nd edition[G43]
PDR for Herbal Medicines 2nd edition[G36]
WHO volume 1 1999[G63]

Legal Category (Licensed Products)

GSL (for external use only)[G37]

Constituents[G22,G44,G60,G64]

Amino acids Alanine and serine (major components), aminobutyrate, aspartate, glutamate, histidine, lysine and threonine.[1] The root contains greater quantities than the herb.[1]

Flavonoids Quercetin, kaempferol and various glycosides.[2–4]

Terpenoids Triterpenes, asiaticoside, centelloside, madecassoside, brahmoside and brahminoside (saponin glycosides). Aglycones are referred to as hydrocotylegenin A–E;[5] compounds A–D are reported to be esters of the triterpene alcohol R_1-barrigenol.[5,6] Asiaticentoic acid, centellic acid, centoic acid and madecassic acid.

Volatile oils Various terpenoids including β-caryophyllene, *trans*-β-farnesene and germacrene D (sesquiterpenes) as major components, α-pinene and β-pinene. The major terpenoid is stated to be unidentified.

Other constituents Hydrocotylin (an alkaloid), vallerine (a bitter principle), fatty acids (e.g. linoleic acid, linolenic acid, lignocene, oleic acid, palmitic acid, stearic acid), phytosterols (e.g. campesterol, sitosterol, stigmasterol),[7] resin and tannin.

The underground plant parts of hydrocotyle have been reported to contain small quantities of at least 14 different polyacetylenes.[8–10]

Food Use

Hydrocotyle is not used in foods.

Herbal Use

Hydrocotyle is stated to possess mild diuretic, antirheumatic, dermatological, peripheral vasodilator and vulnerary properties. Traditionally it has been used for rheumatic conditions, cutaneous affections, and by topical application, for indolent wounds, leprous ulcers, and cicatrisation after surgery.[G7,G64]

Dosage

Dried leaf 0.6 g or by infusion three times daily.[G7]

Pharmacological Actions

In vitro and animal studies

The triterpenoids are regarded as the active principles in hydrocotyle.[7] Asiaticoside is reported to possess wound-healing ability, by having a stimulating effect on the epidermis and promoting keratinisation.[11] Asiaticoside is thought to act by an inhibitory action on the synthesis of collagen and mucopolysaccharides in connective tissue.[11]

Both asiaticoside and madecassoside are documented to be anti-inflammatory, and the total saponin fraction is reported to be active in the carrageenan rat paw oedema test.[12]

In vivo studies in rats have shown that asiaticoside exhibits a protective action against stress-induced gastric ulcers, following subcutaneous administration,[13] and accelerates the healing of chemical-induced duodenal ulcers, after oral administration.[14] It was thought that asiaticoside acted by increasing the ability of the rats to cope with a stressful situation, rather than via a local effect on the mucosa.[13]

In vivo studies in mice and rats using brahmoside and brahminoside, by intraperitoneal injection, have shown a CNS-depressant effect.[15] The compounds were found to decrease motor activity, increase hexobarbitone sleeping time, slightly decrease body temperature, and were thought to act via a cholinergic mechanism.[15] A hypertensive effect in rats was also observed, but only following large doses.[15] *In vitro* studies with brahmoside and brahminoside indicated a relaxant effect on the rabbit duodenum and rat uterus, and an initial increase, followed by a decrease, in the amplitude and rate of contraction of the isolated rabbit heart.[15] Higher doses were found to cause cardiac arrest, although subsequent intravenous administration in dogs caused no marked change in an ECG.[15]

In vitro antifertility activity against human and rat sperm has been described for the total saponin fraction.[16] Asiaticoside and brahminoside are thought to be the active components, although no spermicidal or spermostatic action could be demonstrated for the pure saponins.[16] A crude hydrocotyle extract has been reported to significantly reduce the fertility of female mice when administered orally.[10] No mechanism of action was investigated.

Teratogenicity studies in the rabbit have reported negative findings for a hydrocotyle extract containing asiatic acid, madecassic acid, madasiatic acid and asiaticoside.[17]

Fresh plant juice is reported to be devoid of antibacterial activity,[18] although asiaticoside has been reported to be active versus *Mycobacterium tuberculosis*, *Bacillus leprae* and *Entamoeba histolytica*, and oxyasiaticoside was documented to be active against tubercle bacillus.[16,18] The fresh plant juice is also stated not to exhibit antitumour or antiviral activities, but to possess a moderate cytotoxic action in human ascites tumour cells.[18]

Clinical studies

Several studies describing the use of hydrocotyle to treat wounds and various skin disorders have been documented. A cream containing a hydrocotyle extract was found to be successful in the treatment of psoriasis in seven patients to whom it was applied.[19] An aerosol preparation, containing a hydrocotyle extract, was reported to improve the healing in 19 of 25 wounds that had proved refractory to other forms of treatment.[11] A hydrocotyle extract containing asiaticoside (40%), asiatic acid (29–30%), madecassic acid (29–30%) and madasiatic acid (1%) was stated to be successful as both a preventive and curative treatment, when given to 227 patients with keloids or hypertrophic scars.[17] The effective dose in adults was reported to be between 60 and 90 mg. It was proposed that the triterpene constituents in the hydrocotyle extract act in a similar manner to cortisone, with respect to wound healing, and interfere with the metabolism of abnormal collagen.[17]

The triterpene constituents are reported to be metabolised primarily in the faeces in a period of 24–76 hours, with a small percentage metabolised via the kidneys.[17] An extract containing asiatic acid, madecassic acid, madasiatic acid and asiaticoside reached peak plasma concentrations in 2–4 hours, irrespective of whether it is administered in tablet, oily injection or ointment formulations.[17]

Hydrocotyle has been used in the treatment of patients with chronic lesions such as cutaneous ulcers, surgical wounds, fistulas and gynaecological wounds.[G44,G45] Hydrocotyle has also been reported to improve the blood circulation in the lower limbs. Stimulation of collagen synthesis in the vein wall resulted in an increase in vein tonicity and a reduction in the capacity of the vein to distend.[10]

The juice of the leaves or the whole plant is documented to be effective for relieving the itching associated with prickly heat.[G51]

Asiaticoside has also been documented to improve the general ability and behavioural pattern of 30 mentally retarded children, when given over a period of 12 weeks. It also increased the mean concentrations of blood sugar, serum cholesterol and total protein, and lowered blood urea and serum acid phosphatase concentrations, in 43 adults.[16] Vital capacity was also increased.

Side-effects, Toxicity

A burning sensation was reported by 4 of 20 patients during the period of application of an aerosol preparation containing hydrocotyle.[11] However, it is not clear whether other components in the formulation contributed to this reaction. Ingestion of hydrocotyle is stated to have produced pruritus over the whole body.[G51]

Contra-indications, Warnings

It is stated that hydrocotyle may produce photosensitisation.[G7] Excessive doses may interfere with existing hypoglycaemic therapy and increase serum cholesterol concentrations; hyperglycaemic and hypercholesterolaemic activities have been reported for asiaticoside in humans. Brahmoside and brahminoside have been reported to exert a CNS-depressant action in animal studies.[15]

Pregnancy and lactation Hydrocotyle is reputed to be an abortifacient and to affect the menstrual cycle.[G30] Relaxation of the isolated rat uterus has been documented for brahmoside and brahminoside.[15] Triterpene constituents have been reported to lack any teratological effects in rabbits.[17] In view of the lack of toxicity data, the use of hydrocotyle during pregnancy should be avoided. Excessive use should be avoided during lactation.

Pharmaceutical Comment

The chemistry of hydrocotyle is well studied and its pharmacological activity seems to be associated with the triterpenoid constituents. Documented clinical and animal data support the herbal use of hydrocotyle as a dermatological agent, and warrants further research into the potential role of hydrocotyle in wound management. In view of the lack of toxicity data, excessive ingestion of hydrocotyle should be avoided.

References

See also General References G7, G22, G30, G31, G36, G37, G43, G51, G60, G63 and G64.

1 George VK, Gnanarethinam JL. Free amino acids in *Centella asiatica*. *Curr Sci* 1975; **44**: 790.

2 Rzadkowska-Bodalska H. Flavonoid compounds in herb pennywort (*Hydrocotyle vulgaris*). *Herba Pol* 1974; **20**: 243–246.

3 Voigt G *et al*. Zur Struktur der Flavonoide aus *Hydrocotyle vulgaris* L. *Pharmazie* 1981; **36**: 377–379.

4 Hiller K *et al*. Isolierung von Quercetin-3-O-(6-O-α-L-arabinopyranosyl)-β-D-galaktopyranosid, einem neuen Flavonoid aus *Hydrocotyle vulgaris* L. *Pharmazie* 1979; **34**: 192–193.

5 Hiller K *et al*. Saponins of *Hydrocotyle vulgaris*. *Pharmazie* 1971; **26**: 780.

6 Hiller K *et al*. Zur Struktur des Hauptsaponins aus *Hydrocotyle vulgaris* L. *Pharmazie* 1981; **36**: 844–846.

7 Asakawa Y *et al*. Mono- and sesquiterpenoids from *Hydrocotyle* and *Centella* species. *Phytochemistry* 1982; **21**: 2590–2592.

8 Bohlmann F, Zdero C. Polyacetylenic compounds. 230. A new polyyne from Centella species. *Chem Ber* 1975; **108**: 511–514.

9 Schulte KE *et al*. Constituents of medical plants. XXVII. Polyacetylenes from *Hydrocotyle asiatica*. *Arch Pharm (Weinheim)* 1973; **306**: 197–209.

10 Gotu Kola. *Lawrence Review of Natural Products*, 1988.

11 Morisset T *et al*. Evaluation of the healing activity of hydrocotyle tincture in the treatment of wounds. *Phytother Res* 1987; **1**: 117–121.

12 Jacker H-J *et al*. Zum antiexsudativen Verhalten einiger Triterpensaponine. *Pharmazie* 1982; **37**: 380–382.

13 Ravokatra A, Ratsimamanga AR. Action of a pentacyclic triterpenoid, asiaticoside, obtained from *Hydrocotyle madagascariensis* or *Centella asiatica* against gastric ulcers of the Wistar rat exposed to cold (2°). *C R Acad Sci (Paris)* 1974; **278**: 1743–1746.

14 Ravokatra A *et al*. Action of asiaticoside extracted from hydrocyte on duodenal ulcers induced with mercaptoethylamine in male Wistar rats. *C R Acad Sci (Paris)* 1974; **278**: 2317–2321.

15 Ramaswamy AS *et al*. Pharmacological studies on *Centella asiatica* Linn. (*Brahma manduki*) (N.O. Umbelliferae). *J Res Indian Med* 1970; **4**: 160–175.

16 Oliver-Bever B. *Medicinal Plants in Tropical West Africa*. Cambridge: Cambridge University Press, 1986.

17 Bossé J-P *et al*. Clinical study of a new antikeloid agent. *Ann Plast Surg* 1979; **3**: 13–21.

18 Lin Y-C *et al*. Search for biologically active substances in Taiwan medicinal plants. 1. Screening for anti-tumor and anti-microbial substances. *Chin J Microbiol* 1972; **5**: 76–81.

19 Natarajan S, Paily PP. Effect of topical *Hydrocotyle asiatica* in psoriasis. *Indian J Dermatol* 1973; **18**: 82–85.

Ispaghula

Species (Family)

Plantago ovata Forsk. (Plantaginaceae)

Synonym(s)

Blond Psyllium, Indian Plantago, Ispagol, Pale Psyllium, Spogel

Part(s) Used

Seed, husk

Pharmacopoeial and Other Monographs

BHC 1992[G6]
BHP 1996[G9]
BP 2001[G15]
Complete German Commission E (Psyllium, Blonde)[G3]
ESCOP 1996[G52]
Martindale 32nd edition[G43]
PDR for Herbal Medicines 2nd edition[G36]
Ph Eur 2002[G28]
WHO volume 1 1999[G63]

Legal Category (Licensed Products)

GSL[G37]

Constituents[G2,G6,G41,G52,G59,G64]

Alkaloids Monoterpene-type. (+)-Boschniakine (indicaine), (+)-boschniakinic acid (plantagonine) and indicainine.

Mucilages 10–30%. Mucopolysaccharide consisting mainly of a highly branched arabinoxylan with a xylan backbone and branches of arabinose, xylose and 2-O-(galacturonic)-rhamnose moieties. Present mainly in the seed husk.

Other constituents Aucubin (iridoid glucoside), sugars (fructose, glucose, sucrose), planteose (trisaccharide), protein, sterols (campesterol, β-sitosterol, stigmasterol), triterpenes (α- and β-amyrin), fatty acids (e.g. linoleic, oleic, palmitic, stearic), tannins.

Food Use

In food manufacture, ispaghula may be used as a thickener or stabiliser.[G41]

Herbal Use[G2,G4,G6,G7,G8,G32,G43,G52,G64]

Ispaghula is stated to possess demulcent and laxative properties. Traditionally, ispaghula has been used in the treatment of chronic constipation, dysentery, diarrhoea and cystitis. Topically, a poultice has been used for furunculosis. The German Commission E approved use for chronic constipation and disorders in which bowel movements with loose stool are desirable, e.g. patients with anal fistulas, haemorrhoids, pregnancy, secondary medication in the treatment of various forms of diarrhoea and in the treatment of irritable bowel syndrome.[G3]

The European Medicine Evaluation Agency (EMEA) Herbal Medicinal Products Working Group (HMPWG) has proposed a core SPC (Sumristics) for ispaghula.[G23] The core SPC includes the following indications: (a) treatment of habitual constipation; conditions in which easy defecation with soft stools is desirable, e.g. in cases of painful defecation after rectal or anal surgery; (b) adjuvant symptomatic therapy in cases of diarrhoea from various causes; (c) conditions which need an increased daily fibre intake, e.g. as an adjuvant in irritable bowel syndrome.

Dosage

Seeds 5–10 g (3 g in children) three times daily;[G6,G7] 12–40 g per day, husk 4–20 g;[G3] 3–5 g.[G43] Children 6–12 years, half adult dose. Children under 6 years, treat only under medical supervision.[G52] Seeds should be soaked in warm water for several hours before taking.

Liquid extract 2–4 mL (1 : 1 in 25% alcohol) three times daily.[G6,G7]

Husk 3–5 g.[G46] Seeds and husk should be soaked in warm water for several hours before administration.

7–11 g in one to three doses for indication (a) and (c); 7–20 g in one to three doses for indication (b).[G23]

Pharmacological Actions

The principal pharmacological actions of ispaghula can be attributed to the mucilage component.

In vitro and animal studies

An alcoholic extract lowered the blood pressure of anaesthetised cats and dogs, inhibited isolated rabbit and frog hearts, and stimulated rabbit, rat and guinea-pig ileum.[G41] The extract exhibited cholinergic activity.[G41] A mild laxative action has also been reported in mice administered iridoid glycosides, including aucubin.[1] Four-week supplementation of a fibre-free diet with isphagula seeds (100 or 200 g/kg) was compared with that of the husks and wheat bran in rats.[2] The seeds increased faecal fresh weight by up to 100% and faecal dry weight by up to 50%. Total faecal bile acid secretion was stimulated, and β-glucuronidase activity reduced, by ispaghula. The study concluded that ispaghula acts as a partly fermentable, dietary fibre supplement increasing stool bulk, and that it probably has metabolic and mucosa-protective effects.

Ispaghula husk depressed the growth of chickens by 15% when added to their diet at 2%.[G41]

Ispaghula seed powder is stated to have strongly counteracted the deleterious effects of adding sodium cyclamate (2%), FD & C Red No. 2 (2%), and polyoxyethylene sorbitan monostearate (4%) to the diet of rats.[G41]

Clinical studies

Ispaghula is used as a bulk laxative.[G3,G43,G52] The swelling properties of the mucilage enable it to absorb water in the gastrointestinal tract, thereby increasing the volume of the faeces and promoting peristalsis. Bulk laxatives are often used for the treatment of chronic constipation and when excessive straining must be avoided following anorectal surgery or in the management of haemorrhoids. Ispaghula is also used in the management of diarrhoea and for adjusting faecal consistency in patients with colostomies and in patients with diverticular disease or irritable bowel syndrome.

Laxative effect Ispaghula increases water content of stools and total stool weight in patients,[3] thus promoting peristalsis and reducing mouth-to-rectum transit time.[4] In a short-term study, 42 adults with constipation (⩽ 3 bowel movements per week) received either ispaghula (7.2 g/day) or ispaghula plus senna (6.5 g + 1.5 g/day).[5] Both treatments increased defecation frequency, and wet and dry stool weights, improved stool consistency, and gave subjective relief.

A randomised, double-blind, double-dummy, multicentre study involved 170 subjects with chronic idiopathic constipation.[6] The study included a two-week baseline (placebo) phase, followed by two weeks' treatment with ispaghula (Metamucil) 5.1 g, twice daily or docusate sodium 100 mg twice daily. Compared with docusate, ispaghula significantly increased stool water content (0.01% versus 2.33% for docusate and ispaghula, respectively; $p = 0.007$), and total stool output (271.9 g/week versus 359.9 g/week for docusate and ispaghula, respectively; $p = 0.005$). Furthermore, bowel movement frequency was significantly greater for ispaghula, compared with docusate. It was concluded that isphaghula has greater overall laxative efficacy than docusate in patients with chronic constipation.[6]

Antidiarrhoeal effect An open, randomised, crossover trial involving 25 patients with diarrhoea compared the effects of loperamide with those of ispaghula and calcium.[7] Nineteen patients completed both periods of treatment. The results indicated that both treatments halved stool frequency. Ispaghula and calcium were reported to be significantly better than loperamide with regard to urgency and stool consistency.[7]

Nine volunteers with phenolphthalein-induced diarrhoea were treated in random sequence with placebo, ispaghula (Konsyl), calcium polycarbophil or wheat bran.[8] Wheat bran and calcium polycarbophil had no effect on faecal consistency or on faecal viscosity. By contrast, ispaghula made stools firmer and increased faecal viscosity. In a dose–response study involving six subjects, 9, 18 and 30 g ispaghula per day caused a near-linear increase in faecal viscosity.[8]

The effects of ispaghula have been explored in children. In an open, uncontrolled study, 23 children with chronic non-specific diarrhoea were treated with an unrestricted diet for one week, and then treated with ispaghula (Metamucil) for two weeks (one tablespoonful twice daily). Seven patients responded to the unrestricted diet and 13 were said to respond to ispaghula treatment.[9]

Hypocholesterolaemic effects In a double-blind, placebo-controlled, parallel-group study, 26 men with mild-to-moderate hypercholesterolaemia (serum cholesterol concentration: 4.86–8.12 mmol/L) received ispaghula (Metamucil) 3.4 g, or cellulose placebo, three times daily at meal times for eight weeks.[10] At the end of the study, serum cholesterol concentrations were reduced by 14.8% in the treated group, low-density lipoprotein (LDL) cholesterol by 20.2% and ratio of LDL to high-density lipoprotein (HDL) cholesterol by 14.8%, compared with baseline values. There were no significant changes in serum lipid concentrations with placebo treatment, compared with baseline values. Differences in serum cholesterol concentrations between the two groups were statistically significant after four weeks (p-value not reported).

A double-blind, placebo-controlled, parallel trial study compared the effects of ispaghula (Metamucil 5.1 g, daily) and placebo in 118 patients (aged 21–70 years old) with primary hypercholesterolaemia (total serum cholesterol $\geqslant 5.7$ mmol/L).[11] Thirty-seven participants maintained a high-fat diet and 81 a low-fat diet. Treated patients in both low- and high-fat diet groups showed small significant decreases ($p < 0.05$) in total cholesterol and LDL cholesterol levels (5.8 and 7.2%, respectively, for high-fat diets; 4.2% and 6.4%, respectively, for low-fat diets). No significant differences were seen in LDL cholesterol response for treated patients on either diet.

In a randomised, double-blind, crossover study, 20 males (mean (SD) age 44 (4) years) with moderate hypercholesterolaemia (mean (SD) total cholesterol concentration 265 (17) mg/dL, LDL 184 (15) mg/dL) were randomised to receive a 40-day course of ispaghula (Metamucil) 15 g daily, or placebo (cellulose).[12] There was a wash-out period of more than 10 days between treatments. Ispaghula lowered LDL cholesterol (168 mg/dL) more than did cellulose placebo (179 mg/dL), decreased relative cholesterol absorption, and increased the fractional turnover of both chenodeoxycholic acid and cholic acid. Bile acid synthesis increased in subjects whose LDL cholesterol was lowered by more than 10%. It was concluded that ispaghula lowers LDL cholesterol primarily by stimulation of bile acid synthesis.[12]

A meta-analysis of eight published and four unpublished studies carried out in four countries reviewed the effect of consumption of ispaghula-enriched cereal products on blood cholesterol, and LDL and HDL cholesterol concentrations.[13] Overall, the trials included 404 adults with mild-to-moderate hypercholesterolaemia (5.17–7.8 mmol/L) who consumed low-fat diets. The meta-analysis indicated that subjects who consumed ispaghula cereal had lower total cholesterol and LDL cholesterol than subjects who ate control cereal concentrations (differences of 0.31 mmol/L (5%) and 0.35 mmol/L (9%), respectively). HDL cholesterol concentrations were not affected in subjects eating ispaghula cereal.

Another meta-analysis included eight studies involving a total of 384 patients with hypercholesterolaemia who received ispaghula and 272 subjects who received cellulose placebo.[14] Compared with placebo, consumption of 10.2 g ispaghula per day for $\geqslant 8$ weeks lowered serum total cholesterol concentrations by 4% ($p < 0.0001$) and LDL cholesterol by 7% ($p < 0.0001$), but did not affect serum HDL cholesterol or triacyl glycerol concentrations. The ratio of apolipoprotein (apo) B to apo A-1 was lowered by 6% ($p < 0.05$), relative to placebo, in subjects consuming a low-fat diet.[14] It was concluded that ispaghula is a useful adjunct to a low-fat diet in individuals with mild-to-moderate hypercholesterolaemia.

A randomised, placebo-controlled, multicentre study evaluated the long-term effectiveness of ispaghula husk as an adjunct to diet in treatment of primary hypercholesterolaemia.[15] Men and women with hypercholesterolaemia followed the American Heart Association Step 1 diet for eight weeks prior to treatment. Individuals with LDL cholesterol concentrations between 3.36 and 4.91 mmol/L were randomly assigned to receive either ispaghula (Metamucil 5.1 g) or cellulose placebo twice daily for 26 weeks whilst continuing diet therapy. Overall, 163 participants completed the full protocol, 133 receiving ispaghula and 30 receiving cellulose placebo. Serum total and LDL cholesterol concentrations were 4.7% and 6.7% lower, respectively, in the ispaghula group than in the placebo group after 24–26 weeks ($p < 0.001$).

A randomised, double-blind, placebo-controlled crossover trial assessed the effects of ispaghula in lowering elevated LDL cholesterol concentrations in 20 children (aged 5–17 years).[16] Children with LDL cholesterol concentrations of >2.84 mmol/L after three months on a low-fat, low-cholesterol diet received five weeks' treatment with a ready-to-eat cereal containing water-soluble ispaghula husk (6 g/day) or placebo. The results indicated that there were no significant differences in total cholesterol, LDL cholesterol or HDL cholesterol concentrations between the two groups.

In a similar 12-week study, 50 children (aged 2–11 years) with LDL cholesterol concentrations $\geqslant 110$ mg/dL received either cereal enriched with ispaghula (3.2 g soluble fibre per day) or plain cereal whilst maintaining a low-fat diet.[17] Total cholesterol decreased by 21 mg/dL for the ispaghula group in comparison with 11.5 mg/dL for the control group ($p < 0.001$). LDL cholesterol also decreased by 23 mg/dL for the treated group in comparison with 8.5 mg/dL for the placebo group ($p < 0.01$).

The effect of adding water-soluble fibre to a diet low in total fats, saturated fat and cholesterol to treat hypercholesterolaemic children and adolescents has been reviewed.[18] The review summarised that reductions in LDL cholesterol concentrations ranged from 0 to 23%. This wide range may be related to dietary intervention and to clinical trial conditions. It was proposed that additional trials with larger numbers of well-defined subjects are needed.

Hypoglycaemic effect Several studies have shown that ispaghula husk lowered blood glucose concentrations due to delayed intestinal absorption.[G52] In one crossover study, 18 patients with non-insulin-dependent diabetes received ispaghula (Metamucil) or placebo twice (immediately before breakfast and dinner) during each 15-hour crossover phase.[19] For meals eaten immediately after ispaghula ingestion, maximum postprandial glucose elevation was reduced by 14% at breakfast and 20% at dinner, relative to placebo. Postprandial serum insulin concentrations measured after breakfast were reduced by 12%, relative to placebo. Second-meal effects after lunch showed a 31% reduction in postprandial glucose elevation, relative to placebo. No significant differences in effects were noted between patients whose diabetes was controlled by diet alone and those whose diabetes was controlled by oral hypoglycaemic drugs. It was concluded that the results indicate that ispaghula as a meal supplement reduces proximate and second-meal postprandial glucose and insulin in non-insulin dependent diabetics.[19]

Other effects Ispaghula husk has been used to treat small numbers of patients with left-sided diverticular disease.[4] Marked motility was observed for the right colon, but was not as pronounced for the left colon. The effects of ispaghula in this condition may be worth further investigation.

In an open, randomised, multicentre trial, 102 patients with ulcerative colitis (three months in remission, salicylate-treated, colitis over 20 cm) received ispaghula (10 g twice daily; $n = 35$), oral mesalazine (500 mg three times daily; $n = 37$) or ispaghula plus mesalazine ($n = 30$) for one year.[20] Assessment, including endoscopy, was carried out at 3, 6, 9 and 12 months. The results suggested that ispaghula may be equivalent to mesalazine in maintaining remission in ulcerative colitis. However, this requires further investigation in a randomised, double-blind study.

In China, the seeds of related *Plantago* species have been used to treat hypertension.[G41]

Side-effects, Toxicity

In common with all bulk laxatives, ispaghula may temporarily increase flatulence and abdominal distension, and may cause intestinal obstruction. If swallowed dry, ispaghula may cause oesophageal obstruction. In rare cases, allergic reactions may occur.[G3,G23]

Contra-indications, Warnings

In common with all bulk laxatives, ispaghula should not be gven to patients with intestinal obstruction or conditions that may lead to intestinal obstruction, such as spastic bowel conditions. Ispaghula should always be taken with plenty of fluid to avoid oesophageal obstruction or faecal impaction. Bulk laxatives lower the transit time through the gastrointestinal tract and therefore may affect the absorption of other drugs.[G45] Absorption of currently administered drugs may be delayed. There may be a need to reduce insulin dosage in diabetics who are insulin dependent.[G3]

The EMEA HMPWG proposed core SPC for ispaghula includes the following information.[G23] Ispaghula husk is not to be used by patients with faecal impaction and undiagnosed abdominal symptoms, abdominal pain, nausea and vomiting (unless advised by a doctor), a sudden change in bowel habit that persists for more than two weeks, rectal bleeding, and failure to defecate following the use of a laxative. Ispaghula husk is also not to be used by patients suffering from abnormal constrictions in the gastrointestinal tract, diseases of the oesophagus and cardia, potential or existing intestinal blockage (ileus), or megacolon, diabetes mellitus which is difficult to regulate, or by patients with known hypersensitivity to ispaghula or any other constituents of the product. The husk should be taken with at least 150 mL of water or other fluid. Taking this product without adequate fluid may cause it to swell and block the throat or oesophagus and may cause choking. Intestinal obstructions may occur if an adequate fluid intake is not maintained. Ispaghula should not be taken by anyone who has had difficulty in swallowing or any throat problems. If chest pain, vomiting or difficulty in swallowing or breathing is experienced after taking the product, immediate medical attention should be sought. The treatment of the debilitated requires medical supervision. The treatment of elderly patients should be supervised. In the case of diarrhoea, sufficient intake of water and electrolytes is important.

Interaction with other medicinal products and other forms of interaction[G23]   Enteral absorption of concomitantly administered medicines such as minerals (e.g. calcium, iron, lithium, zinc), vitamins (B_{12}), cardiac glycosides and coumarin derivatives may be delayed. For this reason the product should not be taken 0.5–1 hour before, or after, intake of other drugs. If the product is taken together with meals in the case of insulin-dependent diabetics, it may be necessary to reduce the insulin dose.

Pregnancy and lactation Ispaghula may be used during pregnancy and lactation.

Pharmaceutical Comment

The characteristic component of ispaghula is the mucilage which provides it with its bulk laxative action. Many of the herbal uses are therefore supported although no published information was located to justify the use of ispaghula in cystitis or infective skin conditions. Adverse effects and precautions generally associated with bulk laxatives apply to ispaghula. Clinical evidence exists for hypocholesterolaemia effects but it has been recommended that reduction in dietary fat intake is preferable to food supplements.[21]

References

See also General References G2, G3, G6, G9, G12, G15, G28, G31, G36, G37, G41, G43, G52, G54, G56, G59, G63 and G64.

1   Inouye H *et al.* Purgative activities of iridoid glycosides. *Planta Med* 1974; **25**: 285–288.
2   Leng-Peschlow E. *Plantago ovata* seeds as dietary fibre supplement: physiological and metabolic effects in rats. *Br J Nutr* 1991; **66**: 331–349.
3   Stevens J *et al.* Comparison of the effects of psyllium and wheat bran on gastrointestinal transit time and stool characteristics. *J Am Diet Assoc* 1988; **88**: 323–326.
4   Thorburn HA *et al.* Does ispaghula husk stimulate the entire colon in diverticular disease? *Gut* 1992; **33**: 352–356.
5   Marlett JA *et al.* Comparative laxation of psyllium with and without senna in an ambulatory constipated population. *Am J Gastroenterol* 1987; **82**: 333–337.
6   McRorie JW *et al.* Psyllium is superior to docusate sodium for treatment of chronic constipation. *Aliment Pharmacol Ther* 1998; **12**: 491–497.
7   Qvitzau S *et al.* Treatment of chronic diarrhoea: loperamide versus isphaghula husk and calcium. *Scand J Gastroenterol* 1988; **23**: 1237–1240.
8   Eherer AJ *et al.* Effect of psyllium, calcium polycarbophil, and wheat bran on secretory diarrhea induced by phenolphthalein. *Gastro-*

enterology 1993; **104**: 1007–1012.
9   Smalley JR *et al.* Use of psyllium in the management of chronic nonspecific diarrhea of childhood. *J Pediatr Gastroenterol Nutr* 1982; **1**: 361–363.
10 Anderson JW *et al.* Cholesterol-lowering effects of psyllium hydrophilic mucilloid for hypercholesterolemic men. *Arch Intern Med* 1988; **148**: 292–296.
11 Sprecher DL *et al.* Efficacy of psyllium in reducing serum cholesterol levels in hypercholesterolemic patients on high- or low-fat diets. *Ann Intern Med* 1993; **119**: 545–554.
12 Everson GT *et al.* Effects of psyllium hydrophilic mucilloid on LDL-cholesterol and bile acid synthesis in hypercholesterolemic men. *J Lipid Res* 1992; **33**: 1183–1192.
13 Olson BH *et al.* Psyllium-enriched cereals lower blood total cholesterol and LDL cholesterol, but not HDL cholesterol, in hypercholesterolemic adults: results of a meta-analysis. *J Nutr* 1997; **127**: 1973–1980.
14 Anderson JW *et al.* Cholesterol-lowering effects of psyllium intake adjunctive to diet therapy in men and women with hypercholesterolemia: meta-analysis of 8 controlled trials. *Am J Clin Nutr* 2000; **71**: 472–479.
15 Anderson JW *et al.* Long-term cholesterol-lowering effects of psyllium as an adjunct to diet therapy in the treatment of hypercholesterolaemia. *Am J Clin Nut* 2000; **71**: 1433–1438.
16 Dennison BA, Levine DM. Randomized, double-blind, placebo-controlled, two-period crossover clinical trial of psyllium fiber in children with hypercholesterolemia. *J Pediatr* 1993; **123**: 24–29.
17 Williams CL *et al.* Soluble fiber enhances the hypocholesterolemic effect of the step I diet in childhood. *J Am College Nutr* 1995; **14**: 251–257.
18 Kwiterovich Jr PO. The role of fiber in the treatment of hypercholesterolemia in children and adolescents. *Pediatrics* 1995; **96**: 1005–1009.
19 Pastors JG *et al.* Psyllium fiber reduces rise in postprandial glucose and insulin concentrations in patients with non-insulin-dependent diabetes. *Am J Clin Nutr* 1991; **53**: 1431–1435.
20 Fernández-Bañares F *et al.* Randomised clinical trial of *Plantago ovata* efficacy as compared to mesalazine in maintaining remission in ulcerative colitis. *Gastroenterology* 1997; **112**: A971.
21 Pearson TA, Patel RV. The quest for a cholesterol-decreasing diet: should we substract, substitute, or supplement? *Ann Intern Med* 1993; 119: 627–628.

Jamaica Dogwood

Species (Family)

Piscidia erythrina L. (Leguminosae)

Synonym(s)

Fish Poison Bark, *Ichthymethia piscipula* (L.) A.S. Hitchc. ex Sarg., *Piscidia communis* Harms, *Piscidia piscipula* (L.) Sarg., West Indian Dogwood

Part(s) Used

Root bark

Pharmacopoeial and Other Monographs

BHC 1992[G6]
BHP 1996[G9]
PDR for Herbal Medicines 2nd edition[G36]

Legal Category (Licensed Products)

GSL[G37]

Constituents[G6,G22,G40,G41,G64]

Acids Piscidic acid (*p*-hydroxybenzyltartaric) and its mono and diethyl esters,[1] fukiic acid and the 3'-O-methyl derivative; malic acid, succinic acid, and tartaric acid.

Isoflavonoids Ichthynone, jamaicin, piscerythrone, piscidone and others. Milletone, isomillettone, dehydromillettone, rotenone and sumatrol (rotenoids), and lisetin.[2–5]

Glycosides Piscidin, reported to be a mixture of two compounds, saponin glycoside (unidentified).[6]

Other constituents Alkaloid (unidentified, reported to be from the stem), resin, volatile oil 0.01%, β-sitosterol, tannin (unspecified).[6]

Food Use

Jamaica dogwood is stated by the Council of Europe to to be toxicologically unacceptable for use as a natural food flavouring.[G16]

Herbal Use

Jamaica dogwood is stated to possess sedative and anodyne properties. Traditionally, it has been used for neuralgia, migraine, insomnia, dysmenorrhoea, and specifically for insomnia due to neuralgia or nervous tension.[G6,G7,G8,G64]

Dosage

Dried root bark 1–2 g or by decoction three times daily.[G6,G7]

Liquid extract 1–2 mL (1 : 1 in 30% alcohol) three times daily.[G6,G7]

Liquid Extract of Piscidia (BPC 1934) 2–8 mL.

Pharmacological Actions

In vitro and animal studies

Results of early studies reported Jamaica dogwood to possess weak cannabinoid and sedative activities in the mouse, guinea-pig and cat.[6–8] In addition, *in vitro* antispasmodic activity on rabbit intestine, and guinea-pig and rat uterine muscle[6,9,10] were noted and *in vivo* utero-activity in the cat and monkey were documented.[6,7,10,11] In some instances, *in vitro* antispasmodic activity was found to be comparable to, or greater than, that observed for papaverine.

More recent work has supported these findings and reported that the antispasmodic activity of Jamaica dogwood on uterine smooth muscle is attributable to two isoflavone constituents, one being equipotent to papaverine.[11]

Jamaica dogwood extracts have also been documented to exhibit antitussive, antipyretic, and anti-inflammatory activities in various experimental animals.[7]

Rotenone is an insecticide that has been used in agriculture for the control of lice, fleas, and as a larvicide.[G45] Jamaica dogwood has been used extensively throughout Central and South America as a fish poison;[6] the wood contains two piscicidal principles, rotenone and ichthynone. Rotenone is relatively harmless to warm-blooded animals.[12]

Rotenone has reported exhibited anticancer activity towards lymphocytic leukaemia and human epidermoid carcinoma of the nasopharynx.[G22] It is also documented to be carcinogenic.[G22]

Side-effects, Toxicity

Symptoms of overdose are stated to include numbness, tremors, salivation and sweating.[G22] Jamaica dogwood has been found to be toxic when administered parenterally to rats and rabbits, but non-toxic when given orally, with doses exceeding 90 g dried extract/kg tolerated.[6] An LD$_{50}$ (mice, intravenous injection) of an unidentified saponin constituent has been reported as 75 µg/kg body weight.[9] Oral doses of up to 1.5 mg/kg were stated to have no effect.[6]

Jamaica dogwood is stated to be irritant and toxic to humans.[G51]

Contra-indications, Warnings

It is recommended that Jamaica dogwood should be used with great care, and only by trained practitioners.[G49] Jamaica dogwood may potentiate sedative effects of existing therapy.

Pregnancy and lactation Jamaica dogwood has been reported to exhibit a potent depressant action on the uterus both *in vitro* and *in vivo*. In view of this and the general warnings regarding the use of Jamaica dogwood, it should not be used during pregnancy and lactation.

Pharmaceutical Comment

Jamaica dogwood is characterised by various isoflavone constituents, to which the antispasmodic properties described for the wood have been attributed. In addition, sedative and narcotic activities have been documented that justify the reputed herbal uses. Although Jamaica dogwood is reported to be of low toxicity in various animal species, it is also documented as toxic to humans[G51] and is recommended to be used with great care.[G49] In view of this, excessive use of Jamaica dogwood should be avoided.

References

See also General References G6, G9, G16, G22, G31, G36, G37, G40, G41, G45, G49, G51 and G64.

1 Bridge W *et al.* Constituents of 'Cortex Piscidiae Erythrinae'. Part I. The structure of piscidic acid. *J Chem Soc* 1948; 257.
2 Falshaw CP *et al.* The Extractives of Piscidia Erythrina L. III. The constitutions of lisetin, piscidone and piscerythrone. *Tetrahedron* 1966; Suppl 7: 333–348.
3 Redaelli C, Santaniello E. Major isoflavonoids of the Jamaican dogwood *Piscidia erythrina*. *Phytochemistry* 1984; **23**: 2976–2977.
4 Delle Monache F *et al.* Two isoflavones from *Piscidia erythrina*. *Phytochemistry* 1984; **23**: 2945–2947.
5 Harborne JB, Mabry TJ, eds. *The Flavonoids*. New York: Chapman and Hall, 1982: 606.
6 Costello CH, Butler CL. An investigation of *Piscidia erythrina* (Jamaica Dogwood). *J Am Pharm Assoc* 1948; **37**: 89–96.
7 Aurousseau M *et al.* Certain pharmacodynamic properties of *Piscidia erythrina*. *Ann Pharm Fr* 1965; **23**: 251–257.
8 Della-Loggia R *et al.* Evaluation of the activity on the mouse CNS of several plant extracts and a combination of them. *Riv-Neurol* 1981; **51**: 297–310.
9 Pilcher JD *et al.* The action of the so-called female remedies on the excised uterus of the guinea-pig. *Arch Intern Med* 1916; **18**: 557–583.
10 Pilcher JD, Mauer RT. The action of female remedies on the intact uteri of animals. *Surg Gynecol Obstet* 1918; 97–99.
11 Della Loggia R *et al.* Isoflavones as spasmolytic principles of *Piscidia erythrina*. *Prog Clin Biol Res* 1988; **280**: 365–368.
12 Claus E *et al.*, eds. Pesticides. In: *Pharmacognosy*. Philadelphia: Lea and Febiger, 1970; 486–487.

Java Tea

Species (Family)

Orthosiphon stamineus Benth. (Lamiaceae)

Synonym(s)

Kumis Kucing (Indonesian, Malay), *Orthosiphon aristatus* Miq., *Orthosiphon spicatus* (Thundb.) Bak.

Part(s) Used

Fragmented dried leaves, tops of stems

Pharmacopoeial and Other Monographs

BHP 1996[G9]
BP 2001[G15]
Complete German Commission E[G3]
ESCOP 1997[G52]
Martindale 32nd edition[G43]
PDR for Herbal Medicines 2nd edition[G36]
Ph Eur 2002[G28]

Legal category (Licensed Products)

Java tea is not included in the GSL.

Constituents[G2,G52]

Benzochromenes Orthochromene A,[1] methylripariochromene A[2] and acetovanillochromene.[1]

Diterpenes Isopimarane-type diterpenes (orthosiphonones A and B,[1] orthosiphols A and B,[3] orthosiphols F, G, H and I[4]), pimarane-type diterpenes (neoorthosiphols A and B)[5] and staminol A.[4]

Essential oil 0.02–0.7%. Various compounds including β-elemene, β-caryophyllene, α-humulene, β-caryophyllene oxide, can-2-one and palmitic acid.[6]

Flavonoids Sinensetin, tetramethylscutellarein and other tetramethoxyflavones, eupatorin, salvigenin, cirsimaritin, pilloin, rhamnazin, trimethylapigenin and tetramethylluteolin.[7–11] These lipophilic flavonoids are present in concentrations of approximately 0.2–0.3%;[10] flavonoid glycosides are also present.

Other constituents Caffeic acid and derivatives (e.g. rosmarinic acid), inositol, phytosterols (e.g. β-sitosterol)[11,12] and potassium salts.

Food Use

Java tea is not used in foods.

Herbal Use[G35]

Java tea has traditionally been used in Java for the treatment of hypertension and diabetes.[1,5,13] It has also been used in folk medicine for bladder and kidney disorders, gallstones, gout and rheumatism. Java tea is stated to have diuretic properties.[14]

Dosage

Dried material 2–3 g in 150 mL water two to three times daily as an infusion.[G52]

Pharmacological Actions

In vitro and animal studies

Diuretic effects Several studies in rats have reported diuretic activity of extracts of *O. stamineus* and *O. aristatus*[14–16] and of flavonoids (sinensetin and a tetramethoxyflavone) isolated from *O. aristatus*.[17] Intraperitoneal administration of a hydroalcoholic extract of *O. stamineus* to rats caused a significant diuresis over the following 2–24 hours compared with controls.[14] The effect was similar to that observed following intraperitoneal administration of hydrochlorothiazide (10 mg/kg).[14] Oral administration of an aqueous extract of *O. aristatus* increased ion excretion to a similar extent as did furosemide (frusemide), although no diuretic action was noted.[16]

Oral administration of methylripariochromene A (100 mg/kg) has been shown to increase urinary volume in fasted rats for three hours after oral administration; the increase in urine volume was similar to that observed with oral administration of hydrochlorothiazide (25 mg/kg).[13] Sodium, potassium and chloride ion excretion was increased with methylripariochromene A (100 mg/kg), although urinary sodium ion excretion did not increase. A mechanism for the diuretic action of methylripariochromene A has not yet been elucidated, although it appears to have a different mode of action to that of hydrochlorothiazide.[13]

Hypoglycaemic effects In normoglycaemic rats, oral administration of an aqueous extract of *O. stamineus* (0.5 g/kg) had no significant effect on fasting blood glucose concentrations over a 7-hour period, although administration of 1 g/kg produced a significant decrease in blood glucose concentration compared with that in a control group.[18] A hypoglycaemic effect was also observed following administration of *O. stamineus* extract (1 g/kg) to rats loaded with glucose (1.5 g/kg) and in streptozotocin-induced diabetic rats; the effect of *O. stamineus* extract in streptozotocin-induced diabetic rats was similar to that observed with glibenclamide (10 mg/kg).[18]

Antihypertensive effects Methylripariochromene A has been reported to have several pharmacological actions related to antihypertensive activity.

In stroke-prone, spontaneously hypertensive rats, subcutaneous administration of methylripariochromene A (100 mg/kg) produced a continuous reduction in systolic blood pressure and a decrease in heart rate. Methylripariochromene A also suppressed agonist-induced contractions in the rat thoracic aorta and decreased the contractile force in isolated guinea-pig atria without significantly affecting the beating (heart) rate. The mechanism of action for these antihypertensive effects of methylripariochromene A is, however, unclear.[13]

Migrated pimarane-type diterpenes (neoorthosiphols A and B), isopimarane-type diterpenes (orthosiphols A and B, orthosiphonones A and B), benzochromenes (methylripariochromene, acetovanillochromene, orthochromene A) and flavones (tetramethylscutellarein, sinensetin) isolated from *O. aristatus* have been reported to exhibit a suppressive effect on contractile responses in the rat thoracic aorta.[19]

Cytostatic effects Sinensetin and tetramethylscutellarein have been reported to demonstrate *in vitro* cytostatic activity towards Ehrlich ascites tumour cells.[10] Growth inhibition appears to be dose dependent, with 50% inhibition occurring at concentrations of approximately 30 and 15 µg/mL for sinensetin and tetramethylscutellarein, respectively. Orthosiphols A and B have been reported to inhibit inflammation induced by the tumour promoter

12-O-tetradecanoylphorbol-13-acetate (TPA) on mouse ears.[3]

Fractions of *O. stamineus* leaves have been reported to have activity against a melanoma cell line *in vitro*.[20]

Antimicrobial effects An aqueous extract of *O. aristatus* has demonstrated antibacterial activity against two serotypes of *Streptococcus mutans* (MIC 7.8–23.4 mg/mL).[21] Other *in vitro* studies have reported a lack of antibacterial activity for flavonoids (sinensetin, tetramethylscutellarein and a tetramethoxyflavone in concentrations of 10 and 100 µg/mL) isolated from *O. aristatus* leaves against *Escherichia coli*, *Proteus mirabilis*, *Pseudomonas aeruginosa*, *Staphylococcus aureus* and *Enterococcus*.[17]

O. stamineus extract has also been shown to inhibit spore germination in six out of nine fungal species tested: *Saccharomyces pastorianus*, *Candida albicans*, *Rhizopus nigricans*, *Penicillium digitatum*, *Fusarium oxysporum* and *Trichophyton mentagrophytes*.[22]

Other effects *In vitro*, *O. spicatus* has been shown to inhibit 15-lipoxygenase, an enzyme thought to be involved in the development of atherosclerosis.[11] Furthermore, the flavonoids sinensetin and tetramethylscutellarein demonstrate dose-dependent inhibition with IC_{50} values of 114 ± 5 and 110 ± 3 µmol/L, respectively, although other flavonoids from *O. spicatus* appear to be less efficient inhibitors of 15-lipoxygenase. The inhibitory activity of the whole extract was greater than could be expected from the activities of each of its flavonoid constituents, and it has been suggested that synergism may be occurring.[11] More recent *in vitro* studies have shown that flavonoids from *O. spicatus* prevent oxidative inactivation of 15-lipoxygenase, with trimethylapigenin, eupatorin and tetramethylluteolin showing the strongest enzyme-stabilising effects.[23] However, there was no correlation between enzyme stabilisation and enzyme inhibition.[23]

Clinical studies

Early studies reported increases in diuresis in subjects following the oral administration of extracts of *Orthosiphon*.[G52] A randomised, double-blind, placebo-controlled, crossover study reported no effect on 12- and 24-hour urine output or on sodium excretion in 40 healthy volunteers who received 600 mL of an infusion of *Orthosiphon* leaves daily (equivalent to 10 g dried leaves) for four days.[24] A study involving six healthy volunteers who drank

Orthosiphon tea (250 mL) every 6 hours for one day reported an increase in urine acidity 6 hours after ingestion.[25]

A study involving 67 patients with uratic diathesis who received Java tea for three months reported that no effects were observed on diuresis, glomerular filtration, osmotic concentration, urinary pH, plasma content and excretion of calcium, inorganic phosphorus and uric acid.[26]

Side-effects, Toxicity

None documented.

Contra-indications, Warnings

None known. In view of the lack of clinical data on the use of Java tea, excessive or long-term use should be avoided. Adequate fluid intake (2 L or more per day) should be ensured whilst using Java tea.[G35]

Pregnancy and lactation There are no data available on the use of Java tea in pregnancy and lactation. In view of the lack of toxicity data, use of Java tea during pregnancy and lactation should be avoided.

Pharmaceutical Comment

The reported pharmacological activities of Java tea are mainly associated with the lipophilic flavonoids, benzochromene and, to a lesser extent, diterpene constituents.

Documented scientific evidence from *in vitro* and animal studies provides some supportive evidence for some of the traditional uses of Java tea. However, there is a lack of clinical data and well-designed, controlled clinical trials involving adequate numbers of patients are required. Furthermore, studies investigating the active principles responsible for specific pharmacological activities and their mechanisms of action are necessary.

There have been reports of adulteration/botanical substitution occurring with *Orthosiphon*.[27,28,G2]

In view of the lack of toxicity and safety data, excessive use of Java tea should be avoided.

References

See also General References G2, G3, G9, G15, G28, G36, G43 and G52.

1 Shibuya H *et al*. Indonesian medicinal plants. XXII. 1) Chemical structures of two new iso-pimarane-type diterpenes, orthosiphonones A and B, and a new benzochromene, orthochromene A from the leaves of *Orthosiphon aristatus* (Lamiaceae). *Chem Pharm Bull* 1999; **47**: 695–698.

2 Guerin J-C, Reveillere H-P. *Orthosiphon stamineus* as a potent source of methylripariochromene A. *J Nat Prod* 1989; **52**: 171–173.

3 Masuda T *et al*. Orthosiphol A and B, novel diterpenoid inhibitors of TPA (12-O-tetradeca-noylphorbol-13-acetate)-induced inflammation, from *Orthosiphon stamineus*. *Tetrahedron* 1992; **48**: 6787–6792.

4 Stampoulis P *et al*. Staminol A, a novel diterpene from *Orthosiphon stamineus*. *Tetrahedron Lett* 1999; **40**: 4239–4242.

5 Shibuya H *et al*. Two novel migrated pimarane-type diterpenes, neoorthosiphols A and B, from the leaves of *Orthosiphon aristatus* (Lamiaceae). *Chem Pharm Bull* 1999; **47**: 911–912.

6 Schut G, Zwaving JH. Content and composition of the essential oil of *Orthosiphon aristatus*. *Planta Med* 1986; **52**: 240–241.

7 Bombardelli E *et al*. Flavonoid constituents of *Orthosiphon stamineus*. *Fitoterapia* 1972; **43**: 35.

8 Schneider G, Tan HS. Die lipophilen Flavone von *Folia Orthosiphonis*. *Dtsch Apoth Ztg* 1973; **113**: 201.

9 Wollenweber E, Mann K. Weitere Flavonoide aus *Orthosiphon spicatus*. *Planta Med* 1985; **51**: 459–460.

10 Malterud KE *et al*. Flavonoids from *Orthosiphon spicatus*. *Planta Med* 1989; **55**: 569–570.

11 Lyckander IM, Malterud KE. Lipophilic flavonoids from *Orthosiphon spicatus* as inhibitors of 15-lipoxygenase. *Acta Pharm Nord* 1992; **4**: 159–166.

12 Sumaryono W *et al*. Qualitative and quantitative analysis of the phenolic constituents from *Orthosiphon aristatus*. *Planta Med* 1991; **57**: 176–180.

13 Matsubara T *et al*. Antihypertensive actions of methylripariochromene A from *Orthosiphon aristatus*, an Indonesian traditional medicinal plant. *Biol Pharm Bull* 1999; **22**: 1083–1088.

14 Beaux D *et al*. Effect of extracts of *Orthosiphon stamineus* Benth, *Hieracium pilosella* L., *Sambucus nigra* L., and *Arctostaphylos uva-ursi* (L.) Spreng. in rats. *Phytother Res* 1998; **12**: 498–501.

15 Casadebaig-Lafon J. Elaboration d'extraits végétaux adsorbés, réalisation d'extraits secs d'*Orthosiphon stamineus* Benth. *Pharm Acta Helv* 1989; **64**: 220–224.

16 Englert J, Harnischfeger G. Diuretic action of aqueous *Orthosiphon* extract in rats. *Planta Med* 1992; **58**: 237–238.

17 Schut GA, Zwaving JH. Pharmacological investigation of some lipophilic flavonoids from *Orthosiphon aristatus*. *Fitoterapia* 1993; **64**: 99–102.

18 Mariam A *et al*. Hypoglycaemic activity of the aqueous extract of *Orthosiphon stamineus*. *Fitoterapia* 1996; **67**: 465–468.

19 Ohashi K *et al*. Indonesian medicinal plants. XXIII. 1) Chemical structures of two new migrated pimarane-type diterpenes, neoorthosiphols A and

B, and suppressive effects on rat thoracic aorta of chemical constituents isolated from the leaves of *Orthosiphon aristatus* (Lamiaceae). *Chem Pharm Bull* 2000; **48**: 433–435.

20 Estevez NA. Fractions of *Orthosiphon stamineus* Benth. leaves with antitumour activity. Preliminary results. *Rev Cuba Farm* 1980; **14**: 21.

21 Chen C-P *et al.* Screening of Taiwanese drugs for antibacterial activity against *Steptococcus mutans*. *J Ethnopharmacol* 1989; **27**: 285–295.

22 Guerin J-C, Reveillere H-P. Antifungal activity of plant extracts used in therapy. II. Study of 40 plant extracts against 9 fungi species. *Ann Pharm Franc* 1985; **43**: 77–81.

23 Lyckander IM, Malterud KE. Lipophilic flavonoids from *Orthosiphon spicatus* prevent oxidative inactivation of 15-lipoxygenase. *Prostaglandins Leukot Essent Fatty Acids* 1996; **54**: 239–246.

24 Du Dat D *et al.* Studies on the individual and combined diuretic effects of four Vietnamese traditional herbal remedies (*Zea mays, Imperata cylindrica, Plantago major* and *Orthosiphon stamineus*). *J Ethnopharmacol* 1992; **36**: 225–231.

25 Nirdnoy M, Muangman V. Effects of *Folia orthosiphonis* on urinary stone promoters and inhibitors. *J Med Assoc Thailand* 1991; **74**: 319–321.

26 Tiktinsky OL, Bablumyan YA. The therapeutic effect of Java tea and *Equisetum arvense* in patients with uratic diathesis. *Urol Nefrol* 1983; **48**: 47–50.

27 Schier W, Schultze W. Current falsifications of drugs. Part 5: *Betulae folium, Orthosiphonis folium, Sarothamni scoparii flos, Chenopodii ambrosiodis herba* and *Lichen islandicus*. *Dtsch Apoth Ztg* 1994; **134**: 25–26, 29–32.

28 Van Eijk JL. *Eupatorium riparii* as a falsification for *Orthosiphon stamineus*. *Pharm Week* 1980; **115**: 13.

Juniper

Species (Family)

Juniperus communis L. (Pinaceae)

Synonym(s)

Baccae Juniperi, Genièvre, Wacholderbeeren, Zimbro

Part(s) Used

Fruit (berry)

Pharmacopoeial and Other Monographs

BHP 1996[G9]
BP 2001[G15]
Complete German Commission E[G3]
ESCOP 1997[G52]
Martindale 32nd edition[G43]
PDR for Herbal Medicines 2nd edition[G36]
Ph Eur 2002[G28]

Legal Category (Licensed Products)

GSL[G37]

Constituents[G2,G22,G41,G53,G58,G62,G64]

Acids Diterpene acids, ascorbic acid and glucuronic acid.

Flavonoids Amentoflavone,[1] quercetin, isoquercitrin, apigenin and various glycosides.

Tannins Proanthocyanidins (condensed), gallocatechin and epigallocatechin.[2]

Volatile oils 0.2–3.42%. Primarily monoterpenes (about 58%) including α-pinene, myrcene and sabinene (major), and camphene, camphor, 1,4-cineole, *p*-cymene, α- and γ-cadinene, limonene, β-pinene, γ-terpinene, terpinen-4-ol, terpinyl acetate, α-thujene, borneol; sesquiterpenes including caryophyllene, epoxydihydrocaryophyllene and β-elemem-7α-ol.[3,4]

Other constituents Geijerone (C_{12} terpenoid), junionone (monocyclic cyclobutane monoterpenoid),[5] desoxypodophyllotoxin (lignan),[6] resins and sugars.

Food Use

Juniper berries are widely used as a flavouring component in gin. Juniper is listed by the Council of Europe as a natural source of food flavouring (fruit N2, leaf and wood N3). Category N2 indicates that the berries can be added to foodstuffs in small quantities, with a possible limitation of an active principle (as yet unspecified) in the final product. Category N3 indicates that there is insufficient information available for an adequate assessment of potential toxicity to be made.[G16] In the USA, extracts and oils of juniper are permitted for food use.[G65]

Herbal Use[G2,G7,G64]

The German Commission E approved use for dyspepsia.[G321,53>] Juniper is stated to possess diuretic, antiseptic, carminative, stomachic and antirheumatic properties. Traditionally, it has been used for cystitis, flatulence, colic, and applied topically for rheumatic pains in joints or muscles.

Dosage

Dried ripe fruits 100 mL as an infusion (1 : 20 in boiling water) three times daily.[G7]

Fruit 1–2 g or equivalent three times daily; 2–10 g (equivalent to 20–100 mg of volatile oil).[G3]

Liquid extract 2–4 mL (1 : 1 in 25% alcohol) three times daily.[G7]

Tincture 1–2 mL (1 : 5 in 45% alcohol) three times daily.[G7]

Oil 0.03–0.2 mL (1 : 5 in 45% alcohol) three times daily.

Pharmacological Actions

Pharmacological actions that have been documented for juniper are primarily associated with the volatile oil components.

In vitro and animal studies

The volatile oil is documented to possess diuretic, gastrointestinal antiseptic and irritant properties.[G41]

The diuretic activity of juniper has been attributed to the volatile oil component, terpinen-4-ol, which is reported to increase the glomerular filtration rate.[G60] Terpenin-4-ol is also stated to be irritant to the kidneys although in a later review by the same author there is no such statement and the oil is stated to represent no hazards.[G58]

An antifertility effect has been described for a juniper extract, administered to rats (300/500 mg, by mouth) on days 1–7 of pregnancy.[7]. An abortifacient effect was also noted at both dose levels when the extract was administered on days 14–16.[7] No evidence of teratogenicity was reported. Anti-implantation activity has been reported as 60 to 70%[8] and as dose dependent.[7] Juniper is reported to have both a significant[9] and no[8] antifertility effect. A uterine stimulant activity has been documented for the volatile oil.[G30]

A potent and non-toxic inhibition of the cytopathogenic effects of herpes simplex virus type 1 in primary human amnion cell culture has been described for a juniper extract.[6,10] The active component isolated from the active fraction was identified as a lignan, desoxypodophyllotoxin.[6] Antiviral activities documented for the volatile oil have also been partly attributed to the flavonoid amentoflavone.[1]

Anti-inflammatory activity of 60% compared to 45% for the indomethacin control has been reported for juniper berry extract.[11] Both test and control were administered orally to rats (100 mg/kg and 5 mg/kg respectively) one hour before eliciting foot oedema.

A transient hypertensive effect followed by a more prolonged hypotensive effect has been reported for a juniper extract in rats (25 mg/kg, intravenous injection).[12]

A fungicidal effect against *Penicillium notatum* has been documented.[13]

Astringent activity is generally associated with tannins, which have been documented as components of juniper. An aqueous decoction of the berries has a hypoglycaemic effect in rats.[14] In rats, oral administration of an aqueous infusion (5 mL) increased chloride ion secretion by 119% and by 45% in similar experiments with rabbits.[G52]

Side-effects, Toxicity

The volatile oil is reported to be generally non-sensitising and non-phototoxic, although slightly irritant when applied externally to human and animal skin.[G41,G58] Excessive doses of terpinen-4-ol, the diuretic principle in the volatile oil, may cause kidney irritation.[G22]

Dermatitic reactions have been recognised with juniper and positive patch test reactions have been documented.[15,G51] The latter are attributed to the irritant nature of the juniper extract.[15]

Symptoms of poisoning following external application of the essential oil are described as burning, erythema, inflammation with blisters and oedema.[G22] Internally, symptoms from overdose are documented as pain in or near the kidneys, strong diuresis, albuminuria, haematuria, purplish urine, tachycardia, hypertension, and rarely convulsions, metrorrhagia and abortion.[G22]

The acute toxicity of juniper has been investigated in rats who were administered extracts for seven days.[11] An oral dose of 2.5 g/kg was tolerated with no mortalities or side-effects noted. A dose of 3 g/kg induced hypothermia and mild diarrhoea in 10–30% of animals.[11] An LD_{50} value (mice, intraperitoneal injection) has been stated as 3 g/kg.[4]

Contra-indications, Warnings

Juniper is contra-indicated in individuals with existing renal disease.[G7,G42,G49,G52] The internal use of the oil should be restricted to professionals.[G42] External application of the oil may cause an irritant reaction. However, this has been refuted and the oil is stated to have no hazards and is not contra-indicated.[G58] Juniper has been confused with savin (*Juniperus sabina*) in the literature and this may be the reason for believing that the oil is toxic.[G58] Juniper may potentiate existing hypoglycaemic and diuretic therapies; prolonged use may result in hypokalaemia.

Pregnancy and lactation Juniper is contra-indicated in pregnancy.[G7,G22,G49] It is reputed to be an abortifacient and to affect the menstrual cycle.[G30]

A juniper fruit extract has exhibited abortifacient, antifertility and anti-implantation activities (*see In vitro and animal studies*).

Pharmaceutical Comment

Many of the traditional uses documented for juniper can be supported by documented pharmacological actions or known constituents. There is evidence that the berries are abortifacient and since this is believed not to be due to the oil there must be other toxic constituents present. It is recommended that use should not exceed levels specified in food legislation.

References

See also General References G2, G3, G5, G9, G10, G16, G22, G30, G31, G32, G36, G37, G41, G42, G43, G49, G51, G52, G53, G58, G60, G62 and G64.

1   Chandler RF. An inconspicuous but insidious drug. *Rev Pharm Can* 1986; 563–566.
2   Friedrich H, Engelshowe R. Tannin producing monomeric substances in *Juniperus communis*. *Planta Med* 1978; **33**: 251–257.
3   Wagner H, Wolff P, eds. *New Natural Products and Plant Drugs with Pharmacological, Biological or Therapeutical Activity*. Berlin: Springer-Verlag, 1977.
4   *Fenaroli's Handbook of Flavor Ingredients*, 2nd edn. Boca Raton: CRC Press, 1975.
5   Thomas AF, Ozainne M. 'Junionone' [1-(2,2-Dimethylcyclobutyl)but-1-en-3-one], the first vegetable monocyclic cyclobutane monoterpenoid. *J C S Chem Commun* 1973; 746.
6   Markkanen T *et al*. Antiherpetic agent from juniper tree (*Juniperus communis*), its purification, identification, and testing in primary human amnion cell cultures. *Drugs Exp Clin Res* 1981; 7: 691–697.
7   Agrawal OP *et al*. Antifertility effects of fruits of *Juniperus communis*. *Planta Med* 1980; 40(Suppl.): 98–101.
8   Prakash AO *et al*. Anti-implantation activity of some indigenous plants in rats. *Acta Eur Fertil* 1985; **16**: 441–448.
9   Prakash AO. Biological evaluation of some medicinal plant extracts for contraceptive efficacy. *Contracept Deliv Syst* 1984; **5**: 9.
10 Marrkanen T. Antiherpetic agent(s) from juniper tree (*Juniperus communis*). Preliminary communication. *Drugs Exp Clin Res* 1981; 7: 69–73.
11 Mascolo N *et al*. Biological screening of Italian medicinal plants for anti-inflammatory activity. *Phytother Res* 1987; **1**: 28–31.
12 Lasheras B *et al*. Étude pharmacologique préliminaire de *Prunus spinosa* L. Amelanchier ovalis Medikus, *Juniperus communis* L. et *Urtica dioica* L. *Plant Méd Phytothér* 1986; **20**: 219–226.
13 Hejtmánková N *et al*. The antifungal effects of some Cupressaceae. *Acta Univ Palacki Olomuc Fac Med* 1973; **60**: 15–20.
14 Sanchez de Medina F *et al*. Hypoglycaemic activity of Juniper berries. *Planta Med* 1994; **60**: 197–200.
15 Mathias CGT *et al*. Plant dermatitis – patch test results (1975–78). Note on *Juniperus* extract. *Contact Dermatitis* 1979; **5**: 336–337.

Lady's Slipper

Species (Family)

Cypripedium pubescens Willd. (Orchidaceae) and other related species

Synonym(s)

American Valerian, Cypripedium, *Cypripedium calceolus* var.*pubescens* R.Br., Nerve Root

Related species also referred to as Lady's Slipper include *Calypso bulbosa* (L.) Oakes (*Cypripedium bulbosum* L.) and *Cypripedium parviflorum* Salish

Part(s) Used

Rhizome, root

Pharmacopoeial and Other Monographs

BHP 1983[G7]
PDR for Herbal Medicines 2nd edition (Nerve Root)[G36]

Legal Category (Licensed Products)

GSL (Cypripedium)[G37]

Constituents[G22,G48,G64]

Little chemical information has been documented. Lady's slipper is stated to contain glycosides, resin, tannic and gallic acids (usually associated with hydrolysable tannins), tannins and a volatile oil.

Several quinones have been reported including cypripedin, stated to belong to a group of rare non-terpenoid phenanthraquinones and not previously isolated from natural sources.[1]

Food Use

Lady's slipper is not used in foods.

Herbal Use

Lady's slipper is stated to possess sedative, mild hypnotic, antispasmodic and thymoleptic properties. Traditionally, it has been used for insomnia, hysteria, emotional tension, anxiety states, and specifically for anxiety states with insomnia.[G7,G64]

Dosage

Dried rhizome/root 2–4 g or by infusion three times daily.[G7]

Liquid extract 2–4 mL (1 : 1 in 45% alcohol) three times daily.[G7]

Pharmacological Actions

None documented.

Side-effects, Toxicity

It has been stated that the roots may cause psychedelic reactions and large doses may result in giddiness, restlessness, headache, mental excitement and visual hallucinations.[G22] Lady's slipper is stated to be allergenic and contact dermatitis has been documented.[G51] The sensitising property of lady's slipper has been attributed to the quinone constituents.[1]

Contra-indications, Warnings

Lady's slipper may cause an allergic reaction in sensitive individuals.

Pregnancy and lactation The safety of lady's slipper has not been established. In view of the lack of phytochemical, pharmacological and toxicological information the use of lady's slipper during pregnancy and lactation should be avoided.

Pharmaceutical Comment

Virtually no phytochemical or pharmacological data are available for lady's slipper to justify its use as a herbal remedy. In view of the lack of toxicity data, excessive use should be avoided.

References

See also General References G7, G22, G31, G36, G37, G48, G51 and G64.

1 Schmalle H, Hausen BM. A new sensitizing quinone from lady slipper (*Cypripedium calceolus*). *Naturwissenschaften* 1979; **66**: 527–528.

Lemon Verbena

Species (Family)

Aloysia triphylla (L'Her.) Britton (Verbenaceae)

Synonym(s)

Aloysia citriodora (Cav.) Ort., *Lippia citriodora* (Ort.) HBK, *Verbena citriodora* Cav., *Verbena triphylla* L'Her.

Part(s) Used

Flowering top, leaf

Pharmacopoeial and Other Monographs

PDR for Herbal Medicines 2nd edition[G36]

Legal Category (Licensed Products)

Lemon verbena is not included in the GSL.[G37]

Constituents[G22,G34,G57,G64]

Flavonoids Flavones including apigenin, chryso-eriol, cirsimaritin, diosmetin, eupafolin, eupatorin, hispidulin, luteolin and derivatives, pectolinarigenin and salvigenin.[1]

Volatile oils Terpene components include borneol, cineol, citral, citronellal, cymol, eugenol, geraniol, limonene, linalool, β-pinene, nerol, and terpineol (monoterpenes), and α-caryophyllene, β-caryophyllene, myrcenene, pyrollic acid and isovalerianic acid (sesquiterpenes).[2]

Food Use

In the USA, lemon verbena is listed as GRAS (Generally Recognised As Safe) for human consumption in alcoholic beverages. Lemon verbena is also used in herbal teas.[G57]

Herbal Use

Lemon verbena is reputed to possess antispasmodic, antipyretic, sedative and stomachic properties. It has been used for the treatment of asthma, cold, fever, flatulence, colic, diarrhoea and indigestion.[G38,G57,G64]

Dosage

Decoction 45 mL taken several times daily.[G34]

Pharmacological Actions

None documented.

Side-effects, Toxicity

None documented for lemon verbena. Terpene-rich volatile oils are generally regarded as irritant and may cause kidney irritation during excretion.

Contra-indications, Warnings

Individuals with existing renal disease should avoid excessive doses of lemon verbena in view of the possible irritant nature of the volatile oil.

Pregnancy and lactation In view of the lack of pharmacological and toxicity data, and the potential irritant nature of the volatile oil, excessive doses of lemon verbena are best avoided during pregnancy and lactation.

Pharmaceutical Comment

Limited information is available on lemon verbena. The traditional uses are probably attributable to the volatile oil, for which many components have been identified, and to the flavone constituents. In the UK, lemon verbena is mainly used as an ingredient of herbal teas.

References

See also General References G22, G34, G36, G38, G57 and G64.

1 Skaltsa H, Shammas G. Flavonoids from *Lippia citriodora*. *Planta Med* 1988; **54**: 465.
2 Montes M *et al*. Sur la composition de l'essence d'*Aloysia triphylla* (Cedron). *Planta Med* 1973; **23**: 119–124.

Liferoot

Species (Family)

Senecio aureus L. (Asteraceae/Compositae)

Synonym(s)

Golden Ragwort, Golden Senecio, Squaw Weed

Part(s) Used

Herb

Pharmacopoeial and Other Monographs

BHP 1983[G7]
Martindale 32nd edition[G43]
PDR for Herbal Medicines 2nd edition[G36]

Legal Category (Licensed Products)

Liferoot is not included in the GSL.[G37]

Constituents[G19,G64]

Limited information is documented regarding the constituents of liferoot, although it is well recognised that *Senecio* species contain pyrrolizidine alkaloids.

Pyrrolizidine alkaloids Floridanine, florosenine, otosenine, senecionine.[1,2]

The volatile oil composition of various *Senecio* species (but not *Senecio aureus*) has been investigated.[3]

Food Use

Liferoot is not used as a food, although many *Senecio* species are used as a form of spinach in South Africa.

Herbal Use

Liferoot is stated to possess uterine tonic, diuretic and mild expectorant properties. Traditionally, it has been used in the treatment of functional amenorrhoea, menopausal neurosis and leucorrhoea (as a douche).[G7,G64]

Dosage

Herb 14 g or by infusion three times daily.[G7]

Liquid extract 14 mL (1 : 1 in 25% alcohol) three times daily.[G7]

Pharmacological Actions

No documented studies were located.

Side-effects, Toxicity

Liferoot contains pyrrolizidine alkaloids. The toxicity, primarily hepatic, of this class of compounds is well recognised in both animals and humans[G19] (*see* Comfrey).

Contra-indications, Warnings

In view of the hepatotoxic pyrrolizidine alkaloid constituents, liferoot should not be ingested.[G19]

Pregnancy and lactation In view of the toxic constituents, liferoot is contraindicated during pregnancy and lactation.[G49] Furthermore, liferoot is traditionally reputed to be an abortifacient, emmenagogue, and uterine tonic.[G7,G22] In animals, placental transfer and secretion into breast milk[4] has been documented for unsaturated pyrrolizidine alkaloids.

Pharmaceutical Comment

Little information is documented for liferoot. No pharmacological studies were found to substantiate the traditional uses. The *Senecio* genus is characterised by unsaturated pyrrolizidine alkaloid constituents and the hepatotoxicity of this class of compounds is well recognised (*see* Comfrey). In view of this, liferoot is not suitable for use as a herbal remedy.

References

See also General References G7, G22, G31, G32, G36, G43, G49 and G64.

1 *Pyrrolizidine Alkaloids. Environmental Health Criteria 80*. Geneva: WHO, 1988.
2 Roder E *et al*. Pyrrolizidinalkaloide aus *Senecio aureus*. *Planta Med* 1983; **49**: 57–59.
3 Dooren B *et al*. Composition of essential oils of some *Senecio* species. *Planta Med* 1981; **42**: 385–389.
4 Mattocks AR. *Chemistry and Toxicology of Pyrrolizidine Alkaloids*. London: Academic Press, 1986: 1–393.

Lime Flower

Species (Family)

(i) *Tilia cordata* Mill. (Tiliaceae)
(ii) *Tilia platyphyllos* Scop.
(iii) *Tilia × europaea* – hybrid of (i) and (ii)

Synonym(s)

Lime Tree, Linden Tree

Part(s) Used

Flowerheads

Pharmacopoeial and Other Monographs

BHC 1992[G6]
BHP 1996[G9]
BP 2001[G15]
Complete German Commission E (Linden)[G3]
Martindale 32nd edition[G43]
PDR for Herbal Medicines 2nd edition (Linden)[G36]
Ph Eur 2002[G28]

Legal Category (Licensed Products)

GSL[G37]

Constituents[G2,G6,G22,G49,G62,G64]

Acids Caffeic acid, chlorogenic acid and *p*-coumaric acid.

Amino acids Alanine, cysteine, cystine, isoleucine, leucine, phenylalanine and serine.

Carbohydrates Mucilage polysaccharides (3%). Five fractions identified yielding arabinose, galactose, rhamnose, with lesser amounts of glucose, mannose, and xylose; galacturonic and glucuronic acids;[1] gum.

Flavonoids Kaempferol, quercetin, myricetin and their glycosides.

Volatile oil Many components including alkanes, phenolic alcohols and esters, and terpenes including citral, citronellal, citronellol, eugenol, limonene, nerol, α-pinene and terpineol (monoterpenes), and farnesol (sesquiterpene).

Other constituents Saponin (unspecified), tannin (condensed) and tocopherol (phytosterol).

Food Use

Lime flower is listed by the Council of Europe as a natural source of food flavouring (category N2). This category indicates that lime flower can be added to foodstuffs in small quantities, with a possible limitation of an active principle (as yet unspecified) in the final product.[G16] In the USA, lime flower is listed as GRAS (Generally Recognised As Safe).[G65]

Herbal Use

Lime flower is stated to possess sedative, antispasmodic, diaphoretic, diuretic and mild astringent properties. Traditionally it has been used for migraine, hysteria, arteriosclerotic hypertension, feverish colds, and specifically for raised arterial pressure associated with arteriosclerosis and nervous tension.[G2,G6,G7,G8,G64]

Dosage

Flowerhead 2–4 g by infusion.

Liquid extract 2–4 mL (1 : 1 in 25% alcohol).

Tincture 1–2 mL (1 : 5 in 45% alcohol).

Pharmacological Actions

In vitro and animal studies

In vitro, lime flower has been reported to exhibit antispasmodic activity followed by a spasmogenic effect on rat duodenum.[2] The actions were inhibited by atropine and papaverine, and reinforced by acetylcholine. The diaphoretic and antispasmodic properties claimed for lime flower have been attributed to *p*-coumaric acid and the flavonoids.[G39,G60] In addition, a number of actions have been associated with volatile oils including diuretic, sedative and antispasmodic effects, which may also account for some of the reputed uses of lime flower.[3–5] Volatile oils are not thought to possess any true diuretic activity, but to act as a result of certain terpenoid components having an irritant action on the kidneys during renal excretion.

Lime flower has been documented to possess a restricted range of antifungal activity.[6]

Side-effects, Toxicity

Excessive use of lime flower tea may result in cardiac toxicity.[G60] However, the rationale for this statement is not included by the author.

Contra-indications, Warnings

It is advised that lime flower should be avoided by individuals with an existing cardiac disorder.[G22,G39,G60]

Pregnancy and lactation The safety of lime flower has not been established. In view of the lack of toxicological data, excessive use of lime flower during pregnancy and lactation should be avoided.

Pharmaceutical Comment

The chemistry of lime flower is well documented. Little scientific information was located to justify the reputed herbal uses of lime flower, although some correlation can be made with the known pharmacological activities of the reported constituents. The lack of toxicological data, together with a warning concerning cardiac toxicity, indicates that excessive use of lime flower should be avoided.

References

See also General References G2, G3, G6, G9, G11, G15, G16, G22, G25, G32, G36, G37, G39, G43, G49, G56, G60, G62 and G64.

1 Kram G, Franz G. Structural investigations on the water soluble polysaccharides of lime tree flowers (*Tilia cordata* L.). *Pharmazie* 1985; **40**: 501.

2 Lanza JP, Steinmetz M. Actions comparees des exraits aqueux de graines de *Tilia platyphylla* et de *Tilia vulgaris* sur l'intestin isolé de rat. *Fitoterapia* 1986; **57**: 185.

3 Taddei I *et al*. Spasmolytic activity of peppermint, sage and rosemary essences and their major constituents. *Fitoterapia* 1988; **59**: 463–468.

4 Svendsen AB, Scheffer JJC. *Essential Oils and Aromatic Plants. Proceedings of the 15th International Symposium on Essential Oils*. Dordrecht: Martinus Nijhoff, 1984; 225–226.

5 Sticher O. Plant mono-, di- and sesquiterpenoids with pharmacological and therapeutical activity. In: Wagner H, Wolff P, eds. *New Natural Products with Pharmacological, Biological or Therapeutical Activity*. Berlin: Springer-Verlag, 1977: 137–176.

6 Guerin J-C, Reveillere H-P. Antifungal activity of plant extracts used in therapy. I Study of 41 plant extracts against 9 fungi species. *Ann Pharm Fr* 1984; **B**: 553–559

Liquorice

Species (Family)

Glycyrrhiza glabra L. (Leguminosae)

Synonym(s)

Licorice

Part(s) Used

Root, stolon

Pharmacopoeial and Other Monographs

BHC 1992[G6]
BHP 1996[G9]
BP 2001[G15]
Complete German Commission E[G3]
Martindale 32nd edition[G43]
Mills and Bone[G50]
PDR for Herbal Medicines 2nd edition[G36]
Ph Eur 2002[G28]
WHO volume 1 1999[G63]

Legal Category (Licensed Products)

GSL[G37]

Constituents[G2,G6,G41,G48,G64]

Coumarins Glycyrin, heniarin, liqcoumarin, umbelliferone, GU-7 (3-arylcoumarin derivative).[1]

Flavonoids Flavonols and isoflavones including formononetin, glabrin, glabrol, glabrone, glyzarin, glycyrol, glabridin and derivatives, kumatakenin, licoflavonol, licoisoflavones A and B, licoisoflavanone, licoricone, liquiritin and derivatives, phaseollinisoflavan;[2] chalcones including isoliquiritigenin, licuraside, echinatin, licochalcones A and B, neolicuroside.[3]

Terpenoids Glycyrrhizin glycoside (1–24%) also known as glycyrrhizic or glycyrrhizinic acid yielding glycyrrhetinic (or glycyrrhetic) acid and glucuronic acid following hydrolysis;[4] glycyrrhetol, glabrolide, licoric acid, liquiritic acid and β-amyrin.

Volatile oils 0.047%.[5] More than 80 components identified including anethole, benzaldehyde, butyro-lactone, cumic alcohol, eugenol, fenchone, furfuryl alcohol, hexanol, indole, linalool, γ-nonalactone, oestragole, propionic acid, α-terpineol and thujone[5]

Other constituents Amino acids, amines, gums, lignin, starch, sterols (β-sitosterol, stigmasterol), sugars and wax.

Other plant parts Components documented for the leaves of *G. glabra* include flavonoids (kaempferol and derivatives, isoquercetin, quercetin and derivatives, phytoalexins), coumarins (bergapten, xanthotoxin), phytoestrogen, β-sitosterol and saponaretin.[6]

Food Use

Liquorice is widely used in foods as a flavouring agent. Liquorice root is listed by the Council of Europe as a natural source of food flavouring (category N2). This category indicates that liquorice can be added to foodstuffs in small quantities, with a possible limitation of an active principle (as yet unspecified) in the final product.[G16] In the USA, liquorice is listed as GRAS (Generally Recognised As Safe).[G41]

Herbal Use[G2,G6,G7,G8,G10,G64]

Liquorice is stated to possess expectorant, demulcent, antispasmodic, anti-inflammatory and laxative properties. Traditionally, it is also reported to affect the adrenal glands. It has been used for bronchial catarrh, bronchitis, chronic gastritis, peptic ulcer, colic and primary adrenocortical insufficiency.

Dosage

Powdered root 1–4 g or by decoction three times daily.[G6,G7]

Liquorice Extract (BPC 1973) 0.6–2.0 g.

Pharmacological Actions

The pharmacological actions of liquorice have been reviewed.[7,8]

In vitro and animal studies

Much has been documented regarding the steroid-type actions of liquorice (see Side-effects, Toxicity). Both glycyrrhizin and glycyrrhetinic acid (GA) have been reported to bind to glucocorticoid and mineralocorticoid receptors with moderate affinity, and to oestrogen receptors, sex hormone-binding globulin and corticosteroid-binding globulin with very weak affinity.[9–11] It has been suggested that glycyrrhizin and glycyrrhetinic acid may influence endogenous steroid activity via a receptor mechanism, with displacement of corticosteroids or other endogenous steroids.[9]

The anti-oestrogenic action documented for glycyrrhizin at relatively high concentrations has been associated with a blocking effect that would be caused by glycyrrhizin binding at oestrogen receptors.[9] However, oestrogenic activity has also been documented for liquorice and attributed to the isoflavone constituents.[8] Liquorice exhibits an alternative action on oestrogen metabolism, causing inhibition if oestrogen concentrations are high and potentiation when concentrations are low.[8]

The relatively low affinity of glycyrrhizin and glycyrrhetinic acid for binding to mineralocorticoid receptors, together with the fact that liquorice does not exert its mineralocorticoid activity in adrenalectomised animals, indicates that a direct action at mineralocorticoid receptors is not the predominant mode of action.[12] It has been suggested that glycyrrhizin and glycyrrhetinic acid may exert their mineralocorticoid effect via an inhibition of 11β-hydroxysteroid dehydrogenase (11β-OHSD).[12] 11β-OHSD is a microsomal enzyme complex found predominantly in the liver and kidneys which catalyses the conversion of cortisol (potent mineralocortoid activity) to the inactive cortisone. Deficiency of 11β-OHSD results in increased concentrations of urinary free cortisol and cortisol metabolites. Glycyrrhetinic acid has been shown to inhibit renal 11β-OHSD in rats.[12] It has also been proposed that glycyrrhizin and glycyrrhetinic acid may displace cortisol from binding to transcortin.[13]

Antiplatelet activity in vitro has been documented for a 3-arylcoumarin derivative, GU-7, isolated from liquorice.[1] GU-7 was thought to inhibit platelet aggregation by increasing intraplatelet cyclic AMP concentration.

Isoliquiritigenin has been reported to inhibit aldose reductase, the first enzyme in the polyol pathway which reduces glucose to sorbitol.[14] Isoliquiritigenin was subsequently found to inhibit sorbitol accumulation in human red blood cells in vitro, and in red blood cells, the sciatic nerve and the lens of diabetic rats administered isoliquirigenin intragastrically.[14,15] Many diabetic complications, such as cataracts, peripheral neuropathy, retinopathy and nephropathy have been associated with the polyol pathway and have shown improvement with inhibitors of aldose reductase.[14,15]

Significant anti-inflammatory action is exhibited by glycyrrhetinic acid against UV erythema.[16] 18α-Glycyrrhetinic acid has exhibited stronger anti-inflammatory action compared to its stereoisomer 18β-glycyrrhetinic acid.[17] Chalcones isolated from G. inflata Bat. have been reported to inhibit leukotriene production and increase cyclic AMP concentrations in human polymorphonuclear neutrophils in vitro.[18] Glycyrrhetinic acid derivatives, but not glycyrrhetinic acid, have exhibited inhibitory effects on writhing and vascular permeability tests and on type IV allergy in mice.[19] The dihemiphthalate derivatives were especially active with respect to the two former activities and have previously been found to inhibit lipoxygenase and cyclooxygenase activities, and to prevent formation of gastric ulcer.[19]

Glycyrrhetinic acid is known to inhibit Epstein–Barr virus activation by tumour promotors.[20]

Antimicrobial activity versus Staphylococcus aureus, Mycobacterium smegmatis and Candida albicans has been documented for liquorice and attributed to isoflavonoid constituents (glabridin, glabrol and their derivatives).[2] Antiviral activity has been described for glycyrrhetinic acid, which interacts with virus structures producing different effects according to the viral stage affected.[21] Activity was observed against vaccinia, herpes simplex 1, Newcastle disease and vesicular stomatitis viruses, with no activity demonstrated towards poliovirus 1.[21]

In vitro hepatoprotective activity against CCl₄-induced toxicity has been reported to be greater for glycyrrhizin compared to glycyrrhizin.[22] Glycyrrhetinic acid is thought to act by inhibition of the cytochrome P450 system required for the metabolism of CCl₄ to the highly reactive radical CCl₃.[22] Glycyrrhiza uralensis Fisch is used to treat hepatitis B in China, with a success rate reported to be greater than 70%.[23] Other activities documented for G. uralensis are anti-inflammatory and anti-allergic, treatment of jaundice, inhibition of fibrosis of the liver, corticosteroid-like immunosuppressing effect and a detoxifying effect.[23]

Screening of several plant extracts for antifertility activity reported liquorice to be ineffective following oral administration to rats in days 1–7 of pregnancy.[24]

Clinical studies

Carbenoxolone, an ester derivative of glycyrrhetinic acid, has been used in the treatment of gastric and oesophageal ulcers. It is thought to exhibit a mucosal-protecting effect by beneficially interfering with gastric prostanoid synthesis, and increasing mucous production and mucosal blood flow.[25]

Liquorice is thought to exert its mineralocorticoid effect by inhibition of the enzyme 11β-OHSD, which catalyses the conversion of cortisol to the inactive cortisone (see In vitro and animal studies). Administration of liquorice to healthy volunteers has resulted in a disturbance of cortisol metabolism and a significant rise in urinary free cortisol, despite there being no change in plasma concentrations. These changes are consistent with this hypothesis, being indicative of 11β-OHSD deficiency.[12] Liquorice has also been found to suppress both plasma renin activity and aldosterone secretion.[26–28]

The pharmacokinetic profile of glycyrrhizin in rats has been found to be similar to that observed in humans.[29] Glycyrrhizin is primarily (80%) excreted into the bile from the liver against a concentration gradient.[29] This process is saturable and can therefore affect the excretion rate of glycyrrhizin. In addition, enterohepatic recycling occurs with reabsorption of bile-excreted glycyrrhizin from the intestinal tract.[29] Subjects consuming 100–200 g liquorice/day have been reported to achieve plasma glycyrrhetinic acid concentrations of 80–480 ng/mL.[12]

Side-effects, Toxicity

Apart from confectionery, liquorice can also be ingested from infusions and by chewing tobaccos. Excessive or prolonged liquorice ingestion has resulted in symptoms typical of primary hyperaldosteronism, namely hypertension, sodium, chloride and water retention, hypokalaemia and weight gain, but also in low levels of plasma renin activity, aldosterone and antidiuretic hormone.[13,26,30]

Raised concentrations of atrial natriuretic peptide (ANP), which is secreted in response to atrial stretch and has vasodilating, natriuretic and diuretic properties, have also been observed in healthy subjects following the ingestion of liquorice.[13] Individuals consuming between 10–45 g liquorice/day have exhibited raised blood pressure, together with a block of the aldosterone/renin axis and electrocardiogram changes, which resolved one month after withdrawal of liquorice.[31] Individuals consuming vastly differing amounts of liquorice have exhibited similar side-effect symptoms, indicating that the mineralocorticoid effect of liquorice is not dose dependent and is a saturable process.[31]

Hypokalaemic myopathy has also been associated with liquorice ingestion.[32–36] Severe hypokalaemia

with rhabdomyolysis has been documented in a male patient following the ingestion of an alcohol-free beverage containing only small amounts of glycyrrhetinic acid (0.35 g/day).[32] The patient had known liver cirrhosis due to alcohol consumption and it was suggested that cirrhotic patients may be more susceptible to the mineralocorticoid side-effects of liquorice.[32] In one case,[34] the myoglobinaemia led to glomerulopathy and tubulopathy but with no clinical evidence of acute renal failure (ARF). The latter was attributed to the volume expansion also caused by the liquorice ingestion.

Rhabdomyolysis without myoglobinuria has been described.[37] In addition, severe congestive heart failure and pulmonary oedema have been reported in a previously healthy man who had ingested 700 g liquorice over eight days.[30] Liquorice extract given orally has been reported to have a similar but longer lasting action to intravenous deoxycortone and it has been noted that sodium, chloride and water retention do not have to be accompanied by clinical oedema.[38] Amenorrhoea has been associated with liquorice ingestion (anti-oestrogenic action), with the menstrual cycle re-appearing following the withdrawal of liquorice.[31]

It has been noted that symptoms of hyperaldosteronism often resolve quickly, within a few days to two weeks, following the withdrawal of liquorice, even in individuals who have ingested the substance for many years.[28]

A case has been described where a patient presented with symptoms related to hyperglycaemia and myopathy secondary to liquorice-induced hypokalaemia. An inverse relationship was observed between the concentrations of fasting serum glucose and serum potassium.[39] Interestingly, animal studies have indicated that liquorice may reduce diabetic complications associated with intracellular accumulation of sorbitol.[19]

Contra-indications, Warnings

Numerous instances have been documented where liquorice ingestion has resulted in symptoms of primary hyperaldosteronism, such as water and sodium retention and hypokalaemia. Liquorice should therefore be avoided completely by individuals with an existing cardiovascular-related disorder, and ingested in moderation by other individuals. Hypokalaemia is known to aggravate glucose intolerance and liquorice ingestion may therefore interfere with existing hypoglycaemic therapy. Liquorice may interfere with existing hormonal therapy (oestrogens and antioestrogenic activities documented in vivo).

Pregnancy and lactation In view of the oestrogenic and steroid effects associated with liquorice, which may exacerbate pregnancy-related hypertension, excessive ingestion during pregnancy and lactation should be avoided. In addition, liquorice has exhibited a uterine stimulant activity in animal studies, and is traditionally reputed to be an abortifacient and to affect the menstrual cycle (emmenagogue).[G30]

Pharmaceutical Comment

The phytochemistry is well documented for liquorice and it is particularly characterised by triterpenoid components. Many of the traditional uses of liquorice are supported by documented pharmacological data although limited evidence of antispasmodic activity was found. Carbenoxolone, an ester derivative of a triterpenoid constituent in liquorice, is well known for its use in ulcer therapy. Much has been written concerning the steroid-type adverse effects associated with liquorice ingestion. Liquorice ingestion should therefore be avoided by individuals with an existing cardiovascular disorder and moderate consumption should be observed by other individuals.

References

See also General References G2, G3, G5, G6, G9, G12, G15, G16, G18, G21, G28, G30, G31, G32, G36, G37, G41, G43, G48, G50, G56, G63 and G64.

1 Tawata M *et al.* Anti-platelet action of GU-7, a 3-arylcoumarin derivative, purified from *Glycyrrhizae radix*. *Planta Med* 1990; **56**: 259–263.
2 Mitscher LA *et al.* Antimicrobial agents from higher plants. Antimicrobial isoflavanoids and related substances from *Glycyrrhiza glabra* L. var. *typica*. *J Nat Prod* 1980; **43**: 259–269.
3 Miething H, Speicher-Brinker A. Neolicuroside – A new chalcone glycoside from the roots of *Glycyrrhiza glabra*. *Arch Pharm (Weinheim)* 1989; **322**: 141–143.
4 Takino Y *et al.* Quantitative determination of glycyrrhizic acid in liquorice roots and extracts by TLC-densitometry. *Planta Med* 1979; **36**: 74–78.
5 Kameoka H, Nakai K. Components of essential oil from the root of *Glycyrrhiza glabra*. *Nippon Nogeikagaku Kaishi [J Ag Chem Soc Japan]* 1987; **61**: 1119–1121.
6 Jimenez J *et al.* Flavonoids of *Helianthemum cinereum*. *Fitoterapia* 1989; **60**: 189.
7 Chandler RF. Licorice, more than just a flavour. *Can Pharm J* 1985; **118**: 421–424.
8 Pizzorno JE, Murray AT. *Glycyrrhiza glabra. A Textbook of Natural Medicine*. Seattle, WA: John Bastyr College Publications, 1985 (looseleaf).

9 Tamaya MD *et al.* Possible mechanism of steroid action of the plant herb extracts glycyrrhizin, glycyrrhetinic acid, and paeoniflorin: Inhibition by plant herb extracts of steroid protein binding in the rabbit. *Am J Obstet Gynecol* 1986; **155**: 1134–1139.
10 Armanini D *et al.* Binding of agonists and antagonists to mineralocorticoid receptors in human peripheral mononuclear leucocytes. *J Hypertens* 1985; 3(Suppl.3): S157–159.
11 Armanini D *et al.* Affinity of liquorice derivatives for mineralocorticoid and glucocorticoid receptors. *Clin Endocrinol* 1983; **19**: 609–612.
12 Stewart PM *et al.* Mineralocorticoid activity of liquorice: 11-beta-hydroxysteroid dehydrogenase deficiency comes of age. *Lancet* 1987; **ii**: 821–824.
13 Forslund T *et al.* Effects of licorice on plasma atrial natriuretic peptide in healthy volunteers. *J Intern Med* 1989; **225**: 95–99.
14 Aida K *et al.* Isoliquiritigenin: A new aldose reductase inhibitor from *Glycyrrhizae radix*. *Planta Med* 1990; **56**: 254–258.
15 Yun-ping Z, Jia-qing Z. Oral baicalin and liquid extract of licorice reduce sorbitol levels in red blood cell of diabetic rats. *Chin Med J* 1989; **102**: 203–206.
16 Fujita H *et al.* Antiinflammatory effect of glycyrrhizinic acid. Effects of glycyrrhizinic acid against carrageenin-induced edema, UV-erythema and skin reaction sensitised with DCNB. *Pharmacometrics* 1980; **19**: 481–484.
17 Amagaya S *et al.* Separation and quantitative analysis of 18α-glycyrrhetinic acid and 18β-glycyrrhetinic acid in *Glycyrrhizae radix* by gas-liquid chromatography. *J Chromatogr* 1985; **320**: 430–434.
18 Kimura Y *et al.* Effects of chalcones isolated from licorice roots on leukotriene biosynthesis in human polymorphonuclear neutrophils. *Phytother Res* 1988; **2**: 140–145.
19 Inque H *et al.* Pharmacological activities of glycerrhetinic acid derivatives: Analgesic and anti-type IV allergic effects. *Chem Pharm Bull* 1987; **35**: 3888–3893.
20 Tokuda H *et al.* Inhibitory effects of ursolic and oleandolic acid on skin tumor promotion by 12-O-tetradecanoylphorbol-13-acetate. *Cancer Lett* 1986; **33**: 279–285.
21 Pompei R *et al.* Antiviral activity of glycyrrhizic acid. *Experientia* 1980; **36**: 304.
22 Kiso Y *et al.* Mechanism of antihepatotoxic activity of glycyrrhizin, I: Effect on free radical generation and lipid peroxidation. *Planta Med* 1984; **50**: 298–302.
23 Chang HM *et al. Advances in Chinese Medicinal Materials Research*. Singapore: World Scientific, 1985.

24 Sharma BB *et al.* Antifertility screening of plants. Part I. Effect of ten indigenous plants on early pregnancy in albino rats. *Int J Crude Drug Res* 1983; **21**: 183–187.

25 Guslandi M. Ulcer-healing drugs and endogenous prostaglandins. *Int J Clin Pharmacol Ther Toxicol* 1985; **23**: 398–402.

26 Conn J *et al.* Licorice-induced pseudoaldosteronism. Hypertension, hypokalaemia, aldosteronopenia and suppressed plasma renin activity. *JAMA* 1968; **205**: 492–496.

27 Epstein MT *et al.* Effect of eating liquorice on the renin-angiotensin aldosterone axis in normal subjects. *BMJ* 1977; **1**: 488–490.

28 Mantero F. Exogenous mineralocorticoid-like disorders. *Clin Endocrinol Metab* 1981; **10**: 465–478.

29 Ichikawa T *et al.* Biliary excretion and enterohepatic cycling of glycyrrhizin in rats. *J Pharm Sci* 1986; **75**: 672–675.

30 Chamberlain TJ. Licorice poisoning, pseudoaldosteronism, heart failure. *JAMA* 1970; **213**: 1343.

31 Corrocher R *et al.* Pseudoprimary hyperaldosteronism due to liquorice intoxication. *Eur Rev Med Pharmacol Sci* 1983; **5**: 467–470.

32 Piette AM *et al.* Hypokaliémie majeure avec rhabdomyolase secondaire à l'ingestion de pastis non alcoolisé. *Ann Med Interne (Paris)* 1984; **135**: 296–298.

33 Cibelli G *et al.* Hypokalemic myopathy associated with liquorice ingestion. *Ital J Neurol Sci* 1984; **5**: 463–466.

34 Heidermann HT, Kreuzfelder E. Hypokalemic rhabdomyolysis with myoglobinuria due to licorice ingestion and diuretic treatment. *Klin Wochenschr* 1983; **61**: 303–305.

35 Ruggeri CS *et al.* L. Carnetina cloruro e KCl nel trattamento di un caso di rabdomiolisi atraumatica senza mioglobinuria da ingestione di liquerizia. *Minn Med* 1985; **76**: 725–728.

36 Bannister B *et al.* Cardiac arrest due to liquorice induced hypokalaemia. *BMJ* 1977; **2**: 738–739.

37 Maresca MC *et al.* Low blood potassium and rhabdomyolosis. Description of three cases with different aetiologies. *Minerva Med* 1988; **79**: 79–81.

38 Molhuysen JA. A liquorice extract with deoxycortone-like action. *Lancet* 1950; **ii**: 381–386.

39 Jamil A *et al.* Hyperglycaemia related to licorice-induced hypokalaemia. *J Kwt Med Assoc* 1986; **20**: 69–71.

Lobelia

Species (Family)

Lobelia inflata L. (Campanulaceae)

Synonym(s)

Indian Tobacco

Part(s) Used

Herb

Pharmacopoeial and Other Monographs

BHC 1992[G6]
BHP 1996[G9]
Martindale 32nd edition[G43]
PDR for Herbal Medicines 2nd edition[G36]

Legal Category (Licensed Products)

GSL[G37]

Constituents[G6,G22,G41,G64]

Alkaloids Piperidine-type. 0.48%. Lobeline (major); others include lobelanine, lobelanidine, nor-lobelanine, lelobanidine, norlelobanidine, norlobelanidine and lobinine.

Other constituents Bitter glycoside (lobelacrin), chelidonic acid, fats, gum, resin and volatile oil.

Food Use

Lobelia is not generally used as a food.

Herbal Use

Lobelia is stated to possess respiratory stimulant, antasthmatic, antispasmodic, expectorant, and emetic properties. Traditionally, it has been used for bronchitic asthma, chronic bronchitis, and specifically for spasmodic asthma with secondary bronchitis. It has also been used topically for myositis and rheumatic nodules.[G6,G7,G8,G64]

Dosage

Dried herb 0.2–0.6 g or by infusion or decoction three times daily.[G6,G7]

Liquid extract 0.2–0.6 mL (1:1 in 50% alcohol) three times daily.[G6,G7]

Simple Tincture of Lobelia (BPC 1949) 0.6–2.0 mL.

Tincture Lobelia Acid 1–4 mL (1:10 in dilute acetic acid) three times daily.[G6,G7]

Pharmacological Actions

The pharmacological activity of lobelia can be attributed to the alkaloid constituents, principally lobeline. Lobeline has peripheral and central effects similar to those of nicotine, but is less potent. Hence, lobeline initially causes CNS stimulation followed by respiratory depression. Lobeline is also reported to possess expectorant properties.

Side-effects, Toxicity

Side-effects of lobeline and lobelia are similar to those of nicotine and include nausea and vomiting, diarrhoea, coughing, tremors and dizziness. Symptoms of overdosage are reported to include profuse diaphoresis, tachycardia, convulsions, hypothermia, hypotension and coma, and may be fatal.[G45]

Contra-indications, Warnings

The pharmacological actions of lobeline are similar to those of nicotine.

Pregnancy and lactation Lobelia should not be used during pregnancy or lactation.

Pharmaceutical Comment

The principal constituent of lobelia is lobeline, an alkaloid with similar pharmacological properties to nicotine. Lobelia has previously been used in herbal preparations for the treatment of asthma and bronchitis, and in anti-smoking preparations aimed to lessen nicotine withdrawal symptoms. However, in view of its potent alkaloid constituents, excessive use of lobelia is not recommended.

References

See General References G5, G6, G9, G12, G22, G29, G32, G31, G36, G37, G41, G43, G48, and G64 .

Marshmallow

Species (Family)

Althaea officinalis L. (Malvaceae)

Synonym(s)

Althaea

Part(s) Used

Leaf, root

Pharmacopoeial and Other Monographs

BHC 1992[G6]
BHP 1996[G9]
BP 2001 (root)[G15]
Complete German Commission E[G3]
ESCOP 1996[G52]
Martindale 32nd edition[G43]
PDR for Herbal Medicines 2nd edition[G36]
Ph Eur 2002 (root and leaf)[G28]

Legal Category (Licensed Products)

GSL[G37]

Constituents[G2,G6,G41,G48,G52,G60,G64]

Polysaccharides Mucilage polysaccharides (5–10%), consisting of galacturono-rhamnans, arabinans, glucans, arabinogalactans.[1,G52]

Flavonoids Hyolaetin 8-glucoside, isoscutellarin 4′-methylether-8-glucoside-2″-sulfate.[2]

Phenolic acids Caffeic, *p*-coumaric, ferulic, *p*-hydroxybenzoic and syringic.

Other constituents Asparagine 2%, calcium oxalate, coumarins (scopoletin), pectin, starch and tannin.

Food Use

Marshmallow is listed by the Council of Europe as a natural source of food flavouring (category N2). This category indicates that marshmallow can be added to foodstuffs in small quantities, with a possible limitation of an active principle (as yet unspecified) in the final product.[G16] In the USA, marshmallow is approved for use in foods.[G41]

Herbal Use[G2,G4,G6,G7,G8,G43,G52,G54,G64]

Marshmallow is stated to possess demulcent, expectorant, emollient, diuretic, antilithic and vulnerary properties. Traditionally, it has been used internally for the treatment of respiratory catarrh and cough, peptic ulceration, inflammation of the mouth and pharynx, enteritis, cystitis, urethritis and urinary calculus, and topically for abscesses, boils and varicose and thrombotic ulcers. The German Commission E approved use of root and leaf for irritation of oral and pharyngeal mucosa and associated dry cough and root for mild inflammation of gastric mucosa.[G3] Marshmallow root is used in combination with anise fruit, eucalyptus oil, liquorice and with anise fruit, liquorice and primrose root and with anise fruit and primrose root for catarrh of the upper respiratory tract and resulting dry cough.[G3]

Dosage

Dried leaf 2–5 g or by infusion three times daily;[G6,G7] 5 g.[G3]

Leaf, liquid extract 2–5 mL (1 : 1 in 25% alcohol) three times daily.[G6,G7]

Ointment 5% Powdered althaea leaf in usual ointment base three times daily.[G6,G7]

Dried root 2–5 g or by cold extraction three times daily;[G6,G7] 6 g.[G3]

Root, liquid extract 2–5 mL (1 : 1 in 25% alcohol) three times daily.[G6,G7]

Syrup of Althaea (BPC 1949) 2–10 mL three times daily.[G6,G7]

Pharmacological Actions

In vitro and animal studies

Antimicrobial activity against *Pseudomonas aeruginosa*, *Proteus vulgaris* and *Staphylococcus aureus* has been documented for marshmallow.[3]

The mucilage has demonstrated considerable hypoglycaemic activity in non-diabetic mice.[4]

Inhibition (17%) of mucociliary transport in ciliated epithelium isolated from frog oesophagus was observed with 200 µL of cold macerate of marshmallow root (6.4 g/140 mL).[G52]

Marshmallow root extract is reported to stimulate phagocytosis, and to release oxygen radicals and leukotrienes from human neutrophils.[G52] In addition, release of cytokines, interleukin 6 and tumour necrosis factor from monocytes occurs, demonstrating potential anti-inflammatory and immunomodulatory effects. In mice, intraperitoneal administration of isolated polysaccharide (10 mg/kg) resulted in activity of macrophages in a carbon clearance test, and was indicative of non-specific immunomodulation.[G52] A lack of anti-inflammatory activity has been observed for marshmallow in the carrageenan-induced rat paw oedema test.[5] The anti-inflammatory effect of an ointment containing 0.05% dexamethasone was enhanced by addition of aqueous extract of marshmallow (20%) as assessed in a rabbit ear irritancy test using UV irradiation or furfuryl alcohol.[G52]

A total extract of root and isolated polysaccharide (100 and 50 mg/kg, respectively) have been tested for their antitussive activity in unanaesthetised cats.[6] The polysaccharide gave a statistically significant decrease in the number of cough efforts from laryngopharyngeal and tracheobronchial areas. The root extract was less effective than the isolated polysaccharide.

A polysaccharide enriched extract showed moderate concentration-dependent adhesive properties in porcine buccal membranes *ex vivo*.[7]

Side-effects, Toxicity

None documented.

Contra-indications, Warnings

Marshmallow may interfere with existing hypoglycaemic therapy and the absorption of other drugs taken simultaneously may be retarded.[G52]

Pregnancy and lactation There are no known problems with the use of marshmallow during pregnancy or lactation.

Pharmaceutical Comment

In vitro and animal studies provide some supporting evidence for the use of marshmallow in the treatment of cough, irritation of the throat and gastric inflammation. Antibacterial and anti-inflammatory activities, effects on mucociliary transport, adhesion of polysaccharide to buccal membranes and reduction of cough are reported. However, there is a lack of clinical studies investigating the effects of marshmallow. Although no toxicity data were located, the chemistry of marshmallow and its use in foods indicate that there should not be any reason for concern regarding safety.

References

See also General References G2, G3, G6, G9, G10, G16, G31, G36, G37, G43, G48, G52, G54, G60, G64,

1   Blaschek W, Franz G. A convenient method for the quantitative determination of mucilage polysaccharides in *Althaeae radix*. *Planta Med* 1986; 52(Suppl.): 537.

2   Gudej J. Flavonoids, phenolic acids and coumarins from the roots of *Althaea officinalis*. *Planta Med* 1991; 57: 284–285.

3   Recio MC *et al.* Antimicrobial activity of selected plants employed in the Spanish Mediterranean area Part II. *Phytother Res* 1989; 3: 77–80.

4   Tomodo M *et al.* Hypoglycaemic activity of twenty plant mucilages and three modified products. *Planta Med* 1987; 53: 8–12.

5   Mascolo N *et al.* Biological screening of Italian medicinal plants for anti-inflammatory activity. *Phytother Res* 1987; 1: 28–31.

6   Nosálova G *et al.* Antitussive wirkung des extraktes und der polysaccharide aus eibisch (Althaea officinalis L., var. robusta). *Pharmazie* 1992; 47: 224–226.

7   Schmidgall J *et al.* Evidence for bioadhesive effects of polysaccharides and polysaccharide-containing herbs in an *ex vivo* bioadhesion assay on buccal membranes. *Planta Med* 2000; 66: 48–53.

Maté

Species (Family)

Ilex paraguariensis St. Hil. (Aquifoliaceae)

Synonym(s)

Ilex, Jesuit's Brazil Tea, Paraguay Tea, St. Bartholomew's Tea, Yerba Maté

Part(s) Used

Leaf

Pharmacopoeial and Other Monographs

BHP 1996[G9]
Complete German Commission E[G3]
PDR for Herbal Medicines 2nd edition[G36]

Legal Category (Licensed Products)

GSL[G37]

Constituents[G2,G22,G45,G48,G64]

Alkaloids Xanthine-type. Caffeine 0.2–2.0%, theobromine 0.1–0.2%, theophylline 0.05%.

Flavonoids Kaempferol, quercetin, and their glycosides, including rutin.[1]

Tannins 4–16%.

Terpenoids Ursolic acid (major), β-amyrin, ilexoside A, ilexoside B methyl ester.[2]

Other constituents Choline and trigonellin (amines), amino acids,[1] riboflavine (vitamin B_2), pyridoxine (vitamin B_6), niacin, pantothenic acid, vitamin C and resins.

Other Ilex species Triterpenoid saponins termed ilexsaponins B_1, B_2, and B_3 have been isolated from *Ilex pubescens* Hook. & Arn.[3]

A cyanogenetic glucoside has been isolated from *Ilex aquifolium*.[4]

Food Use

Maté is listed by the Council of Europe as a natural source of food flavouring (category N2). This category indicates that maté can be added to foodstuffs in small quantities, with a possible limitation of an active principle (as yet unspecified) in the final product.[G16] Maté is commonly consumed as a beverage. It is stated to be less astringent than tea.[G45] In the USA, maté is listed as GRAS (Generally Recognised As Safe).[G65]

Herbal Use

Maté is stated to possess CNS-stimulant, thymoleptic, diuretic, antirheumatic and mild analgesic properties. Traditionally, it has been used for psychogenic headache and fatigue, nervous depression, rheumatic pains, and specifically for headache associated with fatigue.[G2,G7,G8,G64]

Dosage

Dried leaf 2–4 g or by infusion three times daily.[G6,G7]

Liquid extract 2–4 mL (1:1 in 25% alcohol) three times daily.[G6,G7]

Pharmacological Actions

In vitro and animal studies

In vivo hypotensive activity in rats has been reported for an aqueous extract of *Ilex pubescens* (commonly referred to as maodongqing or MDQ) It was concluded that intravenous administration of MDQ releases histamine.[5]

Clinical studies

The xanthine constituents, in particular caffeine, are the active principles in maté. The pharmacological actions of caffeine are well documented and include stimulation of the CNS, respiration and skeletal muscle, in addition to cardiac stimulation, coronary dilation, smooth muscle relaxation and diuresis.[G41] Reduction of appetite has been documented for maté.[1]

333

In China, MDQ is used parenterally for the treatment of cardiovascular diseases (hypotensive action).[1]

Side-effects, Toxicity

Side-effects generally associated with xanthine-containing beverages include sleeplessness, anxiety, tremor, palpitations and withdrawal headache.

Veno-occlusive disease of the liver in a young woman has been attributed to the consumption of large quantities of maté over a number of years.[G45] The association between consumption of maté infusions and oesophageal cancer has been investigated in Uruguay, where oesophageal cancer constitutes a major public health problem.[6,7] Heavy consumption was reported to elevate the relative risk of oesophageal cancer by 6.5 and 34.6 in men and women, respectively.

The fatal dose of caffeine in humans is stated to be 10 g.[G41]

Contra-indications, Warnings

Warnings generally associated with caffeine are applicable, such as restricted intake by individuals with hypertension or a cardiac disorder.

Pregnancy and lactation It is generally recommended that caffeine consumption should be restricted during pregnancy, although conflicting results have been documented concerning the association between birth defects and caffeine consumption. In view of this, excessive consumption of maté during pregnancy should be avoided. Caffeine is excreted in breast milk, but at concentrations too low to represent a hazard to breastfed infants.[G45] As with all xanthine-containing beverages, excessive consumption of maté by breastfeeding mothers should be avoided.

Pharmaceutical Comment

Maté is characterised by the xanthine constituents, which also represent the active principles. The herbal uses of maté can be attributed to the pharmacological actions of caffeine, which are well documented. Side-effects and warnings associated with other xanthine-containing beverages, such as tea and coffee, are applicable to maté.

References

See also General References G2, G3, G9, G10, G16, G22, G31, G36, G37, G41, G43, G48 and G64.

1　Ohem N, Holzl J. Some new investigations on *Ilex paraguariensis* – Flavonoids and triterpenes. *Planta Med* 1988; **54**: 576.

2　Inada A. Two new triterpenoid glycosides from the leaves of *Ilex chinensis*. *Chem Pharm Bull* 1987; **37**: 884–885.

3　Hidaka K *et al.* New triterpene saponins from *Ilex pubescens*. *Chem Pharm Bull* 1987; **35**: 524–529.

4　Willems M. Quantification and distribution of a novel cyanogenic glycoside in *Ilex aquifolium*. *Planta Med* 1989; **55**: 114.

5　Yang ML, Pang PKT. The vascular effects of *Ilex pubescens*. *Planta Med* 1986; **52**: 262–265.

6　Morton JF. The potential carcinogenicity of herbal tea. *Environ Carcino Rev. J Environ Sci Health* 1986; **C4**: 203–223.

7　Vassallo A *et al.* Esophageal cancer in Uruguay : a case control study. *J Natl Cancer Inst* 1985; **75**: 1005–1009.

Meadowsweet

Species (Family)

Filipendula ulmaria (L.) Maxim. (Rosaceae)

Synonym(s)

Dropwort, Filipendula, Queen of the Meadow, *Spiraea ulmaria* L.

Part(s) Used

Herb

Pharmacopoeial and Other Monographs

BHC 1992[G6]
BHP 1996[G9]
Complete German Commission E[G3]
Martindale 32nd edition[G43]
PDR for Herbal Medicines 2nd edition[G36]

Legal Category (Licensed Products)

GSL[G37]

Constituents[G2,G6,G22,G42,G62,G64]

Flavonoids Flavonols, flavones, flavanones and chalcone derivatives (e.g. hyperoside[1] and spireoside,[2] kaempferol glucoside[3] and avicularin.[4]

Salicylates Main components of the volatile oil including salicylaldehyde (major, up to 70%), gaultherin, isosalicin, methyl salicylate, monotropitin, salicin, salicylic acid and spirein.[5–8]

Tannins 1% (alcoholic extract), 12.5% (aqueous extract).[5] Hydrolysable type;[9] leaf extracts have also yielded catechols,[1] compounds normally associated with condensed tannins.

Volatile oils Many phenolic components including salicylates (*see above*), benzyl alcohol, benzaldehyde, ethyl benzoate, heliotropin, phenylacetate, vanillin.[4,5]

Other constituents Coumarin (trace),[1] mucilage, carbohydrates and ascorbic acid (vitamin C).

Food Use

Meadowsweet is listed by the Council of Europe as a natural source of food flavouring (category N2). This category indicates that meadowsweet can be added to foodstuffs in small quantities, with a possible limitation of an active principle (as yet unspecified) in the final product.[G16] In the USA, meadowsweet is listed by the Food and Drugs Administration (FDA) as a Herb of Undefined Safety.[G22]

Herbal Use

Meadowsweet is stated to possess stomachic, mild urinary antiseptic, antirheumatic, astringent and antacid properties. Traditionally, it has been used for atonic dyspepsia with heartburn and hyperacidity, acute catarrhal cystitis, rheumatic muscle and joint pains, diarrhoea in children, and specifically for the prophylaxis and treatment of peptic ulcer.[G2,G6,G7,G8,G64]

Dosage

Dried herb 4–6 g or by infusion three times daily.[G6,G7]

Liquid extract 1.5–6.0 mL (1:1 in 25% alcohol) three times daily.[G6,G7]

Tincture 2–4 mL (1:5 in 45% alcohol) three times daily.[G6,G7]

Pharmacological Actions

In vitro and animal studies

Lowering of motor activity and rectal temperature, myorelaxation and potentiation of narcotic action have been documented for meadowsweet.[5] In addition, flower extracts have been reported to prolong life expectancy of mice, lower vascular permeability and prevent the development of stomach ulcers in rats and mice.[5,10,11] However, meadowsweet has also been reported to potentiate the ulcerogenic properties of histamine in the guinea-pig.[10] The anti-ulcer action documented for meadowsweet is associated with the aqueous extract and greatest activity has been observed with the flowers.[9,11] Meadowsweet has been reported to increase bronchial tone in the cat[9] and to potentiate the bronchospastic properties of histamine in the guinea-pig.[9] *In vitro*, meadowsweet has been reported to increase intestinal tone in the guinea-pig and uterine tone in the rabbit.[9]

Bacteriostatic activity against *Staphylococcus aureus*, *Staphylococcus epidermidis*, *Escherichia coli*, *Proteus vulgaris* and *Pseudomonas aeruginosa* has been documented for flower extracts.[12]

Tannins are generally considered to possess astringent properties and have been reported as constituents of meadowsweet. Meadowsweet is stated to promote uric acid excretion.[G42]

Side-effects, Toxicity

None documented.

Contra-indications, Warnings Salicylate constituents have been documented and therefore the usual precautions recommended for salicylates are relevant for meadowsweet (*see* Willow). Meadowsweet is stated to be used for the treatment of diarrhoea in children but in view of the salicylate constituents, this is not advisable.

Bronchospastic activity has been documented and meadowsweet should therefore be used with caution by asthmatics.

Aqueous extracts have been reported to contain high tannin concentrations and excessive consumption should therefore be avoided.

Pregnancy and lactation *In vitro* utero-activity has been documented for meadowsweet. In view of the salicylate constituents and the lack of toxicity data, the use of meadowsweet during pregnancy and lactation should be avoided.

Pharmaceutical Comment

The chemistry of meadowsweet is characterised by a number of phenolic constituents including flavonoids, salicylates and tannins. Documented scientific evidence justifies some of the antiseptic, antirheumatic and astringent actions, although no human data were available. No documented toxicity data were located for meadowsweet and in view of this, excessive use should be avoided.

References

See also General References G2, G3, G5, G6, G9, G16, G22, G31, G36, G37, G42, G43, G50, G56, G62 and G64.

1 Genic AY, Ladnaya LY. Phytochemical study of *Filipendula ulmaria* Maxim. and *Filipendula hexapetala* Gilib. of flora of the Lvov region. *Farm Zh (Kiev)* 1980; **1**: 50–52.

2 Novikova NN. Use of *Filipendula ulmaria* in medicine. *Tr Perm Farm Inst* 1969; 267–270.

3 Scheer T, Wichtl M. Zum Vorkommen von Kämpferol-4′-O-β-D-glucopyranoside in *Filipendula ulmaria* und *Allium cepa*. *Planta Med* 1987 **53**: 573–574.

4 Syuzeva ZF, Novikova NN. Flavonoid composition of *Filipendula ulmaria* queen-of-the meadow. *Nauch Tr Perm Farm Inst* 1973; **5**: 2–26.

5 Barnaulov OD *et al*. Chemical composition and primary evaluation of the properties of preparations from *Filipendula ulmaria* (L.) Maxim flowers. *Rastit Resur* 1977; **13**: 661–669.

6 Saifullina NA, Kozhina IS. Composition of essential oils from flowers of *Filipendula ulmaria*, *F. denudata*, and *F. stepposa*. *Rastit Resur* 1975; **11**: 542–544.

7 Thieme H. Isolierung eines neuen phenolischen glykosids aus den blüten von *Filipendula ulmaria* (L.) Maxim. *Pharmazie* 1966; **21**: 123.

8 Valle MG *et al*. Das ätherische öl aus *Filipendula ulmaria*. *Planta Med* 1988; **54**: 181–182.

9 Barnaulov OD *et al*. Preliminary evaluation of the spasmolytic properties of some natural compounds and galenic preparations. *Rastit Resur* 1978; **14**: 573–579.

10 Barnaulov OD, Denisenko PP. Antiulcerogenic action of the decoction from flowers of *Filipendula ulmaria* (L.). *Pharmakol-Toxicol (Moscow)* 1980; **43**: 700–705.

11 Yanutsh AY *et al*. A study of the antiulcerative action of the extracts from the supernatant part and roots of *Filipendula ulmaria*. *Farm Zh (Kiev)* 1982; **37**: 53–56.

12 Catanicin-Hintz I *et al*. Action of some plant extracts on the bacteria involved in urinary infections. *Clujul-Med* 1983; **56**: 381–384.

Melissa

Species (Family)

Melissa officinalis L. (Labiatae)

Synonym(s)

Balm, Honeyplant, Lemon Balm, Sweet Balm

Part(s) Used

Dried leaves and flowering tops

Pharmacopoeial and Other Monographs

BHP 1996[G9]
BP 2001[G15]
Complete German Commission E (Lemon Balm)[G3]
ESCOP 1996[G52]
Martindale 32nd edition (Lemon Balm)[G43]
Mills and Bone (Lemon Balm)[G50]
PDR for Herbal Medicines 2nd edition[G36]
Ph Eur 2002[G28]

Legal Category (Licensed Products)

GSL[G37]

Constituents[G2,G52,G64]

Volatile oil 0.06–0.375% v/m (volume in mass).[1,G52] Contains at least 70 components,[G2] including: *Monoterpenes* >60%. Mainly aldehydes, including citronellal, geranial, neral; also citronellol, geraniol, nerol, β-ocimene.[2,3] *Sesquiterpenes* >35%. β-Caryophyllene, germacrene D.

Flavonoids 0.5%. Including glycosides of luteolin (e.g. luteolin 3′-O-β-D-glucuronide[4]), quercetin, apigenin and kaempferol.

Polyphenols Protocatechuic acid, hydroxycinnamic acid derivatives,[2] caffeic acid, chlorogenic acid, rosmarinic acid,[2] 2-(3′,4′-dihydroxyphenyl)-1,3-benzodioxole-5-aldehyde.[5]

Food Use

Lemon balm is used to give fragrance to wine, tea and beer. Lemon balm (herb, flowers, flower tips) is listed by the Council of Europe as a natural source of food flavouring (category N2). This category indicates that lemon balm can be added to foodstuffs in small quantities, with a possible limitation of an active principle (as yet unspecified) in the final product.[G16] In the USA, lemon balm is listed as GRAS (Generally Recognised As Safe).[G65]

Herbal Use

Lemon balm has been used traditionally for its sedative, spasmolytic and antibacterial properties.[G54] It is also stated to be a carminative, diaphoretic and a febrifuge,[G64] and has been used for headaches, gastrointestinal disorders, nervousness and rheumatism.[5] Current interest is focused on its use as a sedative, and topically in herpes simplex labialis as a result of infection with herpes simplex virus type 1 (HSV-1). The German Commission E monographs state that lemon balm can be used for nervous sleeping disorders and functional gastrointestinal complaints.[G4]

Dosage

Dried herb 1.5–4.5 g as an infusion in 150 mL water several times daily.[G4]

Topical application Cream containing 1% of a lyophilised aqueous extract of dried leaves of *Melissa officinalis* (70 : 1) two to four times daily.[G52]

Pharmacological Actions

In vitro and animal studies

Antiviral activity Aqueous extracts of *Melissa officinalis* have been reported to inhibit the development of several viruses.[6–8,G52] The virucidal effect of several aqueous extracts of *M. officinalis* against HSV-1 has been demonstrated in a rabbit kidney cell line.[9] However, the extracts appeared to have no activity against experimental HSV-1 infection in the eyes of rabbits.[9]

Anti-human immunodeficiency virus type 1 (HIV-1) activity has been reported for an aqueous extract of *M. officinalis* in *in vitro* studies using MT-4 cells; the ED_{50} (50% effective dose for inhibition of HIV-1-induced cytopathogenicity) was found to be 16 µg/mL.[10] Furthermore, the aqueous extract demonstrated potent inhibitory activity ($ED_{50} = 62\,\mu g/mL$) against HIV-1 replication (KK-1 strain, freshly isolated from a patient with acquired immune deficiency syndrome (AIDS). In other *in vitro* studies, an aqueous extract of *M. officinalis* inhibited giant cell formation in co-cultures of MOLT-4 cells with and without HIV-1 infection, and showed inhibitory activity against HIV-1 reverse transcriptase ($ED_{50} = 1.6\,\mu g/mL$).[10]

Aqueous extracts of *M. officinalis* have been reported to inhibit protein biosynthesis in a cell-free system from rat liver cells, and it has been suggested that this effect may be due to caffeic acid and a component isolated from the glycoside fraction of the extract.[11] The latter component appears to block the binding of the elongation factor EF-2 to ribosomes, thus terminating peptide elongation.[11]

Antimicrobial activity Antimicrobial activity of essential oil extracted from *M. officinalis* by steam distillation, determined using a micro-atmospheric technique, has been reported against the yeasts *Candida albicans* and *Saccharomyces cerevisiae*, and against *Pseudomonas putida*, *Staphylococcus aureus*, *Micrococcus luteus*, *Mycobacterium smegmatis*, *Proteus vulgaris*, *Shigella sonnei* and *Escherichia coli*.[12]

Other activity In studies in mice, a hydroalcoholic extract of *M. officinalis* leaves administered intraperitoneally significantly reduced behavioural activity in two tests, compared with control, suggesting that the extract has sedative effects.[13] In both tests, the effect was maximum at 25 mg/kg. The same extract demonstrated peripheral analgesic activity by reducing acetic acid-induced writhing and stretching in mice when administered intraperitoneally at doses of 25–1600 mg/kg 30 minutes after intraperitoneal administration of 1.2% acetic acid solution.[13] However, no analgesic effects were observed on heat-induced pain (hotplate test) which suggests a lack of central analgesic activity. In other tests, low doses (3 and 6 mg/kg) of a hydroalcoholic extract of *M. officinalis* leaves administered intraperitoneally induced sleep in mice given an infrahypnotic dose of pentobarbital.[13] By contrast, in the same battery of tests, essential oil obtained from *M. officinalis* by distillation did not demonstrate sedative or sleep-inducing effects.[13]

A 30% alcoholic extract of *M. officinalis* demonstrated an antispasmodic effect on rat duodenum *in vitro*.[14]

Aqueous methanolic extracts of the aerial parts of *M. officinalis* demonstrated inhibition of lipid peroxidation *in vitro* in both enzyme-dependent and enzyme-independent systems.[15] The same

tests carried out on the main known phenolic components of *M. officinalis* revealed that rosmarinic acid, caffeic acid, luteolin and luteolin-7-O-glucoside were more potent inhibitors of enzyme-dependent lipid peroxidation than enzyme-independent lipid peroxidation.

Clinical studies

Antiviral effects The effects of a topical preparation of a standardised aqueous extract of *M. officinalis* leaves (drug/extract 70:1) have been investigated in herpes simplex virus (HSV) infection. In an open, multicentre study, 115 patients with HSV infection of the skin or transitional mucosa applied lemon balm leaf extract five times daily for a maximum of 14 days; complete healing of lesions was achieved after eight days of treatment in 96% of participants.[16,17] Subsequently, a randomised, double-blind, placebo-controlled trial involving 116 patients with HSV infection of the skin or transitional mucosa reported statistically significant differences between the treatment (applied locally two to four times daily over 5–10 days) and placebo groups for some (including redness, physician's assessment, patient's assessment), but not all, outcome measures (e.g. extent of scabbing, vesication, pain).[17] Another randomised, double-blind trial involved 66 patients with an acute episode of recurrent (at least four episodes per year) herpes simplex labialis compared verum cream (applied on the affected area four times daily over five days) with placebo.[18] There was a significant difference in the primary outcome measure – symptom score after two days' treatment – between the two groups ($p = 0.042$). However, further investigation is required to determine if time to recurrence is prolonged.

Sedative effects The acute sedative effects of several plant extracts, including a preparation of *M. officinalis* leaves, were explored in a randomised, double-blind, placebo-controlled, crossover study involving 12 healthy volunteers.[19] *M. officinalis* extract 1200 mg was administered orally as a single dose about 2 hours before administration of caffeine 100 mg. Melissa extract was one of the extracts tested that showed least effects on increasing tiredness (i.e. it was no different than placebo) as measured using a visual analogue scale score for alertness.

Several other studies have investigated the sedative effects of combination preparations containing extracts of lemon balm and valerian (*Valeriana officinalis*). A randomised, double-blind trial involving healthy volunteers who received Songha Night (*V. officinalis* root extract 120 mg and *M. officinalis* leaf extract 80 mg) three tablets daily taken as one dose 30 minutes before bedtime for 30 days (n = 66), or placebo (n = 32), found that the proportion of participants reporting an improvement in sleep quality was significantly greater for the treatment group, compared with the placebo group (33.3% versus 9.4%, respectively; p = 0.04).[20] However, analysis of visual analogue scale scores revealed only a slight but statistically non-significant improvement in sleep quality in both groups over the treatment period. Another double-blind, placebo-controlled trial involving patients with insomnia who received Euvegal forte (valerian extract 160 mg and lemon balm extract 80 mg) two tablets daily for 2 weeks reported significant improvements in sleep quality in recipients of the herbal preparation, compared with placebo recipients.[21] A placebo-controlled study involving 'poor sleepers' who received Euvegal forte reported significant improvements in sleep efficiency and in sleep stages 3 and 4 in the treatment group, compared with placebo recipients.[22]

Other studies have investigated the sedative effects of combination preparations of extracts of lemon balm, valerian and hops (*Humulus lupulus*). In an open, uncontrolled, multicentre study, 225 individuals who were experiencing nervous agitation and/or difficulties falling asleep and achieving uninterrupted sleep were treated for two weeks with a combination preparation containing extracts of valerian root, hop grains and lemon balm leaves.[23] Significant improvements in the severity and frequency of symptoms were reported, compared with the pretreatment period. Difficulties falling asleep, difficulties sleeping through the night, and nervous agitation were improved in 89%, 80% and 82% of participants, respectively.

Side-effects, Toxicity

Small-scale, short-term (two weeks' duration) studies investigating the sedative effects of oral combination preparations containing lemon balm extract indicate that these preparations are well-tolerated and do not appear to induce a 'hangover effect'. In an open, uncontrolled, multicentre study, 225 individuals who were experiencing nervous agitation and/or difficulties falling asleep and achieving uninterrupted sleep were treated for two weeks with a combination preparation containing extracts of valerian root, hop grains and lemon balm leaves.[23] The tolerability of the preparation was rated as 'good' or 'very good' by 97% of physicians and 96% of patients. In a randomised, double-blind, placebo-controlled trial involving healthy volunteers who received Songha Night (*V. officinalis* root

120 mg and *M. officinalis* leaf extract 80 mg) three tablets daily for 30 days (n = 66), or placebo (n = 32), the proportion of volunteers reporting adverse events was similar in both groups (around 28%).[20] Sleep disturbances and tiredness were the most common adverse events reported during the study. (N.B. the study was designed to assess the effects of the preparation on sleep quality.) No severe adverse events were reported. A randomised, double-blind, placebo-controlled study involving 48 adults assessed the adverse effects of 2 weeks' treatment with a combination preparation (valerian root extract 95 mg, hops extract 15 mg and lemon balm leaf extract 85 mg) taken alone or with alcohol.[24] Compared with placebo, the herbal combination preparation did not have adverse effects on performance (e.g. concentration, vigilance). Furthermore, co-administration of the combination preparation with alcohol did not have potentiating effects on performance parameters.[24] No serious adverse events were observed during the study.

A randomised, double-blind, placebo-controlled trial of a topical preparation containing 1% dried extract of *M. officinalis* leaves (drug/extract 70 : 1) involving 116 patients with HSV infection of the skin or transitional mucosa reported that there were no statistically significant differences between the treatment and placebo groups with regard to the frequency of adverse effects.[17] Adverse events reported were minor (irritation, burning sensation); there were no reports of allergic contact reactions. However, skin sensitisation may occur with melissa.[G58]

Contra-indications, Warnings

None documented.

Pregnancy and lactation In view of the lack of toxicity data, oral administration of lemon balm during pregnancy and lactation should be avoided. Topical use of lemon balm during pregnancy and lactation is unlikely to be problematic.

Pharmaceutical Comment

Randomised clinical trials have suggested that topical lemon balm extract may have some effects on healing cutaneous lesions resulting from HSV-1 virus infection,[17,18] although further rigorous studies are required to determine whether there is any effect on recurrence of infection.

In the German Commission E monograph, lemon balm is indicated for nervous disturbance of sleep and functional gastrointestinal complaints.[G4] While there is some evidence from randomised controlled trials of combination preparations containing lemon balm leaf extract to support the efficacy of such products in individuals with minor sleep disorders, there has been little investigation of the effects of lemon balm extract alone on sleep quality. Further studies are required to determine the effects of preparations of lemon balm leaf extract in individuals with sleep disorders. Supporting evidence for the use of lemon balm for gastrointestinal complaints is limited to *in vitro* work and requires clinical investigation.

Small-scale, short-term studies indicate that oral combination preparations containing lemon balm extract and topical preparations of lemon balm extract are well tolerated.[17,20] However, there is a lack of research investigating the safety of long-term administration of lemon balm.

References

See also General References G2, G4, G9, G15, G16, G28, G36, G43, G50, G52, G54, G58 and G64.

1 Tittel G *et al*. Über die chemische Zusammensetzung von Melissenölen. *Planta Med* 1982; **46**: 91–98.

2 Carnat AP *et al*. The aromatic and polyphenolic composition of lemon balm (*Melissa officinalis* L. subsp. officinalis) tea. *Pharm Acta Helv* 1998; **72**: 301–305.

3 Sarer E, Kökdil G. Constituents of the essential oil from *Melissa officinalis*. *Planta Med* 1991; **57**: 89–90.

4 Heitz A *et al*. Luteolin 3′-glucuronide, the major flavonoid from *Melissa officinalis* subsp. *officinalis*. *Fitoterapia* 2000; **71**: 201–202.

5 Tagashira M, Ohtake Y. A new antioxidative 1,3-benzodioxole from *Melissa officinalis*. *Planta Med* 1998; **64**: 555–558.

6 Kucera LS, Herrmann ECJr. Antiviral substances in plants of the mint family (Labiatae). I Tannin of *Melissa officinalis*. *Proc Soc Exp Biol Med* 1967; **124**: 865–869.

7 Herrmann ECJr, Kucera LS. Antiviral substances in plants of the mint family (Labiatae). II Nontannin polyphenol of *Melissa officinalis*. *Proc Soc Exp Biol Med* 1967; **124**: 869–874.

8 May G, Willuhn G. Antivirale Wirkung wässriger Pflanzenextrakte in Gewebekulturen. *Arzneimittelforschung* 1978; **28**: 1–7.

9 Dimitrova Z *et al*. Antiherpes effect of *Melissa officinalis* L. extracts. *Acta Microbiol Bulg* 1993; **29**: 65–72.

10 Yamasaki K *et al*. Anti-HIV-1 activity of herbs in Labiatae. *Biol Pharm Bull* 1998; **21**: 829–833.

11 Chlabicz J, Galasinski W. The components of *Melissa officinalis* L. that influence protein biosynthesis in-vitro. *J Pharm Pharmacol* 1986; **38**: 791–794.

12 Larrondo JV *et al*. Antimicrobial activity of essences from labiates. *Microbios* 1995; **82**: 171–2.

13 Soulimani R *et al*. Neurotropic action of the hydroalcoholic extract of *Melissa officinalis* in the mouse. *Planta Med* 1991; **57**: 105–109.

14 Soulimani R *et al*. Recherche de l'activitébiologique de *Melissa officinalis* L. sur le système nerveux central de la souris in vivo et le duodenum de rat in vitro. *Plantes Méd Phytothér* 1993; **26**: 77–85.

15 Hohmann J *et al*. Protective effects of the aerial parts of *Salvia officinalis*, *Melissa officinalis* and *Lavandula angustifolia* and their constituents against enzyme-dependent and enzyme-independent lipid peroxidation. *Planta Med* 1999; **65**: 576–578.

16 Wölbling RH, Milbradt R. Klinik und Therapie des Herpes simplex. *Therapiewoche* 1984; **34**: 1193–1200.

17 Wölbling RH, Leonhardt K. Local therapy of herpes simplex with dried extract from *Melissa officinalis*. *Phytomedicine* 1994; **1**: 25–31.

18 Koytchev R *et al*. Balm mint extract (Lo-701) for topical treatment of recurring Herpes labialis. *Phytomedicine* 1999; **6**: 225–230.

19 Schulz H *et al*. The quantitative EEG as a screening instrument to identify sedative effects of single doses of plant extracts in comparison with diazepam. *Phytomedicine* 1998; **5**: 449–458.

20 Cerny A, Schmid K. Tolerability and efficacy of valerian/lemon balm in healthy volunteers (a double-blind, placebo-controlled, multicentre study). *Fitoterapia* 1999; **70**: 221–228.

21 Dressing H *et al*. Verbesserung der Schlafqualität mit einem hochdosierten Baldrian-Melisse-Präparat. Eine plazebokontrollierte Doppelblindstudie. *Psychopharmakotherapie* 1996; **3**: 123–130.

22 Dressing H *et al*. Baldrian-Melisse-Kombinationen versus Benzodiazepin. Bei Schlafstörungen gleichwertig? *Therapiewoche* 1992; **42**: 726–736.

23 Orth-Wagner S *et al*. Phytosedativum gegen Schlafstärungen. *Z Phytother* 1995; **16**: 147–156.

24 Herberg K-W. Nebenwirkungen pflanzlicher Beruhigungsmittel. *Z Allgemeinmed* 1996; **72**: 234–240.

Milk Thistle

Species (Family)

Silybum marianum (L.) Gaertn. (Asteraceae/Compositae)

Synonym(s)

Carduus marianus L., Lady's Thistle, Marian Thistle, Mediterranean Milk Thistle, St. Mary's Thistle.

Part(s) Used

Fruits (often referred to as 'seeds'), herb

Pharmacopoeial and Other Monographs

BHP 1996[G9]
Complete German Commission E[G3]
Martindale 32nd edition[G43]
Mills and Bone[G50]
PDR for Herbal Medicines 2nd edition[G36]

Legal Category (Licensed Products)

Milk thistle is not included in the GSL.[G37]

Constituents[G2,G43]

Fruit

Flavolignans 1.5–3% silymarin, a mixture containing approximately 50% silibinin (= silybin, silybinin), silichristin and silidianin, as well as silimonin, isosilichristin, isosilibinin, silandrin, silhermin, neosilihermins A and B, 2,3-dehydrosilibinin and tri- to pentamers of silibinin (silybinomers).[1]

Flavonoids Quercetin, taxifolin and dehydrokaempferol.[1]

Lipids 20–30%. Linoleic acid, oleic acid and palmitic acid.

Sterols Cholesterol, campesterol and stigmasterol.

Other constituents Mucilages, sugars (arabinose, rhamnose, xylose, glucose), amines and saponins.[1]

Leaves

Flavonoids Apigenin, luteolin and kaempferol and their glycosides.[1]

Other constituents β-Sitosterol and its glucoside, and a triterpene acetate.[1]
   Silymarin is not found in the leaves.

Food Use

Milk thistle is not used in foods.

Herbal Use[G2,G32,G34,G35,G50,G64]

Traditionally, milk thistle fruits have been used for disorders of the liver, spleen and gall bladder such as jaundice and gall bladder colic. Milk thistle has also been used for nursing mothers for stimulating milk production, as a bitter tonic, for haemorrhoids, for dyspeptic complaints and as a demulcent in catarrah and pleurisy. It is stated to possess hepatoprotective, antioxidant and choleretic properties.[1,2]
   Current interest is focused on the hepatoprotective activity of milk thistle and its use in the prophylaxis and treatment of liver damage and disease.
   The leaves have also been used for the treatment of liver, spleen and gall bladder disorders and as an antimalarial, emmenagogue and for uterine complaints. Milk thistle leaf preparations are available today, although most research has been conducted with preparations of the fruit since the leaf does not contain the pharmacologically active component silymarin.

Dosage

Fruit Crude drug 12–15 g daily in divided doses (equivalent to silymarin 200–400 mg daily).[G3]

Herb Approximately 1.5 g of finely chopped material as a tea, two or three cups daily.

The doses of silymarin used in clinical trials have ranged from 280 to 800 mg/day (equivalent to milk thistle extract 400–1140 mg/day standardised to contain 70% silibinin).[3] For hepatic disorders, doses of up to 140 mg (equivalent to 60 mg silibinin) two or three times daily have been suggested.[G43]

In Germany, the recommended regimen for treatment of *Amanita phalloides* poisoning with a standardised silymarin preparation (Legalon) is a total dose of silibinin (as the disodium dihemisuccinate) (20 mg/kg body weight) over 24 hours, divided into four intravenous infusions each given over a 2-hour period.[G43,G55]

Pharmacological Actions

Several pharmacological activities have been documented for milk thistle fruit, including hepatoprotective, antioxidant, anti-inflammatory, antifibrotic and antitumour properties, as well as inhibition of lipid peroxidation, stimulation of protein biosynthesis and acceleration of liver regeneration. Silymarin (an isomer mixture comprising mainly silibinin, silichristin and silidianin) is the pharmacologically active component of milk thistle fruit; silibinin is the main component of silymarin. There is an extensive literature on the pharmacological effects of silymarin and silibinin, particularly with regard to their hepatoprotective activity which provides supporting evidence for the clinical uses. The pharmacology and clinical efficacy of milk thistle have been reviewed.[1–3,G50,G55] The following represents a summary of selected publications on this subject.

There is a lack of research investigating the pharmacological effects of preparations of milk thistle leaf.[G2,G32,G35]

In vitro and animal studies

Antioxidant activity Silymarin and silibinin (silybin) are antioxidants that react with free radicals (e.g. reactive oxygen species) transforming them into more stable and less reactive compounds.[1,4–6] Silymarin and silybin have been reported to inihibit lipid peroxidation induced by iron-linked systems in rat liver microsomes[7,8] and protect against phenylhydrazine-induced lipid peroxidation in rat erythrocytes.[1] Furthermore, in rats, intraperitoneal silymarin has been shown to increase total glutathione in the liver, intestine and stomach and to improve the reduced glutathione to oxidised glutathione ratio.[9] Silymarin has been shown to inhibit

copper-induced oxidation of human low-density lipoprotein (LDL) *in vitro* in a concentration-dependent manner.[10] Silybin appears to be the constituent of silymarin responsible for the LDL antioxidant effect. In contrast, silichristin and silydianin appeared to act as pro-oxidants, but without significantly reducing the total LDL antioxidant capacity of silymarin.

Free radicals are recognised as having an important role in several pathological processes, including inflammation, necrosis, fibrosis, atherosclerosis, carcinogenesis and ageing and in the hepatotoxic mechanisms of various substances. The antioxidant activity of silymarin is thought to contibute to its hepatoprotective properties.[11,G55]

Hepatoprotective properties *In vitro* studies using isolated hepatocytes have documented the protective activity of silymarin and several of its components against cell damage induced by various cytotoxic substances.[1]

In vivo studies in rats and mice have demonstrated the hepatoprotective activity of silymarin and silybin in acute liver toxicity induced by various toxic agents with different mechanisms of action, including carbon tetrachloride, galactosamine, thioacetamide, ethanol, paracetamol (acetaminophen), thallium, phalloidin and α-amanitin (the main toxic constituents of the mushroom *A. phalloides*).[1] Experimental studies in chronic liver toxicity induced by repeated administration of carbon tetrachloride, heavy metals, thioacetamide and several drugs, including azathioprine and indomethacin, have also demonstrated that administration of silymarin and silybin protects against damage.[1] Other studies have reported protective effects of silymarin against liver injury induced by ischaemia[12] and gamma irradiation.[13]

Studies in rabbits fed a high-fat diet for 12 weeks have shown that histopathological alterations were least advanced in animals which also received a silymarin–phospholipid complex.[14] In rats, silymarin inhibited the development of diet-induced hypercholesterolaemia.[15] The hypocholesterolaemic effects of silymarin may be due to the effects of silymarin on lipoprotein metabolism.[16]

The effects of silymarin on biliary bile salt secretion have been seen in studies in rats.[17] Intraperitoneal silymarin (25, 50, 100 and 150 mg/kg/day) for five days induced a dose-dependent increase in bile flow and bile salt secretion. Stimulation of bile salt secretion was mainly accounted for by an increase in the biliary secretion of the hepatoprotective bile salts β-muricholate and ursodeoxycholate.

Nephroprotective properties Silibinin injected into rats prior to administration of cisplatin afforded protection of glomerular and proximal tubular function.[18,19] Silibinin does not affect the cytotoxic activity of cisplatin.[19] Intraperitoneal silibinin (5 mg/kg) administered to rats 30 minutes before cyclosporin decreased cyclosporin-induced lipid peroxidation but produced no protective effect on the glomerular filtration rate.[20]

Anticancer activity Silybin at concentrations of 0.1–20 μmol/L inhibited the growth of drug-resistant ovarian cancer cells and doxorubicin-resistant breast cancer cells *in vitro*.[21] Furthermore, silybin in the range of 0.1–1.0 μmol/L potentiated the effect of cisplatin and doxorubicin in experimental tumour cell lines. When applied to the skin of SENCAR mice, silymarin gave protection against the effects of the tumour promoters 12-O-tetradecanoylphorbol (TPA) and okaidic acid (OA).[22] Topical application of silymarin prior to that of TPA and OA completely inhibited induction of tumour necrosis factor α (TNFα) mRNA expression in the epidermis. Substantial protection from photocarcinogenesis in mice treated with phorbol ester or 7,12-dimethylbenz(*a*)anthracene has been demonstrated.[23] The antitumour effect is primarily at stage 1 tumour promotion and silymarin acts by inhibiting cyclooxygenase 2 (COX-2) and interleukin 1α (IL-1α).[24] Such effects may involve inhibition of promoter-induced oedema, hyperplasia, the proliferation index and oxidant state.[25]

Treatment of serum-starved human prostate carcinoma DU145 cells with silymarin resulted in significant inhibition of transforming growth factor α (TGFα)-mediated activation of the epidermal growth factor receptor erbB1.[26] There was also a decrease in tyrosine phosphorylation of an immediate downstream target, the adaptor protein SHC, together with a decrease in binding to erbB1. In the silymarin-treated cell lines there was a significant induction of the cyclin-dependent kinase inhibitors (CDKIs) Cip1/p21 and Kip/p27 concomitant with a significant decrease in CDK4 expression, but no changes in the levels of CDK2 and CDK6 and their associated cyclins E and D1, respectively. Additional experiments showed that there was a significant inhibition of constitutive tyrosine phosphorylation of both erbB1 and SHC, but no changes in their protein levels. The results indicated that silymarin may exert a strong anticarcinogenic effect against prostate cancer and that this effect is likely to involve impairment of the erbB1–SHC-mediated signalling pathway, induction of CDKIs and resultant G$_1$ arrest.[26]

There was a significant inhibition of mitogen-activated protein kinase (MAPK) ERK activity at lower doses in epidermal A431 cells treated with silymarin, whereas higher doses activated MAPK/JNK1.[27] Silymarin exerted a strong anticarcinogenic effect against human breast carcinoma cells MDA-MB468 with G$_1$ arrest in cell cycle progression and also induction in protein expression of the CDKI Cip/p21.[28]

The cancer chemoprevention and anticarcinogenic effects of silymarin have been shown to be due to its major constituent silibinin.[29] Silibinin decreases prostate-specific antigen (PSA) in hormone-refractory human prostate carcinoma LNCaP cells and inhibits cell growth via G$_1$ arrest.[30]

Silibinin was fed orally to SENCAR mice and its tissue distribution investigated.[31] Free silibinin mainly accumulated in the liver, although it was also distributed in other organs. Increases in glutathione-*S*-transferase and quinone reductase activities in the liver, lung, stomach, skin and small bowel were observed. The results demonstrated the bioavailability of and phase II enzyme induction of silibinin in different tissues where silymarin has been shown to be a strong cancer chemopreventive agent.

Anti-inflammatory activity Silymarin administered orally reduced foot-pad abscesses in a dose-dependent manner in the carrageenan rat paw oedema test (ED$_{50}$ = 62.4 mg/kg).[32] In the xylene-induced inflammation test, topically applied silymarin was comparable with indomethacin.[32] Silymarin given intraperitoneally to mice resulted in inhibition of leukocyte accumulation in inflammatory exudates and reduced the neutrophil count.[32] Activation of NF-κB induced by TNF, phorbol ester, okaidic acid and ceramide was blocked by silymarin in a dose-dependent manner.[33] Silymarin also inhibited TNF-induced activation of mitogen-activated protein kinase and *c*-Jun N-terminal kinase.[33] The inhibition of activation of NF-κB and the kinases may provide part of the molecular basis for the anti-inflammatory and anticarcinogenic effects of silymarin.[33] Silymarin potently suppressed both NF-κB–DNA binding activity and its dependent gene expression induced by okaidic acid in the hepatoma cell line Hep G2.[34] In addition, silymarin inhibits COX-2 and IL-1α.[24]

Gastric ulcer protective effects Oral administration of silymarin to rats prevented gastric ulceration induced by cold-restraint stress.[35] Gastric secretion volume and acidity were not affected, but histamine concentration was significantly decreased. It was suggested that the anti-ulcerogenic effect of silymarin may be related to inhibition of enzymic peroxidation by the lipoxygenase pathway.[35] The protective effect of silymarin on gastric injury induced in rats by ischaemia–reperfusion and its effects on mucosal myeloperoxidase has been compared with that of allopurinol.[36] The mean ulcer indexes (4.75, 4.50 and 3.63 ui, respectively) of rats treated with 25, 50 and 100 mg/kg silymarin were significantly lower than in control rats, although allopurinol was considerably more potent (2.3 ui; 100 mg/kg).[36]

Other effects   Silymarin has been shown to prevent alloxan-induced diabetes mellitus in rats, possibly due to its antioxidant activity and increases in plasma and pancreatic glutathione concentrations.[37]

It has been reported that *Silybum marianum* and silymarin beneficially affect skin elasticity. A phospholipid–silymarin complex (Silymarin–Phytosome) evaluated for its topical effects against croton oil dermatitis in mice and UV-induced erythema in humans showed reduction of oedema and inhibition of myeloperoxidase activity.[38] A standardised extract of *S. marianum* significantly inhibited porcine elastase *in vitro*.[39] An 80% ethanol extract of *S. marianum* aerial parts showed activity against *Bacillus subtilis*, *Staphylococcus aureus*, *Streptococcus haemolyticus*, *Escherichia coli*, *Klebsiella pneumoniae*, *Proteus mirabilis*, *Pseudomonas aeruginosa* and *Salmonella typhi*.[40]

Clinical studies

Clinical trials with milk thistle preparations have focused on their use in alcoholic liver disease, cirrhosis and acute viral and chronic hepatitis. However, several trials have included patients with liver disease of different aetiology, e.g. alcoholic and non-alcoholic cirrhosis. There is also interest in the use of silymarin in toxin- and drug-induced hepatitis, for example following ingestion of the death cap mushroom *A. phalloides*.

A randomised, double-blind, placebo-controlled, multicentre trial involving 200 alcoholic patients with histologically or laparoscopically proven liver cirrhosis investigated the effects of administration of silymarin (150 mg) three times daily.[41] The results indicated that silymarin had no effect on survival and the clinical course in these patients: 125 patients (silymarin $n = 57$ and placebo $n = 68$) completed the two-year study period, during which 29 died ($n = 15$ and 14 for silymarin and placebo, respectively; no statistically significant difference).

In a randomised, double-blind, placebo-controlled trial, patients with alcoholic ($n = 91$) or non-alcoholic ($n = 79$) cirrhosis received silymarin (140 mg) three

times daily or placebo for two years.[42] The four-year survival rate was significantly higher in silymarin-treated patients than in placebo recipients (58 versus 39%, respectively, $p = 0.036$). Subgroup analysis indicated that the effect of silymarin on mortality was more pronounced in those patients with alcoholic cirrhosis.

Another randomised, double-blind, placebo-controlled trial carried out over four years reported a significantly higher survival rate in patients with alcoholic cirrhosis treated with silymarin (420 mg) daily compared with placebo recipients, although the effect in patients with non-alcoholic cirrhosis was less marked.[43]

Other controlled trials have investigated the effects of silymarin in patients with alcohol-related liver damage. Several of these,[44,45] but not all,[46] reported statistically significant benefits with silymarin, e.g. on serum transaminases, compared with placebo.[1]

In a randomised controlled trial, 60 patients with diabetes caused by alcoholic liver cirrhosis received silymarin (600 mg/day) or no silymarin treatment for six months.[47] At the end of the study period, the mean values for fasting blood glucose, daily blood glucose, daily glycosuria, glycosylated haemoglobin, daily insulin requirement, malondialdehyde and glucagon-stimulated C peptide were significantly lower in silymarin-treated patients than in those who did not receive silymarin treatment.

A pilot study involving 20 patients with chronic active hepatitis randomised to receive a silybin–phosphatidylcholine complex preparation (IdB1016; Silipide) (240 mg) twice daily or placebo for seven days reported significant reductions in the mean serum concentrations of aspartate aminotransferase (AST), alanine aminotransferase (ALT), γ-glutamyl-transpeptidase (GGT) and total bilirubin in silybin complex-treated patients compared with values in placebo recipients.[48] The same preparation has been reported to reduce serum concentrations of liver enzymes (AST and ALT) in 65 patients with chronic persistent hepatitis in a randomised placebo-controlled trial.[49]

The hepatoprotective effects of silymarin in 222 *de novo* tacrine-treated patients with mild to moderate dementia of the Alzheimer type were investigated in a randomised, double-blind (for silymarin), placebo-controlled, multicentre, 12-week trial.[50] Patients received tacrine plus silymarin (420 mg/day) ($n = 110$) or tacrine plus placebo ($n = 112$); silymarin (and placebo) were initiated one week before tacrine (40 mg/day for six weeks then 80 mg/day for six weeks). An intention-to-treat analysis indicated that there was no difference in serum ALT concentrations between the two groups, but that silymarin-treated patients experienced significantly fewer gastrointestinal and cholinergic side-effects without any impact on cognitive status than did placebo recipients.[50]

The effects of silymarin in preventing psychotropic drug-induced hepatic damage have been investigated in a randomised, double-blind, placebo-controlled trial.[51] Sixty women aged 40–60 years who had been taking phenothiazines or butyrophenones for at least five years and who had AST and ALT activity twice normal values were randomised to continued treatment with psychotropic agents or suspension of treatment and to silymarin (800 mg/day) or placebo for 90 days. The findings indicated that treatment with silymarin reduced the lipoperoxidative hepatic damage associated with prolonged administration of butyrophenones and phenothiazines and that the protective effect was greater when treatment with these psychotropic agents was suspended for three months.[51]

There have been numerous case reports, many of which report favourable outcomes, on the therapeutic use of silymarin and silibinin, usually given in combination with standard treatment, in poisoning caused by ingestion of the death cap mushroom *A. phalloides*, although there are no controlled trials in this indication.[1,51–54,G55] Silibinin is usually given intravenously and case reports have indicated that early administration appears to be important.[55,56]

Pharmacokinetics Studies of the pharmacokinetics of silymarin and its components and of a silibinin–phosphatidylcholine complex preparation (IdB 1016; Silipide) in both healthy volunteers and patients with cirrhosis and those who have undergone cholecystectomy have been reviewed.[1,G50,G55] Approximately 20–50% of silymarin is absorbed following oral administration and approximately 80% of the dose, whether administered orally or intravenously, is excreted in the bile.[57] Studies in healthy volunteers have reported an elimination half-life of approximately 6 hours following administration of single doses of silymarin corresponding to approximately 240 mg silibinin.[58,59] Other studies have compared the pharmacokinetics of different silymarin preparations and shown statistically significant differences in bioavailability.[60,61]

The bioavailability of a silybin–phosphatidylcholine complex preparation (IdB 1016) has been shown to be several times greater than that of silymarin in single-dose studies involving healthy volunteers[62] and patients with hepatic cirrhosis.[63]

Side-effects, Toxicity

No adverse events were noted in a pharmacokinetic study involving healthy male volunteers following single oral doses of silymarin corresponding to up to 254 mg silibinin.[59]

Clinical trials involving patients with liver disorders of various origin and who received oral silymarin at doses of up to 600–800 mg/day for up to six months have reported that no adverse effects were observed.[42,47,51]

Data from drug monitoring studies involving more than 3500 patients, including one study involving 2637 patients with various types of chronic liver disease treated with silymarin (Legalon) (560 mg/day) for eight weeks, have indicated that the frequency of adverse effects with silymarin is approximately 1%. Adverse effects are mainly transient, non-serious, gastrointestinal complaints.[4,64,G55] It is stated that silymarin may occasionally produce a mild laxative effect.[G3]

A case report from Australia described a reaction associated with a preparation of milk thistle. The symptoms included episodes of severe sweating, abdominal cramping, nausea, vomiting, diarrhoea and weakness and these were verified by rechallenge.[65] Another report described a case of anaphylactic shock in a 54-year-old man with immediate-type allergy to kiwi fruit.[66] He experienced facial oedema, swelling of the oral mucosa, bronchospasm, respiratory distress and decreased blood pressure after taking a preparation of milk thistle; a skin-prick test of an extract of milk thistle fruit elicited an immediate-type reaction.

The acute toxicity of oral and intravenous silymarin and silibinin has been investigated in various animal species (mice, rats, rabbits and dogs).[1] Oral silymarin administered to mice and dogs at doses of 20 and 1 g/kg, respectively, did not cause adverse effects or mortality. Long-term oral administration of silymarin (100 mg/kg/day) to rats for 16 or 22 weeks did not reveal any adverse effects.

Contra-indications, Warnings

None documented. In view of the lack of long-term safety data, excessive use of milk thistle should be avoided (except where its use may help to prevent toxicity caused by other substances).

Milk thistle is contra-indicated for individuals with hypersensitivity to species of Asteraceae.

Pregnancy and lactation In view of the lack of toxicity data, use of milk thistle preparations during pregnancy and lactation should be avoided unless the expected benefit is thought to outweigh any unknown risks to the fetus.

Pharmaceutical Comment

The chemistry of milk thistle is well-documented and there is good evidence that silymarin and its components, particularly silibinin, are responsible for the pharmacological effects.

Documented scientific evidence from in vitro and animal studies provides supportive evidence for some of the uses of milk thistle, particularly those relating to hepatoprotective properties.

There have been several controlled clinical trials investigating the effects of milk thistle in a range of liver disorders, including acute viral hepatitis, chronic hepatitis, alcoholic liver disease, cirrhosis and toxic liver damage. The results of these studies are not entirely consistent or conclusive. In addition, some trials have methodological shortcomings, for example the inclusion of patients with different liver disorders, small numbers of patients and failure to control or monitor alcohol intake.[67] Further, well-designed, clinical trials in clearly defined patient groups are required in order to establish the efficacy of milk thistle and its components in different liver disorders. In Germany, milk thistle is approved for the treatment of toxic liver disorders and as a supportive treatment in chronic inflammatory liver disease and hepatic cirrhosis.[G3]

Teas prepared from milk thistle fruits or herb are not commonly used as only a small proportion of silymarin gets into the aqueous extract such that pharmacologically active doses are not attained.[68] For this reason, in Germany teas are recommended only as supportive treatment in functional gall bladder disorders and not for antihepatotoxic effects.[G2] In Germany, milk thistle fruit (3–5 g) as an infusion three or four times daily is also indicated for mild digestive disorders.[G2]

There are some toxicity and safety data for milk thistle which, together with data on the adverse effects reported in clinical trials, provide good evidence for the safety of milk thistle when used at recommended doses in the short term. However, further data on the long-term safety of milk thistle use are required.

Patients wishing to use milk thistle should be advised to consult a pharmacist, doctor or other suitably trained healthcare professional for advice.

References

See General References G2, G3, G9, G34, G36, G43, G50 and G64.

1 Morazzoni P, Bombardelli E. Silybum marianum (Carduus marianus). Fitoterapia 1995; 66: 3–42.
2 Awang D. Milk thistle. Can Pharm J 1993; 403–404, 422.
3 Pepping J. Milk thistle: Silybum marianum. Am J Health-Syst Pharm 1999; 56: 1195–1197.
4 Leng-Peschlow E. Properties and medical use of flavolignans (silymarin) from Silybum marianum. Phytother Res 1996; 10: S25–26.
5 Pascual C et al. Effect of silymarin and silybinin on oxygen radicals. Drug Dev Res 1993; 29: 73–77.
6 Mira L et al. Scavenging of reactive oxygen species by silibinin dihemisuccinate. Biochem Pharmacol 1994; 48: 753–759.
7 Bindoli A et al. Biochem Pharmacol 1977; 26: 2045.
8 Valenzuela A et al. Antioxidant properties of the flavonoids silybin and (+)-cyanidanol-3: comparison with butylated hydroxyanisole and butylated hydroxytoluene. Planta Med 1986; 19: 438–440.
9 Valenzuela A et al. Selectivity of silymarin on the increase of the glutathione content in different tissues of the rat. Planta Med 1989; 55: 420–422.
10 Skottova N et al. Activities of silymarin and its flavolignans upon low density lipoprotein oxidizability in vitro. Phytother Res 1999; 13: 535–537.
11 Valenzuela A, Garrido A. Biochemical basis of the pharmacological action of the flavonoid silymarin and its structural isomer silibinin. Biol Res 1994; 27: 105–112.
12 Wu CG et al. Protective effect of silymarin on rat liver injury induced by ischaemia. Virchows Arch B Cell Pathol Mol Pathol 1993; 64: 259–263.
13 Kropacova K et al. Protective and therapeutic effect of silymarin on the development of latent liver damage. Radiat Biol Radioecol 1998; 38: 411–415.
14 Drozdzik M et al. Effect of silymarinphospholipid complex on the liver in rabbits maintained on a high-fat diet. Phytother Res 1996; 10: 406–409.
15 Krecman V et al. Silymarin inhibits the development of diet-induced hypercholesterolemia in rats. Planta Med 1998; 64: 138–142.
16 Skottova N, Krecman V. Silymarin a potential hypocholesterolaemic drug. Physiol Res 1998; 47: 1–7.
17 Crocenzi FA et al. Effect of silymarin on biliary bile salt secretion in the rat. Biochem Pharmacol 2000; 59: 1015–1022.
18 Gaedeke J et al. Cisplatin nephrotoxicity and protection by silibinin. Nephrol Dial Transplant 1996; 11: 55–62.
19 Bokemeyer C et al. Silibinin protects against cisplatin-induced nephrotoxicity without compromising cisplatin or ifosfamide anti-tumour activity. Br J Cancer 1996; 74: 2036–2041.
20 Zima T et al. The effect of silibinin on experi-

mental cyclosporine nephrotoxicity. *Renal Failure* 1998; 20: 471–479.

21 Scambia G *et al*. Antiproliferative effects of silybin on gynaecological malignancies: synergism with cisplatin and doxorubicin. *Eur J Cancer* 1996; 32A: 877–882.

22 Zi X *et al*. Novel cancer chemopreventative effects of a flavonoid constituent silymarin: inhibition of mRNA expression of an endogenous tumour promoter TNFalpha. *Biochem Biophys Res Commun* 1997; 239: 334–339.

23 Katiyar SK *et al*. Protective effects of silymarin against photocarcinogenesis in a mouse skin model. *J Natl Cancer Inst* 1997; 89: 556–566.

24 Zhao J *et al*. Significant inhibition by the flavonoid antioxidant silymarin against 12-O-tetradecanoyl-phorbol 13-acetate caused modulation of antioxidant and inflammatory enzymes and cyclooxygenase 2 and interleukin-1 alpha expression in SENCAR mouse epidermis: implications in the prevention of stage I tumour promotion. *Mol Carcinogen* 1999; 26: 321–333.

25 Lahiri-Chatterjee M *et al*. A flavonoid antioxidant, silymarin, affords exceptionally high protection against tumour promotion in the SENCAR mouse skin tumorigenic model. *Cancer Res* 1999; 59: 622–632.

26 Zi X *et al*. A flavonoid antioxidant, silymarin, inhibits activation of erbB1 signaling and induces cyclin-dependent kinase inhibitors, G_1 arrest and anticarcinogenic effects in human prostate carcinoma DU145 cells. *Cancer Res* 1998; 58: 1920–1929.

27 Zi X, Agarwal R. Modulation of mitogen-activated protein kinase activation and cell cycle regulators by the potent skin cancer preventative agent silymarin. *Biochem Biophys Res Commun* 1999; 263: 528–536.

28 Zi X *et al*. Anticarcinogenic effect of a flavonoid antioxidant, silymarin, in human breast cancer cells MDA-MB468: induction of G_1 arrest through an increase in Cip1/p21 concomitant with a decrease in kinase activity of cyclin-dependent kinases and associated cyclins. *Clin Cancer Res* 1998; 4: 1055–1064.

29 Bhatia N *et al*. Inhibition of human carcinoma cell growth and DNA synthesis by silibinin, an active constituent of milk thistle: comparison with silymarin. *Cancer Lett* 1999; 147: 77–84.

30 Zi X *et al*. Silibinin decreases prostate-specific antigen with cell growth inhibition via G_1 arrest, leading to differentiation of prostate carcinoma cells: implications for prostate cancer intervention. *Proc Natl Acad Sci USA* 1999; 96: 7490–7495.

31 Zhao J, Agarwal R. Tissue distribution of silibinin, the major active constituent of silymarin, in mice and its association with enhancement of phase II

enzymes: implications in cancer chemoprevention. *Carcinogenesis* 1999; 20: 2101–2108.

32 De La Puerta R *et al*. Effect of silymarin on different acute inflammation models and in leukocyte migration. *J Pharm Pharmacol* 1996; 48: 968–970.

33 Manna SK *et al*. Silymarin suppresses TNF-induced activation of NF-kappaB, c-Jun N-terminal kinase and apoptosis. *J Immunol* 1999; 163: 6800–6809.

34 Saliou C *et al*. Selective inhibition of NF-kappaB activation by the flavonoid hepatoprotector silymarin in HepG2. *FEBS Lett* 1998; 440: 8–12.

35 De La Lastra C *et al*. Gastric antiulcer activity of silymarin, a lipoxygenase inhibitor, on rats. *J Pharm Pharmacol* 1992; 44: 929–931.

36 De La Lastra C *et al*. Gastroprotection induced by silymarin, the hepatoprotective principle of *Silybum marianum* in ischaemia–reperfusion mucosal injury: role of neutrophils. *Planta Med* 1995; 61: 116–119.

37 Soto CP *et al*. Prevention of alloxan-induced diabetes mellitus in the rat by silymarin. *Comp Biochem Physiol* 1998; 119C: 125–129.

38 Bombardelli E *et al*. Ageing skin: protective effect of silymarin–Phytosome®. *Fitoterapia* 1991; 62: 115–122.

39 Benaiges A *et al*. Study of the refirming effect of a plant complex. *Int J Cosmet Sci* 1998; 20: 223–233.

40 Izzo AA *et al*. Biological screening of Italian medicinal plants for antibacterial activity. *Phytother Res* 1995; 9: 281–286.

41 Pares A *et al*. Effects of silymarin in alcoholic patients with cirrhosis of the liver: results of a controlled, double-blind, randomized and multicenter trial. *J Hepatol* 1998; 28: 615–621.

42 Ferenci P *et al*. Randomized controlled trial of silymarin treatment in patients with cirrhosis of the liver. *J Hepatol* 1989; 9: 105–113.

43 Benda L *et al*. The influence of therapy with silymarin on the survival rate of patients with liver cirrhosis. *Wien Klin Wschr* 1980; 92: 678–683.

44 Salmi H, Sarna S. Effect of silymarin on the chemical, functional and morphological alterations of the liver. *Scand J Gastroenterol* 1982; 17: 517–521.

45 Feher J *et al*. Hepatoprotective activity of silymarin Legalon® therapy in patients with chronic alcoholic liver disease. *Orv Hetil* 1989; 130: 2723–2727.

46 Trinchet JC *et al*. Traitement de l'hépatite alcoolique par la silymarine. Une étude comparative en double insu chez 116 malades. *Gastroenterol Clin Biol* 1989; 13: 120–124.

47 Velussi M *et al*. Silymarin reduces hyperinsulinaemia, malondialdehyde levels, and daily insulin

need in cirrhotic diabetic patients. *Curr Ther Res* 1993; **53**: 533–545.

48 Buzzelli G *et al*. A pilot study on the liver protective effect of silybin–phosphatidylcholine complex (IdB1016) in chronic active hepatitis. *Int J Clin Pharmacol Ther Toxicol* 1993; **31**: 456–460.

49 Marcelli R *et al*. Cited by Morazzoni P *et al*. *Silybum marianum* (*Carduus marianus*). *Fitoterapia* 1995; **66**: 3–42. *Eur Bull Drug Res* 1992; **1**: 131–135.

50 Allain H *et al*. Aminotransferase levels and silymarin in *de novo* tacrine-treated patients with Alzheimer's disease. *Dementia Geriat Cogn Disord* 1999; **10**: 181–185.

51 Palasciano G *et al*. The effect of silymarin on plasma levels of malon-dialdehyde in patients receiving long-term treatment with psychotropic drugs. *Curr Ther Res* 1994; **55**: 537–545.

52 Klein AS *et al*. Amanita poisoning: treatment and the role of liver transplantation. *Am J Med* 1989; **86**: 187–193.

53 Floersheim GL *et al*. Die Klinische Knollenblatterpilzverg; Ftung: prognostische faktoren und therapeutische massnahmen. *Schweiz Med Wochenschr* 1982; **112**: 1164–1177.

54 Carducci R *et al*. Silibinin and acute poisoning with *Amanita phalloides*. *Minerva Anestesiol* 1996; **62**: 187–193.

55 Hruby K *et al*. Pharmacotherapy of *Amanita phalloides* poisoning using silybin. *Wien Klin Wochenschr* 1983; **95**: 225–231.

56 Hruby K *et al*. Chemotherapy of *Amanita phalloides* poisoning with intravenous silibinin. *Hum Toxicol* 1983; **2**: 183–190.

57 Mennicke WH. Zur biologischen Verfügbarkeit und Verstoffwechselung von Silybin. *Dtsch Apoth Ztg* 1975; **115**: 1205–1206.

58 Lorenz D *et al*. Pharmacokinetic studies with silymarin in human serum and bile. *Meth Find Exp Clin Pharmacol* 1984; **6**: 655–661.

59 Weyhenmeyer R *et al*. Study on the dose-linearity of the pharmacokinetics of silibinin diastereomers using a new stereospecific assay. *Int J Clin Pharmacol Ther Toxicol* 1992; **30**: 134–138.

60 Cho J-Y *et al*. Pharmacokinetic evaluation of two formulations containing silymarin: Legalon 140™ cap and Silymarin™. *J Korean Soc Clin Pharmacol Ther* 1998; **6**: 119–127.

61 Schulz H-U *et al*. Untersuchungen zum Freisetzungsverhalten und zur Bioäquivalenz von Silymarin–Präparaten. *Arzneimittelforschung* 1995; **45**: 61–64.

62 Barzaghi N *et al*. Pharmacokinetic studies on IdB 1016, a silybin–phosphatidylcholine complex, in healthy human volunteers. *Eur J Drug Metab Pharmacokinet* 1990; **15**: 333–338.

63 Orlando R *et al*. Silybin kinetics in patients with liver cirrhosis: a comparative study of silybin–phosphatidylcholine complex and silymarin. *Med Sci Res* 1990; **18**: 861–863.

64 Albrecht M, Fredrick H. Therapy of toxic liver pathologies with Legalon. *Z Klin Med* 1992; **47**: 87–92.

65 Anon. An adverse reaction of the herbal medication milk thistle (*Silybum marianum*). Adverse Drug Reactions Advisory Committee. *Med J Aust* 1999; **170**: 218–219.

66 Geier J *et al*. Anaphylactic shock due to an extract of *Silybum marianum* in a patient with immediate-type allergy to kiwi fruit. *Allergologie* 1990; **13**: 387–388.

67 Flora K *et al*. Milk thistle (*Silybum marianum*) for the therapy of liver disease. *Am J Gastroenterol* 1998; **93**: 139–143.

68 Merfort E, Willuhn G. Cited by ref. G2. *Dtsch Apoth Ztg* 1985; **125**: 695.

Mistletoe

Species (Family)

Viscum album L. (Loranthaceae)

Synonym(s)

Viscum

Part(s) Used

Leaf, fruit (berry), twig

Pharmacopoeial and Other Monographs

BHP 1996[G9]
Complete German Commission E[G3]
Martindale 32nd edition[G43]
PDR for Herbal Medicines 2nd edition[G36]

Legal Category (Licensed Products)

Mistletoe is not included in the GSL.[G37]

Constituents[G2,G22,G64]

Acids Fatty acids (C_{12}–C_{22}), 80% oleic and palmitic;[1] phenolic acids (e.g. anisic, caffeic, *p*-coumaric, ferulic, gentisic, myristic, *p*-hydroxybenzoic, *p*-hydroxyphenylacetic, protocatechuic, shikimic, sinapic, quinic, vanillic).[1,2]

Alkaloids[3] It has been suggested that alkaloids can be passed on from hosts to parasitic plants like mistletoe (e.g. nicotine alkaloids have been isolated from mistletoe growing on Solanaceae shrubs).[4]

Amines Acetylcholine, choline, β-phenylethylamine, histamine, propionylcholine and tyramine.[5]

Flavonoids Flavonol (e.g. quercetin) derivatives,[3] chalcone derivatives[6] and flavonone derivatives.[6]

Lectins Mixture of high molecular weight polypeptides. Quoted molecular weights include 160 000,[7] 115 000 (four chains)[7,8] and 60 000 (two chains).[9] Three lectins have been isolated which possess either two chains (LII, LIII) or four chains (LI).[10]

Terpenoids β-Amyrin, betulinic acid, lupeol and ester combinations, oleanolic acid, resin acids, ursolic acid, β-sitosterol, dihydro-β-sitosterol, stigmasterol, sterol A and phytosterol glucoside.[6,11]

Viscotoxins Mixture of low molecular weight polypeptides including the pure proteins viscotoxins A_2, A_3 and B.[12–14]

Other constituents Mucilage, polyols (e.g. mannitol, dulcitol, xylitol, inositol, pinitol, quebrachitol, quercitol),[15] sugars (e.g. fructose, glucose, raffinose, sucrose),[13] starch, syringin (a phenolic glucoside)[6] and tannin.

Food Use

Mistletoe is not generally used as a food. The branches and berries of mistletoe are listed by the Council of Europe as natural sources of food flavouring (category N3).[G16] This category indicates that mistletoe may be added to foodstuffs in the traditionally accepted manner, although there is insufficient information available for an adequate assessment of potential toxicity.

Herbal Use

Mistletoe is stated to possess hypotensive, cardiac-depressant and sedative properties. Traditionally, it has been used for high blood pressure, arteriosclerosis, nervous tachycardia, hypertensive headache, chorea and hysteria.[G2,G7,G64]

Dosage

Dried leaves 2–6 g or by infusion three times daily.[G7]

Liquid extract 1–3 mL (1 : 1 in 25% alcohol) three times daily.[G7]

Tincture 0.5 mL (1 : 5 in 45% alcohol) three times daily.[G7]

Infusion 40–120 mL (1 : 20 in cold water) daily.[G7]

Soft extract 0.3–0.6 mL (1 : 8 infusion or tincture) three times daily.[G7]

Pharmacological Actions

Documented pharmacological studies for mistletoe have concentrated on the cytotoxic and immunostimulant properties of the plant. The pharmacological actions of mistletoe have been reviewed extensively.[4,5,12,16,17]

In vitro and animal studies

Much has been documented concerning the possible role of mistletoe in the treatment of cancer, in particular, a proprietary product Iscador, which is produced from naturally fermented mistletoe plant juice. The immunostimulant and cytotoxic effects exhibited by mistletoe are thought to play an important role in the cancerostatic action.[18]

Cytotoxic activity Cytotoxic activity has been exhibited both *in vitro* and *in vivo* by the crude plant juice, Iscador, glycoprotein fractions (lectins, viscotoxins) and alkaloid fractions.[3,18,19] Significant antitumour activity has been observed *in vivo* for mistletoe extracts against murine tumours, Lewis lung carcinoma, colon adenocarcinoma 38, and C3H mammary adenocarcinoma 16/C.[4] Researchers in Korea have isolated cytotoxic alkaloids from twigs and leaves of Korean mistletoe (*V. album*) with activity reported against L1210 (*in vitro*) and P388 (*in vivo*) test systems.[3] The authors commented that preliminary studies indicated the presence of some of these cytotoxic alkaloids in the European mistletoe (*V. album*). The anticancer activities of various mistletoe extracts and the contribution of the alkaloidal components towards this activity has been reviewed.[4] Alkaloidal components in mistletoe are thought to form glycoconjugates with lectins and viscotoxins, and help maintain the specific structures of these molecules necessary for therapeutic activity.[4]

The mode of action for cytotoxic activity of mistletoe has been linked to the ability of the basic amino acids present in mistletoe to maintain cell differentiation.[18] Sensitivity to mistletoe extracts has been documented for acute lymphoblastic leukaemia cells resistant to methotrexate and cytarabine.[20]

The optimum dose of Iscador for tumour inhibition in mice weighing approximately 30 g, has been estimated at 0.11 mg and 0.153 mg.[18] The degree of inhibition compared to controls was stated as 20–50%.[18]

Immunostimulant activity *In vivo* immunostimulant activity in mice (humoral and cellular), demonstrated by an enhancement of delayed hypersensitivity and antibody formation to sheep red blood cells, has been documented for the crude plant juice, Iscador and for a polysaccharide fraction isolated from the berries.[21] Activity was attributed to stimulation of the monophagocytic system and to induction of inflammation. The results indicated that the immunostimulant property of mistletoe is not solely attributable to the polysaccharides found in the berries (plant juice also active) or to the lactobacilli content of the fermented plant juice (crude extract also active). Non-specific immunological effects with mistletoe extracts are reported to be dependent on the frequency and quantity of the applied extract.[22]

Agglutinating activity Agglutinating activity that is preferential towards tumour cells over erythrocytes has been exhibited by Iscador and by a lectin fraction.[23–25] The lectins have been shown to bind to a number of cells including erythrocytes (non-specific to blood type),[7,10] lymphocytes, leukocytes, macrophages, glycoproteins and plasma proteins.[9,10] Binding has been found to be stereospecific towards units containing a D-galactose molecule,[8,9,25] although D-galactose units with unmodified hydroxyl groups at C_2, C_3 and C_4 inhibit erythrocyte agglutination.[26] Tyrosine residues are also thought to be involved in the agglutination process.[8] Plasma proteins compete for the lectin receptor site and, therefore, decrease the agglutination of erythrocytes and tumour cells.[27] Unlike many other sugars, lactose units have also been found to inhibit erythrocyte agglutination.[26]

Mistletoe lectins have been reported to prevent viscotoxin- and allergen-stimulated histamine release from human leukocytes.[28]

Hypotensive effect The hypotensive effect documented for mistletoe has been attributed to various biologically active constituents such as acetylcholine, histamine, gamma aminobutyric acid (GABA), tyramine and flavones.[G24] The exact nature of the hypotensive effect of mistletoe seems unclear: it has been reported that activity is mainly due to an inhibitory action on the excitability of the vasomotor centre in the medulla oblongata.[29] However, it has also been stated that the hypotensive action of mistletoe is mainly of a reflex character, exerting a normalising effect on both hypertensive and hypotensive states.[29] The effect of different mistletoe plant parts and host plant on the hypotensive activity has been studied with highest activity reported for mistletoe leaves parasitising on willow.[29]

Clinical studies

Iscador has been administered to patients with cancer of the breast, cervix, colon, rectum and stomach.[18] Treated groups were reported to show a slight improvement over controls, the best results being obtained with cancer of the colon. It has been suggested that the relatively weak antitumour effects of Iscador may provide a useful adjunct to conventional surgery and radiotherapy.[18] Intrapleural instillation of Iscador has been used to dry out malignant pleural exudations[30,31] and it has been reported to increase lifespan in a fatal case of small-cell lung cancer.[32]

Cytolytic activity   Cells responsible for natural killer (NK) cytolytic activity have been shown to be large granular lymphocytes (LGLs).[33] The cytolytic activity of NK cells is regulated by a number of factors including polymorphonuclear leukocytes (PMNs). A significant increase in NK cell cytotoxicity and antibody dependent cell-mediated cytotoxicity, with augmented concentrations of LGLs, has been noted in peripheral blood samples taken from breast cancer patients given a single infusion of Iscador.[34] A decrease in NK and LGL values has been shown to be paralleled by an increase in PMN concentrations in peripheral blood after Iscador infusion.[33] Interferons, interleukin 2 and some other lymphokines have previously been described as modifiers of the spontaneous cytotoxicity of NK cells and of monocytes.[35] The effect of Iscador on immunological parameters is stated to follow a kinetic pattern similar to that seen after treatment with interferon α.[34] Stimulation of cell-mediated immunity has been observed in female patients with arthrosis administered weekly injections (i.c.) of mistletoe extract.[22] A depressive action was observed in patients receiving daily administration of higher doses.[22]

Extracts of mistletoe have been shown to strongly increase the cytolytic activity of NK cells using human peripheral blood mononuclear cells and a human cell line (K562 leukaemia).[35] The active component in the mistletoe extract is stated not to be a protein, thus excluding lectins and viscotoxins, and is thought to be a complex polysaccharide.[35] Mistletoe extract is not itself cytolytic but must be present during the NK cell-mediated tumour cell lysis to elicit enhancement.[35] Galacturonic acid inhibits this enhancement of NK cell cytotoxicity by acting at the effector cell specific site.[35] Two mechanisms have been proposed for the enhancement of NK cell cytotoxicity by mistletoe; one involves a bridging mechanism between the effector (NK) and target (tumour) cells, and another involves an immediate trigger of receptor expression on effector cells for target cell recognition.[35]

A systematic review of controlled clinical trials of mistletoe extracts in the treatment of cancer identified 11 trials involving patients with various cancers (e.g. gastric, colorectal and cervical cancer).[36] Of these, ten trials reported results in favour of mistletoe treatment over control treatment, although most of these trials were deemed to be of poor methodological quality. The remaining, high-quality, trial reported no difference between the treatment and control groups.

Side-effects, Toxicity

Hepatitis has been documented in a woman who had ingested a herbal preparation containing kelp, motherwort, skullcap and mistletoe.[37] Mistletoe was assumed to be the causal factor since it was the only known toxic ingredient in the remedy.[37] However, no other instances of hepatotoxicity have been documented for mistletoe and, more recently, hepatitis has been documented with scullcap (*see* Scullcap).

Symptoms of toxicity documented following the ingestion of mistletoe include hypotension, coma, seizures, myosis, mydriasis and death.[38] Hypertension leading to cardiovascular collapse has been reported for American mistletoe (*Phoradendron* species).[38] It has been stated that no serious side-effects have been reported for Iscador following its administration to at least 1000 patients, although mild pyrexia and mild leukocytosis have been documented.[18] In contrast to the immunosuppression normally associated with cytotoxic therapy, Iscador has exhibited immunostimulant actions.

Toxic actions in animals have been documented for mistletoe lectins and viscotoxins.

Intravenous administration of viscotoxin to cats (35 μg/kg) resulted in a negative inotropic effect on cardiac muscle, reflex bradycardia and hypotension.[39] Viscotoxins A_3 and B have also caused muscle contracture and progressive depolarisation in isolated smooth, skeletal and cardiac muscle preparations (rabbit, frog).[40] The mode of action was thought to involve the displacement of calcium from cell membrane bound sites. The viscotoxins precipitate histamine release from human leucocytes in an irritant manner without destroying the cells.[28] Viscotoxin is toxic on parenteral administration and an LD_{50} value (mice, intraperitoneal injection) has been estimated as 0.7 mg/kg.[41]

Mistletoe lectins inhibit protein synthesis in both cells and cell-free systems.[42] In common with other known toxic lectins (e.g. ricin), mistletoe lectins bind to plasma proteins, are specific towards D-galactose, possess some cytotoxic activity and have caused macroscopic lesions in rats (e.g. ascites, congested intestine, pancreatic haemorrhages).[21] An LD_{50}

(mice) value for mistletoe lectin fraction is reported as 80 µg/kg compared with 3 µg/kg for ricin.[42]

Documented LD_{50} values (mice, intraperitoneal injection) are greater than 2.25 mg for the polysaccharide fraction from the berries, 32 mg for the crude plant juice, and 276 mg for Iscador.[21]

Contra-indications, Warnings

Mistletoe berries are highly poisonous and it is advised that the herb should only be prescribed by a registered herbal practitioner.[G42] Mistletoe may interfere with existing cardiac, immunosuppressant, hypo/hypertensive, antidepressant and anticoagulant/coagulant therapies.

Pregnancy and lactation The use of mistletoe is contra-indicated in view of the toxic constituents. Tyramine and a cardioactive principle isolated from mistletoe have both exhibited uterine stimulant activity in animal studies.

Pharmaceutical Comment

The constituents of mistletoe have been well investigated and to some extent are thought to be dependent on the host plant on which mistletoe is a parasite. Mistletoe is reputed to be a cardiac depressant. Cardioactive constituents are not generally recognised as constituents of mistletoe, although this may depend on the nature of the host plant.

Documented literature for mistletoe has centred primarily on the pharmacological and toxic actions of the lectin and viscotoxin constituents. Much interest has been generated by the immunostimulant and cytotoxic actions documented for mistletoe and its potential role in treating conditions involving the immune system. Mistletoe seems to have the unusual combination of being both cytotoxic and immunostimulating. Further research is required to establish the true usefulness of mistletoe in these therapeutic areas.

The toxic nature of the mistletoe constituents (e.g. alkaloids, lectins, viscotoxins) indicates that it is unsuitable for self-medication. Mistletoe berries may only be supplied from pharmacies.[43]

References

See also General References G2, G3, G5, G9, G10, G16, G22, G31, G36, G42, G43, G56 and G64.

1 Krzaczek T. Pharmacobotanical studies of the subspecies *Viscum album* L. IV. *Ann Univ Mariae Curie-Sklodowska, Sect D* 1977; **32**: 281–291.
2 Becker H, Exner J. Comparative studies of flavonoids and phenylcarboxylic acids of mistle-

toes from different host trees. *Z Pflanzenphysiol* 1980; **97**: 417–428.
3 Khwaja TA *et al.* Isolation of biologically active alkaloids from Korean mistletoe *Viscum album, coloratum. Experientia* 1980; **36**: 599–600.
4 Khwaja TA *et al.* Recent studies on the anticancer activities of mistletoe (*Viscum album*) and its alkaloids. *Oncology* 1986; **43**(Suppl.1): 42–50.
5 Graziano MN *et al.* Isolation of tyramine from five Argentine species of Loranthaceae. *Lloydia* 1967; **30**: 242–244.
6 Fukunaga T *et al.* Studies on the constituents of the European mistletoe, *Viscum album* L. *Chem Pharm Bull* 1987; **35**: 3292–3297.
7 Ziska P *et al.* The lectin from *Viscum album* L. purification by biospecific affinity chromatography. *Experientia* 1978; **34**: 123–124.
8 Ziska P *et al.* Chemical modification studies on the D-galactopyranosyl binding lectin from the mistletoe *Viscum album* L. *Acta Biol Med Ger* 1979; **38**: 1361–1363.
9 Luther P *et al.* The lectin from *Viscum album* L. – isolation, characterization, properties and structure. *Int J Biochem* 1980; **11**: 429–435.
10 Franz H *et al.* Isolation and properties of three lectins from mistletoe (*Viscum album* L.). *Biochem J* 1981; **195**: 481–484.
11 Krzaczek T. Pharmacobotanical studies of the subspecies *Viscum album* L. III. Terpenes and sterols. *Ann Univ Mariae Curie-Sklodowska, Sect D* 1977; **32**: 125–134.
12 Samuelsson G. Mistletoe toxins. *Syst Zool* 1973; **22**: 566–569.
13 Olson T. The disulphide bonds of viscotoxin A2 from the European mistletoe (*Viscum album* L. Loranthaceae). *Acta Pharm Suec* 1974; **11**: 381–386.
14 Samuelsson G, Jayawardene AL. Isolation and characterization of viscotoxin 1-Ps from *Viscum album* L. ssp. austriacum (Wiesb.) Vollmann, growing on *Pinus silvestris*. *Acta Pharm Suec* 1974; **11**: 175–184.
15 Krzaczek T. Pharmacobotanical studies of the subspecies *Viscum album* L. II. Saccharides. *Ann Univ Mariae Curie-Sklodowska Sect D* 1976; **31**: 281–290.
16 Locock RA. Mistletoe. *Can Pharm J* 1986; **119**: 125–127.
17 Anderson LA, Phillipson JD. Mistletoe – the magic herb. *Pharm J* 1982; **229**: 437–439.
18 Evans MR, Preece AW. *Viscum album* – A possible treatment for cancer? *Bristol MedicoChir J* 1973; **88**: 17–20.
19 Konopa J *et al.* Isolation of viscotoxins. Cytotoxic basic polypeptides from *Viscum album* L. *Hoppe-Seyler's Z Physiol Chem* 1980; **361**: 1525–1533.
20 Hülsen H, Mechelke F. *In vitro* effectiveness of a

mistletoe preparation on cytostatic-drug-resistant human leukemia cells. *Naturwissenschaften* 1987; **74**: 144–145.

21 Bloksma N *et al*. Stimulation of humoral and cellular immunity by *Viscum* preparations. *Planta Med* 1982; **46**: 221–227.

22 Coeugniet EG, Elek E. Immunomodulation with *Viscum album* and *Echinacea purpurea* extracts. *Onkologie* 1987; **10**(Suppl.3): 27–33.

23 Luther P, Mehnert WH. Zum serologischen Verhalten einiger handelsüblicher Präparate aus *Viscum album* L., insbesondere des Iscador, in bezug aug menschliche Blutzellen und Aszites-Tumorzellen von Mäusen. *Acta Biol Med Ger* 1974; **33**: 351–357.

24 Luther P *et al*. Isolation and characterization of mistletoe extracts. II. Action of agglutinating and cytotoxic fractions on mouse ascites tumor cells. *Acta Biol Med Ger* 1977; **36**: 119–125.

25 Luther P *et al*. Reaktionen einiger antikörperähnlicher Substanzen aus Insekten (Protektine) und Pflanzen (Lektine) mit Aszites-Tumorzellen. *Acta Biol Med Ger* 1973; **31**: K11–18.

26 Ziska P, Franz H. Studies on the interaction of the mistletoe lectin I with carbohydrates. *Experientia* 1981; **37**: 219.

27 Franz H *et al*. Isolation and characterization of mistletoe extracts. I. Affinity chromatography of mistletoe crude extract on insolubilized plasma proteins. *Acta Biol Med Ger* 1976; **36**: 113–117.

28 Luther P *et al*. Allergy and lectins: Interaction between IgE-mediated histamine release and glycoproteins from *Viscum album* L. (mistletoe). *Acta Biol Med Ger* 1978; **37**: 1623–1628.

29 Petkov V. Plants with hypotensive, antiatheromatous and coronarodilatating action. *Am J Chin Med* 1979; **7**: 197–236.

30 Salzer G. The local treatment of malignant pleural exudations with Iscador (a drug obtained from mistletoe). Preliminary report. *Osterr Z Onkol* 1977; **4**: 13–14.

31 Salzer G. Pleura carcinosis. Cytomorphological findings with the mistletoe preparation Iscador and other pharmaceuticals. *Oncology* 1986; **43**(Suppl.1): 66–70.

32 Bradley GW, Clover A. Apparent response of small cell lung cancer to an extract of mistletoe and homoeopathic treatment. *Thorax* 1989; **44**: 1047–1048.

33 Hajto T, Hostanska K. An investigation of the ability of *Viscum album*-activated granulocytes to regulate natural killer cells *in vivo*. *Clin Trials J* 1986; **23**: 345–357.

34 Hajto T. Immunomodulatory effects of Iscador: a *Viscum album* preparation. *Oncology* 1986; **43**(Suppl.1): 51–65.

35 Mueller EA *et al*. Biochemical characterization of a component in extracts of *Viscum album* enhancing human NK cytotoxicity. *Immunopharmacology* 1989; **17**: 11–18.

36 Kleijnen J, Knipschild P. Mistletoe treatment for cancer: review of controlled trials in humans. *Phytomedicine* 1994; **1**: 255–260

37 Harvey J, Colin-Jones DG. Mistletoe hepatitis. *BMJ* 1981; **282**: 186–187.

38 Hall AH *et al*. Assessing mistletoe toxicity. *Ann Emerg Med* 1986; **15**: 1320–1323.

39 Rosell S, Samuelsson G. Effect of mistletoe viscotoxin and phoratoxin on blood circulation. *Toxicon* 1966; **4**: 107–110.

40 Andersson K-E, Jóhannsson M. Effects of viscotoxin on rabbit heart and aorta, and on frog skeletal muscle. *Eur J Pharmacol* 1973; **23**: 223–231.

41 Samuelsson G. Screening of plants of the family Loranthaceae for toxic proteins. *Acta Pharm Suec* 1966; **3**: 353–362.

42 Stirpe F *et al*. Inhibition of protein synthesis by a toxic lectin from *Viscum album* L. (mistletoe). *Biochem J* 1980; **190**: 843–845.

43 The Medicines (Retail Sale or Supply of Herbal Medicines) Order 1977, SI 1977: 2130.

Motherwort

Species (Family)

Leonurus cardiaca L. and various other *Leonurus* species (Labiatae)

Synonym(s)

Leonurus

Part(s) Used

Herb

Pharmacopoeial and Other Monographs

BHC 1992[G6]
BHP 1996[G9]
Complete German Commission E[G3]
Martindale 32nd edition[G43]
PDR for Herbal Medicines 2nd edition[G36]

Legal Category (Licensed Products)

GSL[G37]

Constituents[G6,G22,G40,G49,G64]

Alkaloids 0.35%. Stachydrine (a pyrrolidine-type alkaloid), betonicine and turicin (stereoisomers of 4-hydroxystachydrine), leonurine 0.0068% (a guanidine derivative),[1] leonuridin, leonurinine. The presence of leonurine in *L. cardiaca* has been disputed, although it has been documented for other *Leonurus* species.

Flavonoids Glycosides of apigenin, kaempferol, and quercetin (e.g. hyperoside, kaempferol-3-D-glucoside, genkwanin, quinqueloside, quercitrin and rutin).[2,3]

Iridoids Ajugol, ajugoside, galiridoside, leonurid and three or four more unidentified glycosides.[4]

Tannins 2–8%. Type not specified. Pseudotannins (e.g. pyrogallol, catechins).

Terpenoids Volatile oil 0.05%, resin, wax, ursolic acid, leocardin (a labdane diterpene)[5] as an epimeric mixture, and a diterpene lactone similar to marrubiin.[2] Cardiac glycosides (bufadienolide/bufanolide

type) have been documented although their presence in motherwort has not been confirmed.

Other constituents Citric acid, malic acid, oleic acid, bitter principles,[6,7] carbohydrates 2.89%, choline and a phenolic glycoside (caffeic acid 4-rutinoside).[8]

A *Cad*-specific lectin has been isolated from the seeds.[9]

Food Use

Motherwort is not used in foods. In the USA, motherwort is listed by the Food and Drugs Administration (FDA) as a Herb of Undefined Safety.[G22]

Herbal Use

Motherwort is stated to possess sedative and antispasmodic properties. Traditionally, it has been used for cardiac debility, simple tachycardia, effort syndrome, amenorrhoea, and specifically for cardiac symptoms associated with neurosis.[G6,G7,G8,G64]

Dosage

Dried herb 2–4 g or by infusion three times daily.[G6,G7]

Liquid extract 2–4 mL (1 : 1 in 25% alcohol) three times daily.[G6,G7]

Tincture 2–6 mL (1 : 5 in 45% alcohol) three times daily.[G6,G7]

Pharmacological Actions

In vitro and animal studies

The uterotonic principle in motherwort is unclear, although leonurine is reported to be the utero-active constituent in various *Leonurus* species. In addition, oxytocic activity documented for *L. cardiaca* has been attributed to another alkaloid constituent, stachydrine.[G30] Uterotonic activity has been reported for leonurine in various *in vitro* preparations including human myometrial strips and isolated rat uterus.[10,11]

In vitro cardioactivity has been documented for motherwort.[12] An alcoholic extract was found to have a direct inhibitory effect on myocardial cells:

antagonistic action towards calcium chloride (provided that the extract was administered before calcium chloride), and towards both α- and β-adrenoceptor stimulation was observed. No significant effect on the cardiac activity of the isolated guinea-pig heart was noted for caffeic acid 4-rutinoside.[8]

A related species, *Leonurus heterophyllus*, has been stated to prevent platelet aggregation, although no such documented action was located for motherwort.[13]

Ursolic acid has been reported to possess antiviral, tumour-inhibitory and cytotoxic activities.[14,15] Ursolic acid was found to inhibit the Epstein–Barr virus *in vitro* and to inhibit tumour production by 12-O-tetradeconoyl phorbol (TPA) in mouse skin, with activity comparable to that of retinoic acid, a known tumour-promoter inhibitor.[15] *In vitro* cytotoxicity was documented in lymphocytic leukaemia (P-388, L-1210), human lung carcinoma (A-549), KB cells, human colon (HCT-8) and mammary tumour (MCF-7).[14]

Side-effects, Toxicity

It has been stated that the leaves of motherwort may cause contact dermatitis and that the lemon-scented oil may result in photosensitisation.[G51] No documented toxicity studies were located. Cytotoxic activities have been reported for ursolic acid (*see In vitro* and animal studies).

Contra-indications, Warnings

Excessive use may interfere with existing therapy for a cardiac disorder (cardiac glycoside constituents, *in vitro* activity). Sensitive individuals may experience an allergic reaction.

Pregnancy and lactation Motherwort is reputed to affect the menstrual cycle.[G22] In view of the lack of toxicity data and the documented *in vitro* uterotonic activity,[G30] the use of motherwort during pregnancy and lactation should be avoided.

Pharmaceutical Comment

The common name motherwort may be applied to one of many *Leonurus* species. *L. cardiaca* is the typical European species utilised, whereas *Leonurus artemisia* is commonly used in traditional Chinese medicine. Other species referred to as motherwort include *Leonurus sibirious* and *L. heterophyllus*. The chemistry of *L. cardiaca* is well studied although the presence of the uterotonic principle leonurine has been disputed. Cardioactive properties in animals have been reported for motherwort (*L. cardiaca*), which thus support some of the stated herbal uses. However, any symptoms of cardiac disorder are not suitable for self-diagnosis and treatment with a herbal remedy. In view of the lack of toxicity data and possible cardioactivity, excessive use of motherwort should be avoided.

References

See also General References G3, G6, G9, G22, G30, G31, G36, G37, G40, G43, G49, G51 and G64.

1 Gulubov AZ. Structure of alkaloids from *Leonurus cardiaca*. *Nauch Tr Vissh Predagog Inst Plovdiv Mat Fiz Khim Biol* 1970; **8**: 129–132.

2 Scott JH *et al*. Components of *Leonurus cardiaca*. *Sci Pharm* 1973; **41**: 149–155.

3 Kartnig T *et al*. Flavonoid-O-glycosides from the herbs of *Leonurus cardiaca*. *J Nat Prod* 1985; **48**: 494–507.

4 Buzogany K, Cucu V. Comparative study between the species of *Leonurus quinquelobatus*. Part II Iridoids. *Clujul Med* 1983; **56**: 385–388.

5 Malakov P *et al*. The structure of leocardin, two epimers of a diterpenoid from *Leonurus cardiaca*. *Phytochemistry* 1985; **24**: 2341–2343.

6 Brieskorn CH, Hofmann R. Labiatenbitterstoffe: Ein clerodanderivat aus *Leonurus cardiaca* L. *Tetrahedron Lett* 1979; **27**: 2511–2512.

7 Brieskorn CH, Broschek W. Bitter principles and furanoid compounds of *L. cardiaca*. *Pharm Acta Helv* 1972; **47**: 123–132.

8 Tschesche R *et al*. Caffeic acid 4-rutinoside from *Leonurus cardiaca*. *Phytochemistry* 1980; **19**: 2783.

9 Bird GWG, Wingham J. Anti-Cad lectin from the seeds of *Leonurus cardiaca*. *Clin Lab Haematol* 1979; **1**: 57–59.

10 Yeung HW *et al*. The structure and biological effect of leonurine – a uterotonic principle from the Chineses drug, I-mu Ts'ao. *Planta Med* 1977; **31**: 51–56.

11 Kong YC *et al*. Isolation of the uterotonic principle from *Leonorus artemisia*, the Chinese motherwort. *Am J Chin Med* 1976; **4**: 373–382.

12 Yanxing X. The inhibitory effect of motherwort extract on pulsating myocardial cells in vitro. *J Trad Chin Med* 1983; **3**: 185–188.

13 Chang CF, Li CZ. Experimental studies on the mechanism of anti-platelet aggregation action of motherwort. *Chung-Hoi-I- Chich-Ho-TSQ Chin* 1986; **6**: 39–40.

14 Kuo-Hsiung L *et al*. The cytotoxic principles of *Prunella vulgaris*, *Psychotria serpens*, and *Hyptis*

capitata: Ursolic acid and related derivatives. *Planta Med* 1988; **54**: 308.

15 Tokuda H *et al*. Inhibitory effects of ursolic and oleanolic acid on skin tumor promotion by 12-*O*-tetradecanoylphorbol-13-acetate. *Cancer Lett* 1986; **33**: 279–285.

Myrrh

Species (Family)

(i) *Commiphora molmol* Engl. (Bursuraceae)
(ii) *Commiphora abyssinica* (Berg) Engl.
(iii) Other *Commiphora* species

Synonym(s)

(i) African Myrrh, Balsamodendron Myrrha, Commiphora, *Commiphora myrrha* (Nees) Engl., Somali Myrrh
(ii) Arabian Myrrh, Yemen Myrrh

Part(s) Used

Oleo-gum-resin

Pharmacopoeial and Other Monographs

BHC 1992[G6]
BHP 1996[G9]
BP 2001[G15]
Complete German Commission E[G3]
ESCOP 1999[G52]
Martindale 32nd edition[G43]
PDR for Herbal Medicines 2nd edition[G36]
Ph Eur 2002[G28]
USP24/NF19[G61]

Legal Category (Licensed Products)

GSL[G37]

Constituents[G2,G6,G41,G48,G52,G64]

Carbohydrates Up to 60% gum yielding arabinose, galactose, xylose, and 4-O-methylglucuronic acid following hydrolysis.

Resins Up to 40% (average 20%) consisting of α-, β- and γ-commiphoric acids, commiphorinic acid, α- and β-heerabomyrrhols, heeraboresene and commiferin.

Steroids Campesterol, cholesterol and β-sitosterol.

Terpenoids α-Amyrin. Furanosesquiterpenes, including furaneudesma-1,3-diene (major), furaneudesma-1,4-diene-6-one, lindestrine, curzerenone, furanodiene, 2-methoxyfuranodiene and 4,5-dihydrofuranodiene-6-one.[1,G52]

Volatile oils 1.5–17%. Main constituents are furanosesquiterpenes. Dipentene, cadinene, heerabolene, limonene, pinene, eugenol, *m*-cresol, cinnamaldehyde, cuminaldehyde, cumic alcohol and others.

Food Use

Myrrh is listed by the Council of Europe as a natural source of food flavouring (category N2). This category indicates that myrrh can be added to foodstuffs in small quantities, with a possible limitation of an active principle (as yet unspecified) in the final product.[G16] In the USA, myrrh is permitted for use in alcoholic beverages.[G65]

Herbal Use[G2,G4,G6,G7,G8,G43,G52,G64]

Myrrh is stated to possess antimicrobial, astringent, carminative, expectorant, anticatarrhal, antiseptic and vulnerary properties. Traditionally, it has been used for aphthous ulcers, pharyngitis, respiratory catarrh, common cold, furunculosis, wounds and abrasions, and specifically for mouth ulcers, gingivitis and pharyngitis. The German Commission E approved topical use for mild inflammation of the oral and pharyngeal mucosa.[G3]

Dosage

Myrrh Tincture (BPC 1973) 2.5–5.0 mL; in a glass of water several times daily as a gargle or a mouthwash. For skin, undiluted or diluted.[G52]

Tincture Myrrh Co (Thompsons) (1 part Capsicum Tincture BPC 1973 to 4 parts Myrrh Tincture BPC 1973) 1.0– 2.5 mL.

Pharmacological Actions

In vitro and animal studies

Anti-inflammatory activity Anti-inflammatory (carrageenan-induced inflammation and cotton pellet granuloma)[2] and antipyretic activities in mice[2,3] have been documented for *C. molmol*.

Hypoglycaemic activity Hypoglycaemic activity in both normal and diabetic rats has been reported for a myrrh extract.[4,5] Together with an aloe gum extract, myrrh was found to be an active component of a multi-plant extract that exhibited antidiabetic activity. The mode of action was thought to involve a decrease in gluconeogenesis and an increase in peripheral utilisation of glucose in diabetic rats.

Myrrh is stated to have astringent properties on mucous membranes[G45] and to have antimicrobial activities *in vitro*.[G41]

Anti-inflammatory activity Anti-inflammatory activities have been reported for an Indian plant, *Commiphora mukul*, commonly known as guggulipid. Anti-inflammatory activity was described for a crystalline steroidal fraction of guggulipid in both acute (carrageenan-induced rat paw oedema test) and chronic (adjuvant arthritis) models of inflammation.[6]

Lipid-lowering effects A ketosteroid has been identified as the active hypocholesterolaemic principle in guggulipid.[7] In some animal species, thyroid suppression is required as well as cholesterol administration in order to achieve experimental hypercholesterolaemia. Results of studies in chicks administered a thyroid suppressant and cholesterol indicated that guggulipid prevents endogenous hypercholesterolaemia via stimulation of the thyroid gland.[7] When fed to rabbits, guggulipid has been found to reverse the decrease in catecholamine concentrations and dopamine-β-decarboxylase activity that are associated with hyperlipidaemia.[8]

Stimulation of phagocytosis Stimulation of phagocytosis has been documented in mice innoculated with *Escherichia coli* and given with extracts of myrrh by intraperitoneal injecton.[G52]

Cytoprotective activity An aqueous suspension of myrrh administered to rats at oral doses of 250–1000 mg/kg gave significant and dose-dependent protection to gastric mucosa against various ulcerogenic agents.[G52]

Analgesic activity In mice, powdered myrrh (1 mg/kg, orally) had significant analgesic activity in the hotplate test.[G52] Isolated furanoeudesma-1,3-dione (50 mg/kg, orally) was significantly more effective than control ($p < 0.01$) in the mouse writhing test, and the effective dose was reversed by naloxone (1 mg/kg).[G52]

Anti-tumour and cytotoxic activities In mice with Ehrlich solid tumours, an aqueous suspension of myrrh (250 or 500 mg/kg, orally) produced significant decreases in tumour weight ($p < 0.05$) after 25 days.[G52] Aqueous suspension of myrrh increased survival time in mice with Erlich ascite tumours.

Clinical studies

Well-designed clinical studies of myrrh are lacking. Guggulipid has been reported to lower the concentration of total serum lipids, serum cholesterol, serum triglycerides, serum phospholipids and β-lipoproteins in 20 patients.[9] This effect was reported to be comparable to that of two other known lipid-lowering drugs also used in the study.

Side-effects, Toxicity

No reported side-effects were located for *C. molmol* or *C. abyssinica*. Hiccup,[9] diarrhoea,[7] restlessness and apprehension,[9] were documented as side-effects for guggulipid when administered to 20 patients.[9] Myrrh has been reported to be non-irritating, non-sensitising and non-phototoxic to human and animal skins.[G41]

Contra-indications, Warnings

Myrrh may interfere with existing antidiabetic therapy, as hypoglycaemic properties have been documented. Thyroid stimulation and lipid lowering properties have been documented for the related species, *Commiphora mukul*.

Pregnancy and lactation Myrrh is reputed to affect the menstrual cycle[G41] and the safety of myrrh taken during pregnancy has not been established. Excessive use of myrrh during pregnancy should be avoided.

Pharmaceutical Comment

The volatile oil, gum and resin components of myrrh are well documented. The anti-inflammatory and antipyretic activities documented in animals support some of the traditional uses. Phenol components of the volatile oil may account for the antimicrobial properties of myrrh, although no documented studies were located. Lipid-lowering properties via a stimulant action on the thyroid gland have been documented for *C. mukul* in both animals and humans. In view of the lack of toxicity data, excessive use of myrrh should be avoided.

References

See also General References G2, G3, G6, G9, G12, G15, G16, G28, G29, G31, G32, G36, G37, G41, G43, G48, G52 and G64.

1 Brieskorn CH, Noble P. Constituents of the essential oil of myrrh. II: Sesquiterpenes and furanosesquiterpenes. *Planta Med* 1982; **44**: 87–90.

2 Tariq M *et al*. Anti-inflammatory activity of *Commiphora molmol*. *Agents Actions* 1986; **17**: 381–382.

3 Mohsin A *et al*. Analgesic, antipyretic activity and phytochemical screening of some plants used in traditional Arab system of medicine. *Fitoterapia* 1989; **60**: 174–177.

4 Al-Awadi FM, Gumaa KA. Studies on the activity of individual plants of an antidiabetic plant mixture. *Acta Diabetol Lat* 1987; **24**: 37–41.

5 Al-Awadi FM *et al*. On the mechanism of the hypoglycaemic effect of a plant extract. *Diabetologia* 1985; **28**: 432–434.

6 Arora RB *et al*. Anti-inflammatory studies on a crystalline steroid isolated from *Commiphora mukul*. *Indian J Med Res* 1972; **60**: 929–931.

7 Tripathi SN *et al*. Effect of a keto-steroid of *Commifora mukul* L. on hypercholesterolemia and hyperlipidemia induced by neomercazole and cholesterol mixture in chicks. *Indian J Exp Biol* 1975; **13**: 15–18.

8 Srivastava M *et al*. Effect of hypocholesterolemic agents of plant origin on catecholamine biosynthesis in normal and cholesterol fed rabbits. *J Biosci* 1984; **6**: 277–282.

9 Malhotra SC, Ahuja MMS. Comparative hypolipidaemic effectiveness of gum guggulu (*Commiphora mukul*) fraction 'A', ethyl-*p*-chlorophenoxyisobutyrate and Ciba-13437-Su. *Indian J Med Res* 1971; **59**: 1621–1632.

Nettle

Species (Family)

Urtica dioica L. (Urticaceae)

Synonym(s)

Stinging Nettle, Urtica

Part(s) Used

Herb

Pharmacopoeial and Other Monographs

BHC 1992[G6]
BHP 1996[G9]
Complete German Commission E[G3]
ESCOP 1996 and 1997[G52]
Martindale 32nd edition[G43]
Mills and Bone[G50]
PDR for Herbal Medicines 2nd edition[G36]

Legal Category (Licensed Products)

GSL[G37]

Constituents[G6,G22,G52,G64]

Acids   Carbonic, caffeic, caffeoylmalic, chlorogenic, formic, silicic, citric, fumaric, glyceric, malic, oxalic, phosphoric, quinic, succinic, threonic and threono-1,4-lactone.[1]

Amines   Acetylcholine, betaine, choline, lecithin, histamine, serotonin[2] and a glycoprotein.[3]

Flavonoids   Flavonol glycosides (e.g. isorhamnetin, kaempferol, quercetin).[4]

Inorganics   Up to 20% minerals, including calcium, potassium and silicon.

Lignans   Several lignans, including (−)-secoisolariciresinol.

Other constituents   Choline acetyltransferase,[5] scopoletin,[4] β-sitosterol and tannin

Other plant parts   The rhizome contains lectin (*Urtica dioica* agglutinin) composed of six isolec-

tins,[6,7] coumarin (scopoletin), triterpenes (β-sitosterol, its glucoside, and six stearyl derivatives),[8,9] two phenylpropane derivatives, and six lignans.[10]

Food Use

Nettle (herbs and leaves) is listed by the Council of Europe as a natural source of food flavouring (category 1) (*see* Appendix 23).[G17] Nettle is used in soups and herbal teas. In the USA, nettle is listed by the Food and Drugs Administration (FDA) as a Herb of Undefined Safety.[G22]

Herbal Use[G2,G4,G6,G7,G8,G32,G43,G50,G52,G54,G64]

Nettle is stated to possess antihaemorrhagic and hypoglycaemic properties. Traditionally, it has been used for uterine haemorrhage, cutaneous eruption, infantile and psychogenic eczema, epistaxis, melaena and specifically for nervous eczema. The German Commission E approved internal use of nettle leaf as supportive therapy for rheumatic ailments and as irrigation therapy for inflammatory disease of the lower urinary tract and prevention of kidney gravel; internal and external use for rheumatic ailments.[G3] The root is approved for difficulty in urination from benign prostatic hyperplasia.[G3]

Dosage

Dried herb   2–4 g or by infusion three times daily;[G6,G7] 8–12 g daily;[G3] fresh juice 10–15 mL three times daily.[G52]

Liquid extract   3–4 mL (1 : 1 in 25% alcohol) three times daily.[G6,G7]

Tincture   2–6 mL (1 : 5 in 45% alcohol) three times daily.[G6,G7]

Pharmacological Actions

In vitro and animal studies
The pharmacological properties of nettle have been reviewed.[G50,G52,G56]   Information   from   these reviews is summarised below.

Anti-inflammatory activity   An   aqueous   ethanol extract and also isolated caffeoylmalic acid partially inhibited the biosynthesis of arachidonic acid *in vitro*.[G52] Nettle extract (0.1 mg/mL) and isolated acid (1 mg/mL) inhibited 5-lipoxygenase-derived biosynthesis of leukotriene B$_4$ by 20.8% and 68.2%, respectively, and inhibited synthesis of cyclooxygenase-derived prostaglandins (IC$_{50}$ 92 µg/mL and 38 µg/mL, respectively). The same extract significantly reduced tumour-necrosis-factor-α (TNFα) and interleukin 1β (IL-1β) concentrations after lipopolysaccharide (LPS)-stimulated secretion of these proinflammatory cytokines in human blood.[G52] An aqueous ethanol extract (0.25 mg/mL) inhibited platelet-activating factor (PAF)-induced exocytosis of elastase from human neutrophils by 93%, but failed to inhibit biosynthesis of prostaglandins from [^{14}C]arachidonic acid.[G52]

In vitro addition of a commercial preparation of nettle leaf (IDS-23) to whole human blood resulted in an inhibition of LPS-stimulated TNFα and IL-1β secretion, correlating with drug ingestion. The same preparation inhibited phytohaemogglutinin-stimulated production of T helper cell 1 (Th1)-specific interleukin-2 (IL-2) and interferon-γ (IFNγ) in culture in a dose-dependent manner up to 50% and 74%, respectively.[11] By contrast, T helper cell 2 (Th2)-specific interleukin-4 (IL-4) production was stimulated. The results suggested that the nettle leaf extract acts by mediating a switch in T helper cell-derived cytokine patterns and may inhibit the inflammatory cascade in autoimmune diseases such as rheumatoid arthritis.[11] The transcription factor NF-κB is elevated in several chronic inflammatory diseases and is responsible for the enhanced expression of some proinflammatory gene products. A nettle leaf extract (IDS 23) potently inhibited NF-κB activation in a number of cells, including human T cells, macrophages, epithelial cells and mouse L929 fibrosarcoma cells *in vitro*.[12] It was proposed that part of the anti-inflammatory effects of nettle may be due to its inhibitory effect on NF-κB activity.

Benign prostatic hyperplasia activity[G50] Several lignans and their metabolites reduce binding activity of human sex hormone-binding globulin (SHBG) *in vitro*. Lignans from nettle are competitive inhibitors of the interaction between SHBG and 5α-dihydrotestosterone.[G50] An aqueous extract of nettle root led to a concentration-dependent (0.6–10 mg/mL) inhibition of SHBG interaction with its receptor on human prostatic membranes. A 20% methanol extract of root inhibited binding capacity of SHBG after preincubation in human serum.[G50]

Subfractions of an aqueous methanol extract of nettle root inhibited cellular proliferation in benign prostatic hyperplasia (BPH) tissue. A root extract had a specific and concentration-dependent inhibition of human leukocyte elastase (HLE) activity *in vitro*. (HLE is an important marker in clinically silent genitourinary tract infection and inflammation.) Root extracts inhibited alternative and classic complementary pathways and significantly inhibited prostate growth in mice with induced BPH (by 51%, compared with control; $p < 0.003$).[G50]

Other activities CNS-depressant activity has been documented for nettle. It has been shown to produce a reduction in spontaneous activity in rats and mice,[13,14] inhibition of drug-induced convulsions, and a lowering of body temperature in rats.[13] Nettle has been reported to have no effect on the blood pressure of mice,[14] whereas in cats it has produced a marked hypotensive effect and bradycardia.[15] Atropine was reported to have no effect on these latter actions and a mode of action via α-adrenoceptors was suggested.[15]

Nettle is stated to contain both hypoglycaemic and hyperglycaemic principles.[16] The hypoglycaemic component has been termed 'urticin' and nettle has been reported to lower the blood sugar concentration in hyperglycaemic rabbits.[16]

An 80% ethanolic and an aqueous extract of nettle administered to mice at a dose of 25 mg/kg orally prior to glucose load, led to hypoglycaemia effects.[17] No diuretic or ion excretion effects were observed in rats after oral administration of an aqueous extract of nettle (1 g/kg).[14,18] Dried nettle had a potassium ion to sodium ion ratio of 63 : 1, whereas an aqueous decoction had a corresponding ratio of 448 : 1.[19] It was suggested that the high potassium ion concentration in aqueous decoctions may contribute to their diuretic activity.

Utero-activity has been documented for nettle in pregnant and non-pregnant mice; betaine and serotonin were stated to be the active constituents.[20] A nettle extract was reported to be devoid of antifertility activity following oral administration to mice (250 mg/kg).[21] Analgesic activity in mice has been documented.[14] Administration of an aqueous extract (1200 mg/kg) to mice showed resistance to stimulation in the hotplate test at 55°C with a 190% increase in reaction time.[14] Conversely, no analgesic activity was noted in the hotplate test on rats given an ethanolic extract, but the same extract did reduce the writing response to phenylquinone after oral (1 g/kg) and intraperitoneal (500 mg/kg) treatment.[18]

The isolectins isolated from the rhizome are reported to cause nonspecific agglutination of erythrocytes, to induce the synthesis of interferon by human lymphocytes,[6,7] and have carbohydrate-binding properties.[6,7]

An extract of nettle at a concentration of 1.2 mg/mL has been reported to be active against L-1210 leukaemic cells in mice.[22]

Clinical studies

Diuretic effect In an open, uncontrolled study, 32 patients with myocardial or chronic venous insufficiency were treated with 15 mL of nettle juice three times daily for two weeks.[G52] A significant increase in daily volume of urine was observed throughout the study, the volume by day 2 being 9.2% ($p < 0.0005$) higher than the baseline value in patients with myocardial insufficiency and 23.9% higher than the baseline value ($p < 0.0005$) in those with chronic venous insufficiency. It has been proposed that the diuretic activity of aqueous extracts of nettle may be attributed to the high potassium content.[19] The reputed diuretic effects of nettle require further investigation.

Arthritis and rheumatism An open, uncontrolled multicentre study involving 152 patients with various, mainly degenerative, rheumatic conditions reported that 70% of participants experienced symptom relief by the end of the three-week treatment period.[G52] In an open, randomised pilot study involving 37 patients with acute arthritis, diclofenac 50 mg plus stewed nettle herb 50 g was compared with diclofenac 200 mg.[23] Assessment was based on the decrease in elevated acute phase C-reactive protein serum concentrations, and clinical signs of acute arthritis. Clinical improvement was observed in both groups to a similar extent. On the basis of the findings, it was suggested that nettle herb administration may enhance the effectiveness of diclofenac in rheumatic conditions. However, this requires further investigation.

Postmarketing surveillance studies involving a total of almost 2000 patients with rheumatoid arthritis treated for three weeks with nettle leaf extract (IDS-23) administered as an adjuvant to non-steroidal anti-inflammatory drugs (NSAIDs), or as monotherapy, have reported that the extract was well-tolerated.[24,25]

In a randomised, double-blind, crossover study, 27 patients with osteoarthritis pain at the base of the thumb and index finger, received stinging nettle leaf (applied for 30 seconds daily for one week to the painful area) or white dead nettle (*Lamium album*) as placebo, followed by a five-week wash-out period before crossing to the other arm of the study.[26] The results indicated that reductions in visual analogue scale scores for pain and in a health assessment questionnaire score for disability were significantly better for the stinging nettle group, compared with the placebo group ($p = 0.026$ and $p = 0.0027$ for pain and disability, respectively).

Benign prostatic hyperplasia Clinical studies of nettle preparations in the treatment of symptoms of benign prostatic hyperplasia (BPH) have been reviewed.[G50] Information from this review is summarised below.

Several uncontrolled trials have reported improvements in urological symptoms, compared with baseline values, following administration of nettle root extract (5 : 1) 600–1200 mg daily for three weeks to 20 months.[G50] Large observational studies involving patients with BPH who received nettle root extract for two to three months have reported improvements in various symptoms, such as urinary frequency, urinary flow and nocturia.[G50] These studies provide justification for further, rigorous investigation of the effects of nettle in BPH.

A placebo-controlled trial involving 79 patients with BPH assessed the effects of nettle root extract 600 mg daily for six to eight weeks. Compared with placebo, nettle root extract administration resulted in greater improvements in urinary flow and urine volume and residual volume.[G50] Another placebo-controlled trial of nettle root extract 600 mg daily for nine weeks in men with BPH ($n = 50$) reported a significant decrease in SHBG concentrations and significant improvement in micturition volume and maximum urinary flow.[G50]

Rhinitis A randomised, double-blind, placebo-controlled study assessed the effects of a freeze-dried preparation of nettle herb in individuals with allergic rhinitis.[27] Participants received nettle herb 600 mg, or placebo, at the onset of symptoms over a one-week period. Assessment was based on daily symptom diaries and global responses recorded at follow-up visits after one week of therapy. Nettle herb was rated more highly than placebo in the global assessment, but was rated less highly on the basis of data from the symptom diaries. It was concluded that there should be further investigation with a larger sample size and involving a longer treatment period.

Side-effects, Toxicity

Consumption of nettle tea has caused gastric irritation, a burning sensation of the skin, oedema and oliguria.[G22] The leaves are extremely irritant in view of their acetylcholine- and histamine-containing glandular hairs. An LD_{50} in mice following intraperitoneal administration of nettle has been reported as 3.625 g/kg.[12] The LD_{50} for intravenous infusion of nettle leaf in mice has been documented as 1.92 g/kg, and the LD_{50} for chronic administration in rats has been stated as 1.31 g/kg.[G50] An ethanolic extract of nettle (plant part unspecified) showed low toxicity in rats and mice after oral and intraperitoneal administration at doses equivalent to 2 g/kg.[18]

Contra-indications, Warnings

In view of the documented pharmacological actions for nettle, excessive use may interact with concurrent therapy for diabetes, high or low blood pressure, and may potentiate drugs with CNS-depressant actions. Gastrointestinal irritation has been documented.

Pregnancy and lactation Nettle is reputed to be an abortifacient and to affect the menstrual cycle.[G30] Utero-activity has been documented in animal studies. In view of this, the use of nettle during pregnancy should be avoided. Excessive use is best avoided during lactation.

Pharmaceutical Comment

The chemistry of nettle is well documented. Limited pharmacological data are available to support the traditional herbal uses although hypoglycaemic activity *in vivo* has been reported. A number of clinical trials have provided some evidence to support the diuretic and anti-inflammatory effects of nettle, and for the effects of nettle in relief of symptoms of allergic rhinitis. Clinical evidence exists to support the efficacy of root extracts in the treatment of benign prostatic hyperplasia. However, further well-designed clinical trials of nettle involving large numbers of patients are required to establish the benefits. Irritant properties have been documented for nettle and excessive use should be avoided.

References

See also General References G2, G3, G5, G6, G9, G16, G22, G30, G31, G32, G36, G37, G43, G50, G52, G54, G56 and G64.

1 Bakke ILF *et al* Water-soluble acids from *Urtica dioica* L. *Medd Nor Farm Selsk* 1978; **40**: 181–188.

2 Adamski R, Bieganska J. Studies on substances present in *Urtica dioica* L. leaves II. Analysis for protein amino acids and nitrogen containing non-protein amino acids. *Herba Pol* 1984; **30**: 17–26.

3 Andersen S, Wold JK. Water-soluble glycoprotein from *Urtica dioica* leaves. *Phytochemistry* 1978; **17**: 1875–1877.

4 Chaurasia N, Wichtl M. Flavonolglykoside aus *Urtica dioica*. *Planta Med* 1987; **53**: 432–434.

5 Barlow RB, Dixon ROD. Choline aceytltransferase in the nettle *Urtica dioica* L. *Biochem J* 1973; **132**: 15–18.

6 Shibuya N *et al*. Carbohydrates binding properties of the stinging nettle (*Urtica dioica*) rhizome lectin. *Arch Biochem Biophys* 1986; **249**: 215–224.

7 Damme EJM *et al*. The *Urtica dioica* agglutinin is a complex mixture of isolectins. *Plant Physiol* 1988; **86**: 598–601.

8 Chaurasia N, Wichtl M. Scopoletin, 3-β-sitosterin und 3-β-D-glucosid aus Brennesselwurzel (*Urticae radix*). *Dtsch Apothek Zeitung* 1986; **126**: 81–83.

9 Chaurasia N, Wichtl M. Sterols and steryl glycosides from *Urtica dioica*. *J Nat Prod* 1987; **50**: 881–885.

10 Chaurasia N, Wichtl M. Phenylpropane und lignane aus der wurzel von *Urtica dioica* L. *Dtsch Apothek Zeitung* 1986; **126**: 1559–1563.

11 Klingelhoefer S *et al*. Antirheumatic effect of IDS 23, a stinging nettle leaf extract, on *in vivo* expression of T helper cytokines. *J Rheumatol* 1999; **26**: 2517–2522.

12 Riehemann K *et al*. Plant extracts from stinging nettle (*Urtica dioica*), an antirheumatic remedy, inhibit the proinflammatory transcription factor NF-κB. *FEBS Lett* 1999; **442**: 89–94.

13 Broncano J *et al*. Estudio de diferentes preparados de *Urtica dioica* L sobre SNC. *An R Acad Farm* 1987; **53**: 284–291.

14 Lasheras B *et al*. Étude pharmacologique préliminaire de *Prunus spinosa* L. Amelanchier ovalis medikus *Juniperus communis* L. et *Urtica dioica* L. *Plant Méd Phytothér* 1986; **20**: 219–226.

15 Broncano FJ *et al*. Étude de l'effet sur le centre cardiovasculaire de quelques préparations de l'*Urtica dioica* L. *Planta Med* 1983; **17**: 222–229.

16 Oliver-Bever B, Zahland GR. Plants with oral hypoglycaemic activity. *Q J Crude Drug Res* 1979; **17**: 139–196.

17 Neef H *et al*. Hypoglycaemic activity of selected European plants. *Phytother Res* 1995; **9**: 45–48.

18 Tita B *et al*. *Urtica dioica* L.: Pharmacological effect of ethanol extract. *Pharmacol Res* 1993; **27**: 21–22.

19 Szentmihályi K *et al*. Potassium-sodium ratio for the characterization of medicinal plants extracts with diuretic activity. *Phytother Res* 1998; **12**: 163–166.

20 Broncano FJ *et al*. Estudio de efecto sobre musculatura lisa uterina de distintos preparados de las hojas de *Urtica dioica* L. *An R Acad Farm* 1987; **53**: 69–76.

21 Sharma BB *et al*. Antifertility screening of plants. Part I. Effect of ten indigenous plants on early pregnancy in albino rats. *Int J Crude Drug Res* 1983; **21**: 183–187.

22 Ilarionova M *et al*. Cytotoxic effect on leukemic

cells of the essential oils from rosemary, wild geranium and nettle and concret of royal bulgarian rose. *Anticancer Res* 1992; **12**: 1915.

23 Chrubasik S *et al*. Evidence for antirheumatic effectiveness of herba *Urtica dioicae* in acute arthritis: a pilot study. *Phytomedicine* 1997; **4**: 105–108.

24 Sommer R-G, Sinner B. Kennen sie den neuen zytokinanatagonisten? *Therapiewoche* 1996; **1**: 44–49.

25 Ramm S, Hansen C. Brennesselblätter-extrakt bei arthrose und rheumatoider arthritis-Multizentrische anwendungsbeobachtung mit rheuma-hek. *Therapiewoche* 1996; **28**: 1575–1578.

26 Randall C *et al*. Randomized controlled trial of nettle sting for treatment of base-of-thumb pain. *J R Soc Med* 2000; **93**: 305–309.

27 Mittman P. Randomized, double-blind study of freeze-dried *Urtica dioica* in the treatment of allergic rhinitis. *Planta Med* 1990; **56**: 44–47.

Parsley

Species (Family)

Petroselinum crispum (Mill.) Nyman (Apiaceae/Umbelliferae)

Synonym(s)

Apium petroselinum L., *Carum petroselinum* (L.) Benth., *Petroselinum sativum* Hoffm.

Part(s) Used

Leaf, root, seed

Pharmacopoeial and Other Monographs

BHC 1992[G6]
BHP 1996[G9]
Complete German Commission E[G3]
Martindale 32nd edition[G43]
PDR for Herbal Medicines 2nd edition[G36]

Legal Category (Licensed Products)

GSL[G37]

Constituents[G2,G6,G22,G41,G48,G64,G58]

Flavonoids Glycosides of apigenin, luteolin (e.g. apiin, luteolin-7-apiosyl-glucoside, apigenin-7-glucoside (leaf only), luteolin-7-diglucoside (leaf only)).

Furanocoumarins Bergapten and oxypeucedanin as major constituents (up to 0.02% and 0.01% respectively); also 8-methoxypsoralen, imperatorin, isoimperatorin, isopimpinellin, psoralen, xanthotoxin (up to 0.003%).[1]

Volatile oils 2–7% in seed, 0.05% in leaf. The seed contains apiole, myristicin, tetramethoxyallylbenzene, various terpene aldehydes, ketones, and alcohols. The leaf contains myristicin (up to 85%), apiole, 1,3,8-*p*-menthatriene, 1-methyl-4-isopropenylbenzene, methyl disulfide, monoterpenes (e.g. α- and β-pinene, β-myrcene, β-ocimene, β-phellandrene, *p*-terpinene, α-terpineol), sesquiterpenes (e.g. α-copaene, carotol, caryophyllene).

Other constituents Fixed oil, oleo-resin, proteins, carbohydrates, and vitamins (especially vitamins A and C).

A detailed vitamin and mineral analysis is given elsewhere.[G22]

Food Use

Parsley is listed by the Council of Europe as natural source of food flavouring (category N2). This category indicates that parsley can be added to foodstuffs in small quantities, with a possible limitation of an active principle (as yet unspecified) in the final product.[G16] Parsley is commonly used in foods. In the USA, parsley is listed as GRAS (Generally Recognised As Safe).[G65]

Herbal Use

Parsley is stated to possess carminative, antispasmodic, diuretic, emmenagogue, expectorant, antirheumatic and antimicrobial properties. Traditionally, it has been used for flatulent dyspepsia, colic, cystitis, dysuria, bronchitic cough in the elderly, dysmenorrhoea, functional amenorrhoea, myalgia and specifically for flatulent dyspepsia with intestinal colic.[G2,G6,G7,G8,G64]

Dosage

Leaf/root 2–4 g or by infusion.

Seed 1–2 g.

Dried root 2–4 g or by infusion three times daily.[G6,G7]

Liquid extract 2–4 mL (1:1 in 25% alcohol) three times daily.[G6,G7]

Pharmacological Actions

In vitro and animal studies

Parsley extract (0.25–1.0 mL/kg, by intravenous injection) has been reported to lower the blood pressure of cats by more than 40%,[2] and to decrease both respiratory movements and blood pressure in anaesthetised dogs.[3] Parsley exhibits a tonic effect on both intestinal and uterine muscle.[3]

365

This uterine effect has been attributed to the apiole content,[G30] but has also been observed with apiole-free aqueous extracts.[3] An aqueous extract of parsley has been documented to contain an antithiamine substance which was unaffected by cooking or contact with gastric juice.[3] Myristicin and apiole are both effective insecticides.[4]

Parsley seed oil has been reported to stimulate hepatic regeneration.[5]

Clinical studies

Myristicin is the hallucinogenic principle present in nutmeg seed. It has been hypothesised that myristicin is converted in the body to amphetamine, to which it is structurally related.[4] Myristicin has a structural similarity with sympathomimetic amines and it is thought that it may compete for monoamine oxidase enzymes, thereby exhibiting a monoamine oxidase inhibitor (MAOI)-like action.[6] Parsley oil has been included in the diet of pregnant women and is reported to increase diuresis, and plasma protein and plasma calcium concentrations.[4]

The diuretic effect associated with the consumption of parsley is probably attributable to the pharmacological activities of myristicin (sympathomimetic action) and apiole (irritant effect).

Side-effects, Toxicity[G58]

Chronic and excessive consumption of fresh parsley (170 g daily for 30 years) has been associated with generalised itching and pigmentation of the lower legs in a 70-year-old woman.[6] The symptoms were attributed to excessive ingestion of parsley in the presence of chronic liver disease. The aetiology of the chronic hepatitis was unknown, but considered possibly related to the chronic exposure to the psoralen constituents in parsley.[6] Apiole and myristicin are also documented to be hepatotoxic.

The ingestion of approximately 10 g apiole has been reported to cause acute haemolytic anaemia, thrombocytopenia purpura, nephrosis and hepatic dysfunction. However, ingestion of 10 g of apiole would require a dose of more than 200 g parsley. The amount of apiole ingested as a result of normal dietary consumption of parsley is not hazardous. Myristicin has been documented to cause giddiness, deafness, hypotension, decrease in pulse rate, and paralysis, followed by fatty degeneration of the liver and kidney.[G22] In addition, myristicin is known to possess hallucinogenic properties. However, when compared to nutmeg, parsley contains a relatively low concentration of myristicin (less than 0.05% in parsley leaf, about 0.4–0.89% in nutmeg); parsley seed is potentially hazardous in view of its higher

volatile oil content (about 2–7%) which contains apiole and myristicin.

Parsley contains phototoxic furanocoumarins (*see* Celery). However, photodermatitis resulting from the oral ingestion of parsley is thought to be unlikely. The ingestion of 50 g parsley provides negligible amounts of bergapten (0.5–0.8 g).[7] The concentration of oxypeucedanin provided was not mentioned. However, a photoactive reaction from topical contact with parsley is possible.

Apiole is an irritant component of the volatile oil and may cause irritation of the kidneys during excretion.

Parsley seed oil has been reported to stimulate hepatic regeneration.[4] Myristicin and apiole are documented to have a similar chemical structure and acute toxicity to safrole, which is known to be carcinogenic and hepatotoxic (*see* Sassafras).[4] The carcinogenic potential of apiole and myristicin has not been evaluated.[4]

LD_{50} (mice, intravenous injection) values for apiole and myristicin have been documented as 50 mg/kg and 200 mg/kg body weight, respectively.[4]

Contra-indications, Warnings

Parsley should not be ingested in excessive amounts in view of the documented toxicities of apiole and myristicin. Parsley may cause a photoactive reaction, especially following external contact, may aggravate existing renal disease, and may potentiate existing MAOI therapy.

Pregnancy and lactation   Parsley is reputed to affect the menstrual cycle.[G7] Utero-activity has been documented in humans and animals,[G30] and parsley is stated to be contra-indicated during pregnancy.[G49,G58] Myristicin has been reported to cross the placenta and can lead to foetal tachycardia.[8] In view of this, parsley should not be taken during pregnancy and lactation in doses that greatly exceed the amounts used in foods.

Pharmaceutical Comment

Parsley is commonly consumed as part of the diet. The pharmacological and toxicological properties of parsley are primarily associated with the volatile oil, particularly the apiole, myristicin and furanocoumarin constituents. Most of the reported uses of parsley are probably due to the volatile oil; no documented information was located regarding antirheumatic and antimicrobial properties. Parsley should not be consumed in doses that greatly exceed the amounts used in foods, as excessive ingestion may result in apiole and myristicin toxicity.

References

See also General References G2, G3, G6, G9, G16, G22, G30, G31, G32, G36, G37, G41, G43, G48, G49, G58 and G64.

1 Chaudhary SK *et al*. Oxypeucedanin, a major furocoumarin in parsley, *Petroselinum crispum*. *Planta Med* 1986; **52**: 462–464.
2 Petkov V. Plants with hypotensive, antiatheromatous and coronarodilatating action. *Am J Chin Med* 1979; **7**: 197–236.
3 Opdyke DLJ. Parsley seed oil. *Food Cosmet Toxicol* 1975; **13**(Suppl.): 897–898.
4 Buchanan RL. Toxicity of spices containing methylenedioxybenzene derivatives: A review. *J Food Safety* 1978; **1**: 275–293.
5 Gershbein LL. Regeneration of rat liver in the presence of essential oils and their components. *Food Cosmet Toxicol* 1977; **15**: 171–181.
6 Cootes P. Clinical curio: liver disease and parsley. *BMJ* 1982; **285**: 1719.
7 Zaynoun S *et al*. The bergapten content of garden parsley and its significance in causing cutaneous photosensitization. *Clin Exp Dermatol* 1985; **10**: 328–331.
8 Lavy G. Nutmeg intoxication in pregnancy. *J Reprod Med* 1987; **32**: 63–64.

Parsley Piert

Species (Family)

Aphanes arvensis L. (Rosaceae)

Synonym(s)

Alchemilla arvensis Scop., Aphanes

Part(s) Used

Herb

Pharmacopoeial and Other Monographs

BHP 1983[G7]
PDR for Herbal Medicines 2nd edition[G36]

Legal Category (Licensed Products)

GSL[G37]

Constituents[G7,G34,G64]

Limited information is available. A related species *Alchemilla vulgaris* (lady's mantle) is reported to contain 6–8% tannins (hydrolysable-type);[G41] none have been documented for parsley piert, although it is stated to contain an astringent principle.[G6]

Food Use

Parsley piert is not used in foods.

Herbal Use

Parsley piert is stated to possess diuretic and demulcent properties, and to dissolve urinary deposits. Traditionally, it has been used for kidney and bladder calculi, dysuria, strangury, oedema of renal and hepatic origin, and specifically for renal calculus.[G7,G64]

Dosage

Dried herb 2–4 g or by infusion three times daily.[G7]

Liquid extract 2–4 mL (1 : 1 in 25% alcohol) three times daily.[G7]

Tincture 2–10 mL (1 : 5 in 45% alcohol) three times daily.[G7]

Pharmacological Actions

None documented.

Side-effects, Toxicity

None documented.

Contra-indications, Warnings

None documented.

Pregnancy and lactation In view of the lack of phytochemical, pharmacological, and toxicity information, the use of parsley piert during pregnancy and lactation should be avoided.

Pharmaceutical Comment

Little chemical information is available on parsley piert. No scientific evidence was found to justify the herbal uses. Parsley piert may exhibit astringent actions. In view of the lack of toxicity data, excessive use of parsley piert should be avoided.

References

See General References G7, G31, G34, G36, G37 and G64.

Passionflower

Species (Family)

Passiflora incarnata L. (Passifloraceae)

Synonym(s)

Apricot Vine, Grenadille, Maypop, Passiflora, Passion Vine

Part(s) Used

Herb

Pharmacopoeial and Other Monographs

BHC 1992[G6]
BHP 1996[G9]
BP 2001[G15]
Complete German Commission E[G3]
ESCOP 1997[G52]
Martindale 32nd edition[G43]
PDR for Herbal Medicines 2nd edition[G36]
Ph Eur 2002[G28]

Legal Category (Licensed Products)

GSL[G37]

Constituents[G2,G6,G22,G41,G64]

Alkaloids Indole-type. Harman (major), harmaline, harmalol, harmine and harmol have been reported. Of 17 different samples examined, only one contained alkaloids with a possible harmine content of 0.1 ppm.[1]

Flavonoids Pharmacopoeial standard, not less than 1.5%.[G15,G28] Vitexin, isovitexin and their C-glycosides, apigenin, luteolin glycosides (e.g. orientin, homoorientin and lucenin); kaempferol, quercetin and rutin.[2–7]

Other constituents Maltol and ethylmaltol (γ-pyrone derivatives), passicol (a polyacetylene),[8] fatty acids (e.g. linoleic acid, linolenic acid, myristic acid, palmitic acid and oleic acid), formic acid, butyric acid, sitosterol, stigmasterol, sugars and gum.

Other plant parts Coumarins (scopoletin and umbelliferone) are found in the root.

Other Passiflora species Cyanogenetic glycosides passibiflorin, epipassibiflorin and passitrifasciatin (*Passiflora biflora*, *Passiflora talamancensis*, *Passiflora trifasciata*),[9] linamarin and lotaustralin (*Passiflora lutea*)[10] and prunasin (*Passiflora edulis*).[11]

Food Use

Passionflower is listed by the Council of Europe as a natural source of food flavouring (category N3). This category indicates that passionflower can be added to foodstuffs in the traditionally accepted manner, but that there is insufficient information available for an adequate assessment of potential toxicity.[G16] In the USA, passionflower is permitted for use in food.[G65]

Herbal Use[G2,G4,G6,G7,G8,G32,G43,G52,G54,G64]

Passionflower is stated to possess sedative, hypnotic, antispasmodic and anodyne properties. Traditionally, it has been used for neuralgia, generalised seizures, hysteria, nervous tachycardia, spasmodic asthma, and specifically for insomnia. The German Commission E approved internal use for nervous restlessness.[G3] Passionflower is used in combination with valerian root and lemon balm for conditions of unrest, difficulty in falling asleep due to nervousness.[G3] Passionflower is used extensively in homeopathy.

Dosage

Dried herb 0.25–1.0 g or by infusion three times daily;[G6,G7] 0.5–2 g three or four times daily;[G52] 4–8 g daily.[G3]

Liquid extract 0.5–1.0 mL (1:1 in 25% alcohol) three times daily.[G6,G7]

Tincture 0.5–2.0 mL (1:8 in 45% alcohol) three times daily.[G6,G7]

Pharmacological Actions

In vitro and animal studies

CNS sedation, potentiation of hexobarbitone-induced sleeping time, anticonvulsant activity (at high doses) and a reduction in spontaneous motor activity (at low doses) have been documented for maltol and ethylmaltol in mice.[12,13] Subsequent research documenting similar activities in mice was unable to attribute the observed activities to either flavonoid or alkaloid components present in the extract tested.[14] An aqueous ethanolic extract of passionflower administered intraperitoneally to rats (160 mg/kg) prolonged sleeping time induced by pentobarbital (50–4000 mg/kg) and reduced spontaneous locomotor activity.[14] The same extract (160 mg/kg, intraperitoneal or oral administration) raised the threshold to nociceptive stimuli in tail flick and hotplate tests.[14]

Rats showed reduced activity in a one-arm radial maze test after one week of daily oral administration of an aqueous ethanolic extract of passionflower (10 mg/kg).[G52] In mice, a 70% ethanol extract (1000 mg/kg, intraperitoneally) administered 10 minutes prior to sodium pentobarbitol (40 mg/kg, intraperitoneally) resulted in a significant prolongation (40%) of sleeping time.[15] When given by gastric tube 1 hour prior to amphetamine (5 mg/kg, subcutaneous), the same extract (500 mg/kg) caused significant reduction in hypermotility. Oral treatment of mice with an ethanol extract of passionflower (25 and 50 mg/kg) reduced exploratory and spontaneous motor activities, prolonged sleeping time induced by pentobarbital, and inhibited aggressiveness and restlessness caused by amphetamines.[G52] The sedative activity was comparable with that of meprobamate (250 mg/kg), and greater than that of diazepam (10 mg/kg) and chlordiazepoxide (10 mg/kg). In another study in mice, sedative action, as assessed by prolongation of hexobarbital-induced sleeping time, was decreased by a 30% aqueous ethanol extract of passionflower (1.75 mg/kg, orally).[16]

A dry extract of passionflower (800 mg/kg, orally) containing 2.6% flavonoids resulted in a significant ($p < 0.01$) anxiolytic effect, as assessed by prolongation of hexobarbital-induced sleeping time, whereas locomotor activity remained unaffected.[G52]

It has been suggested that the sedative effects of maltol and ethylmaltol mask the stimulant actions of harman alkaloids.[12] The CNS-depressant effect exhibited by *P. edulis* has been attributed to alkaloid and flavonoid compounds[17] and to a protein-like substance.[18] The pharmacological evidence generally supports sedative and anxiolytic effects of passionflower, although there are conflicting results. It is not clear which constituents are the active principles, and clinical data are lacking.[19] Maltol is reportedly an artefact and not a relevant constituent.[19]

Passicol exhibits antimicrobial activity towards a wide variety of moulds, yeasts and bacteria.[8] Group

A haemolytic streptococci are stated to be more susceptible than *Staphylococcus aureus*, with *Candida albicans* of intermediate susceptibility.[8]

Side-effects, Toxicity

In mice, the acute toxicity of a fluid extract of passionflower (intraperitoneal injection) was stated as being greater than 900 mg/kg.[14] In rats, subacute oral treatment with an aqueous ethanol extract of passionflower 10 mg/kg for 21 days showed no changes in weight, rectal temperature or motor coordination.[G52]

Cyanogenetic glycosides have been documented for related *Passiflora* species.

Contra-indications, Warnings

Excessive doses of passionflower may cause sedation.

Pregnancy and lactation No other data regarding the use of passionflower during pregnancy or lactation were located. In view of this, excessive use of passionflower during pregnancy and lactation should be avoided.

Pharmaceutical Comment

The active constituents have not been clearly identified. CNS-sedative properties have been documented in animals, thus providing some data to support some of the traditional uses of passionflower. However, well-designed clinical trials assessing the reputed sedative properties of passionflower are lacking. In view of the lack of toxicity data, excessive use of passionflower should be avoided.

References

See also General Reference G2, G3, G5, G6, G9, G15, G16, G22, G28, G30, G31, G32, G36, G37, G41, G43, G48, G52, G54, G56 and G64.

1 Rehwald A *et al.* Trace analysis of harman alkaloids in *Passiflora incarnata* by reversed-phase high performance liquid chromatography. *Phytochem Anal* 1995; 6: 96–100.
2 Quercia V *et al.* Identification and determination of vitexin and isovitexin in *Passiflora incarnata* extracts. *J Chromatogr* 1978; 161: 396–402.
3 Pietta P *et al.* Isocratic liquid chromatographic method for the simultaneous determination of *Passiflora incarnata* L. and *Crataegus monogyna* flavonoids in drugs. *J Chromatogr* 1986; 357: 233–238.
4 Geiger H *et al.* The C-glycosylfavone pattern of *Passiflora incarnata* L. *Z Naturforsch* 1986; Sept/Oct: 949–950.

5 Proliac A, Raynaud J. The presence of C-β-D-6-glucopyranosyl-C-α-L-arabinopyranosyl-8-apigenin in leafy stems of *Passiflora incarnata* L. *Pharmazie* 1986; **41**: 673–674.

6 Congora C *et al.* Isolation and identification of two mono-C-glucosyl-luteolins and of the di-C-substituted 6,8-diglucosyl-luteolin from the leafy stalks of *Passiflora incarnata* L. *Helv Chim Acta* 1986; **69**: 251–253.

7 Proliac A, Raynaud J. O-glucosyl-2″-C-glucosyl-6 apigénine de *Passiflora incarnata* L. (Passifloraceae). *Pharm Acta Helv* 1988; **63**: 174–175.

8 Nicholls JM *et al.* Passicol, an antibacterial and antifungal agent produced by *Passiflora* plant species: qualitative and quantitative range of activity. *Antimicrob Agents Chemother* 1973; **3**: 110–117.

9 Spencer KC, Seigler DS. Passibiflorin, epipassibiflorin and passitrifasciatin: Cyclopentenoid cyanogenic glycosides from *Passiflora*. *Phytochemistry* 1985; **24**: 981–986.

10 Spencer KC, Siegler DS. Co-occurrence of valine/isoleucine derived cyclopentenoid cyanogens in a *Passiflora* species. *Biochem Syst Ecol* 1985; **13**: 303–304.

11 Spencer KC, Seigler DS. Cyanogenesis of *Passiflora edulis*. *J Agric Food Chem* 1983; **31**: 794–796.

12 Aoyagi N *et al.* Studies on *Passiflora incarnata* dry extract. I. Isolation of maltol and pharmacological action of maltol and ethyl maltol. *Chem Pharm Bull* 1974; **22**: 1008–1013.

13 Kimura R *et al.* Central depressant effects of maltol analogs in mice. *Chem Pharm Bull* 1980; **28**: 2570–2579.

14 Speroni E, Minghetti A. Neuropharmacological activity of extracts from *Passiflora incarnata*. *Planta Med* 1988; **54**: 488–491.

15 Capasso A, Pinto A. Experimental investigations of the synergistic-sedative effect of passiflora and kava. *Acta Ther* 1995; **21**: 127–140.

16 Weischer ML, Okpanyi SN. Pharmakologie eines pflanzlichen schlafmittels. *Z Phytother* 1994; **15**: 257–262.

17 Lutomski J *et al.* Pharmacochemical investigation of the raw materials from *Passiflora* genus. *Planta Med* 1975; **27**: 112–121.

18 Dovale NB *et al.* Psychopharmacological effects of preparations of *P. edulis* Passionflower. *Cienc Cult* 1983; **35**: 11–24.

19 Meier B. *Passiflora incarnata* L.-Passionsblume-Portrait einer arzneipflanze. *Z Phytother* 1995; **16**: 115–126.

Pennyroyal

Species (Family)

(i) *Mentha pulegium* L. (Labiatae)
(ii) *Hedeoma pulegoides* (L.) Pers.

Synonym(s)

Pulegium
(i) European Pennyroyal
(ii) American Pennyroyal

Part(s) Used

Herb

Pharmacopoeial and Other Monographs

BHP 1983[G7]
Martindale 32nd edition[G43]
PDR for Herbal Medicines 2nd edition[G36]

Legal Category (Licensed Products)

Pennyroyal is not included in the GSL.[G37]

Constituents[G22,G48,G64,G58]

Volatile oils 1–2%. Pulegone is the principal component (60–90%); others include menthone, *iso*-menthone, 3-octanol, piperitenone and *trans-iso*-pulegone.

Food Use

Pennyroyal is not commonly used in foods. It is listed by the Council of Europe as a natural source of food flavouring (category N3).[G16] This category indicates that there is insufficient information available for an adequate assessment of toxicity (*but see* Side-effects, Toxicity). In the USA, pennyroyal is permitted for use in foods.[G65]

Herbal Use

Pennyroyal is stated to possess carminative, antispasmodic, diaphoretic and emmenagogue properties, and has been used topically as a refrigerant, antiseptic and insect repellent. Traditionally, it has been used for flatulent dyspepsia, intestinal colic, common cold, delayed menstruation, and topically for cutaneous eruptions, formication and gout.[G7]

Dosage

Herb 1–4 g or as infusion three times daily.[G7]

Liquid extract 1–4 mL (1 : 1 in 45% alcohol) three times daily.[G7]

Pharmacological Actions

None documented.

Side-effects, Toxicity

The toxicity of pennyroyal oil is well recognised and human fatalities following its ingestion as an abortifacient have been reported.[1–3] Symptoms reported following ingestion of the oil include abdominal pain, nausea, vomiting, diarrhoea, lethargy and agitation, pyrexia, raised blood pressure and pulse rate, and generalised urticarial rash. Generally, doses required for an abortifacient effect are also toxic and fatalities have involved both nephrotoxicity and hepatotoxicity.[2,3,4,] Doses of one ounce and 30 mL[1–3] have proved fatal, whereas individuals have recovered following unsuccessful abortion attempts involving the ingestion of 7.5 mL oil.[3] The mechanism of hepatotoxicity for pennyroyal is not known.[2] A direct hepatoxic action has been suggested for the ketone component, pulegone.[2] Alternatively, metabolic conversion of pulegone to a reactive intermediate, a furan or epoxide, has been proposed.[2]

Acute LD_{50} values for pennyroyal oil are documented as 0.4 g/kg (oral, rats) and 4.2 g/kg (dermal, rabbits).[4] The oil is non- or moderately irritating, non-sensitising and non-phototoxic.[4] Acute LD_{50} values documented for pulegone, the principal oil component, are, not suprisingly, similar to those for the oil: 0.47 g/kg (oral, rats), 3.09 g/kg (dermal, rabbits).[5] Steroid (pregnenolone-16α-carbonitrile) treatment has reduced hepatotoxicity observed in female rats fed pulegone, whereas triamcinolone has increased it.[5] Toxicity of pulegone is unaffected by partial hepatectomy or ligation of the common bile duct, while partial nephrectomy intensified toxicity.[5]

Contra-indications, Warnings

Pennyroyal oil is irritant and instances of hepatotoxicity and nephrotoxicity have been documented following its ingestion. Both the internal and external use of pennyroyal oil has been contra-indicated.[G58]

Pregnancy and lactation Pennyroyal is contra-indicated in pregnancy.[G7] Traditionally, it has been employed as an abortifacient, this use probably resulting from the irritant action of the oil on the genito-urinary tract. Fatalities have resulted from the doses of oil required to exert an abortifacient effect.

Pharmaceutical Comment

Interest in pennyroyal has focused on the toxicity associated with the volatile oil. No documented reports of the pharmacological actions exhibited by the herb were located. Pennyroyal herb teas have been reported to be used without side-effects,[2] presumably due to lower amounts of oil ingested. In view of its potential toxicity, excessive ingestion of the oil should be avoided. Pennyroyal oil is not suitable for internal or external use.

References

See also General References G7, G19, G22, G31, G32, G36, G37, G43, G48, G58 and G64.

1 Vallance WB. Pennyroyal poisoning. A fatal case. *Lancet* 1955; **ii**: 850–851.
2 Sullivan JB *et al*. Pennyroyal oil poisoning and hepatotoxicity. *JAMA* 1979; **242**: 2873.
3 Gunby P. Plant known for centuries still causes problems today. *JAMA* 1979; **241**: 2246–2247.
4 Opdyke DLJ. Pennyroyal oil european. *Food Cosmet Toxicol* 1974; **12**: 949–950.
5 Opdyke DLJ. Fragrance raw materials monographs: d-pulegone. *Food Cosmet Toxicol* 1978; **16**: 867–868.

Pilewort

Species (Family)

Ranunculus ficaria L. (Ranunculaceae)

Synonym(s)

Ficaria, *Ficaria ranunculoides Moench.*, Lesser Celandine, Ranunculus

Part(s) Used

Herb

Pharmacopoeial and Other Monographs

BHP 1996[G9]
PDR for Herbal Medicines 2nd edition[G36]

Legal Category (Licensed Products)

GSL[G37]

Constituents[G40,G42,G64]

Lactones Anemonin (dimer), protoanemonin (precursor to anemonin).

Triterpenoids Glycosides based on the sapogenins hederagenin and oleanolic acid, with arabinose, glucose and rhamnose, as sugar moieties.[1]

Other constituents Tannin and ascorbic acid (vitamin C).

Food Use

Pilewort is not used in foods.

Herbal Use

Pilewort is stated to possess astringent and demulcent properties. Traditionally, it has been used for haemorrhoids, and specifically for internal or prolapsed piles with or without haemorrhage, by topical application as an ointment or a suppository.[G7,G64]

Dosage

Dried herb 2–5 g or by infusion three times daily.[G7]

Liquid extract 2–5 mL (1 : 1 in 25% alcohol) three times daily.[G7]

Ointment 3% in a suitable basis.

Pilewort Ointment (BPC 1934) 30% fresh herb in benzoinated lard.

Pharmacological Actions

In vitro and animal studies

Local antihaemorrhoidal activity has been documented for the saponin constituents.[1] Antibacterial and antifungal properties have been documented for both anemonin and protoanemonin, although anemonin is reported to exhibit much weaker activity.[G33,G48]

The reported presence of tannin constituents[G42] supports the reputed astringent activity of pilewort, although no pharmacological studies were located.

Side-effects, Toxicity

The sap of pilewort is stated to be irritant.[G51] Protoanemonin is stated to be an acrid skin irritant, although it is readily converted into the inactive dimer anemonin.[G33] Protoanemonin is stated to have a marked ability to combine with sulfhydryl (-SH) groups and it is thought that the toxic subdermal properties of protoanemonin may depend on the inactivation of enzymes containing -SH groups.[G33] An LD_{50} value (mice, intraperitoneal injection) for anemonin has been reported as 150 mg/kg body weight.[G48]

Contra-indications, Warnings

Pilewort is not recommended for internal consumption.[G49] Topical use of pilewort may cause irritant skin reactions.

Pregnancy and lactation The safety of pilewort has not been established. It is not recommended for internal consumption;[G49] in view of this and the potential irritant action, the use of pilewort during pregnancy and lactation is best avoided.

Pharmaceutical Comment

Limited information is available on the chemistry of pilewort. Little scientific information was located to justify the herbal uses, although antihaemorrhoidal activity has been documented for the saponin constituents. In view of the toxic and irritant properties stated for protoanemonin, the excessive use of pilewort is not advisable.

References

See also General References G9, G10, G33, G36, G37, G40, G42, G48, G49, G57 and G64.

1   Texier O *et al*. A triterpenoid saponin from *Ficaria ranunculoides* tubers. *Phytochemistry* 1984; **23**: 2903–2905.

Plantain

Species (Family)

Plantago major L. (Plantaginaceae)

Synonym(s)

Common Plantain, General Plantain, Greater Plantain

Part(s) Used

Leaf

Pharmacopoeial and Other Monographs

BHP 1996[G9]
Complete German Commission E[G3]
Martindale 32nd edition[G43]
PDR for Herbal Medicines 2nd edition[G36]

Legal Category (Licensed Products)

Plantain is not included in the GSL.[G37]

Constituents[G2,G22,G40,G51,G62,G64]

Acids Benzoic acid, caffeic acid, chlorogenic acid, cinnamic acid, *p*-coumaric acid, ferulic acid, fumaric acid, gentisic acid, *p*-hydroxybenzoic acid, neochlorogenic acid, salicylic acid, syringic acid, ursolic acid, vanillic acid;[1,2] oleanolic acid and ascorbic acid.

Alkaloids Trace (unspecified),[3,4] boschniakine and the methyl ester of boschniakinic acid[5]

Amino acids DL-α-Alanine, asparagine, L-histidine, DL-lysine, DL-leucine, serine and tryptophan.[6]

Carbohydrates L-Fructose, D-glucose, planteose, saccharose, stachyose, *d*-xylose, sorbitol, tyrosol, mucilage and gum.[7]

Flavonoids Apigenin, baicalein, scutellarein, baicalin, homoplantaginin, nepitrin, luteolin, hispidulin and plantagoside.[8–10]

Iridoids Aucubin, aucubin derivatives, plantarenaloside, aucuboside and melitoside.[5,11,12]

Tannins 4%. Unspecified.

Other constituents Choline, allantoin, invertin and emulsin (enzymes), fat 10–20%, resin, saponins, steroids[13] and thioglucoside.

Food Use

Plantain leaf is not used in foods. A related species, *Plantago lanceolata* L., is listed by the Council of Europe as a natural source of food flavouring (category N2). This category indicates that *P. lanceolata* can be added to foodstuffs in small quantities, with a possible limitation of an active constituent (as yet unspecified) in the final product.[G16] In the USA, plantain is listed by the Food and Drugs Administration (FDA) as a Herb of Undefined Safety.[G22]

Herbal Use

Plantain is stated to possess diuretic and antihaemorrhagic properties. Traditionally, it has been used for cystitis with haematuria, and specifically for haemorrhoids with bleeding and irritation.[G2,G7,G42,G64]

Dosage

Dried leaf 2–4 g or by infusion three times daily.[G7]

Liquid extract 2–4 mL (1 : 1 in 25% alcohol) three times daily.[G7]

Tincture 2–4 mL (1 : 5 in 45% alcohol) three times daily.[G7]

Pharmacological Actions

In vitro and animal studies

An aqueous extract has been reported to possess bronchodilatory activity in guinea-pigs. It was more effective against acetylcholine-induced contraction, than towards constriction induced by histamine or serotonin.[14] The bronchodilatory activity of plantain in guinea-pigs has been reported to be less active and of shorter duration compared to salbutamol or atropine.[15]

Hypotensive activity in normotensive, anaesthetised dogs has been documented; 125 mg/kg extract was found to decrease arterial blood pressure by 20–40 mmHg.[16]

An aqueous extract, reported to contain flavonoids, saponins, steroids and alkaloids, was shown to possess anti-inflammatory activity in the rat using various models of inflammation, and a strengthening of capillary vessels has also been documented.[13] However, an extract was found to exhibit minimal (11%) inhibition of carrageenan-induced rat paw oedema.[17] Leaf extracts in hexane have shown potent wound-healing activity in rabbits; the effect was primarily attributed to C_{26}–C_{30} alcohols present in the extract.[18] Both the anti-inflammatory and wound-healing activities of plantain have been attributed to the high content of chlorogenic and neo-chlorogenic acids.[2]

Aucubin and a haemolytic saponin fraction have exhibited antibiotic activity towards *Micrococcus flavus* and *Staphylococcus aureus* (aucubin only).[19] Antibacterial activity towards *Bacillus subtilis* has been documented for the fresh plant juice, which was also found to lack activity towards Gram-positive organisms and fungi.[20] A negative response to cytotoxic, antitumour and antiviral activity was also reported for the plant juice.[20]

A mild laxative action has been reported in mice administered iridoid glycosides, including aucubin.[21] Plantain seed is sometimes used as a substitute for ispaghula (a bulk laxative).[G45]

Plantain has been documented to lower concentrations of total plasma lipids, cholesterol, β-lipoproteins and triglycerides in rabbits with experimental atherosclerosis.[22] Plantain has been reported to be useful in lowering plasma cholesterol concentrations.[23]

A tonus-raising effect on isolated guinea-pig and rabbit uterus tissue has been documented for an aqueous extract at a dose of 1–2 mg/cm^3.[24]

Aucubin has been stated to be the active principle responsible for a hepatoprotective effect documented for plantain.[25]

Clinical studies

Plantain has been reported to be effective in the treatment of chronic bronchitis of a spastic or non-spastic nature.[14,26,27] A pronounced improvement in both subjective and objective symptoms of the common cold following treatment with plantain has also been reported.[28] Plantain, in combination with agrimony, German chamomile, peppermint and St. John's wort, has been documented to provide pain relief in patients with chronic gastroduodenitis.[29] Following treatment, previously diagnosed erosions and haemorrhagic mucous changes were stated to have disappeared.

Side-effects, Toxicity

Allergic contact dermatitis to plantain has been reported.[G51] The green parts of the plant are thought to yield a mustard oil-type of thioglucoside, which releases an irritant principle (isothiocyanate) upon enzymatic hydrolysis.[G51] The seed may also cause sensitisation and dermatitis. Plantain is reported to be of low toxicity with LD_{50} values in the rat documented as 1 g/kg (intraperitoneal injection) and greater than 4 g/kg (by mouth).[15]

Contra-indications, Warnings

Plantain may cause a contact allergic reaction; it induces the formation of IgE antibodies, which may cross-react to psyllium.[30] Excessive doses may exert a laxative effect and a hypotensive effect.

Pregnancy and lactation   *In vitro* uterotonic activity has been documented for plantain. In view of this, excessive use of plantain, which may also exert a laxative effect, should be avoided during pregnancy.

Pharmaceutical Comment

The constituents of plantain are well documented and the reputed antihaemorrhagic properties are probably attributable to the tannin constituents. In addition, bronchospastic activity has been documented in both animal and human studies, and may warrant further research. The toxicity of plantain is reported to be low but excessive ingestion should be avoided. The bulk laxative ispaghula consists of the dried seeds of related species *Plantago psyllium*, *P. ovata* and *P. indica*.[G45]

References

See also General References G2, G3, G9, G16, G22, G31, G36, G37, G40, G42, G43, G51, G62 and G64.

1   Andrzejewska-Golec E, Swiatek K. Chemotaxonomic studies on the genus *Plantago* II. Analysis of phenolic acid fraction. *Herba Pol* 1986; **32**: 19–31.
2   Maksyutina NP. Hydroxycinnamic acids of *Plantago major* and *Pl. lanceolata*. *Khim Prirodn Soedin* 1971; 7: 795.
3   Smolenski SJ *et al.* Alkaloid screening. IV. *Lloydia* 1974; **37**: 30–61.
4   Pailer M, Haschke-Hofmeister E. Inhaltsstoffe aus *Plantago major*. *Planta Med* 1969; **17**: 139–145.
5   Popov S *et al.* Cyclopentanoid monoterpenes from *Plantago* species. *Izv Khim* 1981; **14**: 175–180.
6   Maksyutin GV. Amino acids in *Plantago* (plantain) *major* leaves and *Matricaria recutita* inflorescences. *Rastit Resur* 1972; **8**: 110–112.

7 Tomoda M *et al*. Plant mucilages. XXIX. Isolation and characterization of a mucous polysaccharide, plantago-mucilage A, from the seeds of *Plantago major* var. *asiatica*. *Chem Pharm Bull* 1981; **29**: 2877–2884.

8 Lebedev-Kosov VI. Flavonoids of *Plantago major*. *Khim Prirodn Soedin* 1976; **12**: 730.

9 Lebedev-Kosov VI *et al*. Flavonoids of *Plantago major*. *Khim Prirodn Soedin* 1977; **13**: 223.

10 Endo T *et al*. The glycosides of *Plantago major* var. japonica Nakai. A new flavone glycoside, plantagoside. *Chem Pharm Bull* 1981; **29**: 1000–1004.

11 Oshio H, Inouye H. Two new iridoid glucosides of *Plantago asiatica*. *Planta Med* 1982; **44**: 204–206.

12 Andrzejewska-Golec E, Swiatek K. Chemotaxonomic studies on the genus *Plantago* I. Analysis of the iridoid fraction. *Herba Pol* 1984; **30**: 9–16.

13 Lambev I *et al*. Study of the anti-inflammatory and capillary restorative activity of a dispersed substance from *Plantago major* L. *Probl Vatr Med* 1981; **9**: 162–169.

14 Koichev A *et al*. Pharmacologic-clinical study of a preparation from *Plantago major*. *Probl Pneumol Ftiziatr* 1983; **11**: 68–74.

15 Marcov M *et al*. Pharmacologic study of the influence of the disperse substance extracted from *Plantago major* on bronchial smooth muscles. *Probl Vatr Med* 1980; **8**: 132–139.

16 Kyi KK *et al*. Hypotensive property of *Plantago major* Linn. *J Life Sci* 1971; **4**: 167–171.

17 Mascolo N *et al*. Biological screening of Italian medicinal plants for anti-inflammatory activity. *Phytother Res* 1987; **1**: 28–31.

18 Mironov VA *et al*. Physiologically active alcohols of *Plantago major*. *Khim-Farm Zh* 1983; **17**: 1321–1325.

19 Tarle D. Antibiotic effect of aucubin, saponins and extract of plantain leaf – herba or folium *Plantaginis lanceolata*. *Farm Glas* 1981; **37**: 351–354.

20 Lin Y-C *et al*. Search for biologically active substances in Taiwan medicinal plants I. Screening for anti-tumor and anti-microbial substances. *Chin J Microbiol* 1972; **5**: 76–78.

21 Inouye H *et al*. Purgative activities of iridoid glycosides. *Planta Med* 1974; **25**: 285–288.

22 Maksyutina NP *et al*. Chemical composition and hypocholesterolemic action of some drugs from *Plantago major* leaves. Part I. Polyphenolic compounds. *Farm Zh (Kiev)* 1978; **4**: 56–61.

23 Ikram M. Medicinal plants as hypocholesterolemic agents. *J Pak Med Assoc* 1980; **30**: 278–279.

24 Shipochliev T. Extracts from a group of medicinal plants enhancing the uterine tonus. *Vet Med Nauki* 1981; **18**: 94–98.

25 Chang I-M, Yun (Choi) HS. Plants with liver-protective activities: pharmacology and toxicology of aucubin. In: Chang HM *et al*., eds. *Advances in Chinese Medical Material Research*. Singapore: World Scientific, 1985: 269.

26 Koichev A. Complex evaluation of the therapeutic effect of a preparation from *Plantago major* in chronic bronchitis. *Probl Vatr Med* 1983; **11**: 61–69.

27 Matev M *et al*. Clinical trial of *Plantago major* preparation in the treatment of chronic bronchitis. *Vatr Boles* 1982; **21**: 133–137.

28 Koichev A. Study on the therapeutic effect of different doses from the preparation *Plantago major* in cold. *Prob Vatr Med* 1982; **10**: 117–124.

29 Chakarski I *et al*. Clinical study of a herb combination consisting of *Agrimonia eupatoria*, *Hipericum perforatum*, *Plantago major*, *Mentha piperita*, *Matricaria chamomila* for the treatment of patients with gastroduodenitis. *Probl Vatr Med* 1982; **10**: 78–84.

30 Rosenberg S *et al*. Serum IgE antibodies to psyllium in individuals allergic to psyllium and English plantain. *Ann Allergy* 1982; **48**: 294–298.

Pleurisy Root

Species (Family)

Asclepias tuberosa L. (Asclepiadaceae)

Synonym(s)

Asclepias

Part(s) Used

Root

Pharmacopoeial and Other Monographs

BHP 1983[G7]
PDR for Herbal Medicines 2nd edition[G36]

Legal Category (Licensed Products)

GSL[G37]

Constituents[G48,G64]

Little chemical information is available for pleurisy root. Cardiac glycosides of the cardenolide type (e.g. afroside, asclepin, calactin, calotropin, gomphoside, syriogenin, syrioside, uscharidin, uscharin and uzarigenin) have been documented for many *Asclepias* species,[1–4] including *A. tuberosa*.[5] Concentrations of cardiac glycosides are reported to vary between *Asclepias* species[1] and individual plant parts,[4] in descending order of latex, stem, leaf and root.[6]

No other data regarding constituents of the root were located.

Other plant parts Constituents documented for the herb include flavonols (e.g. kaempferol and quercetin) and flavonol glycosides (e.g. rutin and isorhamnetin), amino acids, caffeic acid, chlorogenic acid, choline, carbohydrates (e.g. glucose, fructose and sucrose), β-sitosterol, triterpenes (e.g. α-amyrin and β-amyrin, lupeol, friedelin, viburnitol), volatile oil and resin.[7,8,G48]

Food Use

Pleurisy root is not used in foods.

Herbal Use

Pleurisy root is stated to possess diaphoretic, expectorant, antispasmodic and carminative properties. It has been used for bronchitis, pneumonitis, influenza, and specifically for pleurisy.[G7,G42,G64]

Dosage

Dried root 1–4 g or by infusion three times daily.[G7]

Liquid extract 1–4 mL (1:1 in 45% alcohol) three times daily.[G7]

Tincture 1–5 mL (1 : 10 in 45% alcohol) three times daily.[G7]

Pharmacological Actions

In vitro and animal studies

Low doses of extracts of *Asclepias* species including *A. tuberosa* have been documented to cause uterine contractions (*in vivo*) and to exhibit oestrogenic effects.[5,9,10,G30] No effect was observed on blood pressure or respiration (*in vivo*), or on the isolated heart (frog, turtle).[9] Various activities have been reported for related *Asclepias* species. A positive inotropic action (*in vivo* and *in vitro*) has been reported for asclepin (*Asclepias curassavica*), which was found to be more potent, longer acting and with a wider safety margin when compared with other cardiac glycosides (including digoxin).[11–13] Asclepin was also reported to exhibit a more powerful activity towards weak cardiac muscle.[13] Plant extracts of *A. curassavica*, *Asclepias engelmanniana* and *Asclepias glaucescens* have exhibited a stimulatory effect on the mammalian CNS, causing an increase in serotonin and noradrenaline concentrations.[14]

Antitumour/cytotoxic activities have been documented for *A. albicans* and were attributed to various cardenolide constituents.[15]

Side-effects, Toxicity

Pleurisy root and other *Asclepias* species have been documented to cause dermatitis; the milky latex is reported to be irritant.[G51] Large doses may cause nausea, vomiting and diarrhoea.[G7,G42] Various *Asclepias* species, including *A. tuberosa*, are known to be toxic to livestock, with cardenolides implicated as the toxic constituents.[1,5] Toxic effects on the lungs, gastrointestinal tract, kidneys, brain and spinal cord have been observed in rats and rabbits following intravenous administration of an alcoholic extract.[10]

Toxicity studies involving related *Asclepias* species have also been documented. The cardenolide fraction of *Asclepias eriocarpa* is reported to contain toxic principles. The whole plant, plant extracts, an isolated and purified cardenolide (labriformin) and digoxin were all found to show qualitatively similar signs of toxicity and gross pathology in sheep and guinea-pigs.[16] LD_{50} values (mice, intraperitoneal injection) for cardenolides obtained from *A. curassavica* and *A. eriocarpa* were all estimated at less than 50 mg/kg body weight. Asclepin (*A. curassavica*) was reported to be safe following a three-month toxicity study in rats, using doses of 0.8, 8 and 20 mg/kg (route unspecified).[13] Asclepin has also been documented to have a wider margin of safety than digoxin[11–13] (*see In vitro* and animal studies).

Studies in cats have reported asclepin to be less cumulative compared to digoxin.[13]

Contra-indications, Warnings

Pleurisy root may interfere with existing cardiac drug therapy. Excessive doses of pleurisy root may interfere with drug therapies that affect amine concentrations in the brain (e.g. antidepressants) and with hormonal therapy.

Pregnancy and lactation Uterotonic activity (*in vivo*) has been reported for pleurisy root.[5,G30] In view of this and the potential toxicity of pleurisy root, it is best avoided during pregnancy or lactation.

Pharmaceutical Comment

The chemistry of pleurisy root is poorly documented, but phytochemical studies on pleurisy root and related *Asclepias* species have identified many cardiac glycoside constituents. No scientific evidence was found to justify the herbal uses. In view of the potential toxicity of pleurisy root, excessive use is not recommended.

References

See also General References G7, G30, G36, G37, G42, G48, G51 and G64.

1 Seiber JN *et al*. New cardiac glycosides (cardenolides) from *Asclepias* species. *Proceedings of the Australia/USA Poisonous Plants Symposium. Plant Toxicol* 1985: 427–437.

2 Radford DJ *et al*. Naturally occurring cardiac glycosides. *Med J Aust* 1986; **144**: P540–544.

3 Jolad SD *et al*. Cardenolides and a lignan from *Asclepias subulata*. *Phytochemistry* 1986; **25**: 2581–2590.

4 Seiber JN *et al*. Cardenolides in the latex and leaves of seven *Asclepias* species and *Calotropis procera*. *Phytochemistry* 1982; **21**: 2343–2348.

5 Conway GA, Slocumb JC. Plants used as abortifacients and emmenagogues by Spanish New Mexicans. *J Ethnopharmacol* 1979; **1**: 241–261.

6 Duffey SS, Scudder GGE. Cardiac glycosides in North American Asclepiadaceae, a basis for unpalatability in brightly coloured Hemiptera and Coleoptera. *J Insect Physiol* 1972; **18**: 63–78.

7 Nelson CJ *et al*. Seasonal and intraplant variation of cardenolide content in the California milkweed *Asclepias eriocarpa* and implications for plant defense. *J Chem Ecol* 1981; **7**: 981–1010.

8 Pagani F. Plant constituents of *Asclepias tuberosa* (Asclepiadaceae). *Boll Chim Farm* 1975; **114**: 450–456.

9 Costello CH, Butler CL. The estrogenic and uterine-stimulating activity of *Asclepias tuberosa*. *J Am Pharm Assoc Sci Educ* 1949; **39**: 233–237.

10 Hassan WE, Reed HL. Studies on species of *Asclepias* VI. Toxicology, pathology and pharmacology. *J Am Pharm Assoc Sci Educ* 1952; **41**: 298–300.

11 Patnaik GK, Dhawan BN. Pharmacological investigations on asclepin – a new cardenolide from *Asclepius curassavica*. Part I. Cardiotonic activity and acute toxicity. *Arzneimittelforschung* 1978; **28**: 1095–1099.

12 Patnaik GK, Koehler E. Comparative studies on the inotropic and toxic effects of asclepin, g-strophanthin, digoxin and digitoxin. *Arzneimittelforschung* 1978; **28**: 1368–1372.

13 Dhawan BN, Patnaik GK. Investigation on some new cardioactive glycosides. *Indian Drugs* 1985; **22**: 285–290.

14 Del Pilar Alvarez Pellitero M. Pharmacological action of medicinal plants in the nervous system. *An Inst Farmacol Espan* 1971; **20**: 299–387.

15 Koike K *et al*. Potential anticancer agents. V. Cardiac glycosides of *Asclepias albicans* (Asclepiadaceae). *Chem Pharm Bull* 1980; **28**: 401–405.

16 Benson JM *et al*. Comparative toxicology of cardiac glycosides from the milkweed *Asclepias eriocarpa*. *Toxicol Appl Pharmacol* 1977; **41**: 131–132.

Pokeroot

Species (Family)

Phytolacca americana L. (Phytolaccaceae)

Synonym(s)

Phytolacca decandra L., Pocan, Pokeweed, Red Plant

Part(s) Used

Root

Pharmacopoeial and Other Monographs

BHP 1996[G9]
Mills and Bone[G50]
PDR for Herbal Medicines 2nd edition[G36]

Legal Category (Licensed Products)

GSL [G37]

Constituents[G22,G48,G64]

Alkaloids Betalain-type. Betanidine, betanine, isobetanine, isobetanidine, isoprebetanine, phytolaccine and prebetanine.

Lectins Pokeweed mitogen (PWM) consisting of five glycoproteins Pa^{-1} to Pa^{-5}.

Saponins Triterpenes – phytolaccosides A-1, D_2, and O,[1–3] aglycones include phytolaccagenin, jaligonic acid, phytolaccagenic acid, aesculentic acid,[2,4–6] acinosolic acid methyl ester;[5] monodesmosidic and bidesmosidic compounds with oleanolic acid and phytolaccagenic acids as aglycone in *P. dodecandra*.[7]

Other constituents Isoamericanin A (neo-lignan),[8] PAP, pokeweed antiviral protein)[9], α-spinasterol,[5], histamine and gamma aminobutyric acid (GABA).[10]

Food Use

Pokeroot is not commonly used in foods. In the USA, the Herb Trade Association has recommended that pokeroot should not be sold as a herbal beverage or food.[11]

Herbal Use

Pokeroot is stated to possess antirheumatic, anticatarrhal, mild anodyne, emetic, purgative, parasiticidal and fungicidal properties. Traditionally, it has been used for rheumatism, respiratory catarrh, tonsillitis, laryngitis, adenitis, mumps, skin infections (e.g. scabies, tinea, sycosis, acne), mammary abscesses and mastitis.[G7,G64]

Dosage

Dried root 0.06–0.3 g or by decoction three times daily.[G7]

Liquid extract 0.1–0.5 mL (1:1 in 45% alcohol) three times daily.[G7]

Tincture (BPC 1923) 0.2–0.6 mL.

Pharmacological Actions

In vitro and animal studies

Anti-inflammatory activity has been documented for saponin fractions isolated from *P. americana*.[2,12] Activity comparable or greater than that of cortisone acetate was observed in the carageenan rat paw oedema test when the extract was administered by intraperitoneal injection. The major aglycone, phytolaccagenin, was reported to exhibit greater activity than glycyrrhetic acid and oleanolic acid, which are both known to be effective in acute inflammation. Oral administration required a six-fold increase in dose for comparable activity.[12] Potency of the saponin extract was reduced to one-eighth of that of cortisone when tested against chronic inflammation (granuloma pouch method).[12] The ED_{50} for saponin and phytolaccagenin fractions against carrageenan-induced oedema in the rat (intraperitoneal injection) has been determined as 15.1 and 26 mg/kg respectively.[12]

Isoamericanin A (a neo-lignan) isolated from the seeds of *P. americana* has been reported to increase prostaglandin I_2 (PGI_2) production from the rat aorta by up to about 150% at a concentration of 10^{-5} and to elicit a moderate inductive effect on the *in vivo* release of PGI_2.[8]

Hypotensive properties have been described for a pokeroot extract with the activity attributed to histamine and GABA.[10]

A diuretic effect has been described in rats administered pokeroot extract orally at a dose of 500 mg/kg.[13] The effect was reported to be significantly greater than that observed in the saline-treated group of rats, but less than in the frusemide-treated (150 mg/kg) group.

In vitro contraction of the guinea-pig ileum has been described for pokeroot extracts.[14] Activity was attributed to a single active constituent that proved to be heat resistant.

The properties of pokeweed antiviral protein have been reviewed.[15]

Molluscicidal activity against schistosomiasis-transmitting snails and spermicidal activity have been documented for saponin components obtained from the fruits of the related species, *P. dodecandra*.[7,16,17] An enzyme located in the seeds has been found to be necessary for molluscicidal activity of *P. dodecandra*.[18] Crushing the seeds to release the enzyme is critical for activity. The enzyme is inactivated by heat or alcohol and a cold water extraction of the finely ground fruits was found to provide the greatest molluscicidal activity. The saponin-containing extract of *P. dodecandra* is commonly referred to as 'Endod'.[19] Fruits of *P. americana* also possess molluscicidal properties.[G44]

Abortifacient activity in mice has been exhibited by a related species *P. acinosa* Roxb. with activity strongest in the seed and weakest in the leaf. Activity in the various extracts was destroyed by heat and pepsin suggesting a protein to be the active principle.[20]

Side-effects, Toxicity

Haematological aberrations have been observed in human peripheral blood following oral ingestion of the berries or exposure of broken skin/conjunctival membrane to the berry juice.[21–23] Analysis of peripheral blood revealed plasmacytoid cells, dividing cells and mature plasmacytes. Eosinophilia was also noted. The mitogenic principles in pokeroot, lectins, are reported to be a mixture of agglutinating and non-agglutinating glycoproteins affecting both T cell and B cell lymphocytes.[24]

Pokeroot leaf extracts have been reported to be agglutinating, but lacking in mitogenic activity.[25]

A 43-year-old woman suffered the following symptoms 30 minutes after drinking a cup of herbal tea prepared from half a teaspoon of powdered pokeroot: nausea, vomiting, cramping, generalised abdominal pain followed by profound watery diarrhoea, weakness, haematemesis and bloody diarrhoea, hypotension and tachycardia.[26] Chewing the root for the relief of a sore throat and cough has resulted in severe abdominal cramps, protracted vomiting and profuse watery diarrhoea.[27] Additional symptoms of poisoning that have been documented for pokeroot include difficulty with breathing, spasms, severe convulsions and death.[28]

The clinical symptoms of pokeroot poisoning have been reviewed.[27]

All parts of the pokeroot plant are considered as potentially toxic, with the root generally recognised as the most toxic part.[27] Toxicity is reported to increase with plant maturity although the young green berries are more toxic compared to the more mature red fruits.[27]

High doses of saponin extracts have produced thymolytic effects in rats.[12]

LD_{50} values for the saponin fraction (intraperitoneal injection) have been determined as 181 mg/kg in mice and 208 mg/kg in rats.[12] In contrast, no deaths were observed in rats administered phytolaccagenin intraperitoneal injection up to a dose of 2 g/kg.[12] Oral doses of saponin up to 1.5 g/kg did not produce any mortalities in treated rats.[12]

The mutagenic potential of *P. americana* and *P. dodecandra* fruit extracts has been tested using *Salmonella typhimurium* strain TM677.[19] No activity was found for any of the extracts tested.

Contra-indications, Warnings

Fresh pokeroot is poisonous and the dried root emetic and cathartic.[G42] The toxic effects documented following the ingestion of pokeroot make it unsuitable for internal ingestion. In addition, external contact with the berry juice should be avoided: systemic symptoms of toxicity have occurred following exposure of broken skin and conjunctival membranes to the juice.

In 1979, the American Herb Trade Association declared that pokeroot should no longer be sold as a herbal beverage or food.[11] It further recommended that all packages containing pokeroot carry an appropriate warning regarding the potential toxicity of pokeroot when taken internally. In the UK, manufacturers of licensed medicinal products are permitted to include pokeroot provided that the dose is restricted and that suitable evidence is given to demonstrate the absence of the toxic protein constituents.

Pregnancy and lactation Pokeroot is reputed to affect the menstrual cycle and is documented to exhibit uterine stimulant activity in animals.[G30]

Pharmaceutical Comment

Apart from its traditional use as a herbal remedy, pokeroot is also known to possess molluscicidal properties. Anti-inflammatory activity documented in animal studies support the traditional use of pokeroot in rheumatism. However, pokeroot is also recognised as a toxic plant. The effects of pokeroot intoxication arise from the ingestion of any or all plant parts, liquid preparations of plant extracts such as herbal teas, or through skin contact with the plant.[27] The main toxic agents are the pokeweed mitogen (lectins) and the glycoside saponins. The toxic properties of these two classes of compounds, mitogenic and irritant respectively, are well recognised. Excessive use of pokeroot cannot be supported in the light of these known toxicities.

References

See also General References G9, G10, G18, G20, G22, G30, G32, G36, G37, G42, G43, G48, G50 and G64.

1 Woo WS et al. Triterpenoid saponins from the roots of Phytolacca americana. Planta Med 1978; 34: 87–92.
2 Woo WS et al. Constituents of phytolacca species. (I) Anti-inflammatory saponins. Korean J Pharmacog 1976; 7: 47–50.
3 Kang SK, Woo WS. Two new saponins from Phytolacca americana. Planta Med 1987; 53: 338–340.
4 Kang S, Woo WS. Triterpenes from the berries of Phytolacca americana. J Nat Prod 1980; 43: 510–513.
5 Woo WS et al. Constituents of Phytolacca species (II). Comparative examination on constituents of the roots of Phytolacca americana, P. esculenta and P. insularis. Korean J Pharmacog 1975; 7: 51–54.
6 Woo WS, Kang SS. The structure of Phytolaccoside G. Pharm Soc Korea 1977; 21: 159–162.
7 Dorsaz A-C, Hostettmann K. Further saponins from Phytolacca dodecandra l'Herit. Helv Chim Acta 1986; 69: 2038–2047.
8 Hasegawa T et al. Structure of isoamericanin A, a prostaglandin I2 inducer, isolated from the seeds of Phytolacca americana L. Chem Lett 1987; 2: 329–332.
9 Ready MP et al. Extracellular localization of pokeweed antiviral protein. Proc Natl Acad Sci USA 1986; 83: 5033–5056.
10 Funayama S, Hikino H. Hypotensive principles of Phytolacca roots. J Nat Prod 1979; 42: 672–674.
11 Tyler VE et al. Poke root. In: Pharmacognosy, 8th edn. Philadelphia: Lea and Febiger, 1981: 493–494.
12 Woo WS, Shin KH. Antiinflammatory action of Phytolacca saponin. J Pharm Soc Korea 1976; 20: 149–155.
13 Anokbonggo WW. Diuretic effect of an extract from the roots of Phytolacca dodecandra l'Herit in the rat. Biochem Biol 1975; 11: 275–277.
14 Anokbonggo WW. Extraction of pharmacologically active constituents of the roots of Phytolacca dodecandra. Planta Med 1975; 28: 69–75.
15 Irvin JD. Pokeweed antiviral protein. Pharmac Ther 1983; 21: 371–387.
16 Adewunmi CO, Marzuis VO. Comparative evaluation of the molluscicidal properties of aridan (Tetrapleura tetrapleura) laplapa pupa (Jatropha gossypyfolia) endod (Phytolacca dodecandra) and bayluscide. Fitoterapia 1987; 58: 325–328.
17 Dorsaz A-C, Hostettmann K. Further saponins from Phytolacca dodecandra: their molluscicidal and spermicidal properties. Planta Med 1986; 52: 557–558.
18 Parkhurst RM et al. The molluscicidal activity of Phytolacca dodecandra. I. Location of the activating esterase. Biochem Biophys Res Commun 1989; 158: 436–439.
19 Pezzuto JM et al. Evaluation of the mutagenic potential of endod (Phytolacca dodecandra), a molluscicide of potential value for the control of schistosomiasis. Toxicol Lett 1984; 22: 15–20.
20 Yeung HW et al. Abortifacient activity in leaves, roots and seeds of Phytolacca acinosa. J Ethnopharmacol 1987; 21: 31–35.
21 Barker BE et al. Haematological effects of pokeweed. Lancet 1967; i: 437.
22 Barker BE et al. Peripheral blood plasmacytosis following systemic exposure to Phytolacca americana (pokeweed). Pediatrics 1966; 38: 490–493.
23 Barker BE et al. Mitogenic activity in Phytolacca americana (pokeweed). Lancet 1965; i: 170.
24 McPherson A. Pokeweed and other lymphocyte mitogens. In: Kinghorn AD, ed. Toxic Plants. New York: Columbia University Press, 1979: 84–102.
25 Downing HJ et al. Plant agglutinins and mitosis. Nature 1968; 217: 655.
26 Lewis WH, Smith PR. Pokeroot herbal tea poisoning. JAMA 1979; 242: 2759–2760.
27 Roberge R et al. The root of evil – poke weed intoxication. Ann Emerg Med 1986; 15: 470–473.
28 Hardin JW, Arena JM. Human Poisoning from Native and Cultivated Plants, 2nd edn. Durham: Duke University Press, 1974: 69–73.

Poplar

Species (Family)

Populus tremuloides Michx. (Salicaceae)

Synonym(s)

Populus Alba, Quaking Aspen, White Poplar

Part(s) Used

Bark

Pharmacopoeial and Other Monographs

BHP 1996[G9]
Complete German Commission E[G3]
Martindale 32nd edition[G43]
PDR for Herbal Medicines 2nd edition[G36]

Legal Category (Licensed Products)

GSL[G37]

Constituents[G6,G39,G40,G64]

Glycosides Salicin (about 2.4%), salicortin, salireposide and various benzoate derivatives including populin (salicin-6-benzoate), tremuloidin (salicin-2-benzoate) and tremulacin (salicortin-2-benzoate).

Other constituents Tannins (unspecified), triterpenes including α-amyrin and β-amyrin, carbohydrates including glucose, fructose and various trisaccharides, fats, waxes.

Food Use

Poplar is listed by the Council of Europe as a natural source of food flavouring (category N2). This category indicates that poplar can be added to foodstuffs in small quantities, with a possible limitation of an active principle (as yet unspecified) in the final product.[G16] In the USA, poplar is permitted for use in foods.[G65]

Herbal Use

Poplar is stated to possess antirheumatic, anti-inflammatory, antiseptic, astringent, anodyne and chola-gogue properties. Traditionally, it has been used for muscular and arthrodial rheumatism, cystitis, diarrhoea, anorexia with stomach or liver disorders, common cold, and specifically for rheumatoid arthritis.[G6,G7,G64]

The buds of *Populus tremula* (European white poplar, aspen) and *Populus nigra* (black poplar) are used, reputedly as expectorant and circulatory stimulant remedies, for upper respiratory tract infections and rheumatic conditions.[G49]

Dosage

Dried bark 1–4 g or by decoction three times daily.[G6,G7]

Liquid extract 1–4 mL (1 : 1 in 25% alcohol) three times daily.[G6,G7]

Pharmacological Actions

In vitro and animal studies

None documented for poplar. *See* Willow for the pharmacological actions associated with salicylates.

Clinical studies

None documented for poplar. The pharmacological actions of salicylates in humans are well documented and are applicable to poplar. Salicin is a prodrug that is metabolised to saligenin in the gastrointestinal tract and to salicylic acid following absorption.

Side-effects, Toxicity

None documented. *See* Willow for side-effects and toxicity associated with salicylates.

Contra-indications, Warnings

See Willow for contra-indications and warnings associated with salicylates.

Pregnancy and lactation The safety of poplar taken during pregnancy has not been established. *See*

Willow for contra-indications and warnings regarding the use of salicylates during pregnancy and lactation.

Pharmaceutical Comment

The chemistry of poplar is characterised by the phenolic glycoside components, which support some of the reputed herbal uses. The usual precautions associated with other salicylate-containing drugs are applicable to poplar.

References

See General References G3, G6, G9, G16, G31, G36, G37, G39, G40, G43, G49 and G64.

Prickly Ash, Northern

Species (Family)

Zanthoxylum americanum Miller (Rutaceae)

Synonym(s)

Toothache Bark, Xanthoxylum, Zanthoxylum

Part(s) Used

Bark, berry

Pharmacopoeial and Other Monographs

BHP 1983[G7]
Martindale 32nd edition[G43]
PDR for Herbal Medicines 2nd edition[G36]

Legal Category (Licensed Products)

Northern prickly ash is not included in the GSL.[G37]

Constituents[G6,G41,G64]

Alkaloids Isoquinoline-type. Lauriflorine and nitidine (major constituents), candicine, chelerythrine, magnoflorine and tembetarine.

Coumarins Xanthyletin, xanthoxyletin, alloxanthoxyletin and 8-(3,3-dimethylallyl)alloxanthoxyletin.

Other constituents Resins, tannins and acrid volatile oil.

Other plant parts Two furoquinoline alkaloids (γ-fagarine and skimmianine) have been isolated from the leaves.

Food Use

Prickly ash is listed by the Council of Europe as a natural source of food flavouring (category N3). This category indicates that prickly ash can be added to foodstuffs in the traditionally accepted manner, but that there is insufficient information available for an adequate assessment of potential toxicity.[G16] In the USA, prickly ash is listed as GRAS (Generally Recognised As Safe).[G65]

Herbal Use

Prickly ash is stated to possess circulatory stimulant, diaphoretic, antirheumatic, carminative and sialagogue properties. Traditionally, it has been used for cramps, intermittent claudication, Raynaud's syndrome, chronic rheumatic conditions, and specifically for peripheral circulatory insufficiency associated with rheumatic symptoms. The berries are stated to be therapeutically more active in circulatory disorders.[G6,G7,G64]

Dosage

Dried bark 1–3 g or by decoction three times daily.[G6,G7]

Bark, liquid extract 1–3 mL (1:1 in 45% alcohol) three times daily.[G6,G7]

Bark, tincture 2–5 mL (1:5 in 45% alcohol) three times daily.[G6,G7]

Dried berry 0.5–1.5 g.[G6,G7]

Berry, liquid extract 0.5–1.5 mL (1:1 in 45% alcohol).[G6,G7]

Pharmacological Actions

In vitro and animal studies

None documented for northern prickly ash. *See* Southern Prickly Ash for activities of alkaloid constituents (e.g. chelerythrine and nitidine).

Side-effects, Toxicity

The alkaloid constituents are potentially toxic (*see* Southern Prickly Ash).

Contra-indications, Warnings

Excessive ingestion may interfere with anticoagulant therapy in view of the coumarin constituents (*see* Southern Prickly Ash).

Pregnancy and lactation The safety of northern prickly ash has not been established. In view of the pharmacologically active constituents the use of northern prickly ash during pregnancy and lactation should be avoided.

Pharmaceutical Comment

Northern prickly ash contains similar alkaloid constituents to the southern species but varies with respect to other documented components. No pharmacological studies documented specifically for northern prickly ash were located. However, activities have been reported for individual alkaloid constituents and the monograph for southern prickly ash should be consulted. There is limited scientific evidence to support the traditional herbal uses. In view of the pharmacologically active constituents and potential toxicity associated with the alkaloids, excessive use of northern prickly ash should be avoided.

References

See General References G6, G7, G10, G16, G31, G36, G37, G41, G43 and G64.

Prickly Ash, Southern

Species (Family)

Zanthoxylum clava-herculis L. (Rutaceae)

Synonym(s)

Toothache Bark, Xanthoxylum, Zanthoxylum

Part(s) Used

Bark, berry

Pharmacopoeial and Other Monographs

BHC 1992[G6]
BHP 1996[G9]
Martindale 32nd edition[G43]

Legal Category (Licensed Products)

GSL[G37]

Constituents[G6,G41,G45,G64]

Alkaloids Isoquinoline-type. Chelerythrine and magnoflorine (major constituents), candicine, lauriflorine, nitidine, N-acetylanonaine[1] and tembetarine.

Amides Cinnamamide, herculin and neoherculin.

Lignans (−)-Asarinin, (−)-sesamin, γ,γ-dimethylallyl ether of (−)-pluviatilol.[1]

Other constituents Resins, tannins and an acrid volatile oil (about 3.3%).

Food Use

Southern prickly ash is listed by the Council of Europe as a natural source of food flavouring (category N3). This category indicates that prickly ash can be added to foodstuffs in the traditionally accepted manner, but that there is insufficient information available for an adequate assessment of potential toxicity.[G16]

Herbal Use

Southern prickly ash is stated to possess circulatory stimulant, diaphoretic, antirheumatic, carminative and sialogogue properties. Traditionally, it has been used for cramps, intermittent claudication, Raynaud's syndrome, chronic rheumatic conditions, and specifically for peripheral circulatory insufficiency associated with rheumatic symptoms. The berries are stated to be therapeutically more active in circulatory disorders.[G6,G7,G8,G64]

Dosage

Dried bark 1–3 g or by decoction three times daily.[G6,G7]

Bark, liquid extract 1–3 mL (1:1 in 45% alcohol) three times daily.[G6,G7]

Bark, tincture 2–5 mL (1:5 in 45% alcohol) three times daily.[G6,G7]

Dried berry 0.5–1.5 g.[G6,G7]

Berry, liquid extract 0.5–1.5 mL (1:1 in 45% alcohol).[G6,G7]

Pharmacological Actions

In vitro and animal studies

Southern prickly ash has been reported to act as a reversible neuromuscular blocking agent. Activity was associated with a neutral fraction of the bark that was thought to act primarily by blockade of endplate receptors.[2]

Various activities have been documented for the benzophenanthridine alkaloids (e.g. chelerythrine, nitidine) present in southern prickly ash. Hypotensive properties in mice have been documented for nitidine chloride, a single dose of 2 mg/kg body weight lowered the blood pressure by 20% within 90 minutes and persisted for 6 hours.[3] Nitidine was also found to antagonise the effects of angiotensin-induced hypertension.[3] Antileukaemic activity has been documented for nitidine, although preclinical toxicity prevented further investigations.[4,5] Anti-inflammatory activity in rats has been documented for chelerythrine (10 mg/kg by mouth) comparable to that achieved with indomethacin (5 mg/kg by mouth).[6] Chelerythrine has also been reported to potentiate the analgesic effect of morphine, prolong barbiturate-induced sleep, and cause temporary hypertension followed by hypotension in cats, mice and rabbits.[7]

Significant antimicrobial activity towards Gram-positive bacteria and *Candida albicans* has been documented for chelerythrine, although conflicting activities have been reported regarding Gram-negative bacteria.[6] Chelerythrine has been shown to interact with Na^+K^+ ATPase and to inhibit hepatic L-alanine and L-aspartate aminotransferases in the rat, while nitidine has been reported to inhibit tRNA methyltransferase and catechol-O-methyltransferase.[5]

The lignan component, asarinin, has been reported to possess antitubercular activity.[G41] Neoherculin is reported to possess insecticidal and sialogogic properties.[1]

Pharmacological activities, including anti-inflammatory, cardiovascular and antibacterial properties have been documented for various other *Zanthoxylum* species (or *Fagara/Xanthoxylum* species).[5] For example, the root of *Zanthoxylum zanthoxyloides*, a Nigerian species, is commonly used as a chewing stick. These sticks are believed to possess antimicrobial properties and extracts were found to exhibit antimicrobial activity towards more than 20 organisms, including Gram-positive and Gram-negative bacteria, and *Candida* species.[5] Anti-inflammatory activity (carrageenan rat paw oedema test) has been described for fagaramide (piperonyl-4-acrylic isobutylamide), isolated from *Z. zanthoxyloides*.[8] The activity, approximately 20 times less potent than indomethacin, was thought to be partially mediated by inhibition of prostaglandin synthesis.[8]

The essential oil obtained from the Indian species *Zanthoxylum limonella* has been reported to exhibit *in vitro* anthelmintic activity against earthworms, tapeworms and hookworms that was stated to be superior to that of piperazine phosphate.[9]

Side-effects, Toxicity

None documented in humans. Ingestion of southern prickly ash by cattle, chicken and fish has proved lethal. This was attributed to the neuromuscular blocking properties of the bark.[2] Neoherculin is reported to be the major ichthyotoxic principle in an extract of southern prickly ash bark.

The acute and chronic toxicity of chelerythrine in mice is reported to be low.[4] LD_{50} values were stated as 18.5 mg/kg body weight (intravenous injection) and 95 mg/kg (subcutaneous injection). Oral administration of 10 mg/kg for three days followed by 5 mg/kg for seven days produced no adverse effects.

Contra-indications, Warnings

None documented for southern prickly ash. Chelerythrine has been reported to interact with Na^+K^+ ATPase which may interfere with cardiac glycoside therapy. However the clinical relevance of this with respect to prickly ash is unknown. Hypotensive and sedative activities have been documented in animals. Both chelerythrine and nitidine have been reported to inhibit various hepatic enzymes (*see In vitro* and animal studies). The alkaloid constituents in southern prickly ash are potentially toxic.

Pregnancy and lactation The safety of southern prickly ash has not been established. In view of this and the pharmacologically active compounds, the use of southern prickly ash during pregnancy and lactation is best avoided.

Pharmaceutical Comment

The chemistry of southern prickly ash is well documented and particularly characterised by the alkaloid constituents. Limited pharmacological information has been documented for southern prickly ash, although several properties have been described for individual constituents. With the exception of anti-inflammatory and analgesic properties few data have been documented that support the herbal uses. Limited toxicity data are available and some benzophenanthridine alkaloids are associated with cytotoxicity. In view of this, excessive use of prickly ash should be avoided. Northern prickly ash has been used for similar herbal uses but has a different chemical composition compared to the southern species (*see* Northern Prickly Ash).

References

See also General References G6, G9, G10, G16, G31, G37, G41, G43 and G64.

1 Rao KV, Davies R. The ichthyotoxic principles of *Zanthoxylum clava-herculis. J Nat Prod* 1986; **49**: 340–342.
2 Bowen JM, Cole RJ. Neuromuscular blocking properties of southern prickly ash toxin. *Fedn Proc* 1981; **40**: 696.
3 Addae-Mensah I *et al.* Structure and anti-hypertensive properties of nitidine chloride from *Fagara* species. *Planta Med* 1986; **52**(Suppl.): 58.
4 Krane BD *et al.* The benzophenanthridine alkaloids. *J Nat Prod* 1984; **47**: 1–43.
5 Simánek V. Benzophenanthridine alkaloids. In: Brossi A, ed. *The Alkaloids*, vol 26. New York: Academic Press, 1985: 185–240.
6 Lenfield J *et al.* Antiinflammatory activity of

quaternary benzophenanthridine alkaloids from *Chelidonium majus*. *Planta Med* 1981; **43**: 161–165.

7 Preininger V. In: Manske RHF, ed. *The Alkaloids*, vol 15. New York: Academic Press, 1975: 242.

8 Oriowo MA. Anti-inflammatory activity of piper-onyl-4-acrylic isobutyl amide, an extractive from *Zanthoxylum zanthoxyloides*. *Planta Med* 1982; **44**: 54–56.

9 Kalyani GA *et al*. *In vitro* anthelmintic acitivity of essential oil from the fruits of *Zanthoxylum limonella*. *Fitoterapia* 1989; **60**: 160–162.

Pulsatilla

Species (Family)

(i) *Anemone pulsatilla* L. (Ranunculaceae)
(ii) *Anemone pratensis* L.
(iii) *Anemone patens* L.

Synonym(s)

Pasque Flower, *Pulsatilla nigrans*

Part(s) Used

Herb

Pharmacopoeial and Other Monographs

BHC 1992[G6]
BHP 1996[G9]
Martindale 32nd edition[G43]
PDR for Herbal Medicines 2nd edition[G36]

Legal Category (Licensed Products)

GSL[G37]

Constituents[G6,G22,G48,G64]

Flavonoids Delphinidin and pelargonidin glycosides.

Saponins Hederagenin (as the aglycone).

Volatile oils Ranunculin (a glycoside); enzymatic hydrolysis yields the unstable lactone protoanemonin which readily dimerises to anemonin.

Other constituents Carbohydrates (e.g. arabinose, fructose, galactose, glucose, rhamnose), triterpenes (e.g. β-amyrin) and β-sitosterol.

Food Use

Pulsatilla is not used in foods.

Herbal Use

Pulsatilla is stated to possess sedative, analgesic, antispasmodic and bactericidal properties. Traditionally, it has been used for dysmenorrhoea, orchitis, ovaralgia, epididymitis, tension headache, hyperactive states, insomnia, boils, skin eruptions associated with bacterial infection, asthma and pulmonary disease, earache, and specifically for painful conditions of the male or female reproductive system.[G6,G7,G8,G64] Pulsatilla is widely used in homeopathic preparations as well as in herbal medicine.

Dosage

Dried herb 0.12–0.3 g by infusion or decoction three times daily.[G6,G7]

Liquid extract 0.12–0.3 mL (1 : 1 in 25% alcohol) three times daily.[G6,G7]

Tincture 0.3–1.0 mL (1 : 10 in 40% alcohol) three times daily.[G6,G7]

Pharmacological Actions

In vitro and animal studies

Utero-activity (stimulant and depressant) has been documented for pulsatilla.[1,2,G30] *In vivo* sedative and antipyretic properties in rodents have been documented for anemonin and protoanemonin.[3]

Cytotoxicity (KB tumour system) has been reported for anemonin.[G22]

Side-effects, Toxicity

Fresh pulsatilla is poisonous because of the toxic volatile oil component, protoanemonin. Protoanemonin rapidly degrades to the non-toxic anemonin. Inhalation of vapour from the volatile oil may cause irritation of the nasal mucosa and conjunctiva.[G51] Allergic reactions to pulsatilla have been documented and patch tests have produced vesicular reactions with hyperpigmentation.[G51] Cytotoxicity has been documented for anemonin (*see In vitro* and animal studies).

Contra-indications, Warnings

Fresh pulsatilla is poisonous and should not be ingested. External contact with the fresh plant should be avoided. The toxic principle, protoanemonin, rapidly degrades to the non-toxic anemonin during drying of the plant material. Individuals may experience an allergic reaction to pulsatilla, especially those with an existing hypersensitivity.

Pregnancy and lactation Pulsatilla is reputed to affect the menstrual cycle.[G22] Utero-activity has been documented for pulsatilla (*see In vitro* and animal studies). In view of this, the use of pulsatilla during pregnancy should be avoided. Excessive ingestion is best avoided during lactation.

Pharmaceutical Comment

Pulsatilla is widely used in both herbal and homeopathic preparations, although little documented chemical and pharmacological information is available to assess its true benefit. The fresh plant is known to be irritant; it contains a toxic principle (protoanemonin) and should not be ingested. The dried plant material is not considered to be toxic.

References

See also General References G6, G9, G10, G22, G30, G31, G36, G37, G43, G48, G51 and G64.

1 Pilcher JM *et al*. The action of the so-called female remedies on the excised uterus of the guinea-pig. *Arch Intern Med* 1916; **18**: 557–583.
2 Pilcher JM *et al*. The action of 'female remedies' on intact uteri of animals. *Surg Gynecol Obstet* 1918; **18**: 97–99.
3 Martin ML *et al*. Pharmacological effects of lactones isolated from *Pulsatilla alpina* subsp. *apiifolia. J Ethnopharmacol* 1988; **24**: 185–191.

Quassia

Species (Family)

(i) *Picrasma excelsa* (Sw.) Planch. (Simaroubaceae)
(ii) *Quassia amara* L.

Synonym(s)

Bitterwood, Picrasma
(i) Jamaican Quassia, *Picraena excelsa* Lindl.
(ii) Surinam Quassia

Part(s) Used

Stem wood

Pharmacopoeial and Other Monographs

BHC 1992[G6]
BHP 1996[G9]
Martindale 32nd edition[G43]
PDR for Herbal Medicines 2nd edition[G36]

Legal Category (Licensed Products)

GSL[G37]

Constituents[G2,G6,G22,G41,G64]

Alkaloids Indole-type. Canthin-6-one, 5-methoxy-canthin-6-one, 4-methoxy-5-hydroxycanthin-6-one, N-methoxy-1-vinyl-β-carboline.[1,2]

Terpenoids Isoquassin (picrasmin) in *P. excelsa*, quassin 0.2%, quassinol, quassimarin,[3] 18-hydroxyquassin, neoquassin, a dihydronorneoquassin[4] and simalikalactone D in *Q. amara*.

Coumarins Scopoletin.[1]

Other constituents β-Sitosterol, β-sitostenone; thiamine 1.8% (in *P. excelsa*).

Food Use

Quassia is listed by the Council of Europe as a natural source of food flavouring (category N2). This category indicates that quassia can be added to foodstuffs in small quantities, although the concentration of quassin must not exceed 5 mg/kg; a concentration of 50 mg/kg is permitted in alcoholic beverages and 10 mg/kg in pastilles and lozenges.[G16] In the USA, quassia is regarded by the Food and Drugs Administration (FDA) as GRAS (Generally Regarded As Safe).

Herbal Use

Quassia is stated to possess bitter, orexigenic, sialogogue, gastric stimulant and anthelmintic properties. Traditionally, it has been used for anorexia, dyspepsia, nematode infestation (by oral or rectal administration), pediculosis (by topical application), and specifically for atonic dyspepsia with loss of appetite.[G2,G6,G7,G8,G64]

Dosage

Dried wood 0.3–0.6 g or by cold infusion three times daily.[G6,G7]

Concentrated Quassia Infusion (BPC 1959) 2–4 mL. Quassia Infusion is prepared by diluting one volume of Concentrated Quassia Infusion to eight volumes with water.

Tincture of Quassia (BP 1948) 2–4 mL.

Enema 150 mL per rectum (infusion with cold water, 1 in 20) on three successive mornings together with 16 g magnesium sulfate by mouth.

Pharmacological Actions

The quassinoids are reported to possess bitter properties 50 times greater than quinine.[G22]

In vitro and animal studies

The β-carboline alkaloids have exhibited positive inotropic activity *in vitro*.[1] Canthin-6-one is reported to possess antibacterial and antifungal activity. Cytotoxic and amoebicidal activities (assessed against guinea-pig keratinocyte and *Entamoeba histolytica* test systems, respectively) have been documented for canthin-6-one and quassin (*P. excelsa*).[5] However, later studies have disputed any amoebicidal action. Quassin is reported to be inactive against P388 leukaemia and 9KB test systems. Significant antitumour activity in mice against the P388 lymphatic leukaemia and *in vitro* against human carcinoma of the nasopharynx (KB) has been documented.[3] Quassimarin and simalikalactone were both isolated from the active extract.

Clinical studies

The successful treatment of 454 patients with head-lice has been documented for quassia tincture.[6] Quassia has been used as an enema to expel thread-worms.[G44]

Side-effects, Toxicity

No side-effects have been reported in 454 patients who used quassia tincture as a scalp lotion to treat headlice.[6] Large doses of quassia may irritate the stomach and cause vomiting.[G6]

Contra-indications, Warnings

Excessive doses may interfere with existing cardiac and anticoagulant therapies. However, the coumarin concentrations in quassia are not thought to pose a hazard. In addition, large doses of quassia are emetic and therefore excessive consumption is self-limiting.

Pregnancy and lactation   In view of the reported cytotoxic and emetic activities, the use of quassia during pregnancy and lactation is best avoided.

Pharmaceutical Comment

The chemistry of quassia is well studied and is characterised by bitter terpenoids (quassinoids) and β-carboline indole alkaloids. Limited data have been documented to justify the traditional herbal uses although the bitter principles support the use of quassia as an appetite stimulant in anorexia. However, in view of the documented cytotoxic activities and limited toxicological data, quassia in herbal remedies should not be taken in amounts greatly exceeding those used in foods.

References

See also General References G2, G6, G9, G12, G16, G22, G29, G36, G37, G41, G43, G56 and G64.

1   Wagner H *et al.* New constituents of *Picrasma excelsa*, I. *Planta Med* 1979; **36**: 113–118.
2   Wagner H, Nestler T. *N*-Methoxy-1-vinyl-β-carbolin, ein neues Alkaloid aus *Picrasma excelsa* (Swartz) Planchon. *Tetrahedron Lett* 1978; **31**: 2777–2778.
3   Kupchan SM, Streelman DR. Quassimarin, a new antileukemic quassinoid from *Quassia amara*. *J Org Chem* 1976; **41**: 3481–3482.
4   Grandolini G *et al.* A new neoquassin derivative from *Quassia amara*. *Phytochemistry* 1987; **26**: 3085–3087.
5   Harris A, Phillipson JD. Cytotoxic and amoebicidal compounds from *Picrasma excelsa* (Jamaican Quassia). *J Pharm Pharmacol* 1982; **34**: 43P.
6   Jensen O *et al.* Pediculosis capitis treated with quassia tincture. *Acta Dermat Venereol (Stockholm)* 1978; **58**: 557–559.

Queen's Delight

Species (Family)

Stillingia sylvatica L. (Euphorbiaceae)

Synonym(s)

Queen's Root, Stillingia, *Stillingia treculeana* (Muell. Arg.) Johnst., Yaw Root

Part(s) Used

Root

Pharmacopoeial and Other Monographs

BHP 1996[G9]
PDR for Herbal Medicines 2nd edition[G36]

Legal Category (Licensed Products)

GSL[G37]

Constituents[G41,G48,G64]

Terpenoids Eight compounds, termed stillingia factors S_1–S_8, have been isolated and identified as daphnane-type and tigliane-type esters carrying saturated, polyunsaturated or hydroxylated fatty acids.[1]

Other constituents Volatile oil 3–4%, fixed oil, acrid resin (sylvacrol), resinic acid, stillingine (a glycoside) and tannin.

Other plant parts Hydrocyanic acid (leaf and stem).[1]

Food Use

Queen's delight is not used in foods.

Herbal Use

Queen's delight is stated to possess sialogogue, expectorant, diaphoretic, dermatological, astringent, antispasmodic and, in large doses, cathartic properties. Traditionally, it has been used for bronchitis, laryngitis, laryngismus stridulus, cutaneous eruptions, haemorrhoids, constipation and specifically for exudative skin eruption with irritation and lymphatic involvement, and laryngismus stridulus.[G7,G64]

Dosage

Dried root 1–2 g or by decoction three times daily.[G7]

Liquid extract 0.5–2.0 mL (1 : 1 in 25% alcohol) three times daily.[G7]

Tincture 1–4 mL (1 : 5 in 45% alcohol) three times daily.[G7]

Pharmacological Actions

None documented.

Side-effects, Toxicity

Overdose of queen's delight is reported to cause vertigo, burning sensation of the mouth, throat and gastrointestinal tract, diarrhoea, nausea and vomiting, dysuria, aches and pains, pruritus and skin eruptions, cough, depression, fatigue and perspiration.[G22] The diterpene esters are toxic irritant principles known to cause swelling and inflammation of the skin and mucous membranes.[1,G33]

The leaves and stem are documented to be toxic to sheep because of the hydrocyanic acid content.[2]

Contra-indications, Warnings

In view of the irritant nature of the diterpene esters, queen's delight may cause irritation to the mucous membranes. It is stated that queen's delight should be used with care, and never taken in large doses.[G49] It is recommended that the root should not be used after two years of storage.[G49]

Pregnancy and lactation In view of the irritant and potentially toxic constituents, the use of queen's delight during pregnancy and lactation should be avoided.

Pharmaceutical Comment

The Euphorbiaceae plant family is characterised by the diterpene esters. These compounds, known as phorbol, ingenane or daphnane esters depending on their skeleton type, have been investigated as constituents of genera such as *Euphorbia* and *Croton*, and some of them have been found to be cocarcinogenic and highly irritant to mucous membranes.[G33] No scientific evidence was found to justify the reputed herbal uses. In view of this and the potential toxicity of queen's delight excessive use is not recommended.

References

See also General References G9, G10, G22, G33, G36, G37, G41, G48, G49 and G64.

1   Adolf W, Hecker E. New irritant diterpene-esters from roots of *Stillingia sylvatica* L. (Euphorbiaceae). *Tetrahedron Lett* 1980; **21**: 2887–2890.
2   Lewis WH, Elvin-Lewis MPF. *Medical Botany*. New York: Wiley Interscience, 1977.

Raspberry

Species (Family)

Rubus idaeus L. (Rosaceae)

Synonym(s)

Rubus

Part(s) Used

Leaf

Pharmacopoeial and Other Monographs

BHP 1996[G9]
Martindale 32nd edition[G43]
PDR for Herbal Medicines 2nd edition[G36]

Legal Category (Licensed Products)

GSL[G37]

Constituents[G2,G59,G62,G64]

Limited phytochemical information is available for raspberry. Documented constituents include acids, polypeptides, tannins and flavonoids (e.g. rutin).[1]

Food Use

Both the leaf and fruit are listed by the Council of Europe as natural sources of food flavouring (categories N2 and N1, respectively). Category N2 allows the addition of the leaf to foodstuffs in small quantities, with a possible limitation of an active principle (as yet unspecified) in the final product. Category N1 indicates that no restrictions apply to the fruit.[G16] Raspberry fruit is commonly used in foods.

Herbal Use

Raspberry is stated to possess astringent and *partus praeparator* properties. Traditionally, it has been used for diarrhoea, pregnancy, stomatitis, tonsillitis (as a mouthwash), conjunctivitis (as an eye lotion), and specifically to facilitate parturition.[G2,G7,G64]

Dosage

Dried leaf 4–8 g or by infusion three times daily.[G7]

Liquid extract 4–8 mL (1:1 in 25% alcohol) three times daily.[G7]

Pharmacological Actions

In vitro and animal studies

Utero-activity has been documented for a leaf infusion in both pregnant and non-pregnant rat and human uteri.[2] The extract was reported to have little or no effect on the uterine strips from non-pregnant rats, but inhibited contractions of those from pregnant rats. Similarly, the extract had no effect on strips from non-pregnant human uteri, but initiated contractions in strips from human uteri at 10–16 weeks of pregnancy. The intrinsic rhythm of the uteri in which a pharmacological effect was observed (pregnant rat and human uteri) was reported to become more regular, with contractions, in most cases, less frequent.[2] Aqueous extracts of raspberry leaves have been reported to contain a number of active constituents, including a smooth muscle stimulant, an anticholinesterase, and an antispasmodic that antagonised the stimulant actions of the two previous fractions. The smooth muscle stimulant fraction was more potent towards uterine muscle.[3]

Hypoglycaemic activity has been documented for a related species, *Rubus fructicosus* L., in both non-diabetic and diabetic (glucose-induced and alloxan-induced) rabbits.[4] Greatest activity was observed in the glucose-induced diabetic rabbits. The authors concluded that *R. fructicosus* possesses slight hypoglycaemic activity, which, in part, results from an increase in the liberation of insulin. Tannins are known to possess astringent properties.

In vitro antiviral activity documented for raspberry fruit extract has been attributed to the phenolic constituents, in particular to tannic acid.[5]

Side-effects, Toxicity

None documented.

Contra-indications, Warnings

The excessive ingestion of tannins is not recommended. Hypoglycaemic activity *in vivo* has been documented for a related species.

Pregnancy and lactation Raspberry is traditionally recommended for use during labour to help ease parturition. Animal studies (*in vitro*) have reported that raspberry can reduce and initiate uterine contractions. In view of this, raspberry should not be used during pregnancy and, if taken during labour, should only be done so under medical supervision.

Pharmaceutical Comment

Limited phytochemical information is available for raspberry leaf. However, the documented presence of tannin constituents supports some of the reputed herbal uses, although it is unsuitable to use as a herbal remedy to treat eye infections such as conjunctivitis. Raspberry leaf is widely recommended to be taken during pregnancy to help facilitate easier parturition. Utero-activity has been documented for raspberry leaf and in view of this it should not be taken during pregnancy, unless under medical supervision.

References

See also General References G2, G9, G11, G16, G31, G32, G36, G37, G43, G59, G62 and G64.

1   Khabibullaeva LA, Khalmatov KK. Phytochemical study of raspberry leaves. *Mater Yubileinoi Resp Nauchn Konf Farm Posvyashch* 1972; Sept: 101–102.
2   Bamford DS *et al*. Raspberry leaf tea: a new aspect to an old problem. *Br J Pharmacol* 1970; **40**: 161–162P.
3   Beckett AH *et al*. The active constituents of raspberry leaves. A preliminary investigation. *J Pharm Pharmacol* 1954; **6**: 785–796.
4   Alonso R *et al*. A preliminary study of hypoglycaemic activity of *Rubus fruticosus*. *Planta Med* 1980; **40**(Suppl.): 102–106.
5   Konowalchuk JK, Speirs JI. Antiviral activity of fruit extracts. *J Food Sci* 1976; **41**: 1013–1017.

Red Clover

Species (Family)

Trifolium pratense L. (Leguminosae)

Synonym(s)

Cow Clover, Meadow Clover, Purple Clover, Trefoil

Part(s) Used

Flowerhead

Pharmacopoeial and Other Monographs

BHC 1992[G6]
BHP 1996[G9]
Martindale 32nd edition[G43]
PDR for Herbal Medicines 2nd edition[G36]

Legal Category (Licensed Products)

GSL[G37]

Constituents[G6,G22,G41,G64]

Carbohydrates Arabinose, glucose, glucuronic acid, rhamnose, xylose (following hydrolysis of saponin glycosides); polysaccharide (a galactoglucomannan).

Coumarins Coumarin, medicagol.

Isoflavonoids Biochanin A, daidzein, formononetin, genistein, pratensin, trifoside, calycosine galactoside[1] and pectolinarin.

Flavonoids Isorhamnetin, kaempferol, quercetin, and their glycosides.[2]

Saponins Soyasapogenols B–F (C–F artefacts) and carbohydrates (*see above*) yielded by acid hydrolysis.[3]

Other constituents Coumaric acid, phaseolic acid, salicylic acid, *trans*- and *cis*-clovamide (L-dopa conjugated with *trans*- and *cis*-caffeic acids), resin, volatile oil (containing furfural),[4] fats, vitamins and minerals. Cyanogenetic glycosides have been

documented for a related species, *Trifolium repens*.[G33]

Food Use

Red clover is listed by the Council of Europe as a natural source of food flavouring (category N2). This category indicates that it can be added to foodstuffs in small quantities, with a possible limitation of an active principle (as yet unspecified) in the final product.[G16] In the USA, red clover is listed as GRAS (Generally Recognised As Safe).[G65]

Herbal Use

Red clover is stated to act as a dermatological agent, and to possess mildly antispasmodic and expectorant properties. Tannins are known to possess astringent properties. Traditionally red clover has been used for chronic skin disease, whooping cough, and specifically for eczema and psoriasis.[G6,G7,G8,G64]

Dosage

Dried flowerhead 4 g or by infusion three times daily.[G6,G7]

Liquid extract 1.5–3.0 mL (1 : 1 in 25% alcohol) three times daily.[G6,G7]

Tincture 1–2 mL (1 : 10 in 45% alcohol) three times daily.[G6,G7]

Pharmacological Actions

In vitro and animal studies

Biochanin A, formononetin, and genistein (isofla-oestrogenic properties.[5] The saponin constituents are reported to lack any haemolytic or fungistatic activity.[3] A possible chemoprotective effect has been documented for biochanin A, which has been reported to inhibit carcinogenic activity in cell culture.[6]

Side-effects, Toxicity

Urticarial reactions have been documented.[G51] Infertility and growth disorders have been reported in grazing animals.[G33] These effects have been attributed to the oestrogenic isoflavone constituents, in particular to formononetin.[5]

Contra-indications, Warnings

In view of the oestrogenic constituents, excessive ingestion should be avoided. Large doses may interfere with anticoagulant and hormonal therapies (coumarin and isoflavonoid constituents).

Pregnancy and lactation In view of the oestrogenic components the use of red clover during pregnancy and lactation should be avoided.

Pharmaceutical Comment

The chemistry of red clover is well documented. Limited information is available on the pharmacological properties and no documented scientific evidence was found to justify the herbal uses. Reported oestrogenic side-effects in grazing animals have been attributed to the isoflavone constituents. Little toxicity data are available for red clover. In view of this and the isoflavone and coumarin components, excessive ingestion should be avoided.

References

See also General References G6, G9, G16, G22, G31, G32, G33, G36, G41, G43, G51 and G64.

1 Saxena VK, Jain AK. A new isoflavone glycoside from *Trifolium pratense*. *Fitoterapia* 1987; **58**: 262–263.
2 Jain AK, Saxena VK. Isolation and characterisation of 3-methoxyquercetin 7-O-β-D-glucopyranoside from *Trifolium pratense*. *Natl Acad Sci Lett* **9**: 379–380.
3 Olesek WA, Jurzysta M. Isolation, chemical characterization and biological activity of red clover (*Trifolium pratense* L.) root saponins. *Acta Soc Bot Pol* 1986; **55**: 247–252.
4 Opdyke DLJ. Furfural. *Food Cosmet Toxicol* 1978; **16**: 759–764.
5 Kelly RW *et al.* Formononetin content of 'Grasslands Pawera' red clover and its oestrogenic activity to sheep. *NZ J Exp Agric* 1979; **7**: 131–134.
6 Cassady JM *et al.* Use of a mammalian cell culture benzo(*a*)pyrene metabolism assay for the detection of potential anticarcinogens from natural products: inhibition of metabolism by biochanin A, an isoflavone from *Trifolium pratense* L. *Cancer Res* 1988; **48**: 6257–6261.

Rhubarb

Species (Family)

Rheum officinale Baill. and *R. palmatum* L. (Poly-

Synonym(s)

Chinese Rhubarb, other *Rheum* species, e.g. *Rheum tanguticum* Maxim. & Reg., *Rheum emodi* Wall. (Indian Rhubarb) and *Rheum rhaponticum* L. (Garden Rhubarb)

Part(s) Used

Rhizome, root

Pharmacopoeial and Other Monographs

BHC 1992[G6]
BHP 1996[G9]
BP 2001[G15]
Complete German Commission E[G3]
ESCOP 1999[G52]
Martindale 32nd edition[G43]
PDR for Herbal Medicines 2nd edition[G36]
Ph Eur 2002[G28]
WHO volume 1 1999[G63]

Legal Category (Licensed Products)

GSL[G37]

Constituents[G2,G6,G22,G41,G48,G59,G64]

Hydroxyanthracenes Primarily anthraquinone O-glycosides (anthraglycosides) of aloe-emodin, emodin, chrysophanol and physcion; dianthrone glycosides of rhein (sennosides A and B) and their oxalates; heterodianthrones including palmidin A (aloe-emodin, emodin), palmidin B (aloe-emodin, chrysophanol), palmidin C (chrysophanol, emodin), sennidin C (rhein, aloe-emodin), rheidin B (rhein, chrysophanol), and reidin C (rhein, physcion); free anthraquinones mainly aloe-emodin, chrysophanol, emodin, physcion and rhein.

Tannins Hydrolysable and condensed including glucogallin, free gallic acid, (−)-epicatechin gallate and catechin.

Other constituents Calcium oxalate, fatty acids, rutin, resins, starch (about 16%), stilbene glycosides, carbohydrates, volatile oil (trace) with more than 100 components.

Food Use

Rhubarb is listed by the Council of Europe as a natural source of food flavouring (category N2). This category indicates that it can be added to foodstuffs in small quantities, with a possible limitation of an active principle (as yet unspecified) in the final product.[G16] Rhubarb stems are commonly eaten as a food. In the USA, rhubarb is permitted for food use.[G65]

Herbal Use

Rhubarb has been used traditionally both as a laxative and an antidiarrhoeal agent.[G2,G6,G8,G64]

Dosage

Rhizome/root   0.2–1.0 g.

Pharmacological Actions

The laxative action of anthraquinone derivatives is well recognised (*see* Senna). Rhubarb also contains tannins, which exert an astringent action. At low doses, rhubarb is stated to act as an antidiarrhoeal because of the tannin components, whereas at higher doses it exerts a cathartic action.[G42]

Side-effects, Toxicity

See Senna for side-effects and toxicity associated with anthraquinone-containing drugs. Rhubarb leaves are toxic because of the oxalic acid content and should not be ingested. A case of anaphylaxis following rhubarb ingestion has been documented.[G51]

Contra-indications, Warnings[G20]

See Senna for contra-indications and warnings associated with anthraquinone-containing drugs. The astringent effect of rhubarb may exacerbate, rather than relieve, symptoms of constipation.[1] It has been stated that rhubarb should be avoided by individuals suffering from arthritis, kidney disease or urinary problems.[G42]

Pregnancy and lactation It is stated that rhubarb should be avoided during pregnancy.[G42] *See* Senna for contra-indications and warnings regarding the use of stimulant laxatives during pregnancy and lactation.

Pharmaceutical Comment

The chemistry of rhubarb is characterised by the anthraquinone derivatives. The laxative action of these compounds is well recognised and justifies the use of rhubarb as a laxative. As with all anthraqui-none-containing preparations, the use of non-standardised products should be avoided because their pharmacological effect will be variable and unpredictable.

References

See also General References G2, G3, G6, G9, G12, G15, G16, G20, G22, G25, G29, G31, G36, G37, G41, G42, G43, G48, G51, G52, G56, G63 and G64.

1   Rohrback JA. Some uses of rhubarb in veterinary medicine. *Herbalist* 1983; **1**: 239–241.

Rosemary

Species (Family)

Rosmarinus officinalis L. (Labiatae)

Synonym(s)

–

Part(s) Used

Leaf, twig

Pharmacopoeial and Other Monographs

BP 2001[G15]
BHP 1996[G9]
Complete German Commission E[G3]
ESCOP 1997[G52]
Martindale 32nd edition[G43]
PDR for Herbal Medicines 2nd edition[G36]
Ph Eur 2002[G28]

Legal Category (Licensed Products)

GSL[G37]

Constituents[G2,G41,G52,G58]

Flavonoids Include diosmetin, diosmin, genkwanin and derivatives, luteolin and derivatives, hispidulin, nepetin, nepitrin and apigenin.

Phenols Caffeic, chlorogenic, labiatic, neochlorogenic and rosmarinic acids.

Volatile oil 1–25%. Components vary according to chemotype. Composed mainly of monoterpene hydrocarbons including α- and β-pinenes, camphene and limonene, together with 1,8-cineole, borneol, camphor (20–50% of the oil), linalool, verbinol, terpineol, 3-octanone and isobornyl acetate.

Terpenoids Carnosol, carnosolic acid, rosmanol (diterpenes);[1] oleanolic and ursolic acids (triterpenes).

Food Use

Rosemary herb and oil are commonly used as flavouring agents in foods. Rosemary is listed by the Council of Europe as a source of natural food flavouring (category N2). This category indicates that rosemary can be added to foodstuffs in small quantities, with a possible limitation of an active principle (as yet unspecified) in the final product.[G16] In the USA, rosemary is listed as GRAS (Generally Recognised As Safe).[G65]

Herbal Use[G2,G4,G7,G32,G52]

Rosemary is stated to act as a carminative, spasmolytic, thymoleptic, sedative, diuretic and antimicrobial.[G7] Topically, rubefacient, mild analgesic and parasiticide properties are documented.[G7] Traditionally rosemary is indicated for flatulent dyspepsia, headache, and topically for myalgia, sciatica, and intercostal neuralgia. The German Commission E approved internal use for dyspeptic complaints and external use as supporting therapy for rheumatic diseases and circulatory problems.[G3]

Dosage

Dried leaf/twig 2–4 g or by infusion three times daily;[G7] 4–6 g daily; external use 50 g for one bath.[G3]

Liquid extract 2–4 mL (1 : 1 in 45% alcohol) three times daily.[G7]

Pharmacological Actions

In vitro and animal studies

Antimicrobial activity Antibacterial and antifungal activities *in vitro* have been reported for rosemary oil.[2,G41,G52] Rosemary herb is an effective antimicrobial agent against *Staphylococcus aureus* in meat and against a wide range of bacteria in laboratory media.[1] Antimicrobial activity has been documented for the oil towards moulds, and Gram-positive and Gram-negative bacteria[1] including *S. aureus*, *S. albus*, *Vibrio cholerae*, *Escherichia coli* and corynebacteria.[3] Carnosol and ursolic acid have inhibited a range of food spoilage microbes (*S. aureus*, *E. coli*, *Lactobacillus brevis*, *Pseudomonas fluorescens*, *Rhodotorula glutinis* and *Kluyveromyces bulgaricus*). Activity was comparable to that of known antioxidants butylated hydroxyanisole (BHA) and butylated hydroxytoluene (BHT), and correlated with the respective antioxidant properties of the two compounds (carnosol > ursolic acid).[1]

Antiviral activity A dried 95% ethanol extract of rosemary (2–100 µg/mL) inhibited *in vitro* formation of herpes simplex virus type 2 plaques from 2 to 100% in a concentration-dependent manner. Carnosolic acid had activity against human immunodeficiency virus type 1 (HIV-1) protease (IC$_{50}$ value 0.08 µg/mL) when assayed against HIV-1 virus replication (IC$_{90}$ value 0.32 µg/mL).[4,5] Carnosolic acid was cytotoxic to lymphocytes with a TC$_{90}$ on H9 lymphocytes of 0.36 µg/mL.

Antitumour activity An extract of rosemary (precipitate from aqueous phase of 70% alcohol extract) inhibited KB cells by 87% when applied at a concentration of 50 µg/mL.[G52] The volatile oil (1.2–300 µg/mL) was reported to be toxic to L-1210 leukaemia cells.[6] Topical administration of a methanol extract 5 minutes prior to application of carcinogens to the dorsal surface of CD-1 mice reduced the irritation and promotion of tumours. Application of rosemary extract (1.2 mg and 3.6 mg) prior to [^{3}H]-benzo(*a*)pyrene reduced the formation of metabolite–DNA adducts by 30% and 54%, respectively.[7] In rats, dietary supplementation with 1% rosemary extract for 21 weeks reduced the development of dimethylbenz(*a*)anthracene mammary carcinoma in the treated group, compared with the control group (40% versus 75%, respectively).[8]

Antispasmodic and anticonvulsant activities Rosemary oil, 1,8-cineole, and bornyl acetate have exerted a spasmolytic action in both smooth muscle (guinea-pig ileum) and cardiac muscle (guinea-pig atria) preparations, with the latter more sensitive.[9] In smooth muscle this spasmolytic effect has been attributed to antagonism of acetylcholine,[10] with borneol considered the most active component of the oil.[10] The spasmolytic action of rosemary oil is preceded by a contractile action, which is attributed to the pinene components.[10] α-Pinenes and β-pinenes have exhibited a spasmogenic activity towards smooth muscle, with no effect on cardiac muscle.[9]

Spasmolytic action *in vivo* (guinea-pigs) has been demonstrated by rosemary oil (administered intravenously) via a relaxant action on Oddi's sphincter contracted by morphine. Activity increased with incremental doses of oil until an optimum dose was reached (25 mg/kg) at which the unblocking effect

was immediate.[11] Further increases in dose reintroduced a delayed response time.[11] Smooth muscle-stimulant and analgesic actions have been documented for a rosmaricine derivative.[G41]

The volatile oil of rosemary inhibited contractions of rabbit tracheal smooth muscle induced by acetylcholine, and inhibited contraction of guinea-pig tracheal smooth muscle induced by histamine.[12] The oil also inhibited contractions in both preparations induced by high potassium concentrations. Contractions of rabbit and guinea-pig tracheal smooth muscle induced by acetylcholine and histamine, respectively, were inhibited by rosemary oil in calcium ion-free solution. It was suggested that the oil has calcium antagonist activity.[12] A 30% ethanol extract of rosemary produced a spasmolytic effect on guinea-pig ileum, as demonstrated by measuring the increase in the ED$_{50}$ of acetylcholine (4.9 µg/L after addition of 2.5 mL extract and 25.1 µg/L after addition of 10 mL extract).[G52] An increase in the ED$_{50}$ for histamine from 8.1 µg/L to 44.6 µg/L, respectively, was noted for the same doses of extract.

Noradrenaline (norephinephrine)- and potassium ion-induced contractions of rabbit aortic rings were significantly reduced by rosemary oil 0.48 mg/mL and 0.64 mg/mL, respectively. It was proposed that action was by a direct vascular smooth muscle effect.[13]

Anti-inflammatory activity Complement activation and subsequent triggering of the arachidonic acid cascade are thought to play an important role in the early phase of shock. An intact complement system is required for the formation of vasoactive prostanoids (prostacyclin, thromboxane A$_2$), arterial hypotension and thrombocytopenia.[14] The effect of rosmarinic acid on endotoxin-induced haemodynamic and haematological changes has been studied in a rabbit model of circulatory shock.[14,15] Rosmarinic acid (20 mg/kg, intravenous) was found to suppress the endotoxin-induced activation of complement, formation of prostacyclin, hypotension, thrombocytopenia, and the release of thromboxane A$_2$.[14] Unlike non-steroidal anti-inflammatory drugs (NSAIDs), the mode of action by which rosmarinic acid suppresses prostaglandin formation does not involve interference with cyclooxygenase activity or prostacyclin synthetase.[15] Activity has been attributed to inhibition of complement factor C3 conversion to activated complement components, which mediate the inflammatory process.[15] Rosmarinic acid has inhibited carrageenan-induced rat paw oedema, and passive cutaneous anaphylaxis, also in rats (ID$_{50}$ 1 mg/kg, intravenously; 10 mg/kg, intramuscularly).[16]

Topical application of rosmarinic acid (5%) to rhesus monkeys reduced gingival plaque indices when compared with placebo.[G52] A methanol extract of herb (3.6 mg) applied topically to CD-1 mice twice daily for four days inhibited skin inflammation and hyperplasia caused by 12-O-tetradecanoylphorbol-13-acetate (TPA).[G52] A similar extract inhibited both TPA- and arachidonic acid-induced inflammation as well as TPA-induced hyperplasia.[7]

Anti-hepatotoxic activity A lyophilised aqueous extract of rosemary significantly reduced hepatotoxicity of *t*-butylperoxide to rat hepatocytes *in vitro*, significantly decreasing malonaldehyde formation, release of lactic acid dehydrogenase and aspartate aminotransferase.[17] Pretreatment of rats with an aqueous extract (1 mg of lyophilisate equivalent to 7 mg young shoots) 30 minutes prior to exposure to carbon tetrachloride, resulted in a 72% decrease in plasma glutamic-pyruvic transaminase.[18] Rosemary extract supplementation in the diet of rats enhanced the activity of GSH-transferase and NAD(P)H-quinone reductase.[G52]

Cholagogic activity A lyophilised ethanolic extract (1 mg) of young shoots at doses of 0.1, 1.0 and 2.0 g/kg was injected into the jugular vein of common bile duct-cannulated Sprague–Dawley rats infused with sodium taurocholate.[18] A significant, rapid increase in bile flow (114%) was achieved with maximum effect in 30 minutes. The extract of young shoots was significantly more active in stimulating bile flow than a similar extract of whole plant. A rapid increase in bile secretion was observed (138% in 40 minutes) in cannulated guinea-pigs given an aqueous-ethanol extract (15%).[G52]

Antioxidant activity A number of extracts and constituents of rosemary have been shown to have antioxidant activity.[G52] An antioxidant action, demonstrated by inhibition of chemiluminescence and hydrogen peroxide generation from human granulocytes, has been reported for rosmarinic acid.[15]

Lipophilic and hydrophobic fractions of rosemary showed activity which was attributed to the diterpenes carnosol, carnosolic acid and rosmanol inhibiting superoxide anion production in the xanthine/xanthine oxidase system.[19] These diterpenes at concentrations of 3–30 μmol/L also completely inhibit mitochondrial and microsomal lipid peroxidation induced by NADPH or NADPH oxidation.[19]

The complement-inhibiting and antioxidant properties of rosmarinic acid are not thought to adversely affect the chemotaxic, phagocytic and enzymatic properties of polymorphonuclear leukocytes.[20]

Other activities A hyperglycaemic effect was observed in glucose-loaded rats treated with a solution of rosemary oil (925 mg/kg, intramuscular).[23] In rabbits with alloxan-induced diabetes given rosemary oil (25 mg/kg, intramuscular) 6 hours after fasting, plasma glucose concentrations increased by 17% 6 hours later.

Pretreatment with rosmarinic acid (20 mg/kg and 10 mg/kg, intravenously) has been reported to inhibit the development of adult respiratory distress syndrome (ARDS) in a rabbit model.[20] This action can be attributed to both the antioxidant and anticomplement activities of rosmarinic acid.[20]

The ability to reduce capillary permeability has been described for diosmin.[G41] Activity reportedly exceeds that exhibited by rutin.[G41]

An increase in locomotor activity has been observed in mice following either inhalation or oral administration of rosemary oil.[21] The increase in activity paralleled a dose-related increase in serum 1,8-cineole level. Biphasic elimination of 1,8-cineole from the blood was observed ($t_{1/2} = 6$ minutes, $t_{1/2} = 45$ minutes).[21]

In rats, antigonadotrophic activity has been documented for oxidation products of rosmarinic acid administered intramuscularly.[22] Activity was determined by suppression of pregnant mares' serum-induced increase in ovarian and uterine weights. Concentrations of 10^{-7} mol/L of the flavonoids nepitrin and nepetin inhibited aldose-reductase activity in homogenised rat eye lenses by 31%.[G52]

Side-Effects, Toxicity[G58]

Rosemary oil is stated to be non-irritating and non-sensitising when applied to human skin,[G58] but moderately irritating when applied undiluted to rabbit skin.[G41] Bath preparations, cosmetics and toiletries containing rosemary oil may cause erythema and dermatitis in hypersensitive individuals.[G51] Photosensitivity has been associated with the oil.[G51]

Rosmarinic acid exhibits low toxicity (an LD_{50} in mice is stated as 561 mg/kg for intravenous administration) and is rapidly eliminated from the circulation ($t_{1/2} = 9$ minutes following intravenous administration).[16] Transient cardiovascular actions become pronounced at intravenous doses exceeding 50 mg/kg.[16] Acute LD_{50} values quoted include 5 mL/kg (rat, oral) and >10 mL/kg (rabbit, dermal).[3]

Diosmin is reportedly less toxic than rutin.[G41] No mortality was seen in Wistar rats and Swiss mice given single intraperitoneal doses of 2 g/kg of aqueous alcoholic rosemary extract (15%).[G52]

Contra-indications, Warnings

Topical preparations containing rosemary oil should be used with caution by hypersensitive individuals. Rosemary oil contains 20–50% camphor; orally, camphor readily causes epileptiform convulsions if taken in sufficient quantity.[G58]

Pregnancy and lactation Rosemary is reputed to be an abortifacient[G30] and to affect the menstrual cycle (emmenagogue).[G48] In view of its common culinary use, rosemary should not be ingested in amounts greatly exceeding those normally encountered in foods.

Pharmaceutical Comment

In addition to the well-known culinary uses of rosemary, various medicinal properties are also associated with the herb. Documented antibacterial, anti-inflammatory and spasmolytic actions, which support the traditional uses of the herb, are attributable to the essential oil. Anticomplement and antoxidant activities documented for rosmarinic acid have generated considerable interest in a potential preventative use against endotoxin shock and adult respiratory distress syndrome. A method for the isolation (TLC, thin-layer chromatography) and subsequent identification (HPLC, high-performance liquid chromatography) of rosmarinic acid has been proposed.[24] Rosemary should not be used by epileptic patients in doses greatly exceeding amounts used in food.

References

See also General References G2, G3, G9, G12, G16, G22, G29, G31, G32, G36, G37, G41, G43, G48, G51, G52 and G58.

1 Collin MA, Charles HP. Antimicrobial activity of carnosol and ursolic acid: two anti-oxidant constituents of *Rosmarinus officinalis* L. *Food Microbiol* 1987; **4**: 311–315.
2 Panizzi L *et al.* Composition and antimicrobial properties of essential oils of four Mediterranean Lamiaceae. *J Ethnopharmacol* 1993; **39**: 167–170.
3 Opdyke DLJ. Rosemary oil. *Food Cosmet Toxicol* 1974; **12**: 977–978
4 Pariš A *et al.* Inhibitory effect of carnosolic acid on HIV-1 protease in cell-free assays. *J Nat Prod* 1993; **56**: 1426–1430.
5 Pukl M *et al.* Inhibitory effect of carnosolic acid on HIV-1 protease. *Planta Med* 1992; **58**: A632.
6 Ilarionova M *et al.* Cytotoxic effect on leukemic cells of the essential oils from rosemary, wild geranium and nettle and concret of royal bulgarian rose. *Anticancer Res* 1992; **12**: 1915.
7 Huang M-T *et al.* Inhibition of skin tumorigenesis by rosemary and its constituents carnosol and ursolic acid. *Cancer Res* 1994; **54**: 701–708.
8 Singletary K. Inhibition of DMBA-induced mammary tumorigenesis by rosemary extract. *FASEB J* 1991; **5**: 5A927.
9 Hof S, Ammon HPT. Negative inotropic action of rosemary oil, 1,8-cineole, and bornyl acetate. *Planta Med* 1989; **55**: 106–107.
10 Taddei I *et al.* Spasmolytic activity of peppermint, sage and rosemary essences and their major constituents. *Fitoterapia* 1988; **59**: 463–468.
11 Giachetti D *et al.* Pharmacological activity of essential oils on Oddi's sphincter. *Planta Med* 1988; 389–392.
12 Aqel MB. Relaxant effect of the volatile oil of *Rosmarinus officinalis* on tracheal smooth muscle. *J Ethnopharmacol* 1991; **33**: 57–62.
13 Aqel MB. A vascular smooth muscle relaxant effect of *Rosmarinus officinalis*. *Int J Pharmacog* 1992; **30**: 281–288.
14 Bult H *et al.* Modification of endotoxin-induced haemodynamic and haematological changes in the rabbit by methylprednisolone, F(ab′)2 fragments and rosmarinic acid. *Br J Pharmacol* 1985; **84**: 317–327.
15 Rampart M *et al.* Complement-dependent stimulation of prostacyclin biosynthesis: inhibition by rosmarinic acid. *Biochem Pharmacol* 1986; **35**: 1397–1400.
16 Parnham MJ, Kesselring K. Rosmarinic acid. *Drugs Future* 1985; **10**: 756–757
17 Joyeux M *et al.* Screening of antiradical, antilipoperoxidant and hepatoprotective effects of nine plants extracts used in Caribbean folk medicine. *Phytother Res* 1995; **9**: 228–230.
18 Hoefler C *et al.* Comparative choleretic and hepatoprotective properties of young sprouts and total plant extracts of *Rosmarinus officinalis* in rats. *J Ethnopharmacol* 1987; **19**: 133–143.
19 Haraguchi H *et al.* Inhibition of lipid peroxidation and superoxide generation by diterpenoids from *Rosmarinus officinalis*. *Planta Med* 1995; **61**: 333–336.
20 Nuytinck JKS *et al.* Inhibition of experimentally induced microvascular injury by rosmarinic acid. *Agents Actions* 1985; **17**: 373–374.
21 Kovar KA *et al.* Blood levels of 1,8-cineole and locomotor activity of mice after inhalation and oral administration of rosemary oil. *Planta Med* 1987; 315–318.
22 Gumbinger HG *et al.* Formation of compounds with antigonadotropic activity from inactive phe-

nolic precursors. *Contraception* 1981; **23**: 661–665.

23 Al-Hader AA *et al*. Hyperglycemic and insulin release inhibitory effects of *Rosmarinus officinalis*.

J Ethnopharmacol 1994; 43: 217–221.

24 Verotta L. Isolation and HPLC determination of the active principles of *Rosmarinus officinalis* and *Gentiana lutea*. *Fitoterapia* 1985; **56**: 25–29.

Sage

Species (Family)

Salvia officinalis L. (Labiatae)

Synonym(s)

Dalmatian Sage, Garden Sage, True Sage
Red Sage refers to *Salvia haematodes* Wall.
Greek Sage refers to *Salvia triloba*[1]
Spanish Sage refers to *Salvia lavundaefolia*

Part(s) Used

Leaf

Pharmacopoeial and Other Monographs

BHP 1996[G9]
BP 2001[G15]
Complete German Commission E[G3]
ESCOP 1996[G52]
Martindale 32nd edition[G43]
PDR for Herbal Medicines 2nd edition[G36]
Ph Eur 2002[G28]

Legal Category (Licensed Products)

GSL[G37]

Constituents[G2,G22,G41,G52,G58,G62,G64]

Acids Phenolic – caffeic, chlorogenic, ellagic, ferulic, gallic and rosmarinic.[2]

Flavonoids 5-Methoxysalvigenin.

Terpenes Monoterpene glycosides. Diterpenes, abietanes including carnosic acid and derivatives, e.g. carnasol. Triterpenes, oleanolic acid and derivatives.

Tannins 3–8%. Hydrolysable and condensed.[2,3]

Volatile oil 1–2.8%. Pharmacopoeial standard not less than 1.0% cut herb.[G15,G28] Major components are α- and β-thujones (35–50%, mainly α). Others include 1,8-cineole, borneol, camphor, caryophyllene, linalyl acetate and various terpenes.[4,5]
  It has been noted that commercial sage may be substituted with *Salvia triloba*.[1] In contrast to *S. officinalis*, the principal volatile oil component of *S. triloba* is 1,8-cineole, with α-thujone only accounting for 1–5%.[1] Compared to *S. officinalis*, volatile oil yield of various *Salvia* species is lower, with lower total ketone content and higher total alcohol content.[6]

Food Use

Sage is commonly used as a culinary herb. It is listed by the Council of Europe as a natural source of food flavouring (category N2).[G16] This category indicates that sage can be added to foodstuffs providing the concentration of thujones (α and β) present in the final product does not exceed 0.5 mg/kg, with the exceptions of alcoholic beverages (10 mg/kg), bitters (35 mg/kg), food containing sage (25 mg/kg) and sage stuffing (250 mg/kg).[G16] In the USA, sage is listed as GRAS (Generally Recognised As Safe).[G65]

Herbal Use[G2,G4,G7,G32,G43,G52,G54,G64]

Sage is stated to possess carminative, antispasmodic, antiseptic, astringent and antihidrotic properties. Traditionally, it has been used to treat flatulent dyspepsia, pharyngitis, uvulitis, stomatitis, gingivitis, glossitis (internally or as a gargle/mouthwash), hyperhidrosis, and galactorrhoea. The herbals of Gerard, Culpeper and Hill credit sage with the ability to enhance memory.[7] The German Commission E approved internal use for dyspeptic symptoms and excessive perspiration, and external use for inflammation of mucous membranes of mouth and throat.[G3]

Dosage

Leaf 1–4 g or by infusion three times daily;[G7] 4–6 g daily.[G3]

Liquid extract 1–4 mL (1:1 in 45% alcohol) three times daily.[G7]

Gargles, rinses 2.5 g/100 mL water.[G3]

Pharmacological Actions

In vitro and animal studies

Hypotensive activity in anaesthetised cats, CNS-depressant action (prolonged barbiturate sleep) in anaesthetised mice, and an antispasmodic action *in vitro* (guinea-pig ileum) have been reported for a sage extract[8] and for the essential oil.[9]

Antispasmodic activity Inhibition of contractions induced by acetylcholine, histamine, serotonin and barium chloride by 60–80% has been noted for a total sage extract, with lesser activity exhibited by a total flavonoid extract.[8] An initial spasmogenic action exhibited by low doses of sage oil has been attributed to the pinene content.[9] Antispasmodic activity *in vivo* (guinea-pigs) has been reported for sage oil administered intravenously, which released contraction of Oddi's sphincter induced by intravenous morphine.[5]

Anticholinesterase activity Early herbals claim that sage enhances the memory.[7] The anticholinesterase activity of several *Salvia* species and their constituents have been investigated in the search for new drugs for the treatment of Alzheimer's disease. The inhibition of anticholinesterase *in vitro* by an ethanolic extract of *S. officinalis* (2.5 mg/mL) was 68%, and by oils of *S. officinalis* and *S. lavandulaefolia* (0.1 µg/mL) was 52% and 63%, respectively.[10] The IC_{50} value of *S. lavandulaefolia* oil is reportedly 0.03 µg/mL.[11] The monoterpenes 1,8-cineole and α-pinene from the oil have been identified as the inhibitors of acetylcholinesterase with IC_{50} values of 0.67 and 0.63 mmol/L, respectively.[11] Rats given *S. lavanadulaefolia* oil (20 µL or 50 µL for five days) were sacrificed, and acetylcholinesterase activity assessed for striatum, cortex and hippocampus of brain left hemisphere.[12] At the lower dose, there was a decrease in acetylcholinesterase activity in the striatum, but not in the hippocampus or cortex of treated rats. At the higher dose, there was a decrease in striatal acetylcholinesterase activity. It was concluded that the oil inhibited acetylcholinesterase in selective areas of the brain.

Hypoglycaemic activity Hypoglycaemic activity *in vivo* (rabbits) has been reported for *S. lavandulaefolia*.[13] and for mixed phytotherapy preparations containing various *Salvia* species, including *S. officinalis*.[14] Activity in normoglycaemic, hypoglycaemic and in alloxan-diabetic rabbits was observed, although no change in insulin concentrations was noted.[13]

Antimicrobial and antiviral activity Antimicrobial activity of the volatile oil has been attributed to the thujone content.[4] Antimicrobial activity *in vitro* was noted against *Escherichia coli*, *Shigella sonnei*, *Salmonella* species, *Klebsiella ozanae* (Gram-negative), *Bacillus subtilis* (Gram-positive), and against various fungi (*Candida albicans*, *C. krusei*, *C. pseudotropica-*

lis, *Torulopsis glabrata*, *Cryptococcus neoformans*).[15] No activity was observed versus *Pseudomonas aeruginosa*.[4] Microencapsulation of sage oil into gelatin-acacia capsules introduced a lagtime with respect to antibacterial activity and inhibited antifungal activity.[4] Diterpene constituents of *S. officinalis* are reported to be active against vesicular stomatitis virus.[G52]

Other activities An aqueous ethanolic extract of sage (50%) strongly inhibited collagenolytic activity of *Porphyromonas gingivitis*.[G52] In addition to anticholinesterase activity, other biological activities have relevance in the treatment of Alzheimer's disease. In this context, *S. lavanadulaefolia* and its individual constituents have been assessed for antioxidant, anti-inflammatory and oestrogenic activities.[11] An ethanolic extract of dried herb (5 mg/mL) and the monoterpenes α- and β-pinene and 1,8-cineole (0.1 mol/L) inhibited bovine brain liposome peroxidate activity. Anti-inflammatory activity was demonstrated by weak inhibition of thromboxane B_2 and leukotriene B_4 synthesis, and possible oestrogenic activity of sage oil (0.01 mg/mL) and geraniol (0.1–2 mmol/L), demonstrated by induction of β-galactosidase in yeast cells.

Other species Various activities in rats, mice and rabbits have been reported for a related species, *S. haematodes* Wall. (commonly known as red sage), including wound-healing, anti-inflammatory, analgesic, anticonvulsant and hypotensive, and positive inotropic and chronotropic actions (*in vitro*).[16,17] *In vivo* studies have indicated different activities for *S. triloba* and *S. verbenaca*, compared with *S. officinalis*.[8]

Clinical studies

Excessive sweat induced by pilocarpine was inhibited by a dialysate of an aqueous extract of fresh sage.[G52] In an open study, 40 patients were given dried aqueous extract of sage (440 mg, equivalent to 2.6 g herbs) and 40 were given infusion of sage (4.5 g herb daily). Reduction of sweat (less than 50%) was achieved in both groups of patients with idiopathic hyperhidriosis.[G52] It should be noted, however, that this study did not include a control group.

A double-blind, placebo-controlled, crossover study involving 20 healthy volunteers compared the effects of 50 µL, 100 µL and 150 µL of *S. lavandulaefolia* oil and sunflower oil.[12] Cognitive assessment indicated improvements in both immediate and delayed word recall scores, coupled with decrements in accuracy and speed of attention, with sage oil 50 µL. At this dose, self-related alertness at 2.5 hours and calmness at 4 hours and 6 hours were reported to be reduced. The results suggest that the effects of sage oil in modulating mood and cognition are worth further investigation.

Side-effects, Toxicity

A case of human poisoning has been documented following ingestion of sage oil for acne.[18] Convulsant activity in both humans and animals has been documented for sage oil.[19,20] In rats, the subclinical, clinical and lethal doses for convulsant action of sage oil are estimated as 0.3, 0.5, and 3.2 g/kg.[19] This toxicity has been attributed to the ketone terpenoids in the volatile oil, namely camphor and thujone. Acute LD_{50} values for sage oil are documented as 2.6 g/kg in rats for oral administration and 5 g/kg in rabbits for intradermal administration.[21] S. officianalis has no mutagenic or DNA-damaging activity in either the Ames test or Bacillus rec-assay.[G52]

Sage oil is reported to be a moderate skin irritant[21] and is not recommended for aromatherapy.[G58]

Contra-indications, Warnings

Sage oil is toxic (due to the thujone content) and should not be ingested. S. lavandulaefolia oil has a much lower content of thujone than S. officinalis oil.[12] In view of the toxicity of the essential oil, sage extracts should be used with caution and not ingested in large amounts. Sage may interfere with existing hypoglycaemic and anticonvulsant therapies, and may potentiate sedative effects of other drugs.

Pregnancy and lactation Sage is contra-indicated during pregnancy. Traditionally, it is reputed to be an abortifacient and to affect the menstrual cycle.[G30] The volatile oil contains a high proportion of α- and β-thujones, which are known to be abortifacient and emmenagogic.

Pharmaceutical Comment

The characteristic components of sage to which its traditional uses can be attributed are the volatile oil and tannins. However, the oil contains high concentrations of thujone, a toxic ketone and should not be ingested. Sage is commonly used as a culinary herb and presents no hazard when ingested in amounts normally encountered in foods. However, extracts of the herb should be used with caution and should not be ingested in large amounts or over prolonged periods. S. lavandulaefolia oil is being investigated for symptomatic treatment of Alzheimer's disease.[11] However, at present, there is a lack of well-designed clinical studies investigating the reputed effects of sage.

References

See also General References G2, G3, G9, G10, G15, G16, G22, G28, G30, G31, G32, G36, G37, G41, G43, G52, G54, G58, G62 and G64.

1 Tucker AO *et al.* Botanical aspects of commercial sage. *Econ Bot* 80; **34**: 16–19.
2 Petri G *et al.* Tannins and other polyphenolic compounds in the genus *Salvia. Planta Med* 1988: **54**: 575.
3 Murko D *et al.* Tannins of *Salvia officinalis* and their changes during storage. *Planta Med* 1974; **25**: 295–300.
4 Jalsenjak V *et al.* Microcapsules of sage oil: Essential oils content and antimicrobial activity. *Pharmazie* 1987; **42**: 419–420.
5 Giachetti D *et al.* Pharmacological activity of essential oils on Oddi's sphincter. *Planta Med* 1988: **54**: 389–392.
6 Ivanic R, Savin K. A comparative analysis of essential oils from several wild species of *Salvia. Planta Med* 1976; **30**: 25–31.
7 Perry EK *et al.* Medicinal plants and Alzheimer's disease: integrating ethnobotanical and contemporary scientific evidence. *J Alt Complement Med* 1998; **4**: 419–428.
8 Todorov S *et al.* Experimental pharmacological study of three species from genus *Salvia. Acta Physiol Pharmacol Bulg* 1984; **10**: 13–20.
9 Taddei I *et al.* Spasmolytic activity of peppermint, sage and rosemary essences and their major constituents. *Fitoterapia* 1988; **59**: 463–468.
10 Perry N *et al.* European herbs with cholinergic activities: potential in dementia therapy. *Int J Geriat Psychiat* 1996; **11**: 1063–1069.
11 Perry NSL *et al. In-vitro* inhibition of human erythrocyte acetylcholinesterase by *Salvia lavandulaefolia* essential oil and constituent terpenes. *J Pharm Pharmacol* 2000; **52**: 895–902.
12 Houghton PJ. Personal communication.
13 Jimenez J *et al.* Hypoglycaemic activity of *Salvia lavandulifolia. Planta Med* 1986; **52**: 260–262.
14 Cabo J *et al.* Accion hipoglucemiante de preparados fitoterapicos que contienen especies del genero salvia. *Ars Pharmac* 1985; **26**: 239–249.
15 Recio MC *et al.* Antimicrobial activity of selected plants employed in the Spanish Mediterranean area. Part II. *Phytother Res* 1989; **3**: 77.
16 Akbar A *et al.* Pharmacological studies on *Salvia haematodes* Wall. *Acta Tropica* 1985; **42**: 371–374.
17 Akbar S. Pharmacological investigations on the ethanolic extract of *Salvia haematodes. Fitoterapia* 1989; **60**: 270.
18 Centini F *et al.* A case of sage oil poisoning. *Zacchia*

1987; **60**: 263–174.

19 Millet Y. Experimental study of the toxic convulsant properties of commercial preparations of essences of sage and hyssop. *Electroencephal Clin Neurophysiol* 1980; **49**: 102P.

20 Millet Y *et al.* Toxicity of some essential plant oils – clinical and experimental study. *Clin Toxicol* 1981; **18**: 1485–1498.

21 Opdyke DLJ. Sage oil Dalmatian. *Food Cosmet Toxicol* 1974; **12**: 987–988.

Sarsaparilla

Species (Family)

Smilax species (Liliaceae) including
(i) *Smilax aristolochiifolia* Mill.
(ii) *Smilax regelii* Killip & Morton
(iii) *Smilax ornata* Hook. f.
(iv) *Smilax febrifuga* Kunth

Synonym(s)

Ecuadorian Sarsaparilla, Sarsa, Smilax
(i) Mexican Sarsaparilla
(ii) Honduras Sarsaparilla
(iii) Jamaican Sarsaparilla
(iv) Ecuadorian Sarsaparilla

Part(s) Used

Rhizome, root

Pharmacopoeial and Other Monographs

BHC 1992[G6]
BHP 1996[G9]
Martindale 32nd edition[G43]
PDR for Herbal Medicines 2nd edition[G36]

Legal Category (Licensed Products)

GSL[G37]

Constituents[G6,G22,G41,G48,G62,G64]

Saponins About 2%. Sarsasapogenin (parigenin), smilagenin, diosgenin, tigogenin, asperagenin, laxogenin from various species,[1] sarsasaponin (parillin), smilasaponin (smilacin) and sarsaparilloside.

Other constituents Caffeoylshikimic acid, ferulic acid, shikimic acid, kaempferol, quercetin, phytosterols (e.g. β-sitosterol, stigmasterol, pollinastanol), resin, starch, volatile oil (trace) and cetyl alcohol.

Food Use

Sarsaparilla is listed by the Council of Europe as a natural source of food flavouring (category N4). This category indicates that the use of sarsaparilla as a flavouring agent is recognised but that there is insufficient information available to further classify it into categories N1, N2 or N3.[G16] Sarsaparilla has been used as a vehicle and flavouring agent for medicaments,[G45] and is widely employed in the manufacture of non-alcoholic beverages.[G59] In the USA, sarsaparilla is permitted for food use.

Herbal Use

Sarsaparilla is stated to possess antirheumatic, antiseptic and antipruritic properties. Traditionally, it has been used for psoriasis and other cutaneous conditions, chronic rheumatism, rheumatoid arthritis, as an adjunct to other treatments for leprosy, and specifically for psoriasis.[G6,G7,G8,G64]

Dosage

Dried root 1–4 g or by decoction three times daily.[G6]

Sarsaparilla Liquid Extract (BP 1898) 8–15 mL (1 : 1 in 20% alcohol, 10% glycerol).

Pharmacological Actions

In vitro and animal studies
Anti-inflammatory[2] and hepatoprotective[3] effects have been shown in rats.

Clinical studies
Improvement of appetite and digestion[4] as well as a diuretic[4,5] action have been reported. Limited clinical data utilising extracts indicate improvement in psoriasis;[6] the extract has also been used as an adjuvant for the treatment of leprosy.[7]

Side-effects, Toxicity

None documented for sarsaparilla. Large doses of saponins are reported to cause gastrointestinal irritation resulting in diarrhoea and vomiting. Although haemolytic activity has been documented for the saponins,[G62] they are not harmful when taken by mouth and are only highly toxic if injected into the bloodstream.[G59]

Contra-indications, Warnings

None documented for sarsaparilla. In view of the possible irritant nature of the saponin constituents, excessive ingestion should be avoided.

Pregnancy and lactation   There are no known problems with the use of sarsaparilla during pregnancy and lactation. However, in view of the possible irritant nature of the saponin components, excessive ingestion should be avoided.

Pharmaceutical Comment

Phytochemical studies on sarsaparilla have focused on the nature of the steroidal saponin constituents, with limited information available regarding additional constituents. No documented scientific evidence was found to justify the herbal uses. No toxicity data were located, although large doses may be irritant to the gastrointestinal mucosa and should, therefore, be avoided.

Sarsaparilla saponins have been used in the partial synthesis of cortisone and other steroids. Several related *Smilax* species native to China are used to treat various skin disorders.[G41]

References

See also General References G6, G9, G11, G16, G22, G29, G31, G32, G36, G37, G41, G43, G48, G62 and G64.

1   Sharma SC *et al.* Über Saponine von *Smilax parvifolia* Wall. *Pharmazie* 1980; **35**: 646.
2   Ageel AM *et al.* Experimental studies on antirheumatic crude drugs used in Saudi traditional medicine. *Drugs Exp Clin Res* 1989; **15**: 369–372.
3   Rafatullah S *et al.* Hepatoprotective and safety evaluation studies on sarsaparilla. *Int J Pharmacog* 1991; **29**: 296–301.
4   Harnischfeger G, Stolze H. Smilax species – Sarsaparille. In: *Bewährte Pflanzendrogen in Wissenschaft und Medizin.* Bad Homburg/Melsungen: Notamed Verlag., 1983: 216–225.
5   Hobbs C. Sarsaparilla – a literature review. *Herbalgram* 1988; **17**: 1, 10–15.
6   Thermon FM. The treatment of psoriasis with a sarsaparilla compound. *N Engl J Med* 1942; **227**: 128–133.
7   Rollier R. Treatment of lepromatous leprosy by a combination of DDS and sarsaparilla (*Smilax ornata*). *Int J Leprosy* 1959; **27**: 328–340.

Sassafras

Species (Family)

Sassafras albidum (Nutt.) Nees (Lauraceae)

Synonym(s)

Ague Tree, Cinnamon Wood, Saloop, *Sassafras varifolium* (Salisb.) Kuntze, *Sassafras officinale* Nees & Eberm., Saxifrax

Part(s) Used

Inner root bark

Pharmacopoeial and Other Monographs

BHP 1983[G7]
Martindale 32nd edition[G43]
PDR for Herbal Medicines 2nd edition[G36]

Legal Category (Licensed Products)

Sassafras is not permitted for use in medicinal products.

Constituents[G2,G22,G41,G48,G64]

Alkaloids Isoquinoline-type about 0.02%. Boldine, isoboldine, norboldine, cinnamolaurine, norcinnamolaurine and reticuline.

Volatile oils 5–9%. Safrole as major component (80–90%), others include anethole, apiole, asarone, camphor, caryophyllene, coniferaldehyde, copaene, elemicin, eugenol, 5-methoxyeugenol, menthone, myristicin, α-pinene, α- and β-phellandrene, piperonylacrolein and thujone.

Other constituents Gum, mucilage, lignans (sesamin, desmethoxyaschantin), resin, sitosterol, starch, tannins and wax.

Food Use

Sassafras oil was formerly used as flavouring agent in beverages including root beer.[G58] However, in the 1960s safrole, the major component of the volatile oil, was reported to be carcinogenic.[G58] The use of safrole in foods is now banned, and its use in toilet preparations controlled.[G45] In the USA, safrole-free sassafras extract, leaf and leaf extract are approved for food use. In 1976, the US Food and Drugs Administration (FDA) banned interstate marketing of sassafras for sassafras tea.[G22]

Herbal Use

Sassafras is stated to possess carminative, diaphoretic, diuretic, dermatologic and antirheumatic properties. Traditionally, it has been used for cutaneous eruptions, gout and rheumatic pains.[G2,G7,G64]

Dosage

Bark 2–4 g or by infusion three times daily.[G7]

Liquid extract 2–4 mL (1:1 in 25% alcohol) three times daily.[G7]

Pharmacological Actions

Studies have concentrated on investigating the toxicity associated with the bark. However, aqueous and alcoholic extracts have been reported to elicit ataxia, hypersensitivity to touch, CNS depression and hypothermia in mice.[1] Both inhibition and induction of hepatic microsomal enzymes have been documented for safrole.[2,3] Enzyme-inducing activity was found to be a transient phenomenon, with activity falling after the onset of hepatic toxicity (*see* Side-effects, Toxicity).[2] Safrole is reported to induce both cytochrome P488 and P450 activities. Sassafras oil has been used as a topical antiseptic, pediculicide and carminative.[4]

Side-effects, Toxicity[G58]

The toxicity of sassafras is attributable to the volatile oil, and in particular to the safrole content. It is estimated that a few drops of sassafras oil are sufficient to kill a toddler and as little as one teaspoonful has proved fatal in an adult.[5] Symptoms of poisoning are described as vomiting, stupor and collapse. High doses may cause spasm followed by paralysis.[G58] Large amounts of the oil are reported to be psychoactive with the hallucinogenic effects lasting for several days.[G22] One of the components of the oil is myristicin, the hallucinogenic principle in nutmeg.

Sassafras has traditionally been used as an ingredient of beverages. To put the potential toxicity of sassafras into perspective, the following estimation has been made.[1] Extrapolation of results from animal toxicity studies indicate that 0.66 mg/kg may prove hazardous in humans.[1] By comparison, a cup of sassafras tea, prepared from a 2.5 g teabag, may provide up to 200 mg safrole, representing approximately 3 mg/kg.[1]

Safrole, the principal component of the volatile oil, was first recognised to be a hepatocarcinogen in the 1960s[6] and many animal studies have been documented concerning this toxicity.[7] Both benign and malignant tumours have developed in laboratory animals, depending on the dose of safrole administered.[2]

Both human and animal studies have shown that safrole gives rise to a large number of metabolites.[8] A sulfate ester (formed via a hydroxylated metabolite) has been established as the ultimate carcinogen for safrole with tumour incidence parallelling the rate of conversion to the ester.[9] Induction of cytochrome P450 activity has been associated with mutagenic and carcinogenic activity of the inducing agent.[10] The inducing effect of safrole on certain metabolising enzymes is thought to play a role in the carcinogenic activity of safrole. The liver has a high level of cytochrome P450 activity and is therefore susceptible to induction.[10]

Acute oral LD_{50} values for safrole have been reported as 1.95 g/kg (rats) and 2.35 g/kg (mice).[2] Major symptoms of toxicity are stated as ataxia, depression, diarrhoea, followed by death within 4 hours to seven days.[11] Rats fed safrole in their diet at concentrations of 0.25, 0.5 and 1.0% exhibited reduction in growth, stomach and testicular atrophy, liver necrosis, biliary proliferation and primary hepatomas.[G22] Animals have also developed tumours when fed safrole-free extracts.[G22]

Conflicting results have been reported from studies investigating the mutagenicity of safrole, using the Ames test and DNA repair test.[12,13] Purity of the safrole, test system employed, type of metabolic activation mix, and toxicity of the test system have been suggested as reasons for the observed variations.[12]

Contra-indications, Warnings

Sassafras should not be used internally or externally. Safrole, the major component in the volatile oil of sassafras, is hepatotoxic and even safrole-free extracts have been reported to produce tumours in animals. Sassafras essential oil is contra-indicated in internal and external use.[G58] Sassafras has been reported to inhibit and induce microsomal enzymes.

Pregnancy and lactation Sassafras is contra-indicated during pregnancy and lactation. The oil is reported to be abortifacient.[5]

Pharmaceutical Comment

In addition to its traditional herbal use for treating dermatological and rheumatic ailments, sassafras also used to be a common flavouring ingredient in beverages, in particular root beer. However, animal studies have revealed the carcinogenic and hepatotoxic potential of safrole, the major component of sassafras volatile oil. Consequently, the use of safrole is no longer permitted in foods and sassafras is not permitted as a constituent of licensed medicinal products.

Antiseptic and diuretic properties claimed for sassafras are probably attributable to the volatile oil, although no documented studies were found supporting the antirheumatic claims. Sassafras should not be used as a herbal remedy, either internally or externally.

References

See also General References G2, G7, G11, G18, G21, G22, G31, G32, G36, G41, G43, G48, G58 and G64.

1 Segelman AB *et al.* Sassafras and herb tea. Potential health hazards. *JAMA* 1976; **238**: 477.
2 Opdyke DLJ. Safrole. *Food Cosmet Toxicol* 1974; **12**: 983–986.
3 Jaffe H *et al. In vivo* inhibition of mouse liver microsomal hydroxylating systems by methylenedioxyphenyl insecticidal synergists and related compounds. *Life Sci* 1968; **7**: 1051–1062.
4 International Agency for Research on Cancer. *IARC Monographs on the Evaluation of Carcinogenic Risk of Chemicals to Man. Some Naturally Occurring Substances, vol 10.* Geneva: WHO, 1976.
5 Craig JO. Poisoning by the volatile oils in childhood. *Arch Dis Child* 1953; **28**: 475–483.
6 Homburger F, Boger E. The carcinogenicity of essential oils, flavors, and spices: A review. *Cancer Res* 1968; **28**: 2372–2374.
7 Opdyke DLJ. Sassafras oil. *Food Cosmet Toxicol* 1982; **20**: 825–826.
8 Ioannides C *et al.* Safrole: its metabolism, carcinogenicity and interactions with cytochrome P-450. *Food Cosmet Toxicol* 1981; **19**: 657–666.
9 Bock KW, Schirmer G. Species differences of glucuronidation and sulfation in relation to hepato-

carcinogenesis. *Arch Toxicol* 1987; **10**(Suppl.): 125–135.

10 Iwasaki K *et al*. Induction of cytochrome P-448 activity as exemplified by the O-deethylation of ethoxyresorufin. Effects of dose, sex, tissue and animal species. *Biochem Pharmacol* 1986; **35**: 3879–3884.

11 Jenner PM *et al*. Food flavourings and compounds of related structure. I. Acute oral toxicity. *Food Cosmet Toxicol* 1964; **2**: 327–343.

12 Sekizawa J, Shibamoto T. Genotoxicity of safrole-related chemicals in microbial test systems. *Mutat Res* 1982; **101**: 127–140.

13 Swanson AB *et al*. The mutagenicities of safrole, estragole, eugenol, *trans*-anethole, and some of their known or possible metabolites for *Salmonella typhimurium* mutants. *Mutat Res* 1979; **60**: 143–153.

Saw Palmetto

Species (Family)

Serenoa serrulata Hook., F. (Arecaceae/Palmae)

Synonym(s)

Sabal, *Sabal serrulata* (Michx.) Nutt. & Schult., Serenoa, *Serenoa repens* (Bartram) Small

Part(s) Used

Fruit

Pharmacopoeial and Other Monographs

BHP 1996[G9]
BPC 1934[G10]
Complete German Commission E[G3]
Martindale 32nd edition[G43]
Mills and Bone[G50]
PDR for Herbal Medicines 2nd edition[G36]

Legal Category (Licensed Products)

GSL[G37]

Constituents[G22,G64]

Carbohydrates Invert sugar 28.2%, mannitol, high molecular weight polysaccharides (e.g. MW 100 000) with galactose, arabinose and uronic acid[1] identified as main sugar components for one.

Fixed oils 26.7%. Many free fatty acids and their glycerides. Monoacylglycerides (1-monolaurin, 1-monomyristicin).[2] Oleic acid (unsaturated) and capric acid, caproic acid, caprylic acid, lauric acid, myristic acid, palmitic acid and stearic acid (saturated).

Steroids β-Sitosterol, campesterol, stigmasterol and other compounds.[3–5]

Other constituents Flavonoids (e.g. rutin, isoquercitrin, kaempferol),[5] pigment (carotene), resin, tannin and volatile oil 1.5%.
Most commercial preparations of saw palmetto contain lipophilic extracts.[G56]

Food Use

Saw palmetto is not used in foods. In the USA, saw palmetto is listed by the Food and Drugs Administration (FDA) as a Herb of Undefined Safety.[G41]

Herbal Use

Saw palmetto is stated to possess diuretic, urinary antiseptic, endocrinological and anabolic properties. Traditionally, it has been used for chronic or subacute cystitis, catarrh of the genitourinary tract, testicular atrophy, sex hormone disorders and specifically for prostatic enlargement.[G7,G32,G64] Modern interest in saw palmetto is focused on its use in the treatment of symptoms of benign prostatic hyperplasia (BPH).

Dosage

Dried fruit 0.5–1.0 g or by decoction three times daily.[G7]

Extract 320 mg lipophilic ingredients extracted with lipophilic solvents (hexane or ethanol 90% v/v).[G3]

Clinical trials have assessed the effects of lipophilic extracts (containing lipids and sterols) of saw palmetto usually at a dosage of 160 mg twice daily.

Pharmacological Actions

Several pharmacological activities have been documented for saw palmetto *in vitro* and *in vivo* (animals). Several of these properties, such as inhibition of 5-α-reductase activity, inhibition of androgen binding and spasmolytic activity, are thought to explain, at least in part, the effects of saw palmetto in BPH. However, the clinical significance of the *in vitro* inhibition of 5-α-reductase activity by saw palmetto has not been clearly established (*see* Clinical studies). 5-α-Reductase is the enzyme that catalyses the conversion of testosterone to 5-α-dihydrotestosterone (DHT) in androgen target tissues, including the prostate. DHT is more potent than testosterone, and is thought to be implicated in the development of BPH. There is evidence that 5-α-reductase activity is higher in cells obtained from BPH tissue than from normal prostate tissue.

In vitro and animal studies

A lipidic (liposterolic) extract of saw palmetto was found to inhibit 5-α-reductase-mediated conversion of testosterone to dihydrotestosterone, and 3-ketosteroid reductase-mediated conversion of dihydrotestosterone to an androgen derivative.[5] Other *in vitro* studies have shown that an ethanolic extract of saw palmetto (IDS-89) inhibited 5-α-reductase activity in the epithelium and stroma of human BPH tissue in a concentration-dependent manner.[7] The IC_{50} was around 2.2 mg/mL. This study also demonstrated that the inhibitory effect of IDS-89 was mainly due to the fatty acid constituents of a saponifiable subfraction of the extract, as non-saponifiable and hydrophilic subfractions showed little or no inhibition of 5-α-reductase activity. Inhibition of 5-α-reductase by a liposterolic extract of saw palmetto has also been documented in porcine prostatic microsomes.[8]

There are at least two isoenzymes of 5-α-reductase (5-α-reductase types I and II), and several studies have documented that a liposterolic extract (Permixon) of saw palmetto inhibits both isoenzymes in prostate epithelial cells[9,10] and fibroblast cells.[10] Several other studies have documented inhibition of 5-α-reductase activity by liposterolic extracts of saw palmetto *in vitro*; these studies have been summarised elsewhere.[5,G50] Permixon was reported to inhibit 5-α-reductase activity without affecting the secretion of prostate-specific antigen (PSA) by epithelial cells, suggesting that use of saw palmetto extract should not interfere with PSA measurements for prostate-cancer screening.[9]

Anti-androgenic activity has been documented for a hexane liposterolic extract (Permixon) of saw palmetto. *In vitro* studies in rat prostate tissue and human foreskin fibroblasts indicated that this extract competitively inhibited the binding of dihydrotestosterone to cytosolic and nuclear androgen receptor sites.[6,11] By contrast, an alcoholic extract of saw palmetto appeared to be without androgen receptor-binding activity.[12]

Liposterolic extracts of saw palmetto have also been investigated in animal models of BPH. A liposterolic extract (Permixon) of saw palmetto 50 mg/kg body weight administered for 30 days to castrated rats with oestradiol/testosterone-induced prostate enlargement resulted in significant reductions in the wet weight of the dorsal region of the prostate, compared with control.[13] Another study in rats compared the effects of a liposterolic extract of saw palmetto with those of the 5-α-reductase inhibitor finasteride in rat prostate hyperplasia induced by hyperprolactinaemia.[14] It was reported that the liposterolic extract of saw palmetto inhibited rat prostate hyperplasia in the lateral lobe induced by hyperprolactinaemia, and that finasteride did not antagonise the action of prolactin. By contrast, a study in dogs with BPH reported a lack of effect for saw palmetto extract on prostatic weight, prostatic volume, prostatic histologic scores, prostatic ultrasonographs and serum testosterone concentrations.[15] In the study, 20 dogs with BPH, determined by raised prostatic volume and prostatic volume per kilogram body weight, received saw palmetto extract (type of extract not specified) 1500 mg daily in meatballs (n = 8), 300 mg daily in meatballs (n = 6) or unmedicated meatballs (n = 6), for 91 days. Dogs included in this study did not have clinical signs of BPH (i.e. decreased urinary flow and residual urine volume) that often occur in human males with BPH. Dogs did not appear to be randomly assigned to treatment, and the mean prostatic volume in the control group was higher than that in the active treatment groups before treatment, although it was stated that this was not statistically significant. Assessments and data analysis were carried out by blinded investigators.

In a study using human prostate tissue, a liposterolic extract of saw palmetto (Permixon) 30 µg/mL significantly inhibited basic fibroblast growth factor-induced proliferation of human prostate cell cultures, compared with control, although the extract did not affect basal prostate cell proliferation.[16] An unsaponified fraction of the extract also markedly inhibited basic fibroblast growth factor-induced cell proliferation, but had only a minimal effect on basal cell proliferation. In a study using stromal and epithelial tissue from normal prostate and from patients with BPH, cell numbers and proliferative indices were found to be higher in BPH tissue than in tissue from normal prostates.[17] In tissue from patients with BPH who had been treated with a liposterolic extract of saw palmetto (Permixon), there was significant induction of apoptosis and inhibition of cell proliferation, compared with tissue from patients with BPH who had not received saw palmetto extract. In another *in vitro* study, incubation with Permixon 10 µg/mL also increased the apoptotic index for prostate epithelial cells by 35%.[10]

Other *in vitro* studies have explored the effects of saw palmetto extract and its constituents on human prostatic cancer cells and other tumour cell lines. An extract of saw palmetto fruit, prepared by supercritical fluid extraction with carbon dioxide, induced cell death in LNCaP cells (a hormonal therapy-resistant prostatic cancer cell line) in a concentration-dependent manner.[18] This confirms the findings of previous studies demonstrating the effect of a liposterolic extract of saw palmetto (Permixon) on the mortality rate of LNCaP cells: increased mortality was observed with saw palmetto extract 50 μg/mL, compared with control.[19] Further investigation identified myristoleic acid as a component of saw palmetto extract that caused cell death. The EC_{50} for both the extract and myristoleic acid was around 100 μg/mL.[18] Following incubation of LNCaP cells with saw palmetto extract 130 μg/mL or myristoleic acid 100 μg/mL, the proportions of apoptotic and necrotic cells were 16.5% and 46.8%, respectively, for the extract, and 8.8% and 81.8%, respectively, for myristoleic acid. An extract of saw palmetto obtained by supercritical extraction with carbon dioxide inhibited the invasion of PC-3 cells (derived from human adenocarcinoma of the prostate) into Matrigel *in vitro* in a concentration-dependent manner at concentrations in the range 1–10 μg/mL.[20] However, LNCaP cells and SKRC-1 cells (derived from human renal carcinoma) were unaffected by the extract. The extract was also shown to inhibit the activity of urokinase-type plasminogen activator, a protease enzyme that is necessary for tumour-cell invasion into basement membranes. The monoacylglycerides 1-monolaurin and 1-monomyristicin isolated from saw palmetto demonstrated *in vitro* activity against renal (A-498) and pancreatic (PACA-2) human tumour cells (EC_{50} for 1-monolaurin: 3.77 μg/mL and 2.33 μg/mL, respectively; EC_{50} for 1-monomyristicin: 3.58 μg/mL and 1.87 μg/mL, respectively).[2] However, only borderline cytotoxicity was observed against PC-3 cells (EC_{50} for 1-monomyristicin: 8.84 μg/mL).[2]

Spasmolytic activity has also been documented for saw palmetto and it has been suggested that this may contribute to the herb's effects in BPH. An ethanolic lipidic extract was reported to produce a concentration-dependent relaxation on rat uterus tonic contraction induced by vanadate (EC_{50} 11.41 μg/mL).[21] Further investigation suggested that a mechanism for the observed effect could be interference with intracellular calcium mobilisation, possibly mediated via cyclic AMP. Other *in vitro* studies demonstrated that a lipophilic ethanolic extract of saw palmetto 0.3–0.75 mg/mL reduced norepinephrine (noradrenaline)-induced contractions in rat deferential duct. Further study indicated that the relaxant effect of saw palmetto extract results from either α-adrenoceptor blockade or from calcium-blocking activity.[22]

Other activity *In vivo* oestrogenic activity in the rat has also been documented for an alcoholic extract.[23] Activity was attributed to the high content of β-sitosterol, a known oestrogenic agent, present in saw palmetto.

In vivo anti-oedema activity in the rat has been documented for a hexane extract of saw palmetto, acting by inhibition of histamine-induced increase in capillary permeability.[24] Low doses of an aqueous extract were effective in carrageenan-induced paw oedema and pellet tests in the rat, although the extract was not found to influence the proliferative stage of inflammation.[1,25] The observed anti-inflammatory activity was attributed to a high molecular weight polysaccharide (approximately 100 000). Polysaccharides possessing immunostimulating activity have also been documented for saw palmetto and were stated to contain a high content of glucuronic acid.[1,25]

An extract (SG-291) prepared from saw palmetto fruits by supercritical fluid extraction with carbon dioxide was reported to inhibit both cyclooxygenase and 5-lipoxygenase *in vitro* (IC_{50} 28.1 μg/mL and 18.0 μg/mL, respectively).[26] Further study indicated that the component(s) of saw palmetto extract that inhibits these enzymes must be within the acidic lipophilic fraction. Subsequent studies have documented that a liposterolic extract of saw palmetto (Permixon) significantly inhibited the production of 5-lipoxygenase metabolites, including leukotriene B_4, by human polymorphonuclear neutrophils at concentrations of saw palmetto extract of 5 μg/mL and above.[27]

Clinical studies

Pharmacokinetics Some data on the pharmacokinetics of saw palmetto extracts in healthy male volunteers ($n = 12$) come from an open, randomised, single-dose bioequivalence study of a 320-mg capsule of a liposterolic extract of saw palmetto compared with two capsules of saw palmetto extract 160 mg as the reference preparation.[28] The plasma concentration–time curves were reported to be almost identical for both preparations. The maximum concentration (C_{max}) for saw palmetto extract 320-mg capsule and 2×160-mg capsules was 2.54–2.61 μg/mL and 2.57–2.67 μg/mL, respectively, and time to C_{max} (T_{max}) was 1.58 and 1.5 hours for the 320-mg capsule and 2×160-mg capsules, respectively. Another study explored the bioavailability and pharmacokinetic profile of a rectal formulation of saw palmetto extract 640 mg in healthy male volunteers ($n = 12$).[29] The mean maximum plasma concentration of the second component of saw palmetto was almost 2.6 μg/mL at around 3 hours after drug administration.

Pharmacodynamics The inhibitory effects of saw palmetto extract on 5-α-reductase activity documented *in vitro* (see Pharmacological Actions, *In vitro* and animal studies) have been confirmed in some studies in humans, and refuted by others.

In one study, 25 men with symptomatic, established BPH were randomised to receive either a liposterolic extract of saw palmetto (Permixon) 320 mg/day for three months ($n = 10$), or no treatment ($n = 15$).[30] At the end of the treatment period, analysis of samples of BPH tissue, obtained by suprapubic prostatectomy, showed that dihydrotestosterone concentrations were significantly reduced and that testosterone concentrations were significantly higher in the treatment group, compared with the control group ($p < 0.001$ for both). A significant reduction in concentrations of epidermal growth factor in total BPH tissue was also observed in the treatment group, compared with the control group ($p < 0.01$). The reported biochemical effects were most evident in BPH tissue from the periurethral region.

In another study, biopsy specimens of the prostate were taken from 44 men with symptomatic BPH participating in a randomised, placebo-controlled trial of a herbal combination preparation containing saw palmetto lipoidal extract 106 mg together with nettle root extract, pumpkin seed oil, lemon bioflavonoid extract and vitamin A.[31,32] There were no statistically significant differences in median tissue dihydrotestosterone and testosterone concentrations between the treatment and placebo groups at baseline. At the end of the study, mean tissue dihydrotestosterone concentrations decreased significantly in the treatment group, compared with baseline values ($p = 0.005$), whereas there was no significant change in dihydrotestosterone concentrations in the placebo group. However, in a separate analysis, it was reported that the median change in tissue dihydrotestosterone concentrations for the treatment group (1.38 ng/g) did not differ significantly from the corresponding change in the placebo group (0.87 ng/g). The findings of this study should be interpreted cautiously as it is possible there are other explanations for the observed effect.

Another randomised, double-blind trial involving 18 men with BPH compared saw palmetto extract (IDS-89; Strogen) 640 mg three times daily (i.e. six times the normal dose) for three months with placebo.[33] This high dose of saw palmetto extract achieved only a moderate decrease in 5-α-reductase activity.

An open, randomised, placebo-controlled study involving 32 healthy male volunteers compared the effects of a liposterolic extract of saw palmetto (Permixon) 80 mg twice daily for seven days with those of finasteride 5 mg daily for seven days on inhibition of 5-α-reductase activity.[34] Serum dihydrotestosterone concentrations were reported to decrease significantly with finasteride, compared with baseline values, but no significant changes were observed for the saw palmetto and placebo groups. Thus, this study did not support a mechanism of action for saw palmetto in BPH by inhibition of 5-α-reductase activity.

Alpha-adrenoceptor blocking activity has also been documented for saw palmetto extract *in vitro*,[22] although this has been refuted in a study involving healthy volunteers.[35] In a double-blind, placebo-controlled, four-way, crossover study, 12 healthy male volunteers received three different saw palmetto extract preparations (Prostagutt uno, Prostess uno, Talso uno) 320 mg daily for eight days each, separated by wash-out phases of at least two weeks. It was reported that none of the study medications showed signs of α_1-adrenoceptor subtype occupancy as determined by a radioreceptor assay.

Therapeutic effects Numerous clinical studies have investigated the effects of saw palmetto in men with BPH.

A systematic review and meta-analysis included 18 randomised clinical trials (16 of which were double-blind) of saw palmetto extracts involving a total of 2939 men with BPH.[36] This work has also been published as a Cochrane systematic review.[37] The review included 10 studies which compared saw palmetto extracts alone with placebo, three comparing saw palmetto extracts in combination with other herbals with placebo, two comparing saw palmetto extracts alone with an active control, one comparing saw palmetto extracts in combination with other herbals with an active control, one comparing saw palmetto extract with another herb and with placebo, and one comparing oral saw palmetto extract with a rectal formulation of saw palmetto extract. The mean duration of the included studies was nine weeks (range 4–48 weeks).

Compared with placebo, saw palmetto extracts led to a decrease in urinary symptom scores and nocturia, and improvements in self-rating of urinary symptoms and peak urine flow.[37] Compared with finasteride, saw palmetto extracts achieved similar improvements in urinary symptom scores and peak urine flow. This systematic review was considered to have provided good evidence that saw palmetto is effective in men with symptoms of BPH, although there is scope for further trials.[37,38]

Several other clinical studies of saw palmetto extracts in BPH have now been published since the Cochrane systematic review, although few have comprised rigorous study design capable of testing efficacy, and several have investigated combination preparations of saw palmetto with other herbs.

A short report describes a randomised, double-blind, placebo-controlled trial of saw palmetto extract (LG-166S) 160 mg twice daily for six months in 101 men with BPH.[39] This study reported statistically significant differences in symptom scores between the treatment group and the placebo group at the end of the study ($p < 0.001$).

In a study involving 75 men with mild/moderate BPH according to their International Prostate Symptom Score (IPSS), participants received a liposterolic extract of saw palmetto (Permixon) 160 mg twice daily for nine weeks ($n = 57$).[40] A control group ($n = 18$) did not receive any medical treatment for BPH, and there was no random allocation to treatment, although it was stated that baseline parameters were comparable between the two groups. It was reported that, at the end of the study, IPSS and quality-of-life scores, compared with baseline values, significantly improved in Permixon-treated men ($p < 0.001$). There were no significant differences in these parameters, compared with baseline values, for the control group.

Two randomised studies involving men with symptomatic BPH have compared the effects of different regimens of saw palmetto extract.[41,42] A multicentre, randomised, single-blind trial involving 132 men with BPH compared the effects of saw palmetto extract (Prostaserene) 320 mg once daily with 160 mg twice daily for one year.[41] Another study compared a liposterolic extract of saw palmetto (Permixon) 320 mg daily with 160 mg twice daily for three months in 100 men with symptomatic BPH.[42] For each regimen, both studies reported significant improvements in the mean IPSS, maximum and mean urinary flow rates and residual urine volume, at the end of the studies, compared with baseline values. However, as these studies did not include a placebo-control group, the possibility that the observed effects are placebo effects cannot be excluded.

Several other open, uncontrolled studies of saw palmetto extracts (alone or in combination with other herbs), several of which were drug-monitoring studies which also assessed effectiveness, have reported improvements in symptoms of BPH at the end of treatment, compared with baseline values.[43–47] Doses assessed in these studies were usually 160 mg two or three times daily for up to three years. These studies are discussed in more detail later (see Side-effects, Toxicity).

The effects of a combination herbal preparation containing saw palmetto lipoidal extract 106 mg together with nettle root extract, pumpkin seed oil, lemon bioflavonoid extract and vitamin A, were assessed in a six-month, randomised, double-blind,

placebo-controlled trial involving 44 men with symptomatic BPH.[32] At the end of the treatment period, a slight decrease in symptom score and an increase in urinary flow were observed for both groups, compared with baseline values. These changes were greater in the treatment group, compared with the placebo group, but this difference was not statistically significant. In another randomised, double-blind, controlled trial involving 543 men with BPH, participants received a combination of saw palmetto extract 160 mg and nettle root extract 120 mg (Prostagutt forte) daily, or finasteride 5 mg daily, for 48 weeks.[48] Data from a subgroup of 431 participants with ultrasonographic measurements were analysed. Mean maximum urinary flow and IPSS improved in both groups, compared with baseline values; there were no statistically significant differences between the two groups.

Saw palmetto is one of the eight herbal ingredients contained in a commercial preparation known as PC-SPES; the other herbal ingredients are chrysanthemum, isatis, licorice, *Ganoderma lucidum*, *Panax pseudoginseng*, *Rabdosia rubescens* and *Scutellaria* (scullcap). The combination preparation has been investigated for oestrogenic activity, and is currently of interest for its potential effects in the treatment of hormone-sensitive prostate cancer.[49]

Side-effects, Toxicity

A systematic review and meta-analysis of 18 randomised clinical trials of saw palmetto extracts (see Pharmacological Actions, Clinical studies, Therapeutic effects) reported that adverse effects with saw palmetto were generally mild and comparable to those with placebo.[37] Gastrointestinal effects were reported in 1.3% of men taking saw palmetto extracts, placebo (0.9%) and finasteride (1.5%). Study withdrawal rates for men taking saw palmetto, placebo and finasteride were 9.1%, 7.0% and 11.2%, respectively. The authors of the review concluded that saw palmetto extracts are associated with fewer adverse treatment effects than is finasteride, but that little is known about the long-term safety of saw palmetto extracts.

In a drug-monitoring study involving 1334 men with BPH, the tolerability of saw palmetto extract 160 mg twice daily for 12 weeks was reported to be 'good' or 'excellent' by more than 95% of participants.[46] This is similar to a finding from a three-year prospective, uncontrolled study involving 435 men with BPH, in which the tolerability of saw palmetto extract (IDS-89) 160 mg twice daily was classified as 'good' or 'very good' by both physicians and patients for 98% of participants.[45] A total of 46 adverse events was reported in 34 patients. Of these, 30% were gastrointestinal disturbances. The withdrawal rate from the study was 1.8%, mostly because of digestive disturbances ($n = 3$) and tumours ($n = 3$). Non-serious adverse effects (4.95–6.63%), mainly minor gastrointestinal effects, such as gastralgia, nausea, diarrhoea, constipation and anorexia, as well as vertigo, headache, dry mouth and pruritus, were reported in an open study involving 413 men with BPH who received saw palmetto extract 160 mg twice daily for three months.[44] An observational study involving 2080 patients with BPH who received a combination of saw palmetto extract (WS-1473) and nettle root extract (WS-1031) reported that the tolerability of the preparation was classified by physicians to be 'good' or 'very good' for the majority of participants.[47] Mild adverse effects were reported in 15 patients (0.72%).

Studies assessing the equivalence of two different regimens of saw palmetto extract (320 mg once daily and 160 mg twice daily) report that adverse events occurred with a similar frequency in both groups.[41,42] Most events were deemed to be unrelated or unlikely to be related to treatment with saw palmetto extract.

Toxicity   Incubation of high concentrations of saw palmetto extract (Permixon) 9.0 mg/mL for 48 hours inhibited sperm motility, compared with control.[50]

Contra-indications, Warnings

In view of the reported anti-androgen and oestrogenic activities, saw palmetto may affect existing hormonal therapy, including the oral contraceptive pill and hormone replacement therapy.

Pregnancy and lactation   The safety of saw palmetto has not been established. In view of the lack of toxicity data and the documented hormonal activity, the use of saw palmetto during pregnancy and lactation should be avoided.

Pharmaceutical Comment

Several pharmacological activities have been documented for saw palmetto *in vitro* and *in vivo* (animals). Some of these properties, such as inhibition of 5-α-reductase activity, inhibition of androgen binding and spasmolytic activity, are thought to explain, at least in part, the effects of saw palmetto in benign prostatic hyperplasia (BPH). However, some experimental and clinical studies report conflicting results, particularly with regard to the inhibition of 5-α-reductase activity and α-adrenoceptor blocking activity by saw palmetto extracts. Thus, the mechanism(s)

of action of saw palmetto extracts in BPH remain unclear. This is not surprising, given that, at present, the exact cause of BPH is unknown. In addition to the effects of saw palmetto in experimental models of BPH, immunostimulant and anti-inflammatory activities have been documented in laboratory studies.

Results of clinical studies indicate that saw palmetto is a potential agent for the treatment of BPH. However, this is not an indication suitable for self-diagnosis and self-treatment, and over-the-counter use of saw palmetto extract for BPH should be under medical supervision. Data from randomised clinical trials and drug-monitoring studies indicate that, generally, saw palmetto is well-tolerated;[51] adverse events are mild and relate mainly to gastrointestinal symptoms. However, in view of the lack of toxicity data and the documented pharmacological actions of saw palmetto, excessive use should be avoided.

References

See also General References G3, G5, G9, G10, G22, G31, G32, G36, G41, G50, G56 and G64.

1   Wagner H, Flachsbarth H. A new antiphlogistic principle from *Sabal serrulata*, I. *Planta Med* 1981; **41**: 244–251.
2   Shimada H *et al*. Biologically active acylglycerides from the berries of saw palmetto (*Serenoa repens*). *J Nat Prod* 1997; **60**: 417–418.
3   Schöpflin G *et al*. β-Sitosterin als Möglicher Wirkstoff der Sabalfrüchte. *Planta Med* 1966; **14**: 402–407.
4   Hänsel R *et al*. Eine Dünnschichtchromatographische untersuchung der Sabalfrüchte. *Planta Med* 1964; **12**: 169–172.
5   Bombardelli E, Morazzoni P. *Serenoa repens* (Bartram) J.K. Small. *Fitoterapia* 1997; **68**: 99–113.
6   Sultan C *et al*. Inhibition of androgen metabolism and binding by a liposterolic extract of 'Serenoa repens B' in human foreskin fibroblasts. *J Steroid Biochem* 1984; **20**: 515–519.
7   Weisser H *et al*. Effects of the Sabal serrulata extract IDS 89 and its subfractions on 5-α-reductase activity in human benign prostatic hyperplasia. *Prostate* 1996; **28**: 300–306.
8   Palin M-F *et al*. Inhibitory effects of *Serenoa repens* on the kinetic of pig prostatic microsomal 5α-reductase activity. *Endocrine* 1998; **9**: 65–69.
9   Bayne CW *et al*. Serenoa repens (Permixon®): a 5α-reductase types I and II inhibitor – new evidence in a coculture model of BPH. *Prostate* 1999; **40**: 232–241.
10   Bayne CW *et al*. The selectivity and specificity of the actions of the lipido-sterolic extract of Serenoa repens (Permixon®) on the prostate. *J Urol* 2000;

164: 876–881.

11 Carilla E *et al.* Binding of permixon, a new treatment for prostatic benign hyperplasia, to the cytosolic androgen receptor in the rat prostate. *J Steroid Biochem* 1984; **20**: 521–523.

12 Düker E-M *et al.* Inhibition of 5-α-reductase activity by extracts from Sabal serrulata. *Planta Med* 1989; **55**: 587.

13 Paubert-Braquet M *et al.* Effect of *Serenoa repens* extract (Permixon®) on estradiol/testosterone-induced experimental prostate enlargement in the rat. *Pharmacol Res* 1996; **34**: 171–179.

14 Van Coppenolle F *et al.* Pharmacological effects of the lipidosterolic extract of *Serenoa repens* (Permixon®) on rat prostate hyperplasia induced by hyperprolactinaemia: comparison with finasteride. *Prostate* 2000; **43**: 49–58.

15 Barsanti JA *et al.* Effects of an extract of *Serenoa repens* on dogs with hyperplasia of the prostate gland. *Am J Vet Res* 2000; **61**: 880–885.

16 Paubert-Braquet M *et al.* Effect of the lipidosterolic extract of *Serenoa repens* (Permixon®) and its major components on basic fibroblast growth factor-induced proliferation of cultures of human prostate biopsies. *Eur Urol* 1998; **33**: 340–347.

17 Vachero F *et al.* Induction of apoptosis and inhibition of cell proliferation by the lipidosterolic extract of *Serenoa repens* (LSEr, Permixon®) in benign prostatic hyperplasia. *Prostate* 2000; **45**: 259–266.

18 Iguchi K *et al.* Myristoleic acid, a cytotoxic component in the extract from *Serenoa repens*, induces apoptosis and necrosis in human prostatic LNCaP cells. *Prostate* 2001; **47**: 59–65.

19 Ravenna L *et al.* Effects of the lipidosterolic extract of *Serenoa repens* (Permixon®) on human prostatic cell lines. *Prostate* 1996; **29**: 219–230.

20 Ishii K *et al.* Extract from *Serenoa repens* suppresses the invasion activity of human urological cancer cells by inhibiting urokinase-type plasminogen activator. *Biol Pharm Bull* 2001; **24**: 188–190.

21 Gutiérrez M *et al.* Spasmolytic activity of a lipidic extract from *Sabal serrulata* fruits: further study of the mechanisms underlying this activity. *Planta Med* 1996; **62**: 507–511.

22 Odenthal KP. Phytotherapy of benign prostatic hyperplasia (BPH) with *Cucurbita, Hypoxis, Pygeum, Urtica* and *Sabal serrulata* (*Serenoa repens*). *Phytother Res* 1996; **10**: S141–S143.

23 Elghamry MI, Hänsel R. Activity and isolated phytoestrogen of shrub palmetto fruits (*Serenoa repens* Small), a new estrogenic plant. *Experientia* 1969; **25**: 828–829.

24 Stenger A *et al.* Pharmacology and biochemistry of hexane extract of *Serenoa repens*. *Gazz Med Fr* 1982; **89**: 2041–2048.

25 Wagner H *et al.* A new antiphlogistic principle from *Sabal serrulata* II. *Planta Med* 1981; **41**: 252–258.

26 Breu W *et al.* Antiphlogistic activity of an extract from Sabal serrulata fruits prepared by supercritical carbon dioxide: *in vitro* inhibition of cyclooxygenase and 5-lipoxygenase metabolism. *Arzneimittelforschung* 1992; **42**: 547–551.

27 Paubert-Braquet M *et al.* Effect of the lipidic lipidosterolic extract of *Serenoa repens* (Permixon®) on the ionophore A23187-stimulated production of leukotriene B_4 (LTB_4) from human polymorphonuclear neutrophils. *Prostaglandins Leukot Essent Fatty Acids* 1997; **57**: 299–304.

28 De Bernardi di Valserra M *et al.* *Serenoa repens* capsules: a bioequivalence study. *Acta Toxicol Ther* 1994; **15**: 21–39.

29 De Bernardi di Valserra M, Tripodi AS. Rectal bioavailability and pharmacokinetics in healthy volunteers of *Serenoa repens* new formulation. *Arch Med Intern* 1994; **46**: 77–86.

30 Di Silverio F *et al.* Effects of long-term treatment with *Serenoa repens* (Permixon®) on the concentrations and regional distribution of androgens and epidermal growth factor in benign prostatic hyperplasia. *Prostate* 1998; **37**: 77–83.

31 Marks LS *et al.* Tissue effects of saw palmetto and finasteride: use of biopsy cores for in situ quantification of prostatic androgens. *Urology* 2001; **57**: 999–1005.

32 Marks LS *et al.* Effects of a saw palmetto herbal blend in men with symptomatic benign prostatic hyperplasia. *J Urol* 2000; **163**: 1451–1456.

33 Weisser H *et al.* Enzyme activities in tissue of human benign prostatic hyperplasia after three months' treatment with the *Sabal serrulata* extract IDS 89 (Strogen®) or placebo. *Eur Urol* 1997; **31**: 97–101.

34 Strauch G *et al.* Comparison of finasteride (Proscar®) and *Serenoa repens* (Permixon®) in the inhibition of 5-alpha-reductase in healthy male volunteers. *Eur Urol* 1994; **26**: 247–252.

35 Goepel M *et al.* Do saw palmetto extracts block human α_1-adrenoceptor subtypes *in vivo*? *Prostate* 2001; **46**: 226–232.

36 Wilt TJ *et al.* Saw palmetto extracts for treatment of benign prostatic hyperplasia. A systematic review. *JAMA* 1998; **280**: 1604–1609.

37 Wilt TJ *et al.* *Serenoa repens* for treatment of benign prostatic hyperplasia. In: *The Cochrane Library*, Issue 3, 2001. Oxford: Update Software.

38 Anon. Saw palmetto and prostatic hypertrophy. *Bandolier* 2000; **7**: 1–3.

39 Bauer HW *et al.* Sabalfrucht-Extrakt zur Behandlung der benignen Prostatahyperplasie. Ergebnisse einer plazebokontrollierten Doppelblindstudie. *Fortschritte Med* 1999; **25**: 62.

40 Al-Shukri SH *et al.* Early urodynamic effects of the lipido-sterolic extract of *Serenoa repens* (Per-

mixon®) in patients with lower urinary tract symptoms due to benign prostatic hyperplasia. *Prostate Cancer Prostatic Dis* 2000; **3**: 195–199.

41 Braeckman J *et al*. Efficacy and safety of the extract of *Serenoa repens* in the treatment of benign prostatic hyperplasia: therapeutic equivalence between twice and once daily dosage forms. *Phytother Res* 1997; **11**: 558–563.

42 Stepanov VN *et al*. Efficacy and tolerability of the lipidosterolic extract of *Serenoa repens* (Permixon®) in benign prostatic hyperplasia: a double-blind comparison of two dosage regimens. *Adv Ther* 1999; **16**: 231–241.

43 Gerber GS *et al*. Saw palmetto (*Serenoa repens*) in men with lower urinary tract symptoms: effects on urodynamic parameters and voiding symptoms. *Urology* 1998; **51**: 1003–1007.

44 Braeckman J *et al*. Efficacy and safety of the extract of *Serenoa repens* in the treatment of benign prostatic hyperplasia: an open multicentre study. *Eur J Clin Res* 1997; **9**: 47–57.

45 Bach D, Ebeling L. Long-term drug treatment of benign prostatic hyperplasia – results of a prospective 3-year multicenter study using Sabal extract IDS 89. *Phytomedicine* 1996; **3**: 105–111.

46 Vahlensieck W *et al*. Benigne Prostatahyperplasie – Behandlung mit Sabalfrucht-Extrakt. *Fortschritte Ther* 1993; **18**: 45–48.

47 Schneider H-J *et al*. Behandlung der benignen Prostatahyperplasie. *Fortschritte Ther* 1995; **3**: 37–40.

48 Sökeland J. Combined sabal and urtica extract compared with finasteride in men with benign prostatic hyperplasia: analysis of prostate volume and therapeutic outcome. *BJU Int* 2000; **86**: 439–442.

49 DiPaola RS *et al*. Clinical and biological activity of an estrogenic herbal combination (PC-SPES) in prostate cancer. *N Engl J Med* 1998; **339**: 785–791.

50 Ondrizek RR *et al*. Inhibition of human sperm motility by specific herbs used in alternative medicine. *J Assist Reprod Genet* 1999; **16**: 87–91

51 Gerber GS. Saw palmetto for the treatment of men with lower urinary tract symptoms. *J Urol* 2000; **163**: 1408–1412.

Scullcap

Species (Family)

Scutellaria lateriflora L., *S. baicalensis* Georgi and other *Scutellaria* species (Labiatae)

S. baicalensis Georgi is a species commonly referred to as scullcap in Chinese herbal medicine.

Synonym(s)

Helmet Flower, Hoodwort, Quaker Bonnet, Scutellaria, *Scutellaria galericulata* L., Skullcap

Part(s) Used

Herb

Pharmacopoeial and Other Monographs

BHP 1996[G9]
PDR for Herbal Medicines 2nd edition[G36]

Legal Category (Licensed Products)

GSL[G37]

Constituents[G20,G22,G48,G60,G64]

Limited information has been documented regarding the constituents of *S. lateriflora*, although various related *Scutellaria* species have been investigated.

Flavonoids Apigenin, hispidulin, luteolin, scutellarein, scutellarin (bitter glycoside).

Iridoids Catalpol.

Volatile oils Limonene, terpineol (monoterpenes); *d*-cadinene, caryophyllene, *trans*-β-farnesene, β-humulene (sesquiterpenes).

Other constituents Lignin, resin and tannin.

Other Scutellaria species The related species *S. baicalensis* is reported to contain baicalein, baicalin, chrysin, oroxylin A, skullcapflavone II and wogonin.[1-3]

S. galericulata is stated to contain apigenin, baicalein, baicalin, apigenin-7-glucoside and galeroside (baicalein-β-L-rhamnofuranoside).[4]

Food Use

Scullcap is not used in foods. In the USA, scullcap is listed by the Food and Drugs Administration (FDA) as a Herb of Undefined Safety.[G22]

Herbal Use

Scullcap is stated to possess anticonvulsant and sedative properties.[G34,G64] Traditionally, it has been used for epilepsy, chorea, hysteria, nervous tension states, and specifically for grand mal epilepsy.[G7] In Chinese herbal medicine, the roots of *S. baicalensis* Georgi have been used traditionally as a remedy for inflammation, suppurative dermatitis, allergic diseases, hyperlipidaemia and atherosclerosis.

Dosage

Dried herb 1–2 g or by infusion three times daily.[G7]

Liquid extract 2–4 mL (1 : 1 in 25% alcohol) three times daily.[G7]

Tincture 1–2 mL (1:5 in 45% alcohol) three times daily.[G7]

Pharmacological Actions

In vitro and animal studies

None documented for *Scutellaria lateriflora*.

Many investigations have been undertaken to study the pharmacological actions of *S. baicalensis* root. Documented actions have primarily been attributed to the various flavonoid constituents and include: *in vitro* inhibition of mast cell histamine release comparable to disodium cromoglycate for some flavonoids;[1] *in vitro* cytotoxicity of scullcap flavone II;[5] *in vivo* and *in vitro* inhibition of lipid peroxidation;[6-8] *in vitro* inhibition of lipoxygenase and cyclooxygenase pathways;[9] hypocholesterolaemic activity in rats.[10] This *in vivo* effect has been linked to *in vitro* actions documented for various flavonoids, including prevention of ethanol-induced hyperlipidaemia,[11] catecholamine-induced lipolysis[10,11] and lipogenesis in adipose tissue;[10,11] there is no pronounced effect on blood pressure in cats and rabbits.[12] In addition, the latter study found no CNS-depressant and no antispasmodic activity. However, it did find marked antibacterial activity against various Gram-positive bacteria (e.g. *Bacillus subtilis, Escherichia coli, Sarcina lutea* and *Staphylococcus aureus*).[13]

Clinical studies

Clinical investigation of scutellarin involving 634 cases of cerebral thrombosis, cerebral embolism, and paralysis caused by stroke has been undertaken. An overall effective rate of more than 88% was reported following intramuscular, intravenous or oral administration.[14]

Side-effects, Toxicity[G20]

Symptoms caused by overdosage of scullcap tincture include giddiness, stupor, confusion and seizures.[G20] Hepatotoxic reactions have been reported after ingestion of scullcap-containing preparations.[15,G20] Adulteration of scullcap herb by *Teucrium* is recognised. Several cases of hepatitis have been associated with germander (*Teucrium chamaedrys*).[16]

Contra-indications, Warnings

None documented. In view of the possible hepatotoxicity associated with scullcap, its use is best avoided.

Pregnancy and lactation Scullcap is stated to have been used traditionally to eliminate a mother's afterbirth and to promote menstruation.[G22] Limited information is known regarding the pharmacological activity and toxicity of scullcap. In view of this and concerns over hepatotoxicity, scullcap should not be taken during pregnancy and lactation.

Pharmaceutical Comment

Limited information has been documented regarding the chemistry of scullcap. Most of the pharmacological activities reported for other *Scutellaria* species have been attributed to the flavonoid constituents. Despite the traditional uses of scullcap as a sedative and anticonvulsant, there are no documented scientific data to support these uses. Commercial scullcap is commonly recognised to be adulterated with *Teucrium* species, notably *Teucrium canadense*. Herbal preparations stated to contain scullcap may therefore contain a *Teucrium* species. Few pharmacological studies have been undertaken for *Teucrium* species. Hepatitis has been associated with germander (*Teucrium chamaedrys*). Hepatotoxicity has resulted in humans taking commercially available remedies in the UK which are stated to contain

scullcap. It would seem advisable to avoid ingestion of scullcap.

References

See also General References G5, G9, G10, G18, G20, G22, G31, G32, G34, G36, G37, G48, G60 and G64.

1 Kubo M *et al. Scutellariae radix.* X. Inhibitory effects of various flavonoids on histamine release from rat peritoneal mast cells *in vitro. Chem Pharm Bull* 1984; **32**: 5051–5054.

2 Tomimori T *et al.* Studies on the constituents of Scutellarian species. *Yakugaku Zasshi* 1985; **105**: 148–155.

3 Tomimori T *et al.* Studies on the constituents of *Scutellaria* species. VI. On the flavonoid constituents of the root of *Scutellaria baicalensis* Georgi (5). Quantitative analysis of flavonoids in Scutellaria roots by high-performance liquid chromatography. *Yakugaku Zasshi* 1985; **105**: 148–155.

4 Popova TP *et al.* Chemical composition and medicinal properties of *Scutellaria galericulata. Farm Zh (Kiev)* 1972; **27**: 58–61.

5 Ryn SH *et al.* The cytotoxic principle of *Scutellariae radix* against L1210 cell. *Planta Med* 1985; **51**: 355.

6 Kimura Y *et al.* Studies on *Scutellariae radix*; IX. New component inhibiting lipid peroxidation in rat liver. *Planta Med* 1984; **50**: 290–295.

7 Kimura Y *et al.* Studies on *Scutellariae radix.* IV. Effects on lipid peroxidation in rat liver. *Chem Pharm Bull* 1981; **29**: 2610–2617.

8 Kimura Y *et al.* Studies on *Scutellariae radix.* VI. Effects of flavanone compounds on lipid peroxidation in rat liver. *Chem Pharm Bull* 1982; **30**: 1792–1795.

9 Kimura Y *et al.* Studies on *Scutellariae radix.* XIII. Effects of various flavonoids on arachidonate metabolism in leukocytes. *Planta Med* 1985; **51**: 132–136.

10 Kimura Y *et al.* Studies on *Scutellariae radix.* III. Effects on lipid metabolism in serum, liver and fat cells of rats. *Chem Pharm Bull* 1981; **29**: 2308–2312.

11 Kimura Y *et al.* Studies on *Scutellariae radix.* V. Effects on ethanol-induced hyperlipemia and lipolysis in isolated fat cells. *Chem Pharm Bull* 1982; **30**: 219–222.

12 Kurnakov BA. Pharmacology of skullcap. *Farmakol i Toksikol* 1957; **20**: 79–80.

13 Kubo M *et al.* Studies on *Scutellariae radix.* Part II: The antibacterial substance. *Planta Med* 1981; **43**: 194–201.

14 Peigen X, Keji C. Recent advances in clinical studies of Chinese medicinal herbs. 1. Drugs affecting the cardiovascular system. *Phytother Res* 1987; **1**: 53–57.

15 Perharic L *et al.* Toxicological problems resulting

from exposure to traditional remedies and food supplements. *Drug Safety* 1994; **11**: 284–294.

16 Larrey D *et al*. Hepatitis after germander (*Teu-crium chamaedrys*) administration: another instance of herbal medicine toxicity. *Am Coll Physicians* 1992; **117**: 129–132.

Senega

Species (Family)

Polygala senega L. (Polygalaceae) and other closely related species cultivated in western Canada and Japan.

Synonym(s)

Northern Senega (Canada), Polygala, *Polygala senega* var. *latifolia* (Japan), Rattlesnake Root, Snake Root

Part(s) Used

Root, rootstock

Pharmacopoeial and Other Monographs

BHC 1992[G6]
BHP 1996[G9]
BP 2001[G15]
Complete German Commission E[G3]
ESCOP 1997[G52]
Martindale 32nd edition[G43]
PDR for Herbal Medicines 2nd edition[G36]
Ph Eur 2002[G28]

Legal Category (Licensed Products)

GSL[G37]

Constituents[1,G2,G6,G20,G40,G48,G52,G59,G62,G64]

Acids Salicylic acid and its methyl ester 0.1–0.2%; hydroxycinnamic acids (e.g. caffeic acid, ferulic acid, sinapic acid) free or esterified with saponins.[2]

Carbohydrates Arabinose, fructose, glucose, melibiose, raffinose, saccharose, stachyose, sucrose; 1,5-anhydro-D-glucitol and other D-glucitol derivatives;[3,4] trisaccharides; mucilage, pectin. A series of oligosaccharide esters, senegoses A–O, containing acetic, benzoic, *trans*- and *cis*-ferulic acid moieties linked to glucose and fructose.[5,6] Five acylated sucrose glycosides, tenuifolisides A–E, have been isolated from *P. tenuifolia*.[7,8] The esterifying acids are 3,4,5-trimethoxycinnamic, *p*-hydroxybenzoic, sinapic and ferulic.

Terpenoids A complex mixture of bidesmosidic triterpene saponins (6–10%) based on the aglycone presenegin. The total saponin mixture may be referred to as senegin. The saponins of *P. senega* var. *latifolia* are 3-glucosides of presenegin with tetra-, penta- or hexa-glucosyl groups linked at C-28 and including 4″-methoxy-cinnamoyl or 3″,4″-dimethoxycinnamoyl fucosyl resulting in *E*- and *Z*-cinnamoyl isomers of each saponin.[9–11] Senegins I–IV were the first saponins to be characterised and were *E*-isomers.[12,13] *P. tenuifolia* contains similar saponins named onjisaponins A–G.[14,15]

Xanthones A number of xanthones have been isolated from *P. tenuifolia* including 4-C-[β-D-apiofuranosyl-(1→6)-β-D-glucopyranosyl]-1,3,6-trihydroxy-7-methoxyxanthone.[8]

Other constituents Fat, resin, sterols and valeric acid ester.

Other Polygala species *Polygala paniculata* contains coumarins (aurapten, murrangatin, phebalosin and 7-methoxy-8-(1,4-dihydroxy-3-methyl-2-butenyl) coumarin,[16] pyranocoumarin).[17] *Polygala chamaebuxus* (European species) contains hydroxycinnamic acid esters involving acetic, ferulic and sinapic acids as the ester moieties, saponins, tenuifolin (prosapogenin), rutin (flavonoid glycoside), coniferin and syringen (phenolic glycosides).[2]

Other European species (e.g. *Polygala alpestris*, *Polygala comosa*, *Polygala vayredae*) contain complex mixtures of bidesmosidic saponins, tenuifolin (prosapogenin), hydroxycinnimic acid esters similar to those reported for *P. chamaebuxus*.[18] *Polygala triphylla* contains B-ring oxygen-free trioxygenated- and glucosyloxy-xanthones.[19] *Polygala polygama* contains podophyllotoxin and demethylpodophyllotoxin (lignans).[20]

Food Use

Senega is listed by the Council of Europe as a natural source of food flavouring (category N2). This category indicates that senega can be added to foodstuffs in small quantities, with a possible limitation of an active principle (as yet unspecified) in the final product.[G16]

Herbal Use[G2,G6,G7,G8,G32,G43,G52,G54,G64]

Senega is stated to possess expectorant, diaphoretic, sialogogue and emetic properties. Traditionally, it has been used for bronchitic asthma, chronic bronchitis, as a gargle for pharyngitis, and specifically for chronic bronchitis.

Dosage

Dried root 0.5–1.0 g or by infusion three times daily.[G6,G7]

Senega Liquid Extract (BPC 1968) 0.3–1.0 mL.

Senega Tincture (BPC 1968) 2.5–5.0 mL.

Pharmacological Actions

In vitro and animal studies

Mucosal secretion Polygalic acid and senegin are stated to be irritant to the gastrointestinal mucosa, and to cause a reflex secretion of mucus in the bronchioles.[1,G6,G44,G52] A fluid extract of senega increased respiratory tract fluid secretion in guinea-pig, cat and dog, but not in rabbit.[G52]

CNS-depressant activity CNS-depressant properties in mice (e.g. reduction in spontaneous activity, inhibition of amphetamine stimulation, potentiation of barbiturate-induced sleeping time, and decrease in rectal temperature) have been documented for *Polygala microphylla*.[21] Similar properties have been reported for *Polygala tenuifolia* and have been attributed to the saponin constituents. A methanolic extract of *P. tenuifolia*, various fractions and pure onjisaponins B, F and G prolonged hexobarbital sleeping time in mice.[G52] Onjisaponin F produced sleep times in mice of 33 and 35 minutes for doses of 5 and 20 mg/kg, respectively, compared with 24 minutes for control and 42 minutes for chlorpromazine hydrochloride (2 mg/kg).

Inhibition of alcohol absorption E,Z-senegin II and E,Z-senagasaponins a and b from *P. senega* var. *latifolia* have potent inhibitory effects on alcohol absorption in rats. E,Z-senegasaponins a or b (100 mg/kg) administered orally to rats 1 hour after 20% aqueous ethanol (5 mL/kg, orally) reduced blood alcohol concentrations after 1 hour from 0.5 mg/mL to 0.02 mg/mL.[10] Under similar test conditions, E,Z-

senegin II administration led to a blood ethanol concentration of 0.09 mg/mL.

Hypoglycaemic activity Senegin II and E,Z-senagasaponins a and b have significant hypoglycaemic effects in rodents.[22] Senegin II (2.5 mg/kg, intraperitoneally) reduced blood glucose concentrations in normal mice from 220 mg/dL to 131 mg/dL 4 hours after administration and also significantly lowered blood glucose concentrations in KK-Ay mice from 434 mg/dL to 142 mg/dL under similar test conditions ($p < 0.001$, compared with control, for both studies). In glucose tolerance tests in rats, administration of E,Z-senagasaponins a and b (100 mg/kg, orally) resulted in glucose concentrations of 107–123 mg/mL after 30 minutes compared with 156 mg/mL in control animals ($p < 0.01$).[11]

Hypolipidaemic activity Seven hours after administration of an *n*-butanol fraction of a methanolic extract of *P. senega* var. *latifolia* containing senegin II (5 mg/kg, intraperitoneally), the mean (standard deviation) blood triglyceride concentration was 65 (9) mg/100 mL, compared with 152 (17) mg/mL in control animals ($p < 0.05$).[23] The blood triglyceride concentration in cholesterol-fed mice was also significantly reduced ($p < 0.05$) under the similar test conditions. Pure senegin II at a dose of 5 mg/kg was also reported to lower blood triglyceride concentrations in mice.[23]

Other activities Guinea-pig serum taken 2 hours after administration of lyophilised aqueous extract of *P. tenuifolia* (600 mg, intraperitoneally) inhibited the growth of herpes simplex virus type 1 (HSV-1) in Vero cells.[G52] An unspecified senegin from *P. senega* produced a 34% inhibition of influenza virus (A2/Japan 305) at a concentration of 12.5 µg/mL.[G52] An ethanolic extract of *P. senega* has been reported to inhibit growth of a range of fungi.[G52]

Polygala erioptera and *P. paniculata* have exhibited molluscicidal activity, and *P. paniculata* is reported to possess antifungal activity.[17] A butanol extract of *P. tanuifolia* containing onjisaponins (100 µg/mL) inhibited cyclic adenosine monophosphate (cAMP) diesterase by 73%.[G52] Isolated onjisaponins E, F and G inhibited cAMP phosphodiesterase, with IC_{50} values of 3.1, 2.9, and 3.7×10^{-5} mol/L, respectively, being similar in action to papaverine. A total saponin concentration of *P. senega* var. *latifolia* increased rat plasma concentrations of adrenocorticotrophic hormone (ACTH), corticosterone and glucose 30 minutes after intraperitoneal administration (25 mg/kg). Single doses of a dried methanol (50%) extract of *P.*

senega var. *latifolia* and *P. tanuifolia* administered orally (2 g/kg) to rats produced 62% and 100% inhibition, respectively, of congestive oedema.[G52] Under the same conditions, furosemide 100 mg/kg prodced 100% inhibition of concestive oedema.

Clinical studies

A fluid extract of senega root was reported to reduce the viscosity of sputum in patients with bronchiectasis.[G52] A French patent has stated that a triterpenic acid extracted from senega possesses anti-inflammatory activity and is effective against graft rejection, eczema, psoriasis and multiple sclerosis.[24]

Side-effects, Toxicity[G20]

Saponins are generally regarded as irritant to the gastrointestinal mucosa, and irritant properties have been documented for senega plant and for related *Polygala* species.[G51] Large doses of senega are reported to cause vomiting and purging.[G60]

The haemolytic index (HI) of senega saponins is stated to be between 2500 and 4500.[G62] Haemolytic saponins are toxic to mammals when administered intravenously, but have a low toxicity when given orally because they do not cross the gastrointestinal mucosa.[25] Contact with damaged mucosal areas may cause a problem. Toxicity associated with chronic exposure of the gastrointestinal mucosa to haemolytic saponins has not been established. It has been stated that the suitability of saponins for nutritional and pharmacological use requires further investigation: free saponins in the gastrointestinal tract may interact with the mucosal cells, causing a transient increase in the permeability of the small intestine to intraluminal solutes and inhibiting active nutrient absorption.[25] This action may consequently facilitate the entry of antigens and biologically active food peptides into the blood circulation, with adverse systemic effects.[25] Aqueous and methanol extracts of *P. senega* and *P. tenuifolia* were negative in the rec-assay with *Bacillus subtilis* and in the reversion assay with Ames strains TA98 and TA100 of *Salmonella typhimurium*.[G52] A mixture of senegins given to rats (i.p.) gave an LD_{50} value of 3 mg/kg and inhibited the growth of Walker carcinoma in rats with an ED_{50} value of 1.5 mg/kg.[G52]

Cytotoxic lignans have been documented as constituents of a related species, *P. polygama*.[10]

Contra-indications, Warnings

Senega may exacerbate existing gastrointestinal inflammation and excessive doses may cause vomiting. Senega has hypoglycaemic activity and is contraindicated in diabetic patients.

Pregnancy and lactation Limited information is available on the chemistry, pharmacology and toxicity of senega. In view of this, and the potential irritant properties of senega, its use during pregnancy and lactation should be avoided.

Pharmaceutical Comment

The chemistry and pharmacology of senega has been extensively investigated but there is only limited clinical data. The activity of the saponins in animals supports the herbal use for bronchitis. In view of the lack of toxicity data and uncertainty regarding the risk associated with chronic ingestion of haemolytic saponins, excessive use of senega should be avoided.

References

See also General References G2, G3, G6, G9, G12, G15, G16, G20, G25, G29, G31, G32, G36, G37, G40, G43, G48, G51, G52, G60, G62 and G64.

1 Briggs CJ. Senega Snakeroot – A traditional Canadian herbal medicine. *Can Pharm J* 1988; **121**: 199–201.

2 Hamburger M, Hostettmann K. Hydroxycinnamic acid esters from *Polygala chamaebuxus*. *Phytochemistry* 1985; **24**: 1793–1797.

3 Takiura K *et al.* Studies on oligosaccharides. XIII. Oligosaccharides in *Polygala senega* and structures of glycosyl-1,5-anhydro-D-glucitols. *Yakugaku Zasshi* 1974; **94**: 998–1003.

4 Takiura K *et al.* Studies on oligosaccharides XVI. New trisaccharides found in *Senega radix*. *Yakugaku Zasshi* 1975; **95**: 166–169.

5 Saitoh H *et al.* Senegoses A–E, oligosaccharide multi-esters from *Polygala senega* var. latifia Torr. et Gray. *Chem Pharm Bull* 1993; **41**: 1127–1131.

6 Saitoh H *et al.* Senegoses F–I, oligosaccharide multi-esters from the roots of *Polygala senega* var. latifia Torr. et Gray. *Chem Pharm Bull* 1993; **41**: 2125–2128.

7 Ikeya Y *et al.* Four new phenolic glycosides from *Polygala tenuifolia*. *Chem Pharm Bull* 1991; **39**: 2600–2605.

8 Ikeya Y *et al.* Xanthone C-glycoside and acylated sugar from *Polygala tenuifolia*. *Chem Pharm Bull* 1994; **42**: 2305–2308.

9 Yoshikawa M *et al.* E-Senegasaponins a and b, Z-senegasaponins a and b, Z-senegins II and III, new type inhibitors of ethanol absorption in rats from senegae radix, the roots of *Polygala senega* L. var *latifia* Torrey et Gray. *Chem Pharm Bull* 1995; **43**: 350–352.

10 Yoshikawa M *et al.* Bioactive saponins and glycosides. I. Senegae radix. (1): E-senegasaponins a and

b and Z-senegasaponins a and b, their inhibitory effect on alcohol absorption and hypoglycemic activity. *Chem Pharm Bull* 1995; **43**: 2115–2122.

11 Yoshikawa M *et al*. Bioactive saponins and glycosides. II. Senegae radix. (2): Chemical structures, hypoglycemic activity, and ethanol absorption-inhibitory effect of *E*-senegasaponin c, *Z*-senegasaponins c, and *Z*-senegins II, III, and IV. *Chem Pharm Bull* 1996; **44**: 1305–1313.

12 Tsukitani Y *et al*. Studies on the constituents of Senegae radix. II. The structure of senegin-II, a saponin from *Polygala senega* Linne var. *latifolia* Torry et Gray. *Chem Pharm Bull* 1973; **21**: 791–799.

13 Tsukitani Y, Shoji J. Studies on the constituents of Senegae radix III. The structures of senegin-III and -IV, saponins from *Polygala senega* Linne var. latifolia Torry et Gray. *Chem Bull Pharm* 1973; **21**: 1564–1574.

14 Sakuma S, Shoji J. Studies on the constituents of the root of *Polygala tenuifolia* Willdenow. I. Isolation of saponins and the structures of onjisaponins g and f. *Chem Pharm Bull* 1981; **29**: 2431–2441.

15 Sakuma S, Shoji J. Studies on the constituents of the root of *Polygala tenuifolia* Willdenow. II. On the structures of onjisaponins a, b and e. *Chem Pharm Bull* 1982; **30**: 810–821.

16 Hamburger M *et al*. Coumarins from *Polygala paniculata*. *Planta Med* 1985; **51**: 215–217.

17 Hamburger M *et al*. A new pyranocoumarin diester from *Polygala paniculata* L. *Helv Chim Acta* 1984; **67**: 1729–1733.

18 Hamburger M, Hostettmann K. Glycosidic constituents of some European *Polygala* species. *J Nat Prod* 1986; May–June: 557.

19 Ghosal S *et al*. 1,2,3-Trioxygenated glucosyloxyxanthones. *Phytochemistry* 1981; **20**: 489–492.

20 Hokanson GC. Podophyllotoxin and 4-demethylpodophyllotoxin from *Polygala polygama* (Polygalaceae). *Lloydia* 1978; **41**: 497–498.

21 Carretero ME *et al*. Études pharmacodynamiques préliminaires de *Polygala microphylla* (L.), sur le système nerveux central. *Plant Méd Phytothér* 1986; **20**: 148–154.

22 Kako M *et al*. Effect of senegin-II on blood glucose in normal and NIDDM mice. *Biol Pharm Bull* 1995; **18**(Suppl.8): 1159–1161.

23 Masuda H *et al*. Intraperitoneal administration of senegae radix extract and its main component, senegin-II, affects lipid metabolism in normal and hyperlipidemic mice. *Biol Pharm Bull* 1996; **19**: 315–317.

24 Tubery P. Antiinflammatory triterpenic alcohol acids. *Fr Demande Patent* 2,202,683.

25 Johnson IT *et al*. Influence of saponins on gut permeability and active nutrient transport in vitro. *J Nutr* 1986; **116**: 2270–2277.

Senna

Species (Family)

(i) *Cassia senna* L.
(ii) *Cassia angustifolia* Vahl. (Leguminosae)

Synonym(s)

(i) Alexandrian Senna, *Cassia acutifolia* Delite, Khartoum Senna
(ii) Indian Senna, Tinnevelly Senna

Part(s) Used

Fruit (pod), leaf

Pharmacopoeial and Other Monographs

BHC 1992[G6]
BHP 1996[G9]
BP 2001[G15]
Complete German Commission E[G3]
ESCOP 1997[G52]
Martindale 32nd edition[G43]
PDR for Herbal Medicines 2nd edition[G36]
Ph Eur 2002[G28]
WHO volume 1 1999[G63]

Legal Category (Licensed Products)

GSL[G37]

Constituents[G2,G6,G7,G8,G20,G22,G41,G48,G52,G62,G64]

Hydroxyanthracenes Pharmacopoeial standards not less than 2.5% for leaf, 3.5% for *C. senna* fruit and 2.2% for *C. angustifolia* fruit.[G15,G28] Dianthrone glycosides (1.5–3% leaf; 2–5% fruit), primarily sennosides A and B (rhein dianthrones) with sennosides C and D (rhein aloe-emodin heterodianthrones), aloe-emodin dianthrone. Sennosides A and B yield sennidin A and B respectively. Free anthraquinones including aloe-emodin, chrysophanol and rhein with their glycosides.

Carbohydrates Polysaccharides (about 2.5%)[1] including mucilage (arabinose, galactose, galacturonic acid, rhamnose) and a galactomannan (galactose, mannose);[2] free sugars (e.g. fructose, glucose, pinitol, sucrose).

Flavonoids Flavonols including isorhamnetin and kaempferol.

Glycosides 6-Hydroxymusizin and tinnevellin glycosides.

Other constituents Chrysophanic acid, salicylic acid, saponin, resin, volatile oil (trace).

Food Use

Senna is listed by the Council of Europe as a natural source of food flavouring (Tinnevelly category N2, Alexandrian category N3). Category N2 indicates that senna can be added to foodstuffs in small quantities, with a possible limitation of an active principle (as yet unspecified) in the final product. Category N3 indicates that there is insufficient information available about Alexandrian senna, for an adequate assessment of potential toxicity.[G16] In the USA, senna is permitted for food use.

Herbal Use[G2,G4,G6,G7,G8,G32,G43,G52,G54,G56,G64]

Senna is stated to possess cathartic properties (leaf greater than fruit) and has been used traditionally for constipation. The German Commission E approved use for constipation.[G3] Senna is also used in combination with ispaghula for constipation.[G3] The Committee on Proprietary Medicinal Products (CPMP) has adopted core SPCs (Summary of Product Characteristics) for senna leaf and senna fruit (*C. angustifolia* and *C. acutifolia*) with indications for short-term use in cases of occasional constipation.[3].

Dosage

Dried pods 3–6 pods (Alexandrian) or 4–12 pods (Tinnevelly) steeped in 150 mL warm water for 6–12 hours;[G6,G7] 0.6–0.2 g (equivalent to 20–30 mg hydroxyanthracene glycosides calculated as sennosides B).[G52]

Dried leaflets 0.5–2.0 g[G6,G7] (equivalent to 20–30 mg hydroxyanthracene glycosides calculated as sennoside B).[G52]

Leaf, liquid extract 0.5–2.0 mL (1:1 in 25% alcohol).[G6,G7]

Senna Liquid Extract (BPC 1973) 0.5–2.0 mL.

Herbal drug preparations Equivalent to 15–30 mg hydroxyanthracene derivatives (calculated as sennoside B) to be taken at night.[3]

Pharmacological Actions

The cathartic action of hydroxyanthracene-containing drugs is well recognised and they have been used as laxatives for many years. However, there is still some uncertainty as to the exact mode of action of the hydroxyanthracenes.

It is thought that hydroxyanthracene glycosides are absorbed from the gastrointestinal tract, the aglycones liberated during metabolism and excreted into the colon resulting in stimulation and an increase in peristalsis. However, it has also been suggested that the purgative action of senna is due to the action of intestinal bacteria.[4] Using human intestinal flora, it was found that sennoside A is reduced to 8-glucosyl-rheinanthrone, hydrolysed to rheinanthrone and oxidised to sennidin A. The active principle causing peristaltic movements of the large intestine was thought to be rheinanthrone.[4]

In vitro and animal studies

Sennosides A and B, and their natural metabolites sennidins A and B, have been reported to act specifically on the large intestine in the rat with the acceleration of colonic transport the major component of their laxative effect.[5] Sennosides A and B have also been reported to induce fluid secretion exclusively in the colon, following oral administration of the glycosides to rats.[6]

It has been suggested that the laxative action of the sennosides involves prostaglandins. Indomethacin has been found to partly inhibit the action of sennosides A and B, although a bolus injection of prostaglandins into the caecal lumen was stated to neither influence transit time nor to induce diarrhoea.[5] Pretreatment of mice with indomethacin and a prostaglandin E (PGE) antagonist has been documented to prevent diarrhoea caused by intracaecal administration of rhein, which stimulates the production of PGE-like material specifically in the colon.[7] Indomethacin was found to depress the large intestinal propulsive activity of rhein, but did not suppress PGE_2-induced diarrhoea. The authors suggest that the action of rhein is mediated by prostaglandin biosynthesis and release.[7]

Antihepatotoxic activity has been documented for naphtho-α-pyrone and naphtho-γ-pyrone glycosides, and for the hydroxyanthracene glycosides isolated from a related species *Cassia tora*.[8] Greatest activity

was documented for the naphtho-γ-pyrone glycosides.

Significant inhibitory activity in mice against leukaemia P388 has been documented for aloe-emodin.[G41]

Clinical studies

In a randomised, controlled trial, 91 patients with terminal received senna 12 mg daily, or lactulose, for 27 days.[9] At the end of the study, no differences were found between the two groups in defecation-free intervals, or in days with defecation. The general health of each group was also reported to be similar.

A randomised, double-blind, double-dummy, multicentre, controlled, crossover study involving 77 hospitalised elderly patients with a history of chronic constipation compared the effects of a senna–fibre combination (senna 12.4%, ispaghula 54.2%, 10 mL daily) and lactulose (15 mL twice daily) for two 14-day periods with a three- to five-day wash-out period.[10] Assessments included stool frequency and consistency, ease of evacuation, adverse effects and costs of treatment. The senna–fibre combination was reported to be significantly more effective than lactulose.[10]

Commercial preparations containing senna and ispaghula have been reported to be equally effective for the treatment of constipation in small clinical studies involving elderly hospitalised patients and/or residents in nursing homes.[11]

Side-effects, Toxicity[G20]

Senna may cause mild abdominal discomfort such as colic or cramps. Prolonged use or overdosage can result in diarrhoea with excessive loss of potassium, albuminuria and haematuria.[G3] Potassium deficiency may lead to disorders of the heart and muscular weakness especially with concurrent use of cardiac glycosides, diuretics or corticosteroids. An atonic non-functioning colon may also develop.[G45] Excessive use and abuse of senna has been associated with finger clubbing and with the development of cachexia and reduced serum globulin concentrations.[12]

Sennosides A and B are reported to be most potent with respect to laxative action, but to be the least toxic compared with other hydroxyanthracene fractions in senna. Similarly, fractions with a low laxative activity (e.g. rhein-8-glucoside) are reported to have the highest acute toxicity.[13] LD_{50} values in mice following intravenous injection of sennosides A and B and of rhein-8-glycoside are reported to be 4.1 g/kg and 400 g/kg, respectively.[13] The acute oral toxicity of all senna fractions in mice has been reported to be greater than 5 g/kg, although all of the animals were stated to have died by the following week. The toxicity of total senna extracts is greater than that of the individual sennosides and it has been proposed that the laxative and toxic components of senna could be separated.[7]

In vitro carcinogenicity testing has reported certain anthraquinones, including aloe-emodin, to be active in more than one strain of *Salmonella typhimurium*.[14] Aglycones were documented to exhibit genotoxic activity in a mammalian cell assay.[14]

Sensitising properties have been documented for emodin (*see* Aloes).[G51]

The CPMP core SPCs for senna include the following information.[3] There are no new, systematic preclinical tests for senna leaf or preparations thereof. Most data refer to extracts of senna fruit containing 1.4–3.5% of hydroxyanthacenes, corresponding to 0.9–2.35% of potential rhein, 0.05–0.15% potential aloe-emodin and 0.001–0.006% of potential emodin, or to isolated active constituents, e.g. rhein or sennosides A and B. The acute toxicity of senna fruit and specified extracts thereof, as well as of sennosides in rats and mice was low after oral treatment. As a result of investigations with parenteral application in mice, extracts are supposed to possess a higher toxicity than purified glucosides, possibly due to the content of aglycones.

Sennosides displayed no specific toxicity when tested at doses up to 500 g/kg in dogs for four weeks and up to 100 g/kg in rats for six months. Data for herbal drug preparations are not available. There was no evidence of any embryolethal, teratogenic or fetotoxic actions in rats or rabbits after oral treatment with sennosides. Furthermore, there was no effect on the postnatal development of young rats, on rearing behaviour of dams or on male and female fertility in rats. Data on herbal drug preparations are not available.

An extract and aloe-emodin were mutagenic in *in vitro* tests; sennosides A and B and rhein gave negative results. *In vivo* examinations of a defined extract of senna pods were negative. A specified senna extract given orally for two years was not carcinogenic in male or female rats. The extract investigated contained approximately 40.8% of hydroxyanthracenes from which 35% were sennosides, corresponding to about 25.2% of potential rhein, 2.3% of potential aloe-emodin and 0.007% of potential emodin, and 142 ppm free aloe-emodin and 9 ppm free emodin.

Contra-indications, Warnings

It is recommended that senna should not be given to patients with intestinal obstruction and stenosis, atony, inflammatory colon diseases (e.g. Crohn's disease, ulcerative colitis), appendicitis, with undiagnosed abdominal symptoms; severe dehydration states with water and electrolyte depletion. Prolonged use should be avoided.[3,G20,G45,G52]

The CPMP core SPCs for senna include the following information.[3]

As with all laxatives, senna should not be given when any undiagnosed acute or persistent abdominal symptoms are present. If laxatives are needed every day the cause of the constipation should be investigated. Long-term use of laxatives should be avoided. Use for more than two weeks requires medical supervision. Chronic use may cause pigmentation of the colon (pseudomelanosis coli) which is harmless and reversible after drug discontinuation.

Abuse, with diarrhoea and consequent fluid and electrolyte losses, may cause dependence, with possible need for increased dosages, disturbance of water and electrolyte (mainly hypokalaemia) balance, atonic colon with impaired function. Intake of anthranoid containing laxatives exceeding short-term use may result in an aggravation of constipation.

Hypokalaemia can result in cardiac and neuromuscular dysfunction, especially if cardiac glycosides, diuretics or corticosteroids are also taken. Chronic use may result in albuminuria and haematuria.

In chronic constipation, stimulant laxatives are not an acceptable alternative to a changed diet.

Interaction with other medicaments and other forms of interaction[3] Hypokalaemia (resulting from long-term use of senna) may potentiate the action of cardiac glycosides and interacts with antiarrhythmic drugs, with drugs which induce reversion to sinus rhythm (e.g. quinidine). Concomitant use with other drugs inducing hypokalaemia (e.g. thiazide diuretics, adrenocorticosteroids and liquorice root) may enhance electrolyte imbalance. Abdominal spasms and pain may occur, in particular in patients with irritable colon.[3]

Anthraquinones cause discoloration of the urine which may interfere with diagnostic tests.[G45]

Pregnancy and lactation Non-standardised hydroxyanthracene containing laxative preparations should not be taken during pregnancy or lactation since their pharmacological action is unpredictable. Although hydroxyanthracene derivatives may be excreted in the breast milk, following normal dosage their concentration is usually insufficient to affect the nursing infant.[G45]

The CPMP core SPCs for senna include the following information.[3]

Pregnancy Not recommended during pregnancy. There are no reports of undesirable or damaging effects during pregnancy and on the fetus when used at the recommended dosage schedule. However, experimental data concerning a genotoxic risk of several anthranoids (e.g. emodine and physcione) and senna are not counterbalanced by sufficient studies to eliminate a possible risk.[3]

Lactation Breastfeeding is not recommended as there are insufficient data on the excretion of metabolites in breast milk. Excretion of active principles in breast milk has not been investigated. However, small amounts of active metabolites (e.g. rhein) from other anthranoids are known to be excreted in breast milk. A laxative effect in breastfed babies has not been reported.[3]

Pharmaceutical Comment

The chemistry of senna is characterised by the hydroxyanthracene derivatives. The laxative action of these compounds is well recognised and supports the herbal use of senna as a laxative for the treatment of constipation. However, the use of non-standardised hydroxyanthracene-containing preparations should be avoided since their pharmacological effect will be variable and unpredictable. The sennoside content of many licensed senna products is standardised and generally calculated as sennoside B. Clinical investigations have concluded that senna with ispaghula is more effective than lactulose as a laxative (*see* Clinical studies).

References

See also General References G2, G3, G6, G9, G12, G15, G16, G18, G20, G22, G28, G29, G31, G32, G36, G37, G41, G43, G48, G51, G52, G54, G56, G62, G63 and G64.

1 Müller BM *et al.* Isolation and structural investigation of a polysaccharide from *Cassia angustifolia* leaves. *Planta Med* 1989; **55**: 99.
2 Alam N, Gupta PC. Structure of a water-soluble polysaccharide from the seeds of *Cassia angustifolia*. *Planta Med* 1986; **52**: 308–310.
3 European Commission, CPMP Guidelines on Information on Medical Products: Core SPCs for Sennae Fructus Angustifolia, Sennae Fructus Acutifolia, Sennae Folium, February 1994.
4 Kobashi K *et al.* Metabolism of sennosides by human intestinal bacteria. *Planta Med* 1980; **40**: 225–236.
5 Leng-Peschlow E. Acceleration of large intestine transit time in rats by sennosides and related compounds. *J Pharm Pharmacol* 1986; **38**: 369–373.
6 Leng-Peschlow E. Dual effect orally administered sennosides on large intestine transit and fluid absorption in the rat. *J Pharm Pharmacol* 1986; **38**: 606–610.
7 Yagi T *et al.* Involvement of prostaglandin E-like material in the purgative action of rhein anthrone, the intraluminal active metabolite of sennosides A and B in mice. *J Pharm Pharmacol* 1988; **40**: 27–30.
8 Wong SM *et al.* Isolation and structural elucidation of new antihepatotoxic naphtho-gamma-pyrone glycosides, naphtho-α-pyrone glycoside and anthraquinone glycosides from the seeds of *Cassia tora*. *Planta Med* 1989; **55**: 112.
9 Agra Y *et al.* Efficacy of senna versus lactulose in terminal cancer patients treated with opioids. *J Pain Symptom Management* 1998; **15**: 1–7.
10 Passmore AP *et al.* Chronic constipation in long stay elderly patients: a comparison of lactulose and a senna-fibre combination. *BMJ* 1993; **307**: 769–771.
11 Petticrew M *et al.* Epidemiology of constipation in the general adult population. *Health Technol Assess* 1997; **1**: 1–52.
12 Senna *Lawrence Review of Natural Products*. Levittown, Pennsylvania: Pharmaceutical Information Associates Ltd, 1989.
13 Hietala P *et al.* Laxative potency and acute toxicity of some anthraquinone derivatives, senna extracts and fractions of senna extracts. *Pharmacol Toxicol* 1987; **61**: 153–156.
14 Westendorf J *et al.* Possible carcinogenicity of anthraquinone-containing medical plants. *Planta Med* 1988; **54**: 562.

Shepherd's Purse

Species (Family)

Capsella bursa-pastoris (L.) Medic (Cruciferae)

Synonym(s)

Capsella

Part(s) Used

Herb

Pharmacopoeial and Other Monographs

BHP 1996[G9]
Complete German Commission E[G3]
PDR for Herbal Medicines 2nd edition[G36]

Legal Category (Licensed Products)

GSL[G37]

Constituents[G2,G7,G40,G41,G64]

Amines Acetylcholine, choline, amino acids 2.33% (major component proline), histamine, tyramine and unidentified crystalline alkaloids.[1]

Flavonoids Quercetin, diosmetin, luteolin, hesperetin and their glycosides (e.g. rutin, diosmin, hesperidin).[2]

Volatile oils 0.02%. Camphor (major); at least 74 components identified.[3,4]

Other constituents Carotenoids, fumaric acid, sinigrin (mustard oil glucoside), ascorbic acid (vitamin C) and vitamin K.[4,5,G2]

Food Use

Shepherd's purse is not used in foods.

Herbal Use

Shepherd's purse is stated to possess antihaemorrhagic and urinary antiseptic properties. Traditionally, it has been used for menorrhagia, haematemesis, haematuria, diarrhoea and acute catarrhal cystitis.[G2,G7,G64]

Dosage

Dried herb 1–4 g or by infusion three times daily[G7]

Liquid extract 1–4 mL (1 : 1 in 25% alcohol) three times daily.[G7]

Pharmacological Actions

In vitro and animal studies

A variety of actions have been documented for an ethanolic extract of shepherd's purse in various animal models.[6–9] Anti-inflammatory activity has been exhibited versus carrageenan-induced and dextran-induced rat paw oedema.[7] A reduction in capillary permeability in the guinea-pig, induced by histamine and serotonin, has also been observed,[7] and flavonoid components isolated from shepherd's purse have been reported to reduce blood vessel permeability in mice.[2] Anti-ulcer activity has been documented in rats following intraperitoneal injection. The extract did not affect gastric secretion, but accelerated recovery from stress-induced ulcers.[7] A hypotensive effect observed in cats, dogs, rabbits and rats, following intravenous injection, was inhibited by a β-adrenoceptor blocker but not by atropine, thus dismissing earlier reports that this action was attributable to cholinergic compounds present in shepherd's purse.[8,9]

Diuresis has been reported in mice, following oral or intraperitoneal administration of shepherd's purse. The mode of action was stated to involve an increase in the glomerular filtration rate.[7]

Documented cardiac actions include increased coronary blood flow in dogs following intra-arterial administration, and a slight inhibitory effect on ouabain-induced ventricular fibrillation in the rat following intraperitoneal injection, together with a negative chronotropic effect.[9] Studies on the isolated heart have reported negative chronotropic and inotropic actions in the guinea-pig and rabbit and coronary vasodilatation.[9]

A CNS-depressant action in mice has been demonstrated (potentiation of barbiturate-induced sleeping time).[9]

Weak antibacterial activity mainly towards Gram-positive organisms has been reported.[10]

Antineoplastic activity in rats has been documented for fumaric acid, which prevented the development of hepatic neoplasms when co-administered with the carcinogen 3-MeDAB.[11]

Shepherd's purse seeds are stated to possess rubefacient and vesicant properties because of their isothiocyanate-yielding components.[G51]

In vitro studies have documented stimulatory action in various smooth muscle tissues. Induced contractions of the small intestine in the guinea-pig were reported to be unaffected by atropine and diphenhydramine, but were inhibited by papaverine.[8,9] Induced utero-activity in the rat, equivalent to the effect of oxytocin 0.1 i.u., was unaffected by atropine, but inhibited by competitive inhibitors of oxytocin.[8] Two unidentified alkaloid components of shepherd's purse have also been stated to elicit a physiological activity on the uterus.[1] Induced tracheal contractions in the guinea-pig were unaffected by adrenaline, which did inhibit acetylcholine-induced contractions.[9] These studies concluded that the active substance(s) in shepherd's purse responsible for the observed actions on smooth muscle were neither acetylcholine nor histamine.[8,9]

Side-effects, Toxicity

Shepherd's purse extracts have been reported to exhibit low toxicity in mice. LD_{50} values reported are 1.5 g/kg body weight (mice, intraperitoneal injection) and 31.5 g/kg (mice, subcutaneous injection).[9] Signs of toxicity were described as sedation, enlargement of pupils, paralysis of hind limbs, difficulty in respiration, and death by respiratory paralysis.[9] Following hydrolysis, the constituent sinigrin yields allyl isothiocyanate which is an extremely powerful irritant and produces blisters on the skin.[G41] Isothiocyanates have been implicated in endemic goitre (hypothyroidism with thyroid enlargement) and have been reported to produce goitre in experimental animals.[G41]

Contra-indications, Warnings

Prolonged or excessive use of the herb may interfere with existing therapy for hyper- or hypotension, thyroid dysfunction or cardiac disorder, and may potentiate sedative actions.

Pregnancy and lactation Shepherd's purse is reputed to act as an abortifacient and to affect the menstrual cycle, and tyramine is documented as a utero-active constituent.[G30] In view of this and the reported oxytocin-like activity, the use of shepherd's purse during pregnancy should be avoided. Excessive use should be avoided during lactation.

Pharmaceutical Comment

The chemistry of shepherd's purse is well documented and although a number of actions affecting the circulatory system have been observed in animal studies, these actions do not relate to the traditional herbal uses. Limited toxicity data are available. In view of this together with the demonstrated pharmacological activity of the herb, excessive use of shepherd's purse should be avoided.

References

See also General References G2, G3, G9, G30, G31, G36, G37, G40, G41, G51 and G64.

1   Kuroda K, Kaku T. Pharmacological and chemical studies on the alcohol extract of *Capsella bursa-pastoris*. *Life Sci* 1969; **8**: 151–155.

2   Jurisson S. Flavonoid substances of *Capsella bursa pastoris*. *Farmatsiya (Moscow)* 1973; **22**: 34–35.

3   Miyazawa M *et al*. The constituents of the essential oils from *Capsella bursa-pastoris* Medik. *Yakugaku Zasshi* 1979; **99**: 1041–1043.

4   Park RJ. The occurrence of mustard oil glucosides in *Lepidium hyssopifolium*, L. bonariense, and *Capsella bursa pastoris*. *Aust J Chem* 1967; **20**: 2799–2801.

5   Jurisson S. Vitamin content of shepherd's purse. *Farmatsiya (Moscow)* 1976; **25**: 66–67.

6   Kuroda K, Takagi K. Studies on *Capsella bursa pastoris*. I. General pharmacology of ethanol extract of the herb. *Arch Int Pharmacodyn Ther* 1969; **178**: 382–391.

7   Kuroda K, Takagi K. Studies on capsella bursa pastoris. II. Diuretic, anti-inflammatory and anti-ulcer action of ethanol extracts of the herb. *Arch Int Pharmacodyn Ther* 1969; **178**: 392–399.

8   Kuroda K, Takagi K. Physiologically active substance in *Capsella bursa-pastoris*. *Nature* 1968; **220**: 707–708.

9   Jurisson S. Determination of active substances of *Capsella bursa pastoris*. *Tartu Riiliku Ulikooli Toim* 1971; **270**: 71–79.

10   Moskalenko SA. Preliminary screening of far-eastern ethnomedicinal plants for antibacterial activity. *J Ethnopharmacol* 1986; **15**: 231–259.

11   Kuroda K. Neoplasm inhibitor from *Capsella bursa pastoris*. *Japan Kokai* 1977; **41**: 207.

Skunk Cabbage

Species (Family)

Symplocarpus foetidus (L.) Salisb. (Araceae)

Synonym(s)

Dracontium foetidum L., Skunkweed

Part(s) Used

Rhizome, root

Pharmacopoeial and Other Monographs

BHP 1983[G7]
PDR for Herbal Medicines 2nd edition[G36]

Legal Category (Licensed Products)

GSL[G37]

Constituents[G22,G64]

Reported constituents include starch, gum-sugar, fixed and volatile oils, resin, tannin, an acrid principle and iron.

Other plant parts Large amounts of alkaloids (unspecified), phenolic compounds and glycosides have been isolated from all plant parts of skunk cabbage.[1] The leaves are reported to contain hydroxytryptamine;[G22] three anthocyanin pigments have been isolated from the flowers, namely cyanidin-3-monoglucoside, cyanidin-3-rutinoside and peonidin-3-rutinoside.[2]

Food Use

Skunk cabbage is not used in foods.

Herbal Use

Skunk cabbage is stated to possess expectorant, antispasmodic and mild sedative properties. Traditionally, it has been used for bronchitis, whooping cough, asthma and specifically for bronchitic asthma.[G7,G64]

Dosage

Powdered rhizome/root 0.5–1.0 g in honey or by infusion or decoction three times daily.[G7]

Liquid extract 0.5–1.0 mL (1:1 in 25% alcohol) three times daily.[G7]

Tincture 2–4 mL (1:10 in 45% alcohol) three times daily.[G7]

Pharmacological Actions

In vitro and animal studies

None documented for the rhizome/root. The leaf extract has haemolytic properties.[G22]

Clinical studies

None documented.

Side-effects, Toxicity

The root is reported to be bitter and acrid, with a disagreeable odour. Severe itching and inflammation of the skin has been documented.[G51] No published toxicity studies were located.

Contra-indications, Warnings

It has been stated that the fresh plant can cause blistering.[G42] In view of the acrid principle thought to be present in both the dried and fresh root,[G51] skunk cabbage should be used with caution.

Pregnancy and lactation Skunk cabbage is reputed to affect the menstrual cycle.[G22] In view of the lack of phytochemical, pharmacological, and toxicological information, and the irritant properties, the use of skunk cabbage during pregnancy and lactation should be avoided.

Pharmaceutical Comment

Little is known about the constituents, pharmacological activities or safety of skunk cabbage (even though citings as early as 1817 reported its irritant properties).[G51] No documented evidence was found to justify the herbal uses. In view of the documented irritant properties, excessive use is not recommended.

References

See also General References G7, G22, G31, G36, G37, G42, G51 and G64.

1   Konyukhov VP *et al*. Dynamics of the accumulation of biologically active agents in *Lysichitum camtsochatcense* and *Symplocarpus foetidus*. *Uch Zap Khabarovsk Gos Pedagog Inst* 1970; **26**: 59–62.

2   Chang N *et al*. Anthocyanins in *Symplocarpus foetidus* (L.) Nutt. (Araceae). *Bot J Linn Soc* 1970; **63**: 95–96.

Slippery Elm

Species (Family)

Ulmus fulva Michaux (Ulmaceae)

Synonym(s)

Ulmus rubra Muhl.

Part(s) Used

Bark (inner)

Pharmacopoeial and Other Monographs

BHC 1992[G6]
BHP 1996[G9]
Martindale 32nd edition[G43]
PDR for Herbal Medicines 2nd edition[G36]

Legal Category (Licensed Products)

GSL[G37]

Constituents[G6,G59,G64]

Carbohydrates Mucilage (major constituent) consisting of hexoses, pentoses, methylpentoses, at least two polyuronides, and yielding on hydrolysis galactose, glucose and fructose (trace), galacturonic acid, L-rhamnose and D-galactose.

Other constituents Tannin 3.0–6.5% (type unspecified), phytosterols (β-sitosterol, citrostadienol, dolichol), sesquiterpenes, calcium oxalate and cholesterol.

Food Use

It has been recommended by the FACC (Food Additives and Contaminants Committee) that the use of slippery elm as a flavouring agent in foods should be prohibited.[G44] Slippery elm is listed by the Council of Europe as a natural source of food flavouring (category N3). This category indicates that there is insufficient information available to make an adequate assessment of potential toxicity.[G16]

Herbal Use

Slippery elm is stated to possess demulcent, emollient, nutrient and antitussive properties. Traditionally, it has been used for inflammation or ulceration of the stomach or duodenum, convalescence, colitis, diarrhoea and locally for abcesses, boils and ulcers (as a poultice).[G6,G7,G8,G64]

Dosage

Powdered bark 4–16 mL (1 : 8 as a decoction) three times daily.[G6,G7]

Powdered bark 4 g in 500 mL boiling water as a nutritional supplement three times daily.[G6,G7]

Coarse powdered bark With boiling water as a poultice.[G6,G7]

Liquid extract 5 mL (1 : 1 in 60% alcohol) three times daily.[G6,G7]

Pharmacological Actions

Mucilages are known to have demulcent and emollient properties. Mucilage is the principal constituent of slippery elm. Tannins are known to possess astringent properties.

Side-effects, Toxicity

None documented. In view of the known constituents of slippery elm it would appear to be non-toxic.

Contra-indications, Warnings

Whole bark has been used to procure abortions.

Pregnancy and lactation   There are no known problems with the use of powdered slippery elm during pregnancy.

Pharmaceutical Comment

The primary constituent in slippery elm is mucilage, thereby justifying the herbal use of the remedy as a demulcent, emollient and antitussive. There are no known problems regarding toxicity of slippery elm, although its use as a food flavouring agent has not been recommended. The supply of whole bark is controlled by regulations.[1]

References

See also General References G5, G6, G9, G11, G22, G31, G36, G37, G43, G59 and G64.

1   The Medicines (Retail Sale or Supply of Herbal Medicines) Order 1977, SI 1977: 2130.

Squill

Species (Family)

Drimia maritima (L.) Stearn (Liliaceae)

Synonym(s)

Scilla, Urginea, *Urginea maritima* (L.) Baker, *Urginea scilla* Steinh., White Squill

Part(s) Used

Bulb (red and white varieties)

Pharmacopoeial and Other Monographs

BHC 1992[G6]
BHP 1996[G9]
BP 2001[G15]
Complete German Commission E[G3]
Martindale 32nd edition[G43]
PDR for Herbal Medicines 2nd edition[G36]

Legal Category (Licensed Products)

GSL[G37]

Constituents[1,2,G6,G22,G41,G48,G62,G64]

Cardiac glycosides Scillaren A and proscillaridin A (major constituents); others include glucoscillaren A, scillaridin A, scillicyanoside, scilliglaucoside, scilliphaeoside, scillicoeloside, scillazuroside and scillicryptoside. Scillaren B represents a mixture of the squill glycosides.

Flavonoids Apigenin, dihydroquercetin, isovitexin, iso-orientin, luteolin, orientin, quercetin, taxifolin and vitexin.

Other constituents Stigmasterol, tannin, volatile and fixed oils.

Food Use

The Food Additives and Contaminants Committee (FACC) has recommended that squill be prohibited as a food flavouring.[G45]

Herbal Use

Squill is stated to possess expectorant, cathartic, emetic, cardioactive and diuretic properties. Traditionally, it has been used for chronic bronchitis, asthma with bronchitis, whooping cough, and specifically for chronic bronchitis with scanty sputum.[G6,G7,G8,G64]

Dosage

Dried bulb 60–200 mg or by infusion three times daily.[G6,G7]

Squill Liquid Extract (BPC 1973) 0.06–0.2 mL.

Squill Tincture (BPC 1973) 0.3–2.0 mL.

Squill Vinegar (BPC 1973) 0.6–2.0 mL.

Pharmacological Actions

The aglycone components of the cardiac glycoside constituents possess digitalis-like cardiotonic properties.[G41] However, the squill aglycones are poorly absorbed from the gastrointestinal tract and are less potent than digitalis cardiac glycosides.[1,2]

Expectorant, emetic and diuretic properties have been documented for white squill.[G41] Squill is reported to induce vomiting by both a central action and local gastric irritation.[1,2] Subemetic or near-emetic doses of squill appear to exhibit an expectorant effect, causing an increase in the flow of gastric secretions.[1,2]

Antiseborrhoeic properties have been documented for methanol extracts of red squill which have been employed as hair tonics for the treatment of chronic seborrhoea and dandruff.[G41]

Squill extracts have been reported to exhibit peripheral vasodilatation and bradycardia in anaesthetised rabbits.[1,2]

Side-effects, Toxicity

Excessive use of squill is potentially toxic because of the cardiotonic constituents. However, squill is also a gastric irritant and large doses will stimulate a vomiting reflex. Red squill is toxic to rats and is mainly used as a rodenticide, causing death by a centrally induced convulsant action.[1,2] A squill soft mass (crude extract) has been stated to be toxic in guinea-pigs at a dose of 270 mg/kg body weight. A fatal dose for Indian squill (*Urginea indica* Kunth.) is documented as 36 mg/kg.

Contra-indications, Warnings

Squill may cause gastric irritation and should be avoided by individuals with a cardiac disorder. In view of the cardiotonic constituents, precautions applied to digoxin therapy should be considered for squill.

Pregnancy and lactation Squill is reputed to be an abortifacient and to affect the menstrual cycle.[G30] In addition, cardioactive and gastrointestinal irritant properties have been documented. The use of squill during pregnancy should be avoided; excessive use should be avoided during lactation.

Pharmaceutical Comment

Squill is characterised by its cardiac glycoside components and unusual flavonoid constituents. The reputed actions of squill as an expectorant, emetic and cathartic can be attributed to the cardioactive components and squill has been used as an expectorant for many years. However, in view of the documented cardioactive and emetic properties of the aglycones, excessive should be avoided. Red squill is primarily used as a rodenticide.

References

See also General References G3, G6, G9, G12, G13, G15, G22, G29, G30, G31, G36, G37, G41, G43, G48, G56, G62 and G64.

1 Court WE. Squill – energetic diuretic. *Pharm J* 1985; **235**: 194–197.
2 Squill *Lawrence Review of Natural Products*. Levittown, Pennsylvania: Pharmaceutical Information Associates Ltd, 1989.

St. John's Wort

Species (Family)

Hypericum perforatum L. (Hypericaceae)

Synonym(s)

Hypericum, Millepertuis

Part(s) Used

Herb

Pharmacopoeial and Other Monographs

American Herbal Pharmacopoeia[G1]
BHP 1996[G9]
BP 2001[G15]
Complete German Commission E[G3]
ESCOP 1996[G52]
Martindale 32nd edition[G43]
Mills and Bone[G50]
PDR for Herbal Medicines 2nd edition[G36]
Ph Eur 2002[G28]
USP24/NF19[G61]

Legal Category (Licensed Products)

GSL (for external use only)[G37]

Constituents[1,G1,G2,G22,G40,G48,G52,G62,G64]

Anthraquinone derivatives (naphthodianthrones)
Hypericin, pseudohypericin and isohypericin; proto-hypericin and protopseudohypericin (biosynthetic precursors of hypericin and pseudohypericin, respectively) are present in fresh material. Cyclopseudohypericin is also stated to be present. The hypericin content (approximately 0.1–0.15%) includes both hypericin and pseudohypericin[2] and is sometimes referred to as 'total hypericins'.

Flavonoids Flavonols (e.g. kaempferol, quercetin), flavones (e.g. luteolin) and glycosides (e.g. hyperoside, isoquercitrin, quercitrin, rutin), biflavonoids including biapigenin (a flavone) and amentoflavone (a biapigenin derivative)[3,4] and catechins (flavonoids often associated with condensed tannins).[5,6] The concentrations of rutin, hyperoside and isoquercitrin have been reported as 1.6, 0.9 and 0.3%, respectively.[7]

Prenylated phloroglucinols Hyperforin (2.0–4.5%) and adhyperforin (0.2–1.9%).[5,8,9,G1]

Tannins 8–9%. Type not specified. Proanthocyanidins (condensed type) have been reported.[G2]

Other phenols Caffeic, chlorogenic, *p*-coumaric, ferulic, *p*-hydroxybenzoic and vanillic acids.

Volatile oils 0.05–0.9%. Major component (not less than 30%) is methyl-2-octane (saturated hydrocarbon); others include *n*-nonane and traces of methyl-2-decane and *n*-undecane (saturated hydrocarbons),[10] α- and β-pinene, α-terpineol, geraniol, and traces of myrcene and limonene (monoterpenes), caryophyllene and humulene (sesquiterpenes).[11,12]

Other constituents Acids (isovalerianic, nicotinic, myristic, palmitic, stearic), carotenoids, choline, nicotinamide, pectin, β-sitosterol, straight-chain saturated hydrocarbons (C_{16}, C_{30})[10,13] and alcohols (C_{24}, C_{26}, C_{28}).[10,13]

Food Use

St. John's wort is listed by the Council of Europe as a natural source of food flavouring (herb: category 5) (*see* Appendix 23).[G17]

Herbal Use[G1,G2,G7,G32,G64]

St. John's wort is stated to possess sedative and astringent properties. It has been used for excitability, neuralgia, fibrositis, sciatica, wounds, menopausal neurosis, anxiety and depression and as a nerve tonic. St. John's wort is used extensively in homeopathic preparations as well as in herbal products. Modern interest is focused on its use as an antidepressant.

Dosage

Dried herb 2–4 g or by infusion three times daily.[G7]

Liquid extract 2–4 mL (1:1 in 25% alcohol) three times daily.[G7]

Tincture 2–4 mL (1:10 in 45% alcohol) three times daily.[G7]

The doses of St. John's wort extract used in clinical trials involving patients with mild to moderate depression generally range from 350 to 1800 mg daily (equivalent to 0.4 to 2.7 mg hypericin daily, depending on the extract).[14]

Pharmacological Actions

The major active constituents are considered to be hyperforin (a prenylated phloroglucinol) and hypericin (a naphthodianthrone), although other biologically active constituents, e.g. flavonoids and tannins, are also present.[15] Several pharmacological activities, including antidepressant, antiviral and antibacterial effects, have been documented for extracts of St. John's wort and/or its constituents. The pharmacology and pharmacodynamics of St. John's wort have been reviewed.[1,16,G1,G50,G55]

In vitro and animal studies

Antidepressant activity The precise mechanism of action for the antidepressant effect of St. John's wort is unclear. Initially, attention was focused on hypericin as the constituent of St. John's wort believed to be responsible for the herb's antidepressant effects. Inhibition of monoamine oxidase (MAO) type A and B in rat brain mitochondria *in vitro* was described for hypericin.[17] However, other studies have demonstrated only weak or no MAO inhibition.[18–20]

In vitro receptor binding and enzyme inhibition assays carried out using hypericum extract demonstrated significant receptor affinity for adenosine, GABA$_A$, GABA$_B$, benzodiazepine and MAO types A and B, although, with the exception of GABA$_A$ and GABA$_B$, the concentrations of hypericum required were unlikely to be attained after oral administration in humans.[21] Other biochemical studies have reported that the hypericum extract LI 160 is only a weak inhibitor of MAO-A and MAO-B activity, but that it inhibits the synaptosomal uptake of serotonin (5-hydroxytryptamine or 5-HT), dopamine and noradrenaline (norepinephrine) with approximately equal affinity and also leads to a downregulation of β-receptors and an upregulation of 5-HT$_2$ receptors in the rat frontal cortex.[22] The effects of fluoxetine and hypericin- and flavonoid-standardised hypericum extracts (LI 160, 0.3% hypericin and 6% flavonoids and Ph-50, 0.3% hypericin and 50% flavonoids) on the concentrations of neurotransmitters in brain regions were studied in rats.[23] All three preparations induced a significant increase in 5-HT concentrations in the rat cortex, both LI 160 and Ph-50 caused increases in noradrenaline (norepinephrine) and dopamine in the rat diencephalon and Ph-50 also induced an increase in the noradrenaline (norepinephrine) content in the brainstem, areas that are implicated in depression.[23] In studies using the rat forced swimming test, an experimental model of depression, hypericum extracts induced a significant reduction in immobility.[24]

Hyperforin has now emerged as being one of the major active constituents of importance in antidepressant activity. Hyperforin has been shown to be an uptake inhibitor of 5-HT, dopamine, noradrenaline (norepinephrine), GABA and L-glutamate in synaptosomal preparations[25] and to inhibit 5-HT uptake in rat peritoneal cells in a dose-dependent manner.[26] Studies have also described discrepancies between observed and theoretical IC$_{50}$ values, indicating that hyperforin is not the only component of hypericum extract that is responsible for the observed effects.[26,27] It has been reported that the mode of action of hyperforin in serotonin uptake inhibition seems to be associated with the elevation of free intracellular sodium ion concentrations[28] and that this may be secondary to activation of the Na$^+$/H$^+$ exchange as a result of a decrease in intracellular pH.[29] Hyperforin was shown to inhibit 5-HT reuptake in washed platelets but not in fresh platelet-rich plasma, suggesting that plasma-protein binding could be a limiting factor for 5-HT uptake inhibition *in vivo*.[30]

A commercial extract of St. John's wort has exhibited psychotropic and antidepressant activities in mice.[31] Pure hyperforin and hypericum extracts also demonstrated antidepressant activity in a despair behaviour test in rats.[26]

In other experimental models of depression, including acute and chronic forms of escape deficit induced by stressors, hypericum extract was shown to protect rats from the consequences of unavoidable stress.[32] Flavonoid fractions and flavonoids isolated from these fractions have been reported to have antidepressant activity in experimental studies (forced swimming test) in rats.[33]

Antimicrobial activity A leaf extract has been documented as enhancing the immunity of mice towards *Staphylococcus aureus* and *Bordetella pertussis*;[34] hyperforin is reported to be antibacterial with activity against *S. aureus*.[8] Antibacterial activity of hyperforin against multiresistant *S. aureus* and Gram-positive bacteria, including *Streptococcus pyogenes* and *Corynebacterium diphtheriae*, has been reported.[35] However, it has been emphasised that the antibacterial effects of hyperforin are only observed at high concentrations.[36,37] Hyperforin did not exhibit any growth inhibitory effect against Gram-negative bacteria, such as *Enterococcus faecalis*, *Escherichia coli* and *Pseudomonas aeruginosa* or against *Candida albicans*.[35] Further antibiotic constituents have been isolated from St. John's wort: imanine and novoimanine.[38,39] Novoimanine was reported to be the most effective topical agent against *S. aureus*.[38] Herb extracts are reported to exhibit more pronounced activity against staphylococci, shigellae and *E. coli* than are decoctions.[39,40]

Antiviral activity Flavonoid and catechin-containing fractions have exhibited antiviral activity, inhibiting the influenza virus by 83–100%.[41] Hypericin and pseudohypericin have been reported to inhibit several encapsulated viruses *in vitro*, including herpes simplex types 1 and 2[42,43] and human immunodeficiency virus type 1 (HIV-1).[44–47] Hypericin has also been reported to inactivate murine cytomegalovirus (MCMV) and Sindbis virus.[47] The antiviral activity of hypericin appears to involve a photoactivation process.[47,G1]

Other effects *In vitro* studies using a hamster vas deferens smooth muscle cell line demonstrated that hyperforin induces the release of calcium ions from mitochondrial or other sources followed by activation of cellular metabolism.[48] It is not known whether this activity contributes to the antidepressant effects of hyperforin.

Oral administration of a single dose of St. John's wort (100, 200, 400, 600 or 800 mg/kg) to two strains of alcohol-preferring rats significantly reduced alcohol intake in both strains.[49] In another study in experimental alcoholism, acute intraperitoneal administration of St. John's wort (10–40 mg/kg), fluoxetine (1–10 mg/kg) and imipramine (3–30 mg/kg) reduced alcohol intake in a dose-dependent manner in a 12-hour, limited access, two-bottle choice (ethanol/water) procedure.[24] Depression and alcoholism are thought to have some neurochemical similarities, such as low brain serotonin concentrations.[50]

It has been suggested that biflavonoids may be the sedative principles in St. John's wort since CNS activity has been documented for biflavonoid constituents in another plant, *Taxus baccata*.[3]

An extract of St. John's wort was found to suppress inflammation and leukocyte infiltration induced by carrageenan and prostaglandin E_1 (PGE₁) in mice.[51] *In vitro*, hypericin has been shown to inhibit tumour necrosis factor-induced activation of the transcription factor NF-κB,[52] specific growth factor-regulated protein kinases[53–55] and the release of arachidonic acid and leukotriene B_4.[56] In a rabbit model of proliferative vitreoretinopathy (PVR), intravitreal injection of hypericin 0.1 mL (10 or 100 µmol/L, but not 1 µmol/L) inhibited the progression of PVR when compared with severity in control eyes five days after hypericin administration.[57] It was suggested that, as protein kinase C is important in the cellular reactions occurring in PVR, modulation of protein kinase C by hypericin may be a factor in this system. Hypericin and pseudohypericin have been reported to inhibit 12-lipoxygenase activity; the products of lipoxygenase-catalysed reactions, such as leukotrienes, may be involved in inflammatory reactions.[58]

Other compounds may contribute to the anti-inflammatory properties of St. John's wort.[37] Anti-inflammatory and anti-ulcerogenic properties have been documented for amentoflavone, a biapigenin derivative.[4] Analgesic activity in mice has been reported for the total flavonoid fraction;[59] the active principle was stated to be of the quercetin type.

Both water-soluble imanine and imanine were reported to reduce blood pressure and increase the frequency and depth of breathing following intravenous administration (50 mg/kg) to rabbits.[38] A study of the vasoconstrictor action of water-soluble imanine and imanine on the isolated rabbit ear indicated that their hypotensive action was not due to a direct effect on the vasculature.[38] When perfused through the isolated frog heart, both water-soluble imanine and imanine were found to cause cardiac systolic arrest at a dilution of 1×10^{-5}.[38] Proanthocyanidin-containing fractions isolated from St. John's wort have been reported to inhibit contractions of the isolated guinea-pig heart induced by histamine, $PGF_{2\alpha}$ and potassium chloride.[60]

A tonus-raising effect on isolated guinea-pig and rabbit uteri has been documented for a crude aqueous extract.[61] Of the group of plants investigated, St. John's wort was reported to exhibit the weakest uterotonic activity.

Tannins isolated from St. John's wort are stated to have mild astringent activity.[62] The anthraquinone derivatives documented for St. John's wort do not possess any purgative action.[G62]

In vitro cytotoxicity against human colon carcinoma cells (CO 115) has been described for hyperforin-related constituents isolated from *Hypericum calycinum* and *Hypericum revolutum*.[63]

Clinical studies

Clinical trials with extracts of St. John's wort have focused mainly on its effects in patients with depression, although there have been several studies exploring its use in other conditions, including seasonal affective disorder, chronic fatigue and premenstrual syndrome.

Depression Initially, hypericin was thought to be responsible for the antidepressant activity of St.

John's wort, although, more recently, experimental[25,26] and clinical evidence[64] has emerged to indicate that hyperforin is one of the major constituents required for antidepressant activity.

The precise mechanism of action of St. John's wort's antidepressant effect remains unclear (*see* Pharmacological Actions, *In vitro* and animal studies). A double-blind, placebo-controlled, crossover study in 12 healthy male volunteers investigated the effects of a single dose of St. John's wort extract (LI 160) (2700 mg, 9 × 300-mg tablets standardised to 0.3% hypericin) on plasma concentrations of growth hormone, prolactin and cortisol.[65] A significant increase in plasma growth hormone concentration and a significant decrease in plasma prolactin concentration were observed following St. John's wort administration relative to placebo administration. Plasma cortisol concentrations were unchanged. These findings suggest that this dose of St. John's wort extract may increase aspects of brain dopamine function in humans, although further studies are required to confirm this, assess dose–response relationships and determine whether there is evidence for effects on dopaminergic systems in patients with depression treated with St. John's wort.[65] Another study, which used a randomised, three-way, crossover design, investigated the effects of a single dose of St. John's wort extract (LI 160S) (600 or 300 mg) or placebo on hormone concentrations in 12 healthy male volunteers.[66] Compared with placebo, St. John's wort extract (600 mg) increased cortisol secretion between 30 and 90 minutes after dosing, indicating an influence of St. John's wort on certain CNS neurotransmitters. There was no difference between the three groups with regard to adrenocorticotrophic hormone (ACTH), growth hormone and prolactin secretion.[66]

A systematic review and meta-analysis of randomised controlled trials of preparations of St. John's wort extract included 23 trials involving a total of 1757 patients with depressive disorders.[67] This has been updated to include new studies and published as a Cochrane review of 27 randomised controlled trials of St. John's wort extract in patients with 'neurotic depression' and mild to moderately severe depressive disorders.[14] Seventeen of these trials (involving 1168 patients) compared St. John's wort preparations with placebo (16 studies used preparations containing St. John's wort extract as the sole herbal ingredient and one involved a combination product of St. John's wort extract with four other herbal ingredients); the ten other trials (involving 1123 patients) compared St. John's wort extracts with conventional antidepressant or sedative drugs, including amitriptyline, imipramine, desipramine and maprotiline (eight trials used

single-ingredient preparations and two used combinations of St. John's wort and valerian). St. John's wort extracts were administered at doses ranging from 350 to 1800 mg; the hyperforin content of the preparations tested was not known. Most trials lasted for 4–6 weeks, although some studies were conducted for three months.

The results of the meta-analysis showed that St. John's wort preparations were significantly superior to placebo in the short-term treatment of mild to moderately severe depressive disorders (rate ratio 2.47 and 95% confidence interval (95% CI) 1.69–3.61). St. John's wort preparations were found to be as effective as conventional antidepressant agents (single preparations, rate ratio 1.01 and 95% CI 0.87–1.16), although for several reasons – for example, the use of low doses of conventional antidepressants and the trials involving small numbers of patients – this evidence was considered inadequate for establishing whether St. John's wort was as effective as conventional antidepressant drugs.[14] Further studies comparing St. John's wort preparations with standard antidepressant agents in well-defined patient groups and over longer periods were considered necessary.[14]

Another meta-analysis employed tighter inclusion criteria for trials in an effort to increase the validity of the analysis.[68] It included only randomised, blinded, controlled trials of St. John's wort as a single preparation, which involved patients with depressive disorders as defined by the standard criteria ICD-10 (International Statistical Classification of Diseases and Related Health Problems), DSM-IIIR (Diagnostical Manual) or DSM-IV and which used the Hamilton Depression (HAMD) Scale for measuring clinical outcomes. Six such trials involving 651 patients with mainly mild to moderately severe depressive disorders were included; two trials were placebo controlled and four compared St. John's wort with standard antidepressants. The studies lasted for 4–6 weeks and the doses of St. John's wort extract ranged from 200 to 900 mg daily; the range for total hypericin administered was 0.75–2.7 mg daily.

This meta-analysis showed that the response rate for St. John's wort was significantly greater than that for placebo (73.2 versus 37.9%, respectively, relative risk 1.48 and 95% CI 1.03–1.92) and similar to that observed with tricyclic antidepressants (64 versus 6.4% for St. John's wort and tricyclic antidepressants, respectively, relative risk 1.11 and 95% CI 0.92–1.29).[68] Despite the stringent inclusion criteria for trials in this meta-analysis, it was concluded that further studies are required in order to address methodological problems before it can be concluded that St. John's wort is an effective antidepressant.[68]

At least four randomised, controlled trials of monopreparations of St. John's wort involving patients with depressive disorders[64,69-71] have been published since the Cochrane review.[14] Two trials compared St. John's wort against placebo only,[64,69] one compared St. John's wort with fluoxetine[70] and one was a three-arm study comparing St. John's wort with imipramine and placebo.[71]

In a randomised, double-blind, multicentre study, 162 patients with mild to moderate depression received St. John's wort extract (ZE117) (250 mg) twice daily (equivalent to 1 mg hypericin daily) or placebo for six weeks.[69] At the end of the study, 56% of St. John's wort-treated patients compared with 15% of placebo recipients were classified as responders according to recognised criteria. The proportions of patients reporting adverse events were similar between groups (7.4 and 6.2% for St. John's wort and placebo, respectively).

Another randomised, double-blind, multicentre trial compared two different extracts of St. John's wort with placebo in 147 patients with mild or moderate depression according to DSM-IV criteria.[64] Patients received St. John's wort extract (300 mg, WS 5573, containing 0.5% hyperforin or 300 mg, WS 5572, containing 5% hyperforin) or placebo three times daily for six weeks. Patients who received the extract containing 5% hyperforin showed the largest reduction in Hamilton Rating Scale for Depression scores from baseline values. Furthermore, 49% of these patients were classified as treatment responders (according to recognised criteria), whereas 38.8 and 32.7% of patients who received 0.5% hyperforin and placebo recipients, respectively, were classified as responders. The proportions of patients reporting adverse events were similar (28.6 versus 28.6 versus 30.6% for 5% hyperforin, 0.5% hyperforin and placebo, respectively). These findings were the first to show that the therapeutic effect of St. John's wort in mild to moderate depression depends on its hyperforin content.[64]

In a study comparing St. John's wort with a selective serotonin reuptake inhibitor, 161 patients aged 60–80 years with mild or moderate depression according to ICD-10 criteria were randomised to receive St. John's wort extract (LoHyp-57) (400 mg) twice daily or fluoxetine (10 mg) twice daily for six weeks.[70] Neither the hypericin nor the hyperforin content of the St. John's wort extract were stated in a published report of the study. At the end of the treatment period, 71.4% of St. John's wort recipients and 72.2% of fluoxetine recipients were classified as responders according to recognised, pre-defined criteria. Similar efficacy for both St. John's wort and fluoxetine was demonstrated when data from sub-groups of patients with mild and moderate depression were analysed. The numbers of patients developing adverse reactions with a possible or probable relationship to treatment were 12 and 17 for St. John's wort and fluoxetine, respectively, leading to cessation of treatment in six and eight cases, respectively.[70]

In a randomised, double-blind, multicentre trial in a primary care setting, 263 patients with moderate depression received St. John's wort extract (350 mg) three times daily (STEI 300, containing 0.2–0.3% hypericin and 2–3% hyperforin, $n = 106$), imipramine (100 mg) daily (in three divided doses of 50, 25 and 25 mg, titrated from 50 mg on day 1 and 75 mg on days 2–4, $n = 110$) or placebo ($n = 47$) for eight weeks.[71] Hypericum was found to be more effective than placebo after six weeks of treatment and to be as efficacious as imipramine after 8 weeks of treatment. In addition, both St. John's wort and imipramine were shown to improve quality of life, as measured by the SF-36, to a greater extent than placebo. Adverse events were reported by 22% of St. John's wort recipients, 46% of imipramine recipients and 19% of placebo recipients.

This study was criticised for its use of a relatively low dose of imipramine, such that the trial shows only that a comparatively high dose of St. John's wort seems to be as effective as a comparatively low dose of imipramine.[72] Nevertheless, this[71] and other new trials[64,69] have confirmed that St. John's wort extracts are more effective than placebo in mild to moderately severe depression.[72] However, further trials comparing St. John's wort with standard antidepressants, particularly newer classes of agents such as the selective serotonin reuptake inhibitors, are still required. A large placebo-controlled trial comparing St. John's wort extract (900–1800 mg daily) with the selective serotonin reuptake inhibitor sertraline (50–150 mg daily) in patients with major depression according to DSM-IV criteria is ongoing in the United States.[73] Published abstracts of randomised, double-blind, controlled trials have reported superiority of St. John's wort extract over placebo[74] and equivalent efficacy between St. John's wort and fluoxetine (20 mg) daily in mild to moderate depression[75,76] and between St. John's wort and imipramine (150 mg) daily.[76]

In a dose-ranging trial involving 348 patients with mild to moderate depression according to ICD-10 criteria, patients were randomised to receive St. John's wort extract three times daily equivalent to either 1 mg ($n = 119$), 0.33 mg ($n = 115$) or 0.17 mg ($n = 114$) hypericin for six weeks.[77] At the end of the treatment period, there was a significant reduction in HAMD scores compared with baseline values. The response rates (according to recognised criteria) were

68, 65 and 62% for 1, 0.33 and 0.17 mg hypericin, respectively; the differences between groups were not statistically significant. Thus, the study showed that there was no dose-dependent effect of hypericin in St. John's wort extracts.

Seasonal affective disorder The effects of St. John's wort extracts have been investigated in studies involving subjects with seasonal affective disorder (SAD),[78,79] although as yet there have not been any trials that have included a placebo control group. Twenty individuals with SAD were randomised to receive St. John's wort (LI 160) (300 mg) three times daily (equivalent to 0.9 mg hypericin) with or without bright light therapy.[78] After four weeks, there were significant reductions in HAMD scores in both groups compared with baseline values and there were no statistically significant differences between groups. Another study evaluated data from individuals with mild to moderate SAD who had used St. John's wort (300 mg) three times daily (equivalent to 0.9 mg hypericin) with ($n = 133$) or without light therapy ($n = 168$) for eight weeks.[79] The study was not randomised and involved data collection by postal questionnaires. Data from 301 returned questionnaires were suitable for analysis. Significant reductions in the mean SAD scores were observed in both groups compared with baseline values; the differences in the SAD scores between groups were statistically non-significant.

Antiviral activity Antiviral activity has been reported for hypericin against human immunodeficiency virus (HIV) and hepatitis C.[80,81,82,] Several uncontrolled studies in HIV-positive patients who received St. John's wort extract have reported immunologic and clinical benefits, including increases in CD4 cell counts in some patients.[83,84] In a phase I, dose-escalating study, 30 HIV-positive patients with CD4 cell counts <350 cells/mm^3 received intravenous synthetic hypericin twice weekly (0.25 or 0.5 mg/kg body-weight), three times weekly (0.25 mg/kg) or oral hypericin daily (0.5 mg/kg).[85] Sixteen patients discontinued treatment early because of toxic effects, and phototoxicity in several other patients prevented completion of dose escalation. Antiretroviral activity as assessed by significant changes in HIV p24 antigen level, HIV titre, HIV RNA copies and CD4 cell counts was not observed.

Other studies The potential for the use of St. John's wort in 20 individuals presenting with fatigue[86] and in 19 women with self-reported premenstrual syndrome[87] has also been explored in uncontrolled pilot studies. Significant improvements in perceived

fatigue and in symptoms of depression and anxiety were seen after six weeks' treatment with St. John's wort (equivalent to 0.9 mg hypericin daily) compared with baseline values[86] and in overall premenstrual syndrome scores after treatment with St. John's wort (equivalent to 0.9 mg hypericin daily) for two menstrual cycles.[87] Thus, there is scope for conducting randomised controlled trials of St. John's wort in these conditions.[86,87]

In a randomised, double-blind, placebo-controlled trial, 179 women with menopause-related psychovegetative symptoms received a combination preparation of St. John's wort and black cohosh (*Cimicifuga racemosa*) or placebo for six weeks.[88] The results indicated that the combination product had a significantly greater effect on the symptoms than did placebo. Postmarketing surveillance studies have been carried out with extracts of St. John's wort in patients with psychovegetative disorders[89] and in women with menopausal symptoms of psychological origin[90] (*see* Side-effects, Toxicity). Improvements in symptom scores compared with baseline values following treatment with St. John's wort extracts were reported in all studies; these studies did not involve a control group.

A randomised, double-blind, phase I study involving 55 healthy volunteers who received St. John's wort (900 mg) daily (containing 0.5% hyperforin), St. John's wort (900 mg) daily (containing 5.0% hyperforin) or placebo for eight days investigated the effects on quantitative electroencephalogram as an indicator of drug-induced pharmacological action.[91] Reproducible central pharmacodynamic effects were apparent in both groups of St. John's wort recipients compared with placebo recipients. The effects were greater in subjects who received extract containing 5.0% hyperforin than in those who received extract containing 0.5% hyperforin.

Placebo-controlled, crossover studies investigating the effects of St. John's wort (0.9 and 1.8 mg) on the sleep polysomnogram of healthy subjects reported that both doses of St. John's wort significantly increased rapid eye movement (REM) sleep latency compared with placebo, but had no effect on REM sleep duration or other parameters of sleep architecture.[92]

In a randomised, double-blind, placebo-controlled trial involving 23 overweight but otherwise healthy adults, subjects who received treatment with St. John's wort (900 mg) daily, *Citrus aurantium* extract (975 mg) daily and caffeine (528 mg) daily lost significantly more body weight than did subjects in the placebo and no-treatment control groups.[93]

A placebo-controlled, crossover study in 19 healthy volunteers who received St. John's wort for

15 days either alone or in combination with ethanol (to achieve a blood alcohol concentration of 0.05%) reported that there were no differences between the two groups in sense of well-being or adverse events.[94]

A randomised, double-blind, placebo-controlled, six-week trial involving 72 long-distance runners and triathletes reported significant improvements in endurance capacity in subjects who received vitamin E with St. John's wort compared with subjects who received vitamin E alone or placebo.[95]

Pharmacokinetics Detailed pharmacokinetic studies have been carried out with the hypericin-standardised St. John's wort extract LI 160.[96] Administration of single oral doses of LI 160 (300, 900 and 1800 mg) to healthy male volunteers resulted in peak plasma hypericin concentrations of 1.5, 7.5 and 14.2 ng/mL for the three doses, respectively. Peak plasma concentrations were seen with hypericin after 2.0–2.6 hours and with pseudohypericin after 0.4–0.6 hours. The elimination half-life of hypericin was between 24.8 and 26.5 hours. Repeated doses of LI 160 (300 mg) three times daily resulted in steady-state concentrations after four days.[96] Oral administration of the St. John's wort extract WS 5572 (300 mg, equivalent to 14.8 mg hyperforin) resulted in peak plasma concentrations of 150 ng/mL being reached 3.5 hours after administration.[97] The elimination half-life was 9 hours. Following repeated doses of 300 mg three times daily, the estimated steady-state plasma hyperforin concentrations were 100 ng/mL. Other studies investigating the pharmacokinetics of hypericum and hypericin have been summarised.[1,G1]

Side-effects, Toxicity

A review of safety data for St. John's wort obtained from reports of randomised controlled trials, drug monitoring and postmarketing surveillance studies[98–101] and national and international drug safety monitoring bodies has been published.[102] Collectively, the data indicate that St. John's wort is well-tolerated. Adverse effects are generally mild; the most common adverse effects reported are gastrointestinal symptoms, dizziness, confusion and tiredness/sedation. In placebo-controlled trials, the frequency of adverse effects with St. John's wort is similar to that for placebo.[102] Photosensitivity appears to be an extremely rare event with recommended doses of St. John's wort (*see below*).[102]

Several postmarketing surveillance studies of the St. John's wort extracts HYP811,[89,103] LI 160[90,104] and Neuroplant[105] have since been published. These studies provide further confirmation of the tolerability of St. John's wort extracts taken at recommended

doses for short-term treatment (usually 4–6 weeks, although one study monitored 111 women for 12 weeks[90]). The frequency of adverse reactions in 6382 patients with mild depression who took St. John's wort for six weeks was reported to be 0.125% (mainly skin reactions).[105]

A systematic review and meta-analysis of randomised controlled trials of St. John's wort in patients with mild to moderately severe depressive disorders reported that, in the trials comparing St. John's wort with standard antidepressants, the proportions of patients reporting side-effects were 26.3 and 44.7%, respectively (rate ratio 0.57 and 95% CI 0.4–0.69).[14] However, further studies investigating the long-term safety of St. John's wort were advised. Another meta-analysis which employed tighter inclusion criteria reported that tricyclic antidepressants were associated with a higher proportion of side-effects than were St. John's wort preparations (47 versus 26.4%, respectively, relative risk 1.72 and 95% CI 1.30–2.14).[68] Randomised controlled trials[64,69–71] published since the Cochrane meta-analysis[14] and published abstracts[74–76] have also reported that St. John's wort has a more favourable short-term safety profile than standard antidepressants[70,71,75,76] and that the frequency of adverse events seen with St. John's wort is similar to that for placebo[64,69,71,74] (*see* Clinical studies). In a comparative trial of St. John's wort and fluoxetine, the frequency of adverse reactions associated with St. John's wort was higher than expected, although it was stated that the effects reported were similar to those known to occur with fluoxetine.[70] The observation that the frequency of adverse effects is lower in placebo-controlled trials of St. John's wort than in comparative trials with standard antidepressants has been made previously.[102] A review has attempted to compare the safety profile of St. John's wort systematically with that of several conventional antidepressants.[106]

Photosensitivity Sensitivity to sunlight following the ingestion of hypericum or hypericin is known as hypericism.

Delayed hypersensitivity or photodermatitis has been documented for St. John's wort following the ingestion of a herbal tea made from the leaves.[107] Hypericin is stated to be the photosensitising agent present in St. John's wort.[82,G33,G47] A review of the photodynamic actions of hypericin has been published.[108] In a double-blind, crossover, single-dose study in 13 healthy volunteers who received placebo or St. John's wort extract (LI 160) (900, 1800 and 3600 mg containing 0, 2.81, 5.62 and 11.25 mg total hypericin, respectively), no evidence of photosensitivity was observed with or without St. John's wort following skin irradiation with both UV-A and UV-B light 4 hours after dosing.[109] In a multiple-dose study in which 50 volunteers received St. John's wort (LI 160) (600 mg) three times daily (equivalent to 5.6 mg total hypericin daily) for 15 days, a moderate increase in UV-A sensitivity was observed.[109] However, the doses used were higher than those recommended therapeutically. In another single-dose study, administration of St. John's wort (LI 160) (1800 mg, equivalent to 5.4 mg total hypericin) to 12 healthy volunteers resulted in a mean serum total hypericin concentration of 43 ng/mL and a mean skin blister fluid concentration of 5.3 ng/mL.[110] After administration of St. John's wort (300 mg) three times daily for seven days in order to achieve steady-state concentrations, the mean serum total hypericin concentration was 12.5 ng/mL and the mean skin blister fluid concentration was 2.8 ng/mL; these concentrations are below those estimated to be phototoxic (>100 ng/mL).[110]

The consumption of large quantities of St. John's wort by grazing animals has been associated with the development of photosensitivity.[111,G22,G51] Mice given 0.2–0.5 mg of the herb were found to develop severe photodynamic effects.[G22] Studies using cell cultures of human keratinocytes incubated with hypericin or St. John's wort extract and exposed to UV-A resulted in a reduction in the LC_{50} (lethal concentration) with hypericin, but only a mild reduction with hypericum.[112] From these findings it has been estimated that at least 30 times the therapeutic dose would be necessary to produce phototoxic effects in humans.[112] Experimental evidence has suggested that a solution of hypericin can react with visible and UV light to produce free radical species and that this may lead to damage of proteins in the lens of the eye.[113] There are no reports of cataract formation in individuals who have taken St. John's wort.

A study reported that HIV-positive patients treated with oral hypericin (0.05 mg/kg) for 28 days developed mild symptoms of photosensitivity on exposure to sunlight and that two patients developed intolerable symptoms of photosensitivity when the dose was increased to 0.16 mg/kg.[114] In a dose-escalating study involving 30 HIV-infected patients treated with oral (0.5 mg/kg daily) or intravenous hypericin (starting dosage 0.25 mg/kg twice or three times weekly), 16 patients discontinued treatment before completing eight weeks of therapy because of moderate or severe phototoxicity; severe cutaneous phototoxicity was observed in 11 out of 23 evaluable patients.[85] Other serious clinical or laboratory adverse events were infrequent: elevation of alkaline phosphatase and hepatic aminotransferase concentrations to more than five times normal values was noted in two and three patients, respectively.

Other effects *In humans* A case of subacute toxic neuropathy possibly related to the use of St. John's wort and subsequent exposure to sunlight has been reported.[115] A woman developed stinging pains in areas exposed to the sun (face and hands) four weeks after starting treatment with St. John's wort (500 mg/day, extract and hypericin content not stated); the report did not state whether the woman was using any other products. Her symptoms improved three weeks after stopping St. John's wort and disappeared over the next two months.

There have been reports of sensory nerve hypersensitivity occurring in individuals who have taken St. John's wort preparations (tablets or tinctures).[116]

Cases of mania[117,118] and hypomania[119,120] have been reported in individuals taking St. John's wort preparations. Two cases of mania were reported in patients with bipolar depression who began self-treatment with standardised St. John's wort extract (900 mg) daily[118] and one in a patient experiencing a moderate depressive episode who was taking both sertraline and St. John's wort (dosage not known).[117] A case of hypomania was reported in a woman with panic disorder and unipolar major depression who had discontinued sertraline treatment one week before starting St. John's wort tincture.[119] Two cases of hypomania were reported in individuals with no history of bipolar disorder.[120] A man who had received electroconvulsive therapy and who had previously taken various antidepressant drugs, including venlafaxine, fluvoxamine, moclobemide and nortriptyline, experienced a hypomanic episode six weeks after starting St. John's wort (dosage not stated). A man with symptoms of post-traumatic stress disorder was diagnosed with an acute manic episode after three months of self-treatment with St. John's wort (dosage not stated).[120]

Several of these reports stated that the symptoms had resolved after stopping treatment with St. John's wort, although in one case the patient improved but remained agitated despite cessation of St. John's wort.[120] None of the cases involved rechallenge with St. John's wort and, in all cases, there were other pharmacological factors and/or underlying illnesses that could have been responsible for or contributed to the precipitation of mania.

In animals and in vitro studies Experimental studies investigating the genotoxic potential and mutagenic activity of St. John's wort extracts *in vitro* and *in vivo* have been summarised.[G1,G52] *In vivo* studies and most *in vitro* studies provided negative results, indicating a lack of mutagenic potential with defined St. John's wort extracts.[G52] Mutagenic activity observed in an *in vitro* Ames test was attributed to the presence of quercetin, although other studies have found no mutagenic potential with a St. John's wort extract and it has been stated that there is no valid evidence for the carcinogenicity of quercetin in humans.[G1,G52]

Dietary administration of St. John's wort to rats was found to have no affect on various hepatic drug-metabolising enzymes (e.g. aminopyrine, N-demethylase, glutathione S-transferase and epoxide hydrolase) or on copper concentrations in the liver (see Contra-indications, Warnings, Drug interactions). No major effects were observed on hepatic iron or zinc concentrations and no significant tissue lesions were found in four rats fed St. John's wort in their daily diet for 119 days (10% for first 12 days and 5% thereafter because of unpalatability).[121]

Cytotoxic constituents related to hyperforin have been isolated from two related *Hypericum* species (see *In vitro* and animal studies).

Contra-indications, Warnings

Individuals with sensitivity towards St. John's wort may experience allergic reactions. The use of St. John's wort is not advised in known cases of photo-sensitivity and, in view of the potential of hypericin as a photosensitising agent, therapeutic UV treatment should be avoided whilst using St. John's wort.[G1]

It has previously been suggested that excessive doses of St. John's wort may potentiate monoamine oxidase inhibitor therapy.[122] However, as mono-amine oxidase inhibitory activity has not been reported *in vivo* with St. John's wort, this warning is no longer considered necessary. In addition, avoidance of foodstuffs, such as those containing tyramine (e.g. cheese, wine, meat and yeast extracts) and medicines containing sympathomimetic agents (e.g. cough/cold remedies), which interact with MAOIs, is not considered necessary.

Drug interactions Recent evidence has emerged from spontaneous reports[123] and published case reports[124–127] of interactions between St. John's wort and certain prescribed medicines, leading to a loss of or reduction in the therapeutic effect of these prescribed medicines. Drugs that may be affected include indinavir, warfarin, cyclosporin, digoxin, theophylline and oral contraceptives. Drug inter-action studies in healthy volunteers have provided supporting evidence of interactions between St. John's wort and phenprocoumon[128] and digoxin[129] and have provided evidence that St. John's wort may induce some cytochrome P450 (CYP) drug-metabolising enzymes in the liver,[128,130,131] namely CYP3A4, CYP1A2 and

CYP2CP, as well as affecting P-glycoprotein (a transport protein). Other studies have failed to find significant effects on CYP isoenzymes,[132–134] although the numbers of volunteers may have been too small and the duration of St. John's wort administration too short to exclude an inductive effect truly.[133,134]

There have been other reports of increased serotonergic effects in patients taking St. John's wort concurrently with selective serotonin reuptake inhibitors (e.g. sertraline, paroxetine).[135,136]

Also of concern is that the content of active constituents can vary between different preparations of St. John's wort; thus, the degree of enzyme induction may vary.

Collectively, these data led the UK Committee on Safety of Medicines (CSM) to issue advice to pharmacists, doctors and patients on the use of St. John's wort with certain drugs.[137,138] The CSM's advice for healthcare professionals for patients taking St. John's wort and certain drugs can be summarised as follows.

Warfarin, cyclosporin, digoxin, theophylline and anticonvulsants (carbamazepine, phenobarbitone and phenytoin) There is a risk of reduced therapeutic effect, e.g. risk of transplant rejection, seizures and loss of asthma control. Advice is to check plasma drug concentrations (with warfarin, the patient's International Normalised Ratio should be checked) and to stop St. John's wort therapy. In addition, dose adjustment may be necessary.

HIV protease inhibitors (indinavir, nelfinavir, ritonavir and saquinavir) and HIV non-nucleoside reverse transcriptase inhibitors (efavirenz and nevirapine) There is a risk of reduced blood concentrations with possible loss of HIV suppression. Advice is to measure HIV RNA viral load and to stop St. John's wort.

Oral contraceptives There is a risk of reduced blood concentrations, breakthrough bleeding and unintended pregnancy. Advice is to stop St. John's wort.

Triptans (sumatriptan, naratriptan, rizatriptan and zolmitriptan) and selective serotonin reuptake inhibitors (citalopram, fluoxetine, fluvoxamine, paroxetine and sertraline) There is a risk of increased serotonergic effects with the possibility of an increased risk of adverse reactions. Advice is to stop St. John's wort.

Patients already taking any of the above drugs should be advised not to start taking St. John's wort and users of other medicines should be advised to seek professional advice before using St. John's wort. Topical medicines and non-psychotropic medicines that are excreted renally are not likely to interact with St. John's wort. In addition, topical or homeopathic preparations of St. John's wort are not likely to interact with prescribed medicines.

Pregnancy and lactation Slight *in vitro* uterotonic activity has been reported for St. John's wort (*see In vitro* and animal studies).

There is a report of a 38-year-old woman who started taking St. John's wort (900 mg/day) at her 24th week of pregnancy, taking the last dose 24 hours before delivery.[139] The pregnancy was unremarkable except for late onset of thrombocytopenia. Another report described a 43-year-old woman who discontinued fluoxetine and methylphenidate upon becoming pregnant and started taking St. John's wort (900 mg/day). The report does not state the outcome of the pregnancy,[139] although it is assumed that had adverse events occurred, they would have been stated. In view of the lack of toxicity data, St. John's wort should not be used during pregnancy and lactation.

Pharmaceutical Comment

The chemical composition of St. John's wort has been well studied. Documented pharmacological activities provide supporting evidence for several of the traditional uses stated for St. John's wort. Many pharmacological activities appear to be attributable to hypericin and to the flavonoid constituents; hypericin is also reported to be responsible for the photosensitive reactions that have been documented for St. John's wort. With regard to the antidepressant effects of St. John's wort, hyperforin rather than hypericin, as originally thought, has emerged as one of the major constituents responsible for antidepressant activity. However, further research is required in order to determine which other constituents contribute to the antidepressant effect.

Evidence from randomised, controlled trials has confirmed the efficacy of St. John's wort extracts over placebo in the treatment of mild to moderately severe depression.[14] Other randomised controlled studies have provided some evidence that St. John's wort extracts are as effective as some standard antidepressants in mild to moderate depression. However, there is still a need for further trials in order to assess the efficacy of St. John's wort extracts compared with that of standard antidepressants, particularly newer antidepressant agents such as the selective serotonin reuptake inhibitors. In addition, there is generally a need for further studies in well-defined groups of patients, in different types of depression and conducted over longer periods in order to determine

long-term safety.[14] St. John's wort does appear to have a more favourable short-term safety profile than standard antidepressants, a factor that is likely to be important in patients continuing to take medication. Concerns have been raised over interactions between St. John's wort and certain prescribed medicines (including warfarin, cyclosporin, theophylline, digoxin, HIV protease inhibitors, anticonvulsants, selective serotonin reuptake inhibitors, triptans and oral contraceptives); advice is that patients taking these medicines should stop taking St. John's wort, generally after seeking professional advice as dose adjustment may be necessary. With the exception of oral contraceptives, patients taking these prescribed medicines should not be self-treating with over-the-counter medicines, including herbal medicines, without first seeking professional advice.

In view of the lack of long-term safety data for St. John's wort and its reported photosensitising ability, excessive use of St. John's wort should be avoided.

References

See also General References G1, G2, G3, G5, G7, G9, G15, G16, G18, G22, G28, G31, G32, G33, G36, G37, G40, G43, G45, G46, G48, G50, G51, G52, G56, G61, G62 and G64.

1　Bombardelli E, Morazzoni P. *Hypericum perforatum. Fitoterapia* 1995; **66**: 43–68.

2　Vanhaelen M, Vanhaelen-Fastre R. Quantitative determination of biologically active constituents in medicinal plant crude extracts by thin-layer chromatography-densitometry. *J Chromatogr* 1983; **281**: 263–271.

3　Berghöfer R, Hölzl J. Biflavonoids in *Hypericum perforatum*; part 1. Isolation of 13,II8-biapigenin. *Planta Med* 1987; **53**: 216–17.

4　Berghöfer R, Hölzl J. Isolation of I3′,II8-biapigenin (amentoflavone) from *Hypericum perforatum*. *Planta Med* 1989; **55**: 91.

5　Ollivier B *et al.* Separation et identification des acides phenols par chromatographie liquide haute performance et spectroscopie ultra-violette. Application à la pariétaire (*Parietaria officinalis* L.) et au millepertuis (*Hypericum perforatum* L.). *J Pharm Belg* 1985; **40**: 173–177.

6　Hoelzl J, Ostrowski E. St John's wort (*Hypericum perforatum* L.). HPLC analysis of the main components and their variability in a population. *Dtsch Apoth Ztg* 1987; **127**: 1227–1230.

7　Dorossiev I. Determination of flavonoids in *Hypericum perforatum*. *Pharmazie* 1985; **40**: 585–586.

8　Brondz I *et al.* The relative stereochemistry of hyperforin – an antibiotic from *Hypericum perforatum* L. *Tetrahedron Lett* 1982; **23**: 1299–1300.

9 Ayuga C, Rebuelta M. A comparative study of phenolic acids of *Hypericum caprifolium* Boiss and *Hypericum perforatum* L. *An Real Acad Farm* 1986; **52**: 723–728.

10 Brondz I *et al*. *n*-Alkanes of *Hypericum perforatum*: a revision. *Phytochemistry* 1983; **22**: 295–296.

11 Mathis C, Ourisson G. Étude chimio-taxonomique du genre *Hypericum* – II. Identification de constituants de diverses huiles essentielles d'*Hypericum*. *Phytochemistry* 1964; **3**: 115–131.

12 Mathis C, Ourisson G. Étude chimio-taxonomique du genre *Hypericum* – IV. Repartition des sesquiterpenes, des alcools monoterpeniques et des aldehydes satures dans les huiles essentielles d'*Hypericum*. *Phytochemistry* 1964; **3**: 377–378.

13 Mathis C, Ourisson G. Étude chimio-taxonomique du genre *Hypericum* – V. Identification de quelques constituants non volatils d'*Hypericum perforatum* L. *Phytochemistry* 1964; **3**: 379.

14 Linde K, Mulrow CD. St John's wort for depression (Cochrane Review). In: *The Cochrane Library*, Issue 1, 2000. Oxford: Update Software.

15 Nahrstedt A, Butterweck V. Biologically active and other chemical constituents of the herb of *Hypericum perforatum* L. *Pharmacopsychiatry* 1997; **30**(Suppl.): 129–134.

16 Nathan PJ. The experimental and clinical pharmacology of St John's wort (*Hypericum perforatum* L). *Mol Psychiatr* 1999; **4**: 333–338.

17 Suzuki O *et al*. Inhibition of monoamine oxidase by hypericin. *Planta Med* 1984; **50**: 272–274.

18 Bladt S, Wagner H. Inhibition of MAO by fractions and constituents of *Hypericum* extract. *J Geriat Psychiatr Neurol* 1994; **7**: S57–59.

19 Demisch L *et al*. Identification of MAO-type-A inhibitors in *Hypericum perforatum* L. (Hyperforat). *Pharmacopsychiatry* 1989; **22**: 194.

20 Thiede HM, Walper A. Inhibition of MAO and COMT by *Hypericum* extracts and hypericin. *J Geriat Psychiatr Neurol* 1994; **7**: S54–56.

21 Cott JM. *In vitro* receptor binding and enzyme inhibition by *Hypericum perforatum* extract. *Pharmacopsychiatry* 1997; **30**(Suppl.): 108–112.

22 Müller WE *et al*. Effects of hypericum extract (LI 160) in biochemical models of antidepressant activity. *Pharmacopsychiatry* 1997; **30**(Suppl.): 102–107.

23 Calapai G *et al*. Effects of *Hypericum perforatum* on levels of 5-hydroxytryptamine, noradrenaline and dopamine in the cortex, diencephalon and brainstem of the rat. *J Pharm Pharmacol* 1999; **51**: 723–728.

24 De Vry J *et al*. Comparison of hypericum extracts with imipramine and fluoxetine in animal models of depression and alcoholism. *Eur Neuropsychopharmacol* 1999; **9**: 461–468.

25 Chatterjee SS *et al*. Hyperforin as a possible antidepressant component of hypericum extracts. *Life Sci* 1998; **63**: 499–510.

26 Chatterjee SS *et al*. Antidepressant activity of *Hypericum perforatum* and hyperforin: the neglected possibility. *Pharmacopsychiatry* 1998; **31**(Suppl.): 7–15.

27 Gobbi M *et al*. *Hypericum perforatum* L. extract does not inhibit 5-HT transporter in rat brain cortex. *Naunyn-Schmiedebergs Arch Pharmacol* 1999; **360**: 262–269.

28 Singer A *et al*. Hyperforin, a major antidepressant constituent of St. John's wort, inhibits serotonin uptake by elevating free intracellular Na$^+$. *J Pharmacol Exp Ther* 1999; **290**: 1363–1368.

29 Singer A *et al*. Hyperforin alters free intracellular H$^+$ and Na$^+$ concentration in human platelets (abstract). Paper presented at the Biocenter Symposium on Drug Therapy. Pharmacology of St. John's Wort (*Hypericum perforatum* L.) and its Constituents, February 2000, Frankfurt, Germany.

30 Uebelhack R, Franke L. *In vitro* effects of hypericum extract and hyperforin on 5HT uptake and efflux in human blood platelets (abstract). Paper presented at the Biocenter Symposium on Drug Therapy. Pharmacology of St. John's Wort (*Hypericum perforatum* L.) and its Constituents, February 2000, Frankfurt, Germany.

31 Okpanyi SN, Weischer ML. Animal experiments on the psychotropic action of a *Hypericum* extract. *Arzneimittelforschung* 1987; **37**: 10–13.

32 Gambarana C *et al*. Efficacy of an *Hypericum perforatum* (St John's wort) extract in preventing and reverting a condition of escape deficit in rats. *Neuropsychopharmacology* 1999; **21**: 247–257.

33 Butterwech V *et al*. Flavonoids from *Hypericum perforatum* show antidepressant activity in the forced swimming test. *Planta Med* 2000; **66**: 3–6.

34 Zakharova NS *et al*. Action of plant extracts on the natural immunity indices of animals. *Zh Mikrobiol Epidemiol Immunobiol* 1986; **4**: 71–75.

35 Schempp C *et al*. Antibacterial activity of hyperforin from St John's wort, against multiresistant *Staphylococcus aureus* and Gram-positive bacteria. *Lancet* 1999; **353**: 2129.

36 Voss A, Verweij PE. Antibacterial activity of hyperforin from St John's wort. *Lancet* 1999; **354**: 777.

37 Fiebich B *et al*. Antibacterial activity of hyperforin from St John's wort. *Lancet* 1999; **354**: 777.

38 Negrash AK *et al*. Comparative study of chemotherapeutic and pharmacological properties of antimicrobial preparations from common St John's wort. *Fitontsidy Mater Soveshch* 1969; 198–200.

39 Sakar MK *et al*. Antimicrobial activities of some *Hypericum* species growing in Turkey. *Fitoterapia* 1988; **59**: 49–52.

40 Kolesnikova AG. Bactericidal and immunocorrec-

tive properties of plant extracts. *Zh Mikrobiol Epidemiol Immunobiol* 1986; **3**: 75–78.

41 Mishenkova EL *et al*. Antiviral properties of St John's wort and preparations produced from it. *Tr S'ezda Mikrobiol Ukr* 1975; 222–223.

42 Weber ND *et al*. The antiviral agent hypericin has *in vitro* activity against HSV-1 through non-specific association with viral and cellular membranes. *Antiviral Chem Chemother* 1994; **5**: 83–90.

43 Wood S *et al*. Antiviral activity of naturally occurring anthraquinones and anthraquinone derivatives. *Planta Med* 1990; **56**: 651–652.

44 Lavie G *et al*. Studies of the mechanisms of the antiretroviral agents hypericin and pseudohypericin. *Proc Natl Acad Sci USA* 1989; **86**: 5963–5967.

45 Lopez-Bazzocchi I *et al*. Antiviral activity of the photoactive plant pigment hypericin. *Photochem Photobiol* 1991; **54**: 95–98.

46 Meruelo D *et al*. Therapeutic agents with dramatic antiretroviral activity and little toxicity at effective doses: aromatic polycyclic diones hypericin and pseudohypericin. *Proc Natl Acad Sci USA* 1988; **85**: 5230–5234.

47 Hudson JB *et al*. Antiviral activities of hypericin. *Antiviral Res* 1991; **15**: 101–112.

48 Koch E, Chatterjee SS. Hyperforin stimulates intracellular calcium mobilisation and enhances extracellular acidification in DDT1-MF2 smooth muscle cells (abstract). Paper presented at the Biocenter Symposium on Drug Therapy. Pharmacology of St. John's Wort (*Hypericum perforatum* L.) and its Constituents, February 2000, Frankfurt, Germany.

49 Rezvani AH *et al*. Attenuation of alcohol intake by extract of *Hypericum perforatum* (St John's wort) in two different strains of alcohol-preferring rats. *Alcohol Alcoholism* 1999; **34**: 699–705.

50 Ballenger JC *et al*. Alcohol and central serotonin metabolism in man. *Arch Gen Psych Scand* 1979; **57**: 224–227. Cited by Rezvani AH *et al*. *Alcohol Alcoholism* 1999; **34**: 699–705.

51 Shipochliev T *et al*. Anti-inflammatory action of a group of plant extracts. *Vet Med Nauki* 1981; **18**: 87–94.

52 Bork PS *et al*. Hypericin as a non-oxidant inhibitor of NF-κB. *Planta Med* 1999; **65**: 297–300.

53 Takahashi I *et al*. Hypericin and pseudohypericin specifically inhibit protein kinase C: possible relation to their antiretroviral activity. *Biochem Biophys Res Commun* 1989; **165**: 1207–1212.

54 Agostinis P *et al*. Photosensitized inhibition of growth factor regulated protein kinases by hypericin. *Biochemical Pharmacol* 1995; **49**: 1615–1622.

55 De Witte P *et al*. Inhibition of epidermal growth factor receptor tyrosine kinase activity by hypericin. *Biochemical Pharmacol* 1993; **46**: 1929–1936.

56 Panossian AG *et al*. Immunosuppressive effects of hypericin on stimulated human leucocytes: inhibition of the arachidonic acid release, leukotriene B$_4$ and interleukin-1 production and activation of nitric oxide formation. *Phytomedicine* 1996; **3**: 19–28.

57 Tahara Y *et al*. The antidepressant hypericin inhibits progression of experimental proliferative vitreoretinopathy. *Curr Eye Res* 1999; **19**: 323–329.

58 Bezáková L *et al*. Effect of dianthrones and their precursors from *Hypericum perforatum* L. on lipoxygenase activity. *Pharmazie* 1999; **54**: 711.

59 Vasilchenko EA *et al*. Analgesic action of flavonoids of *Rhododendron luteum* Sweet, *Hypericum perforatum* L., *Lespedeza bicolor* Turcz. and *L. hedysaroides* (Pall.) Kitag. *Rastit Resur* 1986; **22**: 12–21.

60 Melzer R *et al*. Proanthocyanidins from *Hypericum perforatum*: effects on isolated pig coronary arteries. *Planta Med* 1988; **54**: 572–573.

61 Shiplochliev T. Extracts from a group of medicinal plants enhancing the uterine tonus. *Vet Med Nauki* 1981; **18**: 94–98.

62 Grujic-Vasic J *et al*. The examining of isolated tannins and their astringent effect. *Planta Med* 1986; **52**(Suppl.): 67–68.

63 Decosterd LA *et al*. Isolation of new cytotoxic constituents from *Hypericum revolutum* and *Hypericum calycinum* by liquid–liquid chromatography. *Planta Med* 1988; **54**: 560.

64 Laakman G *et al*. St John's wort in mild to moderate depression: the relevance of hyperforin for the clinical efficacy. *Pharmacopsychiatry* 1998; **31**(Suppl.): 54–59.

65 Franklin M *et al*. Neuroendocrine evidence for dopaminergic actions of hypericum extract (LI 160) in healthy volunteers. *Biol Psychiatr* 1999; **46**: 581–584.

66 Laakman G *et al*. Effects of hypericum extract on adenohypophysial hormone secretion and catecholamine metabolism (abstract). Paper presented at the Biocenter Symposium on Drug Therapy. Pharmacology of St. John's Wort (*Hypericum perforatum* L.) and its Constituents, February 2000, Frankfurt, Germany.

67 Linde K *et al*. St John's wort for depression – an overview and meta-analysis of randomised clinical trials. *BMJ* 1996; **313**: 253–258.

68 Kim HL *et al*. St John's wort for depression. A meta-analysis of well-defined clinical trials. *J Nerv Ment Dis* 1999; **187**: 532–539.

69 Schrader E *et al*. Hypericum treatment of mild–moderate depression in a placebo-controlled study. A prospective, double-blind, randomized, placebo-controlled, multicentre study. *Human Psychopharmacol* 1998; **13**: 163–169.

70 Harrer G *et al*. Comparison of equivalence between

the St John's wort extract LoHyp-57 and fluox-etine. *Arzneimittelforschung* 1999; **49**: 289–296.

71 Philipp M *et al.* Hypericum extract versus imipra-mine or placebo in patients with moderate depres-sion: randomised multicentre study of treatment for eight weeks. *BMJ* 1999; **319**: 1534–1539.

72 Linde K, Berner M. Commentary: has hypericum found its place in antidepressant treatment? *BMJ* 1999; **319**: 1539.

73 Vitiello B. *Hypericum perforatum* extracts as potential antidepressants. *J Pharm Pharmacol* 1999; **51**: 513–517.

74 Kalb R *et al.* Hypericum extract WS 5572 is effective and safe in the treatment of mild to moderate depression (abstract). Paper presented at the Biocenter Symposium on Drug Therapy. Phar-macology of St. John's Wort (*Hypericum perfor-atum* L.) and its Constituents, February 2000, Frankfurt, Germany.

75 Friede M *et al.* Differential therapy of mild to moderate depressive episodes (ICD-10 F 32.0; F32.1) with *Hyperici herba* (abstract). Paper pre-sented at the Biocenter Symposium on Drug Therapy. Pharmacology of St. John's Wort (*Hyper-icum perforatum* L.) and its Constituents, February 2000, Frankfurt, Germany.

76 Käufeler R *et al.* Efficacy and tolerability of the St John's wort extract (Ze 117) in comparison with placebo, imipramine and fluoxetine for the treatment of mild to moderate depression accord-ing to ICD-10 (abstract). Paper presented at the Biocenter Symposium on Drug Therapy. Pharma-cology of St. John's Wort (*Hypericum perforatum* L.) and its Constituents, February 2000, Frank-furt, Germany.

77 Lenoir S *et al.* No dose-dependent effect of hypericin in hypericum extracts for depression. *Phytomedicine* 1999; **6**: 141–146.

78 Kasper S. Treatment of seasonal affective disorder (SAD) with hypericum extract. *Pharmacopsychia-try* 1997; **30**(Suppl.): 89–93.

79 Wheatley D. Hypericum in seasonal affective disorder (SAD). *Curr Med Res Opin* 1999; **15**: 33–37.

80 Hypericin – a plant extract with anti-HIV activity. *Scrip* 1989; **1415**: 29.

81 Anon. Hypericin improves blood safety? *Scrip* 1995; **2005**: 27.

82 Anon. Hypericin HIV trial in Thailand. *Scrip* 1995; **2019**: 25.

83 Cooper WC, James J. An observational study of the safety and efficacy of hypericin in HIV-positive subjects (abstract). *Int Conf AIDS* 1990; **6**: 369.

84 Steinbeck-Klose A, Wernet P. Successful long-term treatment over 40 months of HIV-patients with intravenous hypericin (abstract). *Int Conf AIDS* 1993; **9**: 470.

85 Gulick RM *et al.* Phase I studies of hypericin, the active compound in St John's wort, as an antiretroviral agent in HIV-infected adults. *Ann Intern Med* 1999; **130**: 510–514.

86 Stevinson C *et al.* Hypericum for fatigue – a pilot study. *Phytomedicine* 1998; **5**: 443–447.

87 Stevinson C, Ernst E. A pilot study of *Hypericum perforatum* for the treatment of premenstrual syndrome. *Br J Obstet Gynaecol* 2000; **107**: 870–876.

88 Boblitz N *et al.* Benefit of a fixed drug combination containing St John's wort and black cohosh for climacteric patients – results of a randomised clinical trial (abstract). *FACT* 2000; **5**: 85.

89 Mueller BM. Effects of hypericum extract HYP811 in patients with psychovegetative disorders. *Adv Ther* 1998; **15**: 255–260.

90 Grube B *et al.* St John's wort extract: efficacy for menopausal symptoms of psychological origin. *Adv Ther* 1999; **16**: 177–186.

91 Schellenberg R *et al.* Pharmacodynamic effects of two different hypericum extracts in healthy volun-teers measured by quantitative EEG. *Pharmaco-psychiatry* 1998; **31**(Suppl.): 44–53.

92 Sharpley AL *et al.* Antidepressant-like effect of *Hypericum perforatum* (St John's wort) on the sleep polysomnogram. *Psychopharmacology* 1998; **139**: 286–287.

93 Colker CM *et al.* Effects of *Citrus aurantium* extract, caffeine, and St John's wort on body fat loss, lipid levels, and mood states in overweight healthy adults. *Curr Ther Res* 1999; **60**: 145–153.

94 Friede M *et al.* Alltagssicherheit eines pflanzlichen Antidepressivums aus Johanniskraut. *Fortschritte Med* 1998; **116**: 131–135.

95 Hottenrot K *et al.* The influence of vitamin E and extract from hypericum on the endurance capacity of competitors. A placebo-controlled double-blind study with long-distance runners and triathletes. *Dtsche Seitschrift Sportmed* 1997; **48**: 22–27.

96 Staffeldt B *et al.* Pharmacokinetics of hypericin and pseudohypericin after oral intake of the *Hypericum perforatum* extract LI 160 in healthy volunteers. *J Geriat Psychiatr Neurol* 1994; **7**: S47–53.

97 Biber A *et al.* Oral bioavailability of hyperforin from hypericum extracts in rats and human volunteers. *Pharmacopsychiatry* 1998; **31**(Suppl.1): 36–43.

98 Grube B *et al.* Use of a hypericum extract in mild, transient depressive mood disorders. *Eur J Clin Res* 1997; **9**: 293–302.

99 Meier B *et al.* Wirksamkeit und Verträglichkeit eines standardisierten Johanniskraut-Vollextraktes (Ze 117) bei Patienten mit depressiver Symptomatik unterschiedlicher Schweregrade – eine Anwen-dungsbeobachtung. *Forsch Komplementärmed* 1997; **4**: 87–93.

100 Woelk H *et al.* Benefits and risks of the hypericum extract LI 160. Drug monitoring study with 3250 patients. *J Geriat Psychiatr Neurol* 1994; 7(Suppl.1): 34–38.

101 Albrecht M *et al.* St John's wort extract in the treatment of depression: observations of the use of Jarsin capsules. *Der Kassenarzt* 1994; 41: 45–54.

102 Ernst E *et al.* Adverse effects profile of the herbal antidepressant St John's wort (*Hypericum perforatum* L.). *Eur J Clin Pharmacol* 1998; 54: 589–594.

103 Mueller BM. St John's wort for depressive disorders: results of an outpatient study with the hypericum preparation HYP811. *Adv Ther* 1998; 15: 109–116.

104 Holsboer-Trachsler E *et al.* Efficacy and tolerability of the hypericum special extract LI 160 in young and elderly outpatients with depressive disorders: a drug monitoring study. *Eur Neuropsychopharmacol* 1999; 9(Suppl.5): S226.

105 Von Lemmer W *et al.* Wirksamkeit im Alter und bei chronischen Verlaufsformen. *Münch Med Wschr Fortschr Med* 1999; 43: 475.

106 Stevinson C, Ernst E. Safety of hypericum in patients with depression. A comparison with conventional antidepressants. *CNS Drugs* 1999; 11: 125–132.

107 Benner MH, Lee HJ. *Med Lett* 1979; 21: 29–30.

108 Durán N, Song P-S. Hypericin and its photodynamic action. *Photochem Photobiol* 1986; 43: 677–680.

109 Brockmöller J *et al.* Hypericin and pseudohypericin: pharmacokinetics and effects on photosensitivity in humans. *Pharmacopsychiatry* 1997; 30(Suppl.): 94–101.

110 Schempp C *et al.* Hypericin levels in human serum and interstitial skin blister fluid after oral single-dose and steady-state administration of *Hypericum perforatum* extract (St John's wort). *Skin Pharmacol Appl Skin Physiol* 1999; 12: 299–304.

111 Giese AC. Hypericism. *Photochem Photobiol* 1980; 5: 229–255.

112 Siegers C *et al.* Zur Frage der Phototoxizität von Hypericum. *Nervenheilkunde* 1993; 12: 320–322.

113 Johnston N. Sun trap. *New Sci* 1999; 24 July: 24.

114 Pitisuttithum P *et al.* Int Conf AIDS 1996; 11: 285. Cited by G50.

115 Bove GM. Acute neuropathy after exposure to sun in a patient treated with St John's wort. *Lancet* 1998; 352: 1121–1122.

116 Baillie N. Hypericum – four hypersensitivity reactions. *Modern Phytother* 1997; 3: 24–26.

117 Barbenel DM *et al.* Mania in a patient receiving testosterone replacement post-orchidectomy taking St John's wort and sertraline. *J Psychopharmacol* 2000; 14: 84–86.

118 Nierenberg AA *et al.* Mania associated with St John's wort. *Biol Psychiatr* 1999; 46: 1707–1708.

119 Schneck C. St John's wort and hypomania. *J Clin Psychiatr* 1998; 59: 689.

120 O'Breasil AM, Argouarch S. Hypomania and St John's wort. *Can J Psychiatr* 1998; 43: 746–747.

121 Garrett BJ *et al.* Consumption of poisonous plants (*Senecio jacobaea, Symphytum officinale, Pteridium aquilinum, Hypericum perforatum*) by rats: chronic toxicity, mineral metabolism, and hepatic drug-metabolizing enzymes. *Toxicol Lett* 1982; 10: 183–188.

122 Newall CA *et al. Herbal Medicines. A Guide for Health-care Professionals*, 1st edn. London: The Pharmaceutical Press, 1996.

123 Yue Q-Y *et al.* Safety of St John's wort (*Hypericum perforatum*). *Lancet* 2000; 355: 576–577.

124 Nebel A *et al.* Potential metabolic interaction between St John's wort and theophylline. *Ann Pharmacother* 1999; 33: 502.

125 Rey J, Walter G. *Hypericum perforatum* (St John's wort) in depression: pest or blessing? *Med J Aust* 1998; 169: 583–586.

126 Piscitelli S *et al.* Indinavir concentrations and St John's wort. *Lancet* 2000; 355: 547–548.

127 Ruschitzka F *et al.* Acute heart transplant rejection due to Saint John's wort. *Lancet* 2000; 355: 548–549.

128 Maurer A *et al.* Interaction of St John's wort extract with phenprocoumon (abstract). *Eur J Clin Pharmacol* 1999; 55: A22.

129 Johne A *et al.* Pharmacokinetic interaction of digoxin with an herbal extract from St John's wort (*Hypericum perforatum*). *Clin Pharmacol Ther* 1999; 66: 338–345.

130 Kerb R *et al.* Urinary 6-beta-hydroxycortisol excretion rate is affected by treatment with hypericum extract. *Eur J Clin Pharmacol* 1992; 52: 607.

131 Roby CA *et al.* St John's wort impact on CYP3A4 activity. Poster no. 129 presented at the 39th Annual Meeting of the New Clinical Drug Evaluation Unit Program, June 1999, Florida.

132 Ereshefsky B *et al.* Determination of St John's wort differential metabolism at CYP2D6 and CYP3A4, using dextromethorphan probe methodology. Poster no. 130 presented at the 39th Annual Meeting of the New Clinical Drug Evaluation Unit Program, June 1999, Florida.

133 Gewertz N *et al.* Determination of the differential effects of St John's wort on the CYP1A2 and NAT2 metabolic pathways using caffeine probe methodology. Poster no. 131 presented at the 39th Annual Meeting of the New Clinical Drug Evaluation Unit Program, June 1999, Florida.

134 Markowitz JS *et al.* Effect of St John's wort (*Hypericum perforatum*) on cytochrome P450 2D6 and 3A4 activity in healthy volunteers. *Life*

Sci 2000; **66**(9): 133–139.

135   Gordon JB. SSRIs and St John's wort: possible toxicity? *Am Family Phys* 1998; **57**: 950–953.

136   Lantz MS *et al.* St John's wort and antidepressant drug interactions in the elderly. *J Geriat Psychiatr Neurol* 1999; **12**: 7–10.

137   Breckenridge A. Important interactions between St John's wort (*Hypericum perforatum*) preparations and prescribed medicines. http://www.open.gov.uk

138   Anon. CSM advice on St John's wort. *Pharm J* 2000; **264**: 358.

139   Grush LR *et al.* St John's wort during pregnancy. *JAMA* 1998; **280**(18): 1566.

Stone Root

Species (Family)

Collinsonia canadensis L. (Labiatae)

Synonym(s)

Heal-All, Knob Root

Part(s) Used

Rhizome, root

Pharmacopoeial and Other Monographs

BHP 1983[G7]
PDR for Herbal Medicines 2nd edition[G36]

Legal Category (Licensed Products)

GSL[G37]

Constituents[G40,G48,G49,G64]

Stone root is stated to contain an unidentified alkaloid, mucilage, resin, saponin glycosides, tannins and volatile oil.

Food Use

Stone root is not used in foods.

Herbal Use

Stone root is stated to possess antilithic, litholytic, mild diaphoretic and diuretic properties. Traditionally, it has been used for renal calculus, lithuria, and specifically for urinary calculus.[G7,G64]

Dosage

Dried root 1–4 g or by decoction three times daily.[G7]

Liquid extract 1–4 mL (1 : 1 in 25% alcohol) three times daily.[G7]

Tincture 2–8 mL (1 : 5 in 40% alcohol) three times daily.[G7]

Tincture of Collinsonia (BPC 1934) 2–8 mL.

Pharmacological Actions

None documented.

Side-effects, Toxicity

None documented.

Contra-indications, Warnings

None documented.

Pregnancy and lactation The safety of stone root has not been established. In view of the lack of phytochemical, pharmacological and toxicological information, the use of stone root during pregnancy and lactation should be avoided.

Pharmaceutical Comment

Information available on the chemistry of stone root is limited and no documented scientific evidence was located to justify the herbal uses. In view of the lack of toxicity data, excessive use of stone root should be avoided.

References

See General References G7, G10, G31, G36, G37, G40, G48, G49 and G64.

Tansy

Species (Family)

Tanacetum vulgare L. (Asteraceae/Compositae)

Synonym(s)

Chrysanthemum vulgare (L.) Bernh., Tanacetum

Part(s) Used

Herb

Pharmacopoeial and Other Monographs

BHP 1983[G7]
PDR for Herbal Medicines 2nd edition[G36]

Legal Category (Licensed Products)

Tansy is not included in the GSL.[G37]

Constituents[G22,G51,G64]

Steroids β-Sitosterol (major), campesterol, cholesterol, stigmasterol and taraxasterol.[1]

Terpenoids α-Amyrin (major), β-amyrin, sesquiterpene lactones including arbusculin-A, tanacetin, germacrene D, crispolide;[2,3] tanacetols A and B.[4,5]

Volatile oils 0.12–0.18%. Major components as β-thujone (up to 95%) and camphor, others include α-pinene, borneol, 1,8-cineole, umbellone and sabinene. At least ten different chemotypes have been identified in which camphor was the most frequently occurring main component and thujone second.[4]

Other constituents Gum, mucilage, resin and tannins.

Food Use

Tansy is listed by the Council of Europe as a natural source of food flavouring (Category N3). This category indicates that tansy can be added to foodstuffs in the traditionally accepted manner, although there is insufficient information for an adequate assessment of potential toxicity. In addition, the Council of Europe recommends that the concentration of thujones present in food products is restricted to 0.5 mg/kg.[G16] Tansy oil is prohibited from use as a food flavouring by the Food Additives and Contaminants Committee (FACC) in view of the thujone content.[G44]

In the USA, tansy is prohibited from sale by botanical dealers or by mail order as the dried herb.[G22]

Herbal Use

Tansy is stated to possess anthelmintic, carminative and antispasmodic properties and to act as a stimulant to abdominal viscera. Traditionally, it has been used for nematode infestation, topically for scabies (as a decoction) and pruritus ani (as an ointment), and specifically for roundworm or threadworm infestation in children.[G7]

Dosage

Dried herb 1–2 g or by infusion three times daily.[G7]

Liquid extract 1–2 mL (1:1 in 25% alcohol) three times daily.[G7]

Pharmacological Actions

In vitro and animal studies

In vitro antispasmodic activity on rabbit intestine, and *in vivo* choleretic activity in the dog have been documented for tansy extracts.[6] It was suggested that the choleretic action might be attributable to caffeic acid, a known bile stimulant that is present in tansy.[6] Anthelmintic activity in dogs has been described for tansy oil, an ether extract of the oil, and for β-thujone.[6] Daily intragastric doses of a tansy extract given to rabbits have been found to reduce serum lipid concentrations and inhibit further development of hypercholesterolaemia.[6] In addition, it was noted that recovery of blood sugar concentrations was inhibited in animals given twice daily doses. *In vitro* antifungal activity in 15 pathogenic and non-pathogenic fungi has been reported.[6]

Clinical studies

Aqueous infusions and alcoholic extracts have been reported to be clinically effective bile stimulants in patients with liver and gall bladder disorders.[6] The treatment alleviated pain and increased appetite and digestion.

Side-effects, Toxicity[(G58)]

Tansy oil contains the toxic ketone β-thujone. Symptoms of tansy oil poisoning are attributable to the thujone content and include rapid and weak pulse, severe gastritis, violent spasms and convulsions.[(G22)] Documented fatalities have mainly been associated with ingestion of the oil, although fatal cases of poisoning have occurred with infusions and powders.[(6,7)] An oral LD_{50} value for tansy oil is stated as 1.15 g/kg body weight.[(7)] The ratio of toxic to therapeutic dose has been reported as 2.5:1 and it was noted that all tansy preparations should be administered with castor oil.[(6)] Tansy yields potentially allergenic sesquiterpene lactones which have been implicated in the aetiology of contact dermatitis. Instances of contact dermatitis to tansy have been documented.[(6,G51)]

In vitro and *in vivo* antitumour activity has been documented for tansy.[(6)]

Contra-indications, Warnings

Tansy oil is toxic and should not be used internally or externally.[(G58)] Fatalities have been reported following ingestion of infusions and extracts. Tansy contains allergenic sesquiterpene lactones and may cause an allergic reaction. Tansy has been reported to affect blood sugar concentrations in animals and may interfere with hypoglycaemic therapy.

Pregnancy and lactation Tansy is contra-indicated in pregnancy and lactation. Tansy is reputed to affect the menstrual cycle and uteroactivity has been documented in animal studies. The volatile oil contains β-thujone, a known hepatotoxin.

Pharmaceutical Comment

Pharmacological activities documented for tansy have been associated with the sterol and triterpene constituents. Tansy yields an extremely toxic volatile oil, which should not be used internally or externally.[(G58)] In view of this, the use of tansy as a herbal remedy is not justified even though documented studies have supported the traditional uses of the herb as a choleretic and anthelmintic agent.

References

See also General References G7, G16, G22, G31, G32, G36, G37, G44, G51, G58 and G64.

1 Chandler RF *et al.* Herbal remedies of the Maritime Indians: Sterols and triterpenes of *Tanacetum vulgare* L. (Tansy). *Lipids* 1982; **17**: 102–106.
2 Chandra A *et al.* Germacranolides and an alkyl glucoside from *Tanacetum vulgare*. *Phytochemistry* 1987; **26**: 1463–1465.
3 Appendino G. Crispolide, an unusual hydroperoxysesquiterpene lactone from *Tanacetum vulgare*. *Phytochemistry* 1982; **21**: 1099–1102.
4 Holopainen M *et al.* A study on tansy chemotypes. *Planta Med* 1987; **53**: 284–287.
5 Appendino G *et al.* Tanacetols A and B, non-volatile sesquiterpene alcohols, from *Tanacetum vulgare*. *Phytochemistry* 1983; **22**: 509–512.
6 Opdyke DLJ. Tansy oil. *Food Cosmet Toxicol* 1976; **14**: 869–871.
7 Hardin JW, Arena JM, eds. *Human Poisoning from Native and Cultivated Plants*, 2nd edn. North Carolina: Duke University, 1974: 150–153.

Thyme

Species (Family)

Thymus vulgaris L., *Thymus zygis* L. (Labiatae)

Synonym(s)

Common Thyme, French Thyme, Garden Thyme, Rubbed Thyme

Part(s) Used

Flowering top, leaf

Pharmacopoeial and Other Monographs

BHP 1996[G9]
BP 2001[G15]
Complete German Commission E[G3]
ESCOP 1996[G52]
Martindale 32nd edition[G43]
Mills and Bone[G50]
PDR for Herbal Medicines 2nd edition[G36]
Ph Eur 2002[G28]
WHO volume 1 1999[G63]

Legal Category (Licensed Products)

GSL[G37]

Constituents[G2,G22,G41,G52,G58,G64]

Volatile oils 0.8–2.6%. Pharmacopoeial standard, not less than 1.2%.[G15] Phenols as major components (20–80%) primarily thymol and carvacrol; others include *p*-cymene and γ-terpinene (monoterpenes), linalool, α-terpineol, and thujan-4-ol (alcohols); biphenyl compounds of monoterpene origin.[G52] A detailed analysis of the volatile oil components is given elsewhere.[G22]

Flavonoids Cirsineol, 8-methoxycirsineol, thymonin and eriodictyol.

Other constituents Caffeic acid, oleanolic acid, ursolic acid, rosmarinic acid, resins, saponins and tannins.

Food Use

Thyme is commonly used as a culinary herb, and thyme oil is used in food flavouring. In the USA, thyme is listed as GRAS (Generally Recognised As Safe).[G65]

Herbal Use[G2,G4,G7,G32,G43,G50,G52,G64]

Thyme is stated to possess carminative, antispasmodic, antitussive, expectorant, secretomotor, bactericidal, anthelmintic and astringent properties. Traditionally, it has been used for dyspepsia, chronic gastritis, asthma, diarrhoea in children, enuresis in children, laryngitis, tonsillitis (as a gargle), and specifically for pertussis and bronchitis. The German Commission E approved internal use for treating symptoms of bronchitis, whooping cough and catarrh of the upper respiratory tract.[G3] Thyme is used in various combinations with anise oil, eucalyptus oil, fennel oil, fennel fruit, Iceland moss, lime flower, liquorice root, marshmallow root, primrose root and star anise fruit for catarrh and diseases of the upper respiratory tract.[G3]

Dosage

Dried herb 1–4 g or by infusion three times daily;[G7] 1–2 g.[G3,G52]

Liquid Extract of Thyme (BPC 1949) 0.6–4.0 mL.

Elixir of Thyme (BPC 1949) 4–8 mL.

Tincture 2–6 mL (1 : 5 in 45% alcohol) three times daily,[G7] four drops.[G3,G52]

Pharmacological Actions

In vitro and animal studies

Antitussive, expectorant and antispasmodic actions are considered to be the major pharmacological properties of thyme,[1] and have been associated with the volatile oils (e.g. thymol, carvacrol) and flavonoid constituents. Thyme oil has produced hypotensive and respiratory stimulant effects in rabbits following oral or intramuscular administration, and in cats following intravenous injection;[G41] an increase in rhythmic heart contraction was also observed in rabbits.[G41] Hypotensive activity in rats has been reported for *Thymus orospedanus*; this action was attributed to adrenaline (epinephrine) antagonism.[2]

462

In vitro antispasmodic activity of thyme and related *Thymus* species has been associated with the phenolic components of the volatile oil[3] and with the flavonoid constituents; their mode of action is thought to involve calcium-channel blockage.[1,4,5] The flavonoids thymonin, circilineol and 8-methoxycircilineol have potent spasmolytic activity in guinea pig trachea preparations *in vitro*.[G52]

Analgesic and antipyretic properties in mice have been reported for a thyme extract.[6]

Thymol possesses anthelmintic (especially hookworms), antibacterial, and antifungal properties.[G41] The antibacterial activity of thymol and thyme oil have been reviewed.[G50] Thymol, carvacrol and thyme oil have antifungal activity against a range of organisms.[G50]

Thyme oil inhibits prostaglandin synthesis; rosmarinic acid has anti-inflammatory activity, inhibiting complement in rats and some of the functions of polymorphonucleocytes.[G52] Rosmarinic acid reduced oedema produced by cobra venom factor in rats, and inhibited passive cutaneous anaphylaxis and impairment of *in vivo* activation of mouse macrophages by heat killed *Corynebacterium parvum*.[G52] Activity may relate to complement inactivation.[G50]

Clinical studies

Generally, well-designed clinical studies assessing the effects of thyme are lacking. A randomised, double-blind, controlled trial involving 60 patients with productive cough compared syrup of thyme and bromhexine over a five-day period. Both groups were similar in self-reported symptom relief.[G50]

Thyme oil has been used for the treatment of enuresis in children.[G44]

Side-effects, Toxicity[G58]

Thyme oil is a dermal and mucous membrane irritant.[G58] Toxic symptoms documented for thymol include nausea, vomiting, gastric pain, headache, dizziness, convulsions, coma, and cardiac and respiratory arrest.[G22] Thymol is present in some toothpaste preparations, and has been reported to cause cheilitis and glossitis. Hyperaemia and severe inflammation have been described for thyme oil used in bath preparations.[G51]

A concentrated extract of thyme decreased locomotor activity and caused a slight slowing down of respiration in mice following oral administration of doses of 0.5–3.0 g/kg, equivalent to 4.3–26.0 g dried plant material.[G52] In rats, oral LD_{50} values stated for thyme oil include 2.84 g/kg[G52] and 4.7 g/kg in rats, and >5 g/kg following dermal administration.[7] In mice, oral administration of a concentrated ethanol extract of herb in subacute toxicity tests resulted in increased weights of liver and testes. Also in mice, a dose of 0.9 g daily for three months resulted in mortality rates of 30% and 10% in males and females, respectively. Thyme oil had no mutagenic or DNA-damaging activity in either the Ames test or *Bacillus subtilis* rec-assay.[G52]

Contra-indications, Warnings

Thyme oil is toxic and should be used with considerable caution. It should not be taken internally and only applied externally if diluted in a suitable carrier oil.

Pregnancy and lactation There are no known problems with the use of thyme during pregnancy and lactation, provided that doses do not greatly exceed the amounts used in foods. Traditionally, thyme is reputed to affect the menstrual cycle and, therefore, large amounts should not be ingested.

Pharmaceutical Comment

Thyme is commonly used as a culinary herb and is characterised by its volatile oil. Documented pharmacological actions support some of the traditional medicinal uses, which have been principally attributed to the volatile oil and flavonoid constituents. However, the oil is also toxic and should not be ingested and only applied externally if diluted in a suitable carrier oil. It has been suggested that standardised thyme extracts based on the phenolic volatile components may not be appropriate because antispasmodic actions previously attributed to these compounds may be attributable to other constituents.[3]

References

See also General References G2, G3, G5, G9, G11, G15, G22, G28, G31, G36, G37, G41, G43, G50, G51, G52, G58, G63 and G64.

1 Van Den Broucke CO. The therapeutic value of *Thymus* species. *Fitoterapia* 1983; 4: 171–174.
2 Jimenez J *et al.* Hypotensive activity of *Thymus orospedanus* alcoholic extract. *Phytother Res* 1988; 2: 152–153.
3 Van Den Broucke CO, Lernli JA. Pharmacological and chemical investigation of thyme liquid extracts. *Planta Med* 1981; 41: 129–135.
4 Cruz T *et al.* The spasmolytic activity of the essential oil of *Thymus baeticus* Boiss in rats. *Phytother Res* 1989; 3: 106–108.
5 Blázquez MA *et al.* Effects of *Thymus* species extracts on rat duodenum isolated smooth muscle contraction. *Phytother Res* 1989; 3: 41–42.

6   Mohsin A *et al*. Analgesic, antipyretic activity and phytochemical screening of some plants used in traditional Arab system of medicine. *Fitoterapia* 1989; **60**: 174.

7   Opdyke DLJ. Thyme oil, red. *Food Cosmet Toxicol* 1974; **12**: 1003–1004.

Uva-Ursi

Species (Family)

Arctostaphylos uva-ursi (L.) Spreng (Ericaceae)

Synonym(s)

Bearberry

Part(s) Used

Leaf

Pharmacopoeial and Other Monographs

BHC 1992[G6]
BHP 1996[G9]
BP 2001[G15]
Complete German Commission E[G3]
ESCOP 1997[G52]
Martindale 32nd edition[G43]
Mills and Bone[G50]
PDR for Herbal Medicines 2nd edition[G36]
Ph Eur 2002[G28]

Legal Category (Licensed Products)

GSL[G37]

Constituents[G2,G6,G22,G41,G62,G64]

Flavonoids Flavonols (e.g. myricetin, quercetin) and their glycosides including hyperin, isoquercitrin, myricitrin and quercitrin.

Iridoids Asperuloside (disputed), monotropein.[1]

Quinones Total content at least 6%, mainly arbutin (5–15%) and methyl-arbutin (glycosides), with lesser amounts of piceoside[2] (a glycoside), free hydroquinone and free *p*-methoxyphenol.[3]

Tannins 6–7% (range 6–40%). Hydrolysable-type (e.g. corilagin pyranoside); ellagic and gallic acids (usually associated with hydrolysable tannins).

Terpenoids α-Amyrin, α-amyrin acetate, β-amyrin, lupeol, uvaol, ursolic acid, and a mixture of mono- and di-ketonic α-amyrin derivatives.[4,5]

Other constituents Acids (malic, quinic), allantoin, resin (e.g. ursone), volatile oil (trace) and wax.

Other plant parts The root is reported to contain unedoside (iridoid glucoside).[6]

Food Use

Uva-ursi is not used in foods.

Herbal Use

Uva-ursi is stated to possess diuretic, urinary antiseptic, and astringent properties. Traditionally, it has been used for cystitis, urethritis, dysuria, pyelitis, lithuria, and specifically for acute catarrhal cystitis with dysuria and highly acidic urine.[G2,G6,G7,G8,G64]

Dosage

Dried leaves 1.5–4.0 g or by infusion three times daily.[G6,G7]

Liquid extract 1.5–4.0 mL (1:1 in 25% alcohol) three times daily.[G6,G7]

Concentrated Infusion of Bearberry (BPC 1934) 2–4 mL.

Fresh Infusion of Bearberry (BPC 1934) 15–30 mL.

Pharmacological Actions

In vitro and animal studies

Uva-ursi has exhibited antimicrobial activity towards a variety of organisms including *Staphylococcus aureus*, *Bacillus subtilis*, *Escherichia coli*, *Mycobacterium smegmatis*, *Shigella sonnei* and *Shigella flexneri*.[7] The antimicrobial activity of arbutin towards bacteria implicated in producing urinary tract infections, has been found to be directly dependent on the β-glucosidase activity of the infective organism.[8] Highest enzymatic activity was shown by *Enterobacter*, *Klebsiella* and *Streptococcus* genera, and lowest by *Escherichia coli*.[8] The minimum inhibitory concentration for arbutin is reported to be 0.4–0.8% depending on the micro-organism.[8] Aqueous and methanolic extracts have demonstrated molluscicidal activity against *Biomphalaria glabrata*,

465

at a concentration of 50 ppm.[9] The activity was attributed to the tannin constituents (condensed and hydrolysable).

Anti-inflammatory activity (rat paw oedema tests) has been documented for uva-ursi against a variety of chemical inducers such as carrageenan, histamine and prostaglandins.[10]

Uva-ursi failed to exhibit any *in vitro* uterotonic action when tested on rabbit and guinea-pig uteri.[11]

Hydroquinone has been reported to show a dose-dependent cytotoxic activity on cultured rat hepatoma cells (HTC line); arbutin was not found to inhibit growth of the HTC cells.[12] It was stated that hydroquinone appeared to have greater cytotoxic activity towards rat hepatoma cells than agents like azauridin or colchicine, but less than valtrate from valerian (*Valeriana officinalis*). The cytoxicity of hydroquinone has also been tested on L1210, CA-755 and S-180 tumour systems.[12]

Clinical studies

A herbal preparation, whose ingredients included uva-ursi, hops and peppermint, has been used to treat patients suffering from compulsive strangury, enuresis and painful micturition.[13] Of 915 patients treated for six weeks, success was reported in about 70%. The antiseptic and diuretic properties claimed for uva-ursi can be attributed to the hydroquinone derivatives, especially arbutin. The latter is absorbed from the gastro-intestinal tract virtually unchanged and during renal excretion is hydrolysed to yield the active principle, hydroquinone, which exerts an antiseptic and astringent action on the urinary mucous membranes.[14,15] The crude extract is reported to be more effective than isolated arbutin as an astringent and antiseptic.[G48] This may be due to the other hydroquinone derivatives, in addition to arbutin, that are present in the crude extract and which will also yield hydroquinone. Furthermore, it has been stated that the presence of gallic acid in the crude extract may prevent β-glucosidase cleavage of arbutin in the gastrointestinal tract before absorption, thereby increasing the amount of hydroquinone released during renal excretion.[G48]

Side-effects, Toxicity

No reported side-effects were located. Hydroquinone is reported to be toxic if ingested in large quantities: 1 g (equivalent to 6–20 g plant material) has caused tinnitus, nausea and vomiting, sense of suffocation, shortness of breath, cyanosis, convulsions, delirium and collapse.[G48] A dose of 5 g (equivalent to 30–100 g of plant material) has proved fatal.[G48] In view of the high tannin content, prolonged use of uva-ursi may cause chronic liver impairment.[G41]

Cytotoxic activity has been documented for hydroquinone (*see In vitro* and animal studies).

Uva-ursi herb can sometimes be adulterated with box leaves (*Buxus sempervirens*), which contain toxic steroidal alkaloids. However, no cases of poisoning as a result of such adulteration have been reported.[G33]

Contra-indications, Warnings

Uva-ursi requires an alkaline urine for it to be effective as a urinary antiseptic; an alkaline reaction is needed to yield hydroquinone from the inactive esters such as arbutin.[14] Patients have been advised to avoid eating highly acidic foods, such as acidic fruits and their juices.[14] The presence of hydroquinone may impart a greenish-brown colour to the urine, which darkens following exposure to air due to oxidation of hydroquinone.

Excessive use of uva-ursi should be avoided in view of the high tannin content and potential toxicity of hydroquinone.

Prolonged use of uva-ursi to treat a urinary tract infection is not advisable. Patients in whom symptoms persist for longer than 48 hours should consult their doctor.

Pregnancy and lactation Large doses of uva-ursi are reported to be oxytocic,[G22] although *in vitro* studies have reported a lack of utero-activity. In view of the potential toxicity of hydroquinone, the use of uva-ursi during pregnancy and lactation is best avoided.

Pharmaceutical Comment

The chemistry of uva-ursi is well documented with hydroquinone derivatives, especially arbutin, identified as the major active constituents. Documented pharmacological actions justify the herbal use of uva-ursi as a urinary antiseptic. However, clinical information is lacking and further studies are required to determine the true usefulness of uva-ursi in the treatment of urinary tract infections. Although hydroquinone has been reported to be toxic in large amounts, concentrations provided by the ingestion of therapeutic doses of uva-ursi are not thought to represent a risk to human health.[G42]

References

See also General References G2, G3, G5, G6, G9, G10, G22, G25, G31, G32, G33, G36, G37, G41, G42, G43, G48, G50, G52, G56, G62 and G64.

1 Jahodár L *et al*. Investigation of iridoid substances in *Arctostaphylos uva-ursi*. *Pharmazie* 1978; **33**:

536–537.

2   Karikas GA *et al.* Isolation of piceoside from *Arctostaphylos uva-ursi. Planta Med* 1987; **53**: 307–308.

3   Jahodár L, Leifertová I. The evaluation of *p*-methoxyphenol in the leaves of *Arctostaphylos uva-ursi. Pharmazie* 1979; **34**: 188–189.

4   Droliac A. Triterpenes of *Arctostaphylos uva-ursi* Spreng. *Plant Méd Phytothér* 1980; **14**: 155–158.

5   Malterud KE. The non-polar components of *Arctostaphylos uva-ursi* leaves. *Medd Nor Farm Selsk* 1980; **42**: 15–20.

6   Jahodár L *et al.* Unedoside in *Arctostaphylos uva-ursi* roots. *Pharmazie* 1981; **36**: 294–296.

7   Moskalenko SA. Preliminary screening of far-Eastern ethnomedicinal plants for antibacterial activity. *J Ethnopharmacol* 1986; **15**: 231–259.

8   Jahodár L *et al.* Antimicrobial action of arbutin and the extract from the leaves of *Arctostaphylos uva-ursi in vitro. Ceskoslov Farm* 1985; **34**: 174–178.

9   Schaufelberger D, Hostettmann K. On the molluscicidal activity of tannin containing plants.

Planta Med 1983; **48**: 105–107.

10 Shipochliev T, Fournadjiev G. Spectrum of the antiinflammatory effect of *Arctostaphylos uva ursi* and *Achillea millefolium*, L. *Probl Vutr Med* 1984; **12**: 99–107.

11 Shipochliev T. Extracts from a group of medicinal plants enhancing the uterine tonus. *Vet Med Nauki* 1981; **18**: 94–98.

12 Assaf MH *et al.* Preliminary study of the phenolic glycosides from *Origanum majorana*; quantitative estimation of arbutin; cytotoxic activity of hydroquinone. *Planta Med* 1987; **53**: 343–345.

13 Lenau H *et al.* Wirksamkeit und Verträglichkeit von Cysto Fink bei Patienten mit Reizblase und/ oder Harninkontinenz. *Therapiewoche* 1984; **34**: 6054–6059.

14 Frohne D. Untersuchungen zur Frage der Harndesinfizierenden Wirkungen von Bärentraubenblatt-Extrakten. *Planta Med* 1970; **18**: 23–25.

15 Natural drugs with glycosides. In: Stahl E, ed. *Drug Analysis in Chromatography and Microscopy*. Ann Arbor: Ann Arbor Scientific Publishers, 1973: 97.

Valerian

Species (Family)

Valeriana officinalis L.s.l. (Valerianaceae)

Synonym(s)

All-Heal, Belgian Valerian, Common Valerian, Fragrant Valerian, Garden Valerian

Part(s) Used

Rhizome, root

Pharmacopoeial and Other Monographs

American Herbal Pharmacopoeia[1,G1]
BHC 1992[G6]
BHP 1996[G9]
BP 2001[G15]
Complete German Commission E[G3]
EMEA HMPWG proposed core SPC[G23]
ESCOP 1997[G52]
Martindale 32nd edition[G43]
Mills and Bone[G50]
PDR for Herbal Medicines 2nd edition[G36]
Ph Eur 2002[G28]
WHO volume 1 1999[G63]

Legal Category (Licensed Products)

GSL[G37]

Constituents[1–5,G1,G2,G6,G21,G22,G29,G41,G64]

Alkaloids Pyridine type. Actinidine, chatinine, skyanthine, valerianine and valerine.

Iridoids (valepotriates) Valtrates (e.g. valtrate, valtrate isovaleroxyhydrin, acevaltrate, valechlorine), didrovaltrates (e.g. didrovaltrate, homodidrovaltrate, deoxydidrovaltrate, homodeoxydidrovaltrate, isovaleroxyhydroxydidrovaltrate) and isovaltrates (e.g. isovaltrate, 7-epideacetylisovaltrate). Valtrate and didrovaltrate are documented as the major components. Valerosidate (iridoid glucoside).[6] The valepotriates are unstable and decompose on storage or processing; the main degradation products are baldrinal and homobaldrinal. The baldrinals may react further and are unlikely to be present in finished products.

Volatile oils 0.5–2%. Not less than 3 mL/kg of essential oil for the cut drug, both calculated with reference to the dried drug.[G28]

Numerous identified components include monoterpenes (e.g. α- and β-pinene, camphene, borneol, eugenol, isoeugenol) present mainly as esters, sesquiterpenes (e.g. β-bisabolene, caryophyllene, valeranone, ledol, pacifigorgiol, patchouli alcohol, valerianol, valerenol and a series of valerenyl esters, valerenal, valerenic acid with acetoxy and hydroxy derivatives).[7–10]

Other constituents Amino acids (e.g. arginine, γ-aminobutyric acid (GABA), glutamine, tyrosine),[1,11,G21] caffeic and chlorogenic acids (polyphenolic), β-sitosterol, methyl 2-pyrrolketone, choline, tannins (type unspecified), gum and resin.

As with other plants, there can be variation in the content of active compounds (e.g. valerenic acid derivatives and valepotriates) found in valerian rhizomes and roots.[12]

Food Use

Valerian is not generally used as a food. Valerian is listed by the Council of Europe as a natural source of food flavouring (root: category 5) (*see* Appendix 23).[G17] In the USA, valerian is permitted for use in food.[G65]

Herbal Use

Valerian is stated to possess sedative, mild anodyne, hypnotic, antispasmodic, carminative and hypotensive properties. Traditionally, it has been used for hysterical states, excitability, insomnia, hypochondriasis, migraine, cramp, intestinal colic, rheumatic pains, dysmenorrhoea, and specifically for conditions presenting nervous excitability.[G2,G6,G7,G8,G32,G64] Modern interest in valerian is focused on its use as a sedative and hypnotic.

A core Summary of Product Characteristics (SPC) proposed by the European Medicines Evaluation Agency Herbal Medicinal Product Working Group (EMEA HMPWG) states the following indications: the relief of temporary mild nervous tension and temporary difficulty in falling asleep.[G23]

Dosage

Dried rhizome/root 1–3 g by infusion or decoction up to three times daily.[G6]

Tincture 3–5 mL (1:5; 70% ethanol) up to three times daily;[G6,G50] 1–3 mL, once to several times daily.[G3]

Extracts Amount equivalent to 2–3 g drug, once to several times daily;[G3] 2–6 mL of 1:2 liquid extract daily.[G50]

Doses given in older texts vary. For example: Valerian Liquid Extract (BPC 1963) 0.3–1.0 mL; Simple Tincture of Valerian (BPC 1949) 4–8 mL; Concentrated Valerian Infusion (BPC 1963) 2–4 mL.

Clinical trials investigating the effects of valerian extracts on sleep parameters have used varying dosages, for example, valerian extract 400 mg/day (drug:extract ratio of 3:1)[13] to 1215 mg/day (drug:extract ratio of 5 to 6:1).[14]

Pharmacological Actions

It remains unclear precisely which of the constituents of valerian are responsible for its sedative properties.[5] Attention had focused on the volatile oil, and then the valepotriates and their degradation products, as the constituents responsible. However, it appeared that the effects of the volatile oil could not account for the whole action of the drug, and the valepotriates, which degrade rapidly, are unlikely to be present in finished products in significant concentrations. Current thinking is that the overall effect of valerian is due to several different groups of constituents and their varying mechanisms of action. Therefore, the activity of different valerian preparations will depend on their content and concentrations of several types of constituent.[4] One mechanism of action is likely to involve increased concentrations of the inhibitory transmitter GABA in the brain. Increased concentrations of GABA are associated with a decrease in CNS activity and this action may, therefore, be involved in the reported sedative activity.

In vitro and animal studies

Sedative properties have been documented for valerian and have been attributed to both the volatile oil and valepotriate fractions.[15,16] Screening of the volatile oil components for sedative activity concluded valerenal and valerenic acid to be the most active compounds, causing ataxia in mice at a dose of 50 mg/kg by intraperitoneal injection.[15] Further studies in mice described valerenic acid as a general CNS depressant similar to pentobarbitone, requiring high doses (100 mg/kg by intraperitoneal injection)

for activity.[17] A dose of 400 mg/kg resulted in muscle spasms, convulsions and death.[17] Valerenic acid was also reported to prolong pentobarbitone-induced sleep in mice, resulting in a hangover effect. Biochemical studies have documented that valerenic acid inhibits the enzyme system responsible for the central catabolism of GABA.[18] An aqueous extract of roots and rhizomes of *V. officinalis* (standardised to 55 mg valerenic acids per 100 g extract) inhibited the uptake and stimulated the release of radiolabelled GABA in isolated synaptosomes from rat brain cortex.[19,20] Further work suggested that this aqueous extract of valerian induces the release of GABA by reversal of the GABA carrier, and that the mechanism is Na^+ dependent and Ca^{2+} independent.[20] The extract contained a high concentration of GABA (about 5 mmol/L) which was shown to be sufficient to induce the release of radiolabelled GABA by this type of mechanism.[21] Aqueous and hydroalcoholic (ethanol) extracts of valerian root displaced radiolabelled muscimol binding to synaptic membranes (a measure of the influence of drugs on $GABA_A$ receptors). However, valerenic acid (0.1 mmol/L) did not displace radiolabelled muscimol in this model.[22] Other *in vitro* studies using rat brain tissue have shown that hydroalcoholic and aqueous total extracts of *V. officinalis* root, and an aqueous fraction derived from the hydroalcoholic extract, show affinity for $GABA_A$ receptors, although far lower than that of the neurotransmitter itself.[23] However, a lipophilic fraction of the hydroalcoholic extract, hydroxyvalerenic acid and dihydrovaltrate did not show any affinity for the $GABA_A$ receptor in this model.

The effects of valerian extracts on benzodiazepine binding to rat cortical membranes have also been explored. Very low concentrations of ethanolic extract of *V. officinalis* had no effect on radiolabelled flunitrazepam binding in this model, although concentrations of 10^{-10} to 10^{-8} mg/mL increased radiolabelled flunitrazepam binding with an EC_{50} of 4.13×10^{-10} mg/mL.[24] However, flunitrazepam binding was inhibited at higher concentrations (0.5–7.0 mg/mL) of valerian extract (IC_{50} 4.82×10^{-1} mg/mL). In other investigations, valerian extract potentiated radiolabelled GABA release from rat hippocampal slices, and inhibited synaptosomal GABA uptake, confirming the effects of valerian extract on $GABA_A$ receptors.[24]

CNS-depressant activities in mice following intraperitoneal injection have been documented for the valepotriates and for their degradation products, although activity was found to be greatly reduced following oral administration.[25] A study explored the effects of a mixture of valepotriates on the behaviour of diazepam-withdrawn male Wistar rats in the elevated plus-maze test (a measure of the anxiolytic or anxiogenic properties of drugs).[26] Rats were given diazepam (up to 5 mg/kg for 28 days) then vehicle only for three days to induce a withdrawal syndrome. Rats given diazepam or a mixture of valepotriates (dihyritoneally (12 mg/kg) spent a significantly greater proportion of time in the 'open' arms of the maze than did those in the control group.

Another specific valepotriate fraction, Vpt$_2$, has been documented to exhibit tranquillising, central myorelaxant, anticonvulsant, coronaro-dilating and anti-arrhythmic actions in mice, rabbits, and cats.[27,28] The fraction was reported to prevent arrhythmias induced by Pituitrin vasopressin and barium chloride, and to exhibit moderate positive inotropic and negative chronotropic effects.

Antispasmodic activity on intact and isolated guinea-pig ileum has been documented for isovaltrate, valtrate and valeranone.[29] This activity was attributed to a direct action on the smooth muscle receptors rather than ganglion receptors. Valerian oil has been reported to exhibit antispasmodic activity on isolated guinea-pig uterine muscle,[30] but proved inactive when tested *in vivo*.[31]

In vitro inactivation of complement activation has been reported for the valepotriates.[32]

In vitro cytotoxicity (inhibition of DNA and protein synthesis, and potent alkylating activity) has been documented for the valepotriates, with valtrate stated to be the most toxic compound.[33] Valepotriates (valtrate and didrovaltrate) isolated from the related species *Valeriana wallichii*, and baldrinal (a degradation product of valtrate) have been tested for their cytotoxic activity *in vitro* using cultured rat hepatoma cells. Valtrate was the most active compound in this system, leading to a 100% mortality of hepatoma cells after 24 hours' incubation at a concentration of 33 μg/mL.[34] More detailed studies using the same system showed that didrovaltrate demonstrated cytotoxic activity when incubated at concentrations higher than 8 μg/mL of culture (1.5×10^{-5} mol/L) and led to 100% cellular mortality with 24 hours of incubation at a concentration of 66 μg/mL. The cytotoxic effect of didrovaltrate was irreversible within 2 hours of incubation with hepatoma cells. In mice, administration of intraperitoneal didrovaltrate led to a regression of Krebs II ascitic tumours, compared with control.[34] A subsequent *in vivo* study, in which valtrate was administered to mice (by intraperitoneal injection and by mouth), did not report any toxic effects on haematopoietic precursor cells when compared with control groups.[35] The valepotriates are known to be unstable compounds in both acidic and alkaline media and it has been suggested that their *in vivo* toxicity is limited due to poor absorption and/or distribution.[2] Baldrinal and homobaldrinal, decomposition products of valtrate and isovaltrate respectively, have exhibited direct mutagenic activity against various *Salmonella* strains *in vitro*.[36]

Clinical studies

Numerous studies have explored the effects of valerian preparations on subjective and/or objective sleep parameters.[13,14,37–45] Collectively, the findings of these studies are difficult to interpret, as different studies have assessed different valerian preparations and different dosages, and some have involved healthy volunteers whereas others have involved patients with diagnosed sleep disorders. In addition, other studies have used different subjective and/or objective outcome measures, and some have been conducted in sleep laboratories, whereas others have assessed participants receiving valerian whilst sleeping at home. Overall, several, but not all, studies have documented a hypnotic effect for valerian preparations with regard to subjective measures of sleep quality, and some have documented effects on objective measures of sleep structure. There is a view that subjective measures of sleep quality may be the most appropriate assessment.[45]

A systematic review of randomised, double-blind, placebo-controlled trials of valerian preparations included nine studies.[46] The review concluded that the evidence for valerian as a treatment for insomnia is inconclusive and that there is a need for further rigorous trials. Several of the studies included in the review, and other studies, are discussed in more detail below.

A placebo-controlled study involving 128 volunteers explored the effects of an aqueous extract of valerian root (400 mg) and a proprietary preparation of valerian and hops (Hova) on subjective measures of sleep quality. Each participant took each of the three preparations at night for three non-consecutive nights.[13] On the basis of participants' self-assessment, valerian significantly reduced sleep latency (time to onset of sleep) and improved sleep quality, compared with placebo ($p < 0.05$). Subgroup analysis suggested that the effects of valerian were most marked among participants who described themselves as 'poor' or 'irregular' sleepers.[13] It was reported that Hova did not significantly affect sleep latency or sleep quality, compared with placebo, only that Hova administration was associated with an increase in the number of reports of 'feeling more sleepy than usual the next morning' (i.e. a 'hangover' effect). The authors were unable to explain this discrepancy in the results for the two preparations.

In a subsequent study, eight volunteers with mild insomnia each received aqueous valerian extract

450 mg, 900 mg or placebo, in a random-order experimental design over almost three weeks.[37] The time to the first period of 5 consecutive minutes without movement, measured using wrist-worn activity meters, was used as an objective measure of sleep latency. For this parameter, valerian 450 mg significantly reduced the mean sleep latency, compared with placebo, although there was no further reduction in sleep latency with valerian 900 mg. Subjective assessments indicated that participants were more likely to experience a 'hangover' effect with valerian 900 mg.[37]

The same dosages of aqueous valerian extract were tested for their effects on sleep latency and wake time after sleep onset in healthy volunteers who were either sleeping at home or in a sleep laboratory.[38] Each participant sleeping at home took valerian 450 mg, 900 mg, or placebo, for two consecutive nights on a double-blind, crossover schedule. Participants sleeping under laboratory conditions were randomly assigned to receive valerian 900 mg on the second or third night of the four nights of the study; placebo was taken on the other nights. Under home conditions, valerian 450 mg and 900 mg significantly reduced subjectively measured sleep latency, compared with placebo. Under laboratory conditions, there were no statistically significant differences between valerian 900 mg and placebo on subjective or objective sleep parameters. It was suggested that the 'more stressful' sleep environment of the laboratory may have masked the hypnotic effects of valerian.[38]

A randomised, double-blind, placebo-controlled, crossover study involving 16 patients with previously established psychophysiological insomnia according to International Classification of Sleep Disorders (ICSD) criteria and confirmed by polysomnography assessed the effects of single-dose and longer term administration of valerian root extract on objective parameters of sleep structure and subjective parameters of sleep quality.[39] Participants received valerian root extract (Sedonium; drug : extract ratio 5 : 1) 600 mg, or placebo, 1 hour before bedtime for 14 days, followed by a wash-out period of 13 days, before crossing over to the other arm of the study. There were no statistically significant effects on objective and subjective parameters of sleep following single-dose valerian administration. After long-term treatment, sleep efficiency (ratio of time spent asleep to time spent in bed) improved in both the valerian and placebo groups, compared with baseline values, although there were no significant differences between groups. There was a statistically significant difference with valerian on parameters of slow-wave

sleep, compared with baseline values, which did not occur with placebo. However, it is not clear if this difference was significantly different for valerian, compared with placebo, as no *p*-value was given.

In a randomised, double-blind, pilot study, 14 elderly women who were poor sleepers received valerian aqueous extract (Valdispert forte; drug : extract ratio 5 to 6 : 1), or placebo, for eight consecutive days.[14] Valerian 405 mg was administered one hour before sleep for one night in the laboratory, then taken three times daily for the following seven days. There was no difference in sleep parameters between valerian extract and placebo after acute administration. Valerian recipients showed an increase in slow-wave sleep, compared with baseline values. However, valerian had no effect on sleep onset time, rapid eye movement (REM) sleep or on self-rated sleep quality.

Aqueous ethanolic valerian extract (Sedonium) was compared with placebo in a randomised, double-blind trial involving 121 patients with insomnia not due to organic causes.[40] Participants received valerian extract, or placebo, 600 mg one hour before bedtime for 28 days. At the end of the study, valerian extract achieved a significantly higher clinical global impression score than did placebo. Sleep quality improved in both groups, compared with baseline values.

The effects of valerian extracts on sleep parameters have been compared with those of the benzodiazepine oxazepam.[41] This randomised, double-blind trial involving people with non-organic and non-psychiatric insomnia compared valerian root extract 600 mg with oxazepam 10 mg; treatment was taken 30 minutes before going to bed for 28 days. At the end of the treatment period, sleep quality had improved significantly ($p < 0.001$) in both groups, compared with baseline values. There was no difference between the two groups with regard to sleep quality.

An open, uncontrolled, multicentre study assessed the effects of a valerian extract (Baldrian-Dispert) 45 mg daily in 11 168 patients with sleep disorders. Valerian was rated as 'good' or 'very good' in 72% of cases of sleep disturbances, 76% of cases of discontinuous sleep, and in 72% of cases of restlessness and tension.[42]

Several other studies have assessed the effects of valerian extract in combination with other herb extracts, such as hops (*Humulus lupulus*) and/or melissa (*Melissa officinalis*), on measures of sleep.[47–50] A randomised, double-blind trial involving healthy volunteers who received Songha Night (*V. officinalis* root extract 120 mg and *M. officinalis* leaf extract 80 mg) three tablets daily taken as one dose 30 minutes before bedtime for 30 days ($n = 66$), or placebo ($n = 32$), found that the proportion of participants reporting an improvement in sleep quality was significantly greater for the treatment group, compared with the placebo group (33.3% versus 9.4%, respectively; $p = 0.04$).[48] However, analysis of visual analogue scale scores revealed only a slight, but statistically non-significant, improvement in sleep quality in both groups over the treatment period. Another double-blind, placebo-controlled trial involving patients with insomnia who received Euvegal forte (valerian extract 160 mg and lemon balm extract 80 mg) two tablets daily for two weeks reported significant improvements in sleep quality in recipients of the herbal preparation, compared with placebo recipients.[49] A placebo-controlled study involving 'poor sleepers' who received Euvegal forte reported significant improvements in sleep efficiency and in sleep stages 3 and 4 in the treatment group, compared with placebo recipients.[50]

Some studies assessing combination valerian preparations have compared the effects with those of benzodiazepines.[51,52] A three-week, randomised, double-blind trial reported that a combination of valerian and hops (200 mg and 45.5 mg dry extract, respectively) was equivalent to bromazepam 3 mg with regard to sleep quality in patients with 'environmental' sleep disorders (temporary dyscoimesis and dysphylaxia) according to Diagnostic and Statistical Manual (DSM)-IV criteria.[51] A study assessing the 'hangover' effects of valerian preparations (valerian syrup and valerian–hops tablets) (see Side-effects, Toxicity) reported that subjective measures of sleep quality improved in both valerian groups, compared with placebo.[52]

In an open, uncontrolled, multicentre study, 225 individuals who were experiencing nervous agitation and/or difficulties falling asleep and achieving uninterrupted sleep were treated for two weeks with a combination preparation containing extracts of valerian root, hop grains and lemon balm leaves.[53] Significant improvements in the severity and frequency of symptoms were reported, compared with the pretreatment period. Difficulties falling asleep, difficulties sleeping through the night, and nervous agitation were improved in 89, 80 and 82% of participants, respectively.

In a single-blind, placebo-controlled, crossover study involving 12 healthy volunteers, two different single doses of valerian-hops (valerian 500 mg, hops 120 mg; valerian 1500 mg, hops 360 mg) were assessed for their effects on EEG recordings.[54] Some slight effects on the quantitative EEG were documented following administration of higher

dose valerian–hops, indicating effects on the central nervous system.

The effects of valerian extract 100 mg (no further details of preparation given) on activation and performance of 48 healthy volunteers under experimental social stress conditions have been assessed, with or without propranolol 20 mg, in a randomised double-blind, placebo-controlled study.[55] Valerian was reported to have no influence on physiological activation and to lead to less intensive subjective feelings of somatic arousal. The effects of a hydroalcoholic extract of valerian have been assessed in a randomised study involving 40 patients with minor symptoms of anxiety and emotional tension.[56] Participants received valerian extract 100 mg three times daily, or placebo, for 21 days. It was reported that valerian was superior to placebo.

Several other studies have assessed the effects of combinations of valerian and St. John's wort (*Hypericum perforatum*) in patients with anxiety or depression.[57–59] In a randomised, double-blind study involving 100 patients with anxiety, a combination of valerian and St. John's wort was reported to be significantly more effective than diazepam according to a physician's rating scale and a patient's self-rating scale.[57] In a randomised, double-blind trial involving 162 patients with dysthymic disorders, the effects of a valerian and St. John's wort combination (Sedariston) were compared with those of amitriptyline 75–150 mg.[58] Another randomised, double-blind trial, involving 100 patients with mild-to-moderate depression compared Sedariston with desipramine 100–150 mg.[59] Pooling the results of these two studies indicated there were 88 (68%) treatment responders in the Sedariston group and 66 (50%) in the group that received standard antidepressants.[60] This difference was not statistically significant.

Several studies have assessed the effects of valerian, or herbal combination products containing valerian, on performance the morning after treatment (see Side-effects, Toxicity).[52,61]

Side-effects, Toxicity

Data relating to the safety of valerian have been reviewed.[G21]

Studies assessing the effects of valerian on measures of performance suggest that there may be slight impairment for a few hours following valerian ingestion. However, studies have shown that 'hangover' effects (impairment of performance the morning following valerian treatment) do not appear to be a concern.

In a randomised, double-blind trial involving 102 healthy volunteers, the effects of single-dose valerian extract (Sedonium) 600 mg on reaction time, alertness and concentration were compared with those of flunitrazepam 1 mg and placebo.[61] The treatment was administered in the evening and psychometric tests were carried out the next morning. After a one-week wash-out period, 91 volunteers continued with the second phase of the study, which comprised 14 days' administration of valerian extract 600 mg or placebo. Single-dose valerian extract administration did not impair reaction time, concentration or co-ordination. A 'hangover' effect was reported by 59% of flunitrazepam recipients, compared with 32% and 30% of placebo and valerian recipients, respectively ($p < 0.05$). At the end of the 14-day study, there was no statistically significant difference ($p = 0.45$) between valerian extract and placebo on mean reaction time (a measure of performance), and valerian recipients showed a trend towards improved sleep quality.

A randomised, double-blind study involving 80 volunteers assessed the 'hangover' effects of tablets containing valerian and hops, and a syrup containing valerian only, given as a single dose, against both placebo and active control (flunitrazepam 1 mg).[52] Performance the morning after treatment, measured both objectively and subjectively, was reported to be impaired only in the flunitrazepam group. Side effects occurred more frequently in the flunitrazepam group (50%), compared with the valerian and placebo groups (10%). A further battery of cognitive psychomotor tests was carried out in another study involving 36 volunteers who received either valerian syrup, valerian–hops tablets, or placebo; tests were conducted 1–2 hours after drug administration to assess acute effects. Compared with placebo, there was a slight, but statistically significant, impairment in vigilance with valerian syrup and impairment in the processing of complex information with valerian–hops tablets.[52]

Few controlled clinical trials of valerian preparations have provided detailed information on safety. Where adverse event data were provided, randomised, placebo-controlled trials involving healthy volunteers or patients with diagnosed insomnia reported that adverse events with valerian were mild and transient, and that the types and frequency of adverse events reported for valerian were similar to those for placebo.[46,61] One study involving small numbers of patients reported a lower frequency of adverse events with valerian than with placebo; the authors did not suggest an explanation for this.[39] Studies comparing valerian preparations with benzodiazepines have reported that valerian root extract (LI-156) 600 mg daily for 14 days[61] or 28 days[41] had a more favourable adverse effect profile than flunitrazepam

1 mg daily for 14 days[61] and oxazepam 10 mg daily for 28 days,[41] respectively.

There is an isolated report of cardiac complications and delirium associated with valerian root extract withdrawal in a 58-year-old man with a history of coronary artery disease, hypertension and congestive heart failure.[62] The man had been taking valerian root extract (530 mg to 2 g, five times daily). It was hypothesised that given the effects of valerian on GABA, withdrawal of valerian root might produce a benzodiazepine-like withdrawal syndrome. However, the man was taking multiple medications and had undergone surgery, and a causal link with valerian could not be made. There have also been isolated reports of hepatotoxic reactions following the use of combination products containing valerian, although these products contained other herbal ingredients, such as scullcap and chaparral, which could have been responsible.[63,G18,G21] Several other reports document hepatotoxic reactions with single-ingredient valerian products, although it is possible that these were idiosyncratic reactions.[64] There is a lack of data on the safety of the long-term use of valerian, and such studies are required.[G21]

Cases of individuals who had taken overdoses of valerian or valerian-containing products have been documented. One case involved an 18-year-old female who ingested 40–50 capsules of powdered valerian root 470 mg, approximately 20 times therapeutic doses.[65] The patient presented 3 hours after ingestion with fatigue, crampy abdominal pain, chest tightness, tremor and lightheadedness. Liver function tests were normal; a urine screen tested positive for tetrahydrocannabinol. The patient was treated with activated charcoal, and symptoms resolved within 24 hours. Several cases ($n = 47$) have been documented of overdose with a combination valerian-containing product ('Sleep-Qik'; valerian dry extract 75 mg, hyoscine hydrobromide 0.25 mg, cyproheptadine hydrochloride 2 mg).[66,67] Individuals had ingested tablets equivalent to 0.5–12 g valerian. Liver function tests were carried out for most patients, all of which were normal.

Toxicological studies documented in the older literature have reported an LD_{50} of 3.3 mg/kg for an ethanolic extract of valerian administered intraperitoneally in rats, and that daily doses of 400–600 mg/kg, administered intraperitoneally for 45 days, did not lead to any changes in weight, blood or urine measurements, compared with controls.[1] Literature cited in a review of the safety of valerian describes an LD_{50} of 64 mg/kg for valtrate, 125 mg/kg for didrovaltrate and 150 mg/kg for acevaltrate in mice after intraperitoneal injection.[G21] Another study in mice reported that valerenic acid 150 mg/kg, given by intraperitoneal injection, caused muscle spasms and that 400 mg/kg caused heavy convulsions.[17] The latter dose was lethal to six of seven mice.

In vitro cytotoxicity and mutagenicity have been documented for the valepotriates. The clinical significance of this is unclear, since the valepotriates are known to be highly unstable and, therefore, probably degrade when taken orally. Also, they are unlikely to be present in high concentrations in finished products. The volatile oil is unlikely to present any hazard in aromatherapy.[G58]

The EMEA HMPWG proposed core SPC states that the total exposure to valepotriates should not exceed the maximum exposure with herbal tea.[G23] Alkylating and cytotoxic properties of valepotriates are not relevant for finished products as valepotriates decompose rapidly and only traces of valepotriates or their degradation products (in part, baldrinals) are found.

Contra-indications, Warnings

The documented CNS-depressant activity of valerian may potentiate existing sedative therapy.

According to the EMEA HMPWG proposed core SPC, patients should seek medical advice if symptoms persist for more than two weeks, or worsen. Intake of valerian preparations immediately (up to 2 hours) before driving a car or operating machinery is not recommended. The effect of valerian preparations may be enhanced by consumption of alcohol.[G23]

Pregnancy and lactation The safety of valerian during pregnancy and lactation has not been established and should, therefore, be avoided.[68]

A study in rats involved the administration of valepotriates (6, 12 and 24 mg/kg administered orally) during pregnancy up to the 19th day when animals were sacrificed.[69] There were no differences between valepotriate-treated rats and control rats as determined by fetotoxicity and external examination studies, although the two highest doses of valepotriates were associated with an increase in retarded ossification evident on internal examination.

The EMEA HMPWG proposed core SPC states that as data on the use of valerian during pregnancy are not available, use is not recommended as a general precaution. No adverse effects have been reported from the common use of valerian root as a medicinal product, but experimental data are lacking.[G23]

Pharmaceutical Comment

The traditional use of valerian as a mild sedative and hypnotic has been supported by actions documented in studies involving both animals and humans.[G62]

The sedative activity of valerian has been attributed to both the volatile oil and iridoid valepotriate fractions, but it is still unclear whether other constituents in valerian represent the active components. The valepotriate compounds are highly unstable and, therefore, are unlikely to be present in significant concentrations in finished products and probably degrade when taken orally. In view of this, the clinical significance of both the sedative and cytotoxic/mutagenic activities of valepotriates documented *in vitro* is unclear.

The acute toxicity of valerian is considered to be very low.[G21] There are isolated reports of adverse effects, mainly hepatotoxic reactions, associated with the use of single-ingredient and combination valerian-containing products. However, causal relationships for these reports could not be established as the cases involved other factors which could have been responsible for the observed effects. Some studies have compared valerian with certain benzodiazepines; the data available appear to suggest that valerian may have a more favourable tolerability profile, particularly in view of its apparent lack of 'hangover' effects. The safety of valerian in comparison with benzodiazepines requires further investigation and documentation.

References

See also General References G2, G3, G5, G6, G9, G15, G18, G21, G22, G28, G31, G32, G36, G41, G43, G50, G52, G56, G58, G63 and G64.

1 Upton R, ed. *American Herbal Pharmacopoeia and Therapeutic Compendium. Valerian root. Valeriana officinalis. Analytical, Quality Control, and Therapeutic Monograph*. Santa Cruz: American Herbal Pharmacopoeia, 1999.

2 Houghton PJ. The biological activity of valerian and related plants. *J Ethnopharmacol* 1988; **22**: 121–142.

3 Morazzoni P, Bombardelli E. *Valeriana officinalis*: traditional use and recent evaluation of activity. *Fitoterapia* 1995; 66: 99–112.

4 Houghton P. The scientific basis for the reputed activity of valerian. *J Pharm Pharmacol* 1999; **51**: 505–512.

5 Houghton PJ, ed. *Valerian. The genus Valeriana*. Amsterdam: Harwood Academic Publishers, 1997.

6 Inouye H *et al*. The absolute configuration of valerosidate and of didovaltrate. *Tetrahedron Lett* 1974; **30**: 2317–2325.

7 Bos R *et al*. Isolation and identification of valerenane sesquiterpenoids from *Valeriana officinalis*. *Phytochemistry* 1986; 25: 133–135.

8 Bos R *et al*. Isolation of the sesquiterpene alcohol (−)-pacifigorgiol from *Valeriana officinalis*.

Phytochemistry 1986; **25**: 1234–1235.

9 Stoll A *et al.* New investigations on Valerian. *Schweiz Apotheker-Zeitung* 1957; **95**: 115–120.

10 Hendricks H *et al.* Eugenyl isovalerate and iso-eugenyl isovalerate in the essential oil of Valerian root. *Phytochemistry* 1977; **16**: 1853–1854.

11 Lapke C *et al.* Free amino acids in commercial preparations of *Valeriana officinalis* L. *Pharm Pharmacol Lett* 1997; **4**: 172–174.

12 Gao XQ, Björk L. Valerenic acid derivatives and valepotriates among individuals, varieties and species of *Valeriana. Fitoterapia* 2000; **71**: 19–24.

13 Leathwood PD *et al.* Aqueous extract of valerian root improves sleep quality in man. *Pharmacol Biochem Behav* 1982; **17**: 65–71.

14 Schulz H *et al.* The effect of valerian extract on sleep polygraphy in poor sleepers: a pilot study. *Pharmacopsychiatry* 1994; **27**: 147–151.

15 Hendricks H *et al.* Pharmacological screening of valerenal and some other components of essential oil of *Valeriana officinalis. Planta Med* 1981; **42**: 62–68.

16 Wagner H *et al.* Comparative studies on the sedative action of *Valeriana* extracts, valepotriates and their degradation products. *Planta Med* 1980; **39**: 358–365.

17 Hendriks H *et al.* Central nervous depressant activity of valerenic acid in the mouse. *Planta Med* 1985; **51**: 28–31.

18 Riedel E *et al.* Inhibition of γ-aminobutyric acid catabolism by valerenic acid derivatives. *Planta Med* 1982; **48**: 219–220.

19 Santos MS *et al.* The amount of GABA present in aqueous extracts of valerian is sufficient to account for [^{3}H]GABA release in synaptosomes. *Planta Med* 1994; **60**: 475–476.

20 Santos MS *et al.* Synaptosomal GABA release as influenced by valerian root extract – involvement of the GABA carrier. *Arch Int Pharmacodyn* 1994; **327**: 220–231.

21 Santos MS *et al.* An aqueous extract of valerian influences the transport of GABA in synaptosomes. *Planta Med* 1994; **60**: 278–279.

22 Cavadas C *et al. In vitro* study on the interaction of *Valeriana officinalis* L. extracts and their amino acids on GABA$_A$ receptor in rat brain. *Arzneimittelforschung/Drug Res* 1995; **45**: 753–755.

23 Mennini T *et al. In vitro* study on the interaction of extracts and pure compounds from *Valeriana officinalis* roots with GABA, benzodiazepine and barbiturate receptors in the brain. *Fitoterapia* 1993; **64**: 291–300.

24 Ortiz JG *et al.* Effects of *Valeriana officinalis* extracts on [^{3}H]flunitrazepam binding, synaptosomal [^{3}H]GABA uptake, and hippocampal [^{3}H]GABA release. *Neurochem Res* 1999; **24**: 1373–1378.

25 Veith J *et al.* The influence of some degradation products of valepotriates on the motor activity of light-dark synchronized mice. *Planta Med* 1986; **52**: 179–183.

26 Andreatini R, Leite JR. Effect of valepotriates on the behavior of rats in the elevated plus-maze during diazepam withdrawal. *Eur J Pharmacol* 1994; **260**: 233–235.

27 Petkov V. Plants with hypotensive, antiatheromatous and coronarodilating action. *Am J Chin Med* 1979; **7**: 197–236.

28 Petkov V, Manolav P. To the pharmacology of iridoids. Paper presented at the 2nd Congress of the Bulgarian Society for Physiological Sciences, Sofia, October 31–November 3, 1974.

29 Hazelhoff B *et al.* Antispasmodic effects of *Valeriana* compounds: an *in vivo* and *in vitro* study on the guinea-pig ileum. *Arch Int Pharmacodyn* 1982; **257**: 274–287.

30 Pilcher JD *et al.* The action of so-called female remedies on the excised uterus of the guinea-pig. *Arch Intern Med* 1916; **18**: 557–583.

31 Pilcher JD, Mauer RT. The action of female remedies on the intact uteri of animals. *Surg Gynecol Obstet* 1918; 97–99.

32 Van Meer JH. Plantaardige stoffen met een effect op het complementsysteem. *Pharm Weekbl* 1984; **119**: 836–942.

33 Bounthanh C *et al.* The action of valepotriates on the synthesis of DNA and proteins of cultured hepatoma cells. *Planta Med* 1983; **49**: 138–142.

34 Bounthanh C *et al.* Valepotriates, a new class of cytotoxic and antitumour agents. *Planta Med* 1981; **41**: 21–28.

35 Braun R *et al.* Influence of valtrate/isovaltrate on the hematopoiesis and metabolic liver activity in mice *in vivo. Planta Med* 1984; **50**: 1–4.

36 Hude W *et al.* Bacterial mutagenicity of the tranquillizing constituents of Valerianaceae roots. *Mutat Res* 1986; **169**: 23–27.

37 Leathwood PD, Chauffard F. Aqueous extract of valerian reduces latency to fall asleep in man. *Planta Med* 1985; **51**: 144–148.

38 Balderer G, Borbely AA. Effect of valerian on human sleep. *Psychopharmacology* 1985; **87**: 406–409.

39 Donath F *et al.* Critical evaluation of the effect of valerian extract on sleep structure and sleep quality. *Pharmacopsychiatry* 2000; **33**: 47–53.

40 Vorbach EU *et al.* Therapie von Insomnien. Wirksamkeit und Verträglichkeit eines Baldrianpräparats. *Psychopharmakotherapie* 1996; **3**: 109–115.

41 Dorn M. (Baldrian versus oxazepam: efficacy and tolerability in non-organic and non-psychiatric insomniacs. A randomised, double-blind, clinical, comparative study). *Forsch Komplement Klass*

Naturheilkd 2000; **7**: 79–84.

42 Schmidt-Voigt J. Treatment of nervous sleep disorders and unrest with a sedative of purely vegetable origin. *Therapiewoche* 1986; **36**: 663–667.

43 Gessner B *et al.* Untersuchung über die Langzeitwirkung von Harmonicum Much® auf den Schlaf von schlafgestörten Personen. *Therapiewoche* 1983; **33**: 5547–5558.

44 Lindhal O, Lindwall L. Double blind study of a valerian preparation. *Pharmacol Biochem Behav* 1989; **32**: 1065–1066.

45 Leathwood PD, Chauffard F. Quantifying the effects of mild sedatives. *J Psychiatr Res* 1983; **17**: 115–122.

46 Stevinson C, Ernst E. Valerian for insomnia: a systematic review of randomized clinical trials. *Sleep Med* 2000; **1**: 91–99.

47 Muller-Limmroth W, Ehrenstein W. Untersuchungen über die Wirkung von Seda-Kneipp auf den Schlaf schlafgestörter Menschen. *Med Klin* 1977; **72**: 1119–1125.

48 Cerny A, Schmid K. Tolerability and efficacy of valerian/lemon balm in healthy volunteers (a double-blind, placebo-controlled, multicentre study). *Fitoterapia* 1999; **70**: 221–228.

49 Dressing H *et al.* Verbesserung der Schlafqualität mit einem hochdosierten Baldrian-Melisse-Präparat. Eine plazebokontrollierte Doppelblindstudie. *Psychopharmakotherapie* 1996; **3**: 123–130.

50 Dressing H *et al.* Baldrian-Melisse-Kombinationen versus Benzodiazepin. Bei Schlafstörungen gleichwertig? *Therapiewoche* 1992; **42**: 726–736.

51 Schmitz M, Jäckel M. (Comparative study investigating the quality of life in patients with environmental sleep disorders (temporary dyscoimesis and dysphylaxia) under therapy with a hop-valerian preparation and a benzodiazepine preparation.) *Wiener Med Wochenschrift* 1998; **148**: 291–298.

52 Gerhard U *et al.* (Effects of two plant-based sleep remedies on vigilance). *Schweiz Runsch Med Prax* 1996; **85**: 473–481.

53 Orth-Wagner S *et al.* Phytosedativum gegen Schlafstörungen. *Z Phytother* 1995; **16**: 147–156.

54 Vonderheid-Guth B *et al.* Pharmacodynamic effects of valerian and hops extract combination (ZE-91019) on the quantitative-topographical EEG in healthy volunteers. *Eur J Med Res* 2000; **5**: 139–144.

55 Kohnen R, Oswald W-D. The effects of valerian, propranolol, and their combination on activation, performance, and mood of healthy volunteers under social stress conditions. *Pharmacopsychiatry* 1988; **21**: 447–448.

56 Delsignore R *et al.* (Placebo-controlled trial of a stabilized valerian extract). *Settimana Med* 1980; **68**: 437–447.

57 Panijel M. Die behandlung mittelschwerer angstzustände. *Therapiewoche* 1985; **41**: 4659–4668.

58 Kneibel R, Burchard JM. Zur Therapie depressiver Verstimmungen in der Praxis. *Z Allgemeinmed* 1988; **64**: 689–696.

59 Steger W. Depressive Verstimmungen. *Z Allgemeinmed* 1985; **61**: 914–918.

60 Linde K *et al.* St John's wort for depression – an overview and meta-analysis of randomised clinical trials. *BMJ* 1996; **313**: 253–258.

61 Kuhlmann J *et al.* The influence of valerian treatment on 'reaction time, alertness and concentration' in volunteers. *Pharmacopsychiatry* 1999; **32**: 235–241.

62 Garges HP *et al.* Cardiac complications and delirium associated with valerian root withdrawal. *JAMA* 1998; **280**: 1566–1567.

63 MacGregor FB *et al.* Hepatotoxicity of herbal medicines. *BMJ* 1989; **299**: 1156–1157.

64 Shaw D *et al.* Traditional remedies and food supplements. A five-year toxicological study (1991–1995). *Drug Safety* 1997; **17**: 342–356.

65 Willey LB *et al.* Valerian overdose: a case report. *Vet Human Toxicol* 1995; **37**: 364–365.

66 Chan TYK *et al.* Poisoning due to an over-the-counter hypnotic, Sleep-Qik (hyoscine, cyproheptadine, valerian). *Postgrad Med J* 1995; **71**: 227–228.

67 Chan TYK. An assessment of the delayed effects associated with valerian overdose. *Int J Clin Pharmacol Ther* 1998; **36**: 569.

68 Houghton PJ. Valerian. *Pharm J* 1994; **253**: 95–96.

69 Tufik S *et al.* Effects of a prolonged administration of valepotriates in rats on the mothers and their offspring. *J Ethnopharmacol* 1994; **41**: 39–44.

Vervain

Species (Family)

Verbena officinalis L. (Verbenaceae)

Synonym(s)

Verbena

Part(s) Used

Herb

Pharmacopoeial and Other Monographs

BHP 1996[G9]
PDR for Herbal Medicines 2nd edition[G36]

Legal Category (Licensed Products)

GSL[G37]

Constituents[G2,G22,G40,G64]

Glycosides Iridoid glycosides: hastatoside, verbenalin (verbanaloside), verbenin (aucubin). Phenylpropanoid glycosides: acetoside (verbascoside) and eukovoside.[1,2]

Volatile oils Monoterpene components include citral, geraniol, limonene and verbenone.

Other constituents Adenosibe, alkaloid (unspecified), bitters, carbohydrates (stachyose, mucilage), β-carotene, invertin (sucrose hydrolytic enzymes), saponin and tannic acid.

Food Use

Vervain is listed by the Council of Europe as a natural source of food flavouring (category N2). This category indicates that vervain can be added to foodstuffs in small quantities, with a possible limitation of an active principle (as yet unspecified) in the final product.[G16] In the USA, vervain is listed by the Food and Drugs Administration (FDA) as a Herb of Undefined Safety.[G22]

Herbal Use

Vervain is stated to possess sedative, thymoleptic, antispasmodic, mild diaphoretic and, reputedly, galactogogue properties. Traditionally, it has been used for depression, melancholia, hysteria, generalised seizures, cholecystalgia, jaundice, early stages of fever, and specifically for depression and debility of convalescence after fevers, especially influenza.[G2,G7,G64]

Dosage

Dried herb 2–4 g or by infusion three times daily.[G7]

Liquid extract 2–4 mL (1:1 in 25% alcohol) three times daily.[G7]

Tincture 5–10 mL (1:1 in 40% alcohol) three times daily.[G7]

Pharmacological Actions

In vitro and animal studies

Galactogogue properties have been documented for vervain and attributed to aucubin.[3] A luteinising action has also been reported, and attributed to inhibition of the gonadotrophic action of the posterior lobe of the pituitary gland.[3] Extracts of vervain fruit have been used to treat dysmenorrhoea and to stimulate lactation.[3] Vervain has been documented to possess weak parasympathetic properties, causing slight contraction of the uterus.[3] Verbenalin has been reported to exhibit uterine stimulant activity.[G30] Sympathetic activity has also been documented: in small doses verbenin has been reported to act as an agonist at sympathetic nerve endings, whereas larger doses result in antagonism.[G22] Verbascoside reportedly acts as an agonist to the antitremor action of levodopa, and as an antihypertensive and analgesic.[3] A slight laxative action in mice has been documented for iridoid glycosides.[4]

Side-effects, Toxicity

None documented for vervain. High doses of verbenalin are stated to paralyse the CNS, resulting in stupor and convulsions.[G22]

Contra-indications, Warnings

None documented. Excessive doses of vervain may interfere with existing hypo- or hypertensive and hormone therapies.

Pregnancy and lactation Vervain is reputed to act as an abortifacient and oxytocic agent[G30] with *in vivo* utero-activity documented (*see In vitro* and animal studies). In view of this, vervain should not be taken during pregnancy.

Vervain may affect lactation in view of the reported galactogogue properties.[3]

Pharmaceutical Comment

Limited chemical, pharmacological and toxicity data are available for vervain. Documented scientific information does not justifiy the herbal uses, although galactogogue properties have been reported. No human data were located. In view of the lack of toxicity data and documented pharmacological actions in animals, excessive use of vervain should be avoided.

References

See also General References G2, G9, G16, G22, G30, G31, G36, G37, G40 and G64.

1 Lahloub MF *et al*. Phenylpropanoid and iridoid glycosides from the Egyptian *Verbena officinalis*. *Planta Med* 1986; **52**: 47.
2 Andary C *et al*. Structures of verbascoside and orobanchoside, caffeic acid sugar esters from *Orobanche rapum-genistae*. *Phytochemistry* 1982; **21**: 1123–1127.
3 Oliver-Bever BEP. *Medicinal Plants in Tropical West Africa*. Cambridge: Cambridge University Press, 1986.
4 Inouye H *et al*. Purgative activities of iridoid glycosides. *Planta Med* 1974; **25**: 285–288.

Wild Carrot

Species (Family)

Daucus carota L. subsp. *carota* (Umbelliferae)

Synonym(s)

Daucus, Queen Anne's Lace

Part(s) Used

Herb

Pharmacopoeial and Other Monographs

BHC 1992[G6]
BHP 1996[G9]
Martindale 32nd edition[G43]
PDR for Herbal Medicines 2nd edition[G36]

Legal Category (Licensed Products)

GSL[G37]

Constituents[G6,G41,G64]

Documented constituents refer to the fruit or seeds obtained from the dried fruit unless stated.

Flavonoids Flavones (e.g. apigenin, chrysin, luteolin), flavonols (e.g. kaempferol, quercetin) and various glycosides.[1]

Furanocoumarin 8-Methoxypsoralen and 5-methoxypsoralen (0.01–0.02 µg/g fresh weight) in fresh plant. Concentrations increased in the diseased plant.[2]

Volatile oils 0.66–1.65%.[3] Many components identified; relative composition varies between different cultivars.[3] Various components include α-pinene, β-pinene, geraniol, geranyl acetate, limonene, α-terpinen, *p*-terpinen, α-terpineol, terpinen-4-ol, *p*-decanolactone (monoterpenes); β-bisabolene, β-elemene, caryophyllene, caryophyllene oxide, carotol, daucol (sesquiterpenes); asarone (phenylpropanoid derivative).[3]

Other constituents Choline,[4] daucine (alkaloid), a tertiary base (uncharacterised),[5] fatty acids (butyric, palmitic), coumarin, xylitol (polyol).

Food Use

Wild carrot should not be confused with the common cultivated carrot, *D. carota* L. subsp. *sativus* (Hoffm.), which has the familiar fleshy orange-red edible root. Wild carrot has an inedible tough whitish root.[G41] Wild carrot is listed by the Council of Europe as a natural source of food flavouring (category N1, N3). Category N1 indicates that for the roots there are no restrictions on use, whereas category N3 indicates that there is insufficient information available for an adequate assessment of potential toxicity.[G16]

Herbal Use

Wild carrot is stated to possess diuretic, antilithic, and carminative properties. Traditionally, it has been used for urinary calculus, lithuria, cystitis, gout, and specifically for urinary gravel or calculus.[G6,G7,G8,G64]

Dosage

Dried herb 2–4 g or by infusion three times daily.[G6,G7]

Liquid extract 2–4 mL (1 : 1 in 25% alcohol) three times daily.[G6,G7]

Pharmacological Actions

In vitro and animal studies

Significant antifertility activity (60%) in rats has been reported for wild carrot.[6] In contrast, insignificant antifertility activity was observed in pregnant rats fed oral doses of up to 4.5 g/kg body weight from day 1 to day 10 of pregnancy.[7] Aqueous, alcoholic and petrol extracts were reported to exhibit 20%, 40% and 10% activities respectively. Weak oestrogenic activity[6,8,9] and inhibition of implantation[6,9] has been documented for seed extracts.[8] Oestrogenic activity, demonstrated by the inhibition of ovarian hypertrophy in hemicastrated rats, has been attributed to the known constituent coumarin (a weak phytooestrogen).[10]

Central effects similar to those of barbiturates have been documented for the seed oil obtained from *D. carota* var.*sativa*.[11] The oil was reported to elicit CNS hypnotic effects in the rat, hypotension in the dog[4] leading to respiratory depression at higher doses, anticonvulsant activity in the frog, *in vitro* smooth muscle relaxant activity reducing acetylcholine-induced contractions (ileum/uterus, rabbit/rat), antagonism of acetylcholine in isolated frog skeletal muscle, direct depressant effect on cardiac muscle in the dog.[4,11] *In vitro* cardiotonic activity[4] and vasodilation of coronary vessels of the isolated cat heart has been reported.[12] Papaverine-like antispasmodic activity has been documented for a tertiary base isolated from wild carrot seeds.[5] Activity of approximately one-tenth that of papaverine was noted in a number of isolated preparations: ileum, uterus, blood vessels and trachea.[5] Cholinergic-type actions have also been reported for wild carrot with *in vitro* spasmodic actions noted in both smooth and skeletal muscle.[4] This cholinergic activity has been attributed to choline.[13] The identity of a second quaternary base isolated was not established.

Terpinen-4-ol is a documented component of the seed oil. This constituent is considered to be the diuretic principle in juniper, exerting its effect by causing renal irritation (*see* Juniper).

Increased resistance to carbon tetrachloride-induced hepatotoxicity has been reported in rats fed wild carrot.[14]

Limited antifungal activity has been documented, with activity exhibited against only one (*Botrytis cinerea*) out of nine fungi tested.[15]

Agglutination of *Streptococcus mutans* cells has been described for wild carrot. The agglutinin, found to be heat and trypsin stable but sensitive to dextranose, was thought to be a dextran.[16]

Side-effects, Toxicity

The oil is reported to be non-toxic.[G41,G58] Acute LD_{50} values in mice (oral) and guinea-pigs (dermal) are reported to exceed 5 g/kg.[17]

The oil contains terpinen-4-ol, which is the component associated with the renal irritancy of juniper oil.

The oil is reported to be generally non-irritating and non-sensitising.[12] However, hypersensitivity reactions, occupational dermatitis and positive patch tests have been reported for wild carrot.[2,G51] Wild carrot is reported to have a slight photosensitising effect.[2] Furanocoumarins are known photosensitisers.

Contra-indications, Warnings

Fruit extracts may cause sensitivity reactions similar to those seen with celery.[2] Excessive doses of the oil may cause renal irritation in view of the terpinen-4-ol content (*see* Juniper). Excessive doses may affect existing hypo- and hypertensive, cardiac and hormone therapies.

Pregnancy and lactation The safety of wild carrot has not been established. Both spasmodic and spasmolytic actions on smooth muscle *in vitro* have been reported. In view of this, the documented mild oestrogenic activity and potentially irritant volatile oil, excessive doses of wild carrot during pregnancy and lactation should be avoided.

Pharmaceutical Comment

Phytochemical studies documented for wild carrot concentrate on the composition of the volatile oil obtained from both the fresh and dried fruits (seeds). The composition of the oil varies between different cultivars. Animal studies have documented a variety of pharmacological actions including CNS-depressant, spasmodic and antispasmodic, hypotensive and cardiac-depressant activities. However, the majority of these actions were observed in *in vitro* preparations. The principal traditional use of wild carrot is as a diuretic. This activity has not been documented in animal studies, but the seed oil of wild carrot does contain terpinen-4-ol, the diuretic principle documented for juniper. Toxicity data only refer to the oil and indicate low toxicity. However, in view of the documented mild oestrogenic activity and potential for internal irritation by the oil, excessive ingestion should be avoided.

References

See also General References G6, G9, G16, G31, G36, G37, G41, G43, G51, G58 and G64.

1 El-Moghazi AM *et al*. Flavonoids of *Daucus carota*. *Planta Med* 1980; **40**: 382–385.

2 Ceska O *et al*. Furocoumarins in the cultivated carrot, *Daucus carota*. *Phytochemistry* 1986; **25**: 81–83.

3 Benecke R *et al*. Vergleichende Untersuchungen über den Gehalt an ätherischem Öl und dessen Zusammensetzung in den Früchten verschiedener Sorten von *Daucus carota* L. ssp. sativus (Hoffm.) Arcang. *Pharmazie* 1987; **42**: 256–259.

4 Gambhir SS *et al*. Studies on *Daucus carota*, Linn. Part I. Pharmacological studies with the water-soluble fraction of the alcoholic extract of the seeds: a preliminary report. *Indian J Med Res* 1966; **54**: 178–187.

5 Gambhir SS *et al*. Antispasmodic activity of the tertiary base of *Daucus carota*, Linn. seeds. *Indian J Physiol Pharmacol* 1979; **23**: 225–228.

6 Prakash AO. Biological evaluation of some medicinal plant extracts for contraceptive efficacy. *Con-*

tracept Deliv Syst 1984; **5**: 9.

7 Lal R *et al*. Antifertility effect of *Daucus carota* seeds in female albino rats. *Fitoterapia* 1986; **57**: 243–246.

8 Kant A *et al*. The estrogenic efficacy of carrot (*Daucus carota*) seeds. *J Adv Zool* 1986; **7**: 36–41.

9 Sharma MM *et al*. Estrogenic and pregnancy interceptory effects of carrot *Daucus carota* seeds. *Indian J Exp Biol* 1976; **14**: 506–508.

10 Kaliwal BB, Rao MA. Inhibition of ovarian compensatory hypertrophy by carrot seed (*Daucus carota*) extract or estradiol-17β in hemicastrated albino rats. *Indian J Exp Biol* 1981; **19**: 1058–1060.

11 Bhargava AK *et al*. Pharmacological investigation of the essential oil of *Daucus carota* Linn. var. sativa DC. *Indian J Pharm* 1967; **29**: 127–129.

12 Carrot seed oil. *Food Cosmet Toxicol* 1976; **14**: 705–706.

13 Gambhir SS *et al*. Studies on *Daucus carota*, Linn. Part II. Cholingergic activity of the quaternary base isolated from water-soluble fraction of alcoholic extracts of seeds. *Indian J Med Res* 1966; **54**: 1053–1056.

14 Handa SS. Natural products and plants as liver protecting drugs. *Fitoterapia* 1986; **57**: 307–351.

15 Guérin J-C, Réveillère H-P. Antifungal activity of plant extracts used in therapy. II Study of 40 plant extracts against 9 fungi species. *Ann Pharm Fr* 1985; **43**: 77–81.

16 Ramstorp M *et al*. Isolation and partial characterization of a substance from carrots, Daucus carota, with ability to agglutinate cells of *Streptococcus mutans*. *Caries Res* 1982; **16**: 423–427.

17 Opdyke DLJ. Carrot seed oil. *Food Cosmet Toxicol* 1974; **14**: 705.

Wild Lettuce

Species (Family)

Lactuca virosa L. (Asteraceae/Compositae)

Synonym(s)

Bitter Lettuce, Lettuce Opium
  Related *Lactuca* species include *Lactuca sativa* (Garden Lettuce), *Lactuca scariola* (Prickly Lettuce), *Lactuca altissima* and *Lactuca canadensis* (Wild Lettuce of America)

Part(s) Used

Leaf, latex

Pharmacopoeial and Other Monographs

BHC 1992[G6]
BHP 1996[G9]
Martindale 32nd edition[G43]
PDR for Herbal Medicines 2nd edition[G36]

Legal Category (Licensed Products)

GSL[G37]

Constituents[G6,G22,G48,G60,G64]

All parts of the plant contain a milky, white latex (sap) which, when collected and dried, forms the drug known as lactucarium.[G33]

Acids Citric, malic and oxalic (up to 1%) acids; cichoric acid (phenolic).[1]

Alkaloids Hyoscyamine, later disputed.[2,G33] *N*-methyl-β-phenethylamine, also disputed.[2]

Coumarins Aesculin, cichoriin.[1]

Flavonoids Flavones (e.g. apigenin, luteolin), flavonols (e.g. quercetin) and their glycosides.[1]

Terpenoids Bitter principles including the sesquiterpene lactones lactucin and lactupicrin (lactucopicrin); β-amyrin, germanicol, and lactucone (lactucerin). Lactucone is a mixture of α- and β-lactucerol acetates, β-lactucerol being identical to taraxasterol.

Other constituents Mannitol, proteins, resins and sugars.

Food Use

Wild lettuce is not used in foods, although the related species *L. sativa* is commonly used as a salad ingredient.

Herbal Use

Wild lettuce is stated to possess mild sedative, anodyne and hypnotic properties. Traditionally, it has been used for insomnia, restlessness and excitability in children, pertussis, irritable cough, priapism, dysmenorrhoea, nymphomania, muscular or articular pains, and specifically for irritable cough and insomnia.[G6,G7,G8,G42,G64]

Dosage

Dried leaves 0.5–3.0 g or by infusion three times daily.[G6]

Liquid extract 0.5–3.0 mL (1 : 1 in 25% alcohol) three times daily.[G6]

Lactucarium (dried latex extract) (BPC 1934) 0.3–1.0 g three times daily.

Soft extract (BPC 1934) 0.3–1.0 g three times daily.

Pharmacological Actions

In vitro and animal studies

Lactucarium has been noted to induce mydriasis.[G6] This effect may be attributable to hyoscyamine, although the dried sap is reportedly devoid of this alkaloid.
  An alcoholic extract of a related species, *L. sativa*, has exhibited a sedative effect in toads, causing a reduction in motor activity and behaviour.[3] Higher doses resulted in flaccid paralysis. In addition, an antispasmodic action on isolated smooth and striated muscle, and *in vitro* negative chronotropic and inotropic effects on normal and stressed (tachycardic) hearts were observed. The antispasmodic action was noted to be antagonised by calcium.

Lactucin, lactupicrin and hyoscyamine have all been proposed as the sedative components in wild lettuce. However in the above study,[3] the active component was uncharacterised and acted mainly peripherally, not readily crossing the blood–brain barrier. The suggested mode of action was via interference with basic excitatory processes common to neural and muscular functions, and not via a neuromuscular block.

Low amounts (nanograms) of morphine have been detected in *Lactuca* species, although the concentrations involved are considered too low to exert any obvious pharmacological effect.[G60]

Side-effects, Toxicity

None documented for *L. virosa*. Wild lettuce contains sesquiterpene lactones which are potentially allergenic.[G19] Occupational dermatitis has been documented for *L. sativa* together with an urticarial eruption after ingestion of the leaves.[4–6,G51] The milky sap of *L. sativa* is reported to be irritant.[G51]

The toxicity of wild lettuce is stated to be low.

Consumption of large amounts of *L. scariola* has caused poisoning in cattle, who developed pulmonary emphysema, severe dyspnoea, and weakness.[7] Only the immature plants were reported to be toxic.

L. sativa has been reported to produce only negative responses when tested for mutagenicity using the Ames test (*Salmonella typhimurium* TA98, TA100).[8]

Contra-indications, Warnings

Overdosage may produce poisoning[G42] involving stupor, depressed respiration, coma and even death. Wild lettuce may cause an allergic reaction in sensitive individuals, in particular those with an existing sensitivity to other members of the Asteraceae/Compositae family.

Pregnancy and lactation The safety of wild lettuce has not been established. In view of the lack of toxicity data and the possibility of allergic reactions, excessive use of wild lettuce during pregnancy and lactation should be avoided.

Pharmaceutical Comment

The chemistry of wild lettuce is well documented although it is not clear which constituents represent the active components. Early reports of hyoscyamine as a constituent have not been substantiated by subsequent study. No published information was found to support the traditional herbal uses of wild lettuce, although a sedative action in toads has been reported for a related species *L. sativa*. In view of the potential allergenicity of wild lettuce and the lack of toxicity data, excessive use should be avoided.

References

See also General References G6, G9, G10, G19, G22, G31, G33, G36, G37, G42, G43, G48, G51, G60 and G64.

1 Rees S, Harborne JB. Flavonoids and other phenolics of *Cichorium* and related members of the Lactuceae (Compositae). *Bot J Linn Soc* 1984; **89**: 313–319.
2 Huang Z-J *et al.* Studies on herbal remedies I: Analysis of herbal smoking preparations alleged to contain lettuce (*Lactuca sativa* L.) and other natural products. *J Pharm Sci* 1982; **71**: 270–271.
3 Gonzálex-Lima F *et al.* Depressant pharmacological effects of a component isolated from lettuce, *Lactuca sativa*. *Int J Crude Drug Res* 1986; **24**: 154–166.
4 Krook G. Occupational dermatitis from *Lactuca sativa* (lettuce) and *Cichorium* (endive). *Contact Dermatitis* 1977; **3**: 27–36.
5 Rinkel HJ, Balyeat RM. Occupational dermatitis due to lettuce. *JAMA* 1932; **98**: 137–138.
6 Zeller W *et al.* The sensitizing capacity of compositae plants 6. Guinea pig sensitization experiments with ornamental plants and weeds using different methods. *Arch Dermatol Res* 1985; **277**: 28–35.
7 Anon *Poisindex* CD-ROM 1995; 85. Denver: Micromedex.
8 White RD *et al.* An evaluation of acetone extracts from six plants in the Ames mutagenicity test. *Toxicol Lett* 1983; **15**: 26–31.

Willow

Species (Family)

Salix species including *Salix alba* L., *Salix fragilis* L., *Salix pentandra* L., *Salix purpurea* L. (Salicaceae)

Synonym(s)

Salix

Part(s) Used

Bark

Pharmacopoeial and Other Monographs

American Herbal Pharmacopoeia[G1]
BHC 1992[G6]
BHP 1996[G9]
BP 2001[G15]
Complete German Commission E[G3]
ESCOP 1997[G52]
Martindale 32nd edition[G43]
PDR for Herbal Medicines 2nd edition[G36]
PH Eur 2002[G28]

Legal Category (Licensed Products)

GSL[G37]

Constituents[G1,G2,G6,G49,G52,G62,G64]

Glycosides (phenolic) Various phenolic glycosides including salicin, salicortin, tremulacin, salireposide, picein and triandrin.[1] Acetylated salicin, salicortin, salireposide, and esters of salicylic acid and salicyl alcohol may also occur.

Salicylates (calculated as salicin) Vary between species, e.g. 0.5% in *S. alba*, 1–10% in *S. fragilis*, 3–9% in *S. purpurea*.[2]

Flavonoids Flavanones, eriodictoyl-7-glucoside; naringenin-5-glucoside; chalcone; isosalipurposide; catechin.[2,G52]

Tannins Condensed.

Other constituents Catechins.

There is reported to be no difference between the phenolic glycoside pattern of the bark and leaf. The latter is also reported to contain flavonoids, catechins and condensed tannins.[2,3]

Food Use

Willow is not used in foods.

Herbal Use[G1,G2,G4,G6,G7,G8,G32,G52,G56,G64]

Willow is stated to possess anti-inflammatory, antirheumatic, antipyretic, antihidrotic, analgesic, antiseptic and astringent properties. Traditionally it has been used for muscular and arthrodial rheumatism with inflammation and pain, influenza, respiratory catarrh, gouty arthritis, ankylosing spondylitis, and specifically for rheumatoid arthritis and other systemic connective tissue disorders characterised by inflammatory changes. The German Commission E approved internal use for diseases accompanied by fever, rheumatic ailments and headaches.[G3]

Dosage

Dry bark 1–3 g or by decoction three times daily[G6,G7] corresponding to 60–120 mg total salicin daily.[G3]

Liquid extract 1–3 mL (1 : 1 in 25% alcohol) three times daily.[G6,G7]

Pharmacological Actions

In vitro and animal studies

Pharmacological actions documented for salicylates include anti-inflammatory, antipyretic, hyperglycaemic/hypoglycaemic and uricosuric/antiuricosuric activities, and increased blood-clotting time and plasma albumin binding.[G46] Anti-inflammatory activity for salicin and tremulacin (isolated from *Populus* spp.) has been assessed in the hen's egg choriollantoic test.[4,G52] The results indicate that the activity may be due to the metabolites of these compounds.[4] Salicin is probably the most active anti-inflammatory compound in willow; it is metabolised to salicylic acid.[5] The enzymatic degradation of salicin, salicortin and tremulacin by β-glucosidase and by esterase has been investigated.[6]

Tannins are known to have astringent properties.

Clinical studies

Willow bark extract (equivalent to 240 mg salicin/day) was compared with placebo in a two-week, randomised, double-blind, controlled trial involving 78 patients with osteoarthritis.[7] A difference in pain dimension in the treated group, compared with placebo, just reached statistical significance ($p = 0.047$). It was concluded that willow bark extract had a moderate analgesic effect in osteoarthritis, and that it was well tolerated.

The pharmacological actions of salicylates in humans are well documented, and are applicable to willow. Salicin is a prodrug which is metabolised to saligenin in the gastrointestinal tract and to salicylic acid after absorption.[2]

Side-effects, Toxicity

Side-effects and signs of toxicity normally associated with salicylates, such as gastric and renal irritation, hypersensitivity, blood in the stools, tinnitus, nausea and vomiting, may occur. Salicin is documented to cause skin rashes.[G44]

Contra-indications, Warnings

Minor adverse effects including stomach ache, nausea, dizziness, sweating and rash have been reported in a small percentage of individuals.[G52] Precautions associated with salicylate therapy are also applicable to willow. Therefore individuals with known hypersensitivity to aspirin, asthma, active peptic ulceration, diabetes, gout, haemophilia, hypoprothrombinaemia, kidney or liver disease should be aware of the possible risks associated with the ingestion of willow.[8,G46] Irritant effects of salicylates on the gastrointestinal tract may be enhanced by alcohol, and barbiturates and oral sedatives have been documented to enhance salicylate toxicity as well as masking the symptoms of overdosage.[G46] Concurrent administration of willow with other salicylate-containing products, such as aspirin, should be avoided. Drug interactions listed for salicylates are also applicable to willow and include oral anticoagulants, methotrexate, metoclopramide, phenytoin, probenecid, spironolactone and valproate.

Pregnancy and lactation The safety of willow has not been established. Conflicting reports have been documented concerning the safety of aspirin taken during pregnancy. In view of this, the use of willow during pregnancy should be avoided. Salicylates excreted in breast milk have been reported to cause macular rashes in breastfed babies.[G46]

Pharmaceutical Comment

Willow is rich in phenolic constituents, such as flavonoids, tannins and salicylates. Pharmacological actions normally associated with salicylates are also applicable to willow which support most of the herbal uses, although no studies were located specifically for willow. In view of the lack of toxicity data on willow, the usual precautions taken with other salicylate-containing drugs are applicable. Products containing willow should preferably be standardised on their salicin content, in view of the considerable variation in salicylate concentrations between different *Salix* species.

References

See also General References G1, G2, G3, G5, G6, G9, G10, G31, G36, G37, G43, G49, G52, G54, G56, G62 and G64.

1 Meier B *et al.* Identifikation und Bestimmung von je acht Phenolglykosiden in *Salix purpurea* und *Salix daphnoides* mit moderner HPLC. *Pharm Acta Helv* 1985; **60**: 269–274.

2 Meier B *et al.* Pharmaceutical aspects of the use of willows in herbal remedies. *Planta Med* 1988: **54**: 559–560.

3 Karl C *et al.* Flavonoide aus *Salix alba*, die Struktur des terniflorins und eines Weiteren Acylflavonoides. *Phytochemistry* 1976; **15**: 1084–1085.

4 Albrecht M *et al.* Anti-inflammatory activity of flavonol glycosides and salicin derivatives from the leaves of *Populus tremuloides*. *Planta Med* 1990; **56**: 660.

5 Meier B, Liebi M. Salicinhaltige pflanzliche Arzneimittel-Überlegungen zu wirksamkeit und unbedenklichkeit. *Z Phytother* 1990; **11**: 50–58.

6 Julkunen-Tiitto R, Meier B. The enzymatic decomposition of salicin and its derivatives obtained from salicaceae species. *J Nat Prod* 1992; **55**: 1204–1212.

7 Schmid B *et al.* Efficacy and tolerability of a standardized willow bark extract in patients with osteoarthritis: randomized placebo-controlled, double blind clinical trial. *Phytother Res* 2001; **15**: 344–350.

8 Baker S, Thomas PS. Herbal medicine precipitating massive haemolysis. *Lancet* 1987; i: 1039–1040.

Witch Hazel

Species (Family)

Hamamelis virginiana L. (Hamamelidaceae)

Synonym(s)

Hamamelis, Witchazel

Part(s) Used

Bark, leaf

Pharmacopoeial and Other Monographs

BHP 1996[G9]
BP 2001[G15]
Complete German Commission E[G3]
ESCOP 1997[G52]
Martindale 32nd edition[G43]
Mills and Bone[G50]
PDR for Herbal Medicines 2nd edition[G36]
Ph Eur 2002[G28]
USP24/NF19[G61]

Legal Category (Licensed Products)

GSL[G37]

Constituents[1,G2,G22,G41,G48,G50,G52,G64]

Flavonoids (leaf) Flavonols (e.g. kaempferol, quercetin) and their glycosides including astragalin, quercitrin, afzelin and myricitrin.

Tannins, catechins Pharmacopoeial standard, not less than 3%.[G15,G28] Hamamelitannin (hydrolysable), lesser amounts of condensed tannins (bark). (+)-catechin, (+)-gallocatechin, (−)-epicatechin gallate, (−)-epigallocatechingallate, proanthocyanidin oligomers of cyanidin and delphinidin type.

Volatile oils About 0.5%. Hexen-2-ol, hexenol, α- and β-ionones, eugenol, safrole and sesquiterpenes.

Other constituents Fixed oil (about 0.6%), resin (hamamelin, hamamamelitannin), wax, saponins, choline, free gallic acid and free hamamelose.

Food Use

Witch hazel is listed by the Council of Europe as a natural source of food flavouring (category N3). This category indicates that there is insufficient information available for an adequate assessment of potential toxicity.[G16]

Herbal Use[1,G2,G4,G6,G32,G43,G52,G54,G56,G64]

Witch hazel is stated to possess astringent, antihaemorrhagic and anti-inflammatory properties. Traditionally, it has been used for diarrhoea, mucous colitis, haemorrhoids, haematemesis, haemoptysis, and externally for external haemorrhoids, bruises and localised inflamed swellings. The German Commission E approved use for minor skin injuries, local inflammation of skin and mucous membranes, haemorrhoids and varicose veins.[G3]

Dosage

Dried leaves 2 g or by infusion three times daily.[G6]

Hamamelis Liquid Extract (BPC 1973) 2–4 mL (1 : 1 in 45% alcohol) three times daily.[G6]

Hamamelis Water (BPC 1973) for local application, undiluted or 1 : 3 dilution for external use.[G3]

Decoction 5–10 g in 250 mL water for compresses.[G3]

Pharmacological Actions

The pharmacological properties of witch hazel have been reviewed.[1,G50,G52]

In vitro and animal studies

Witch hazel is known to possess astringent and haemostatic properties, which have been attributed to the tannin constituents. Vasoconstriction was reduced in the hindquarters of rabbits when arteries were perfused with aqueous or ethanolic extracts of witch hazel leaf. A 70% ethanolic extract of leaf (1 : 5, 200 mg/kg, administered orally) significantly inhibited the chronic phase of carrageenan-induced rat paw oedema over a period of 19 days, compared with control ($p < 0.05$).[2] An aqueous ethanolic extract of witch hazel bark yielded a fraction rich in polymeric proanthocyanins after ultracentrifugation.[3] This fraction was significantly active against herpes simplex virus type 1 (HSV-1). It also showed radical scavenging properties, inhibited β-glucosidase and human leukocyte elastase activity, and was active in the croton oil ear oedema test in mice. In other studies, 3-O-galloyl-epicatechin-(4β,8)-catechin, a catechin oligomer and hamamelitannin isolated from witch hazel bark had IC_{50} values of 6.6, 8.8 and 1.0 μmol/L, respectively, for inhibition of 5-lipoxygenase.[4] The oligomer was active in the microsomal lyso-PAF:acetyl-CoA-acetyltransferase inhibition assay, with an IC_{50} value of 9.4 μmol/L, whereas hamamelitannin was inactive.[4]

Clinical studies

Haemorrhoids Uncontrolled studies have suggested that witch hazel bark distillate (5%) and a salve containing witch hazel bark may be effective in the treatment of haemorrhoids.[G50] A double-blind, controlled trial involving 90 patients with haemorrhoids compared the effects of witch hazel bark salve with those of other salves. Witch hazel was reported to be superior in relief of symptoms.

Dermatology In a study involving 30 volunteers who received topical applications of a hydroglycolic extract of witch hazel leaf, skin temperature was significantly reduced, compared with baseline values. This was interpreted as a possible vasoconstrictor effect of witch hazel.[G52] The effects of an after-sun lotion containing 10% hamamelis distillate were explored in 30 healthy volunteers using a modified UV-B erythema test for inflammation.[5] It was reported that erythema suppression ranged from 20% at 7 hours to 27% at 48 hours.

Witch hazel leaf extract incorporated into a cream formulation was applied twice daily for two weeks to seven children suffering from dermatitis atopica of the feet (chilblains) and to five children with eczema. Improvements in these conditions were reported.[G52]

In a two-week, randomised, double-blind trial, 72 patients with moderately severe eczema were treated with either a hamamelis distillate cream (5.35 g distillate with 0.64 g ketone/100 g), hydrocortisone cream 0.5%, or drug-free cream.[6] All three treatments significantly reduced itching, erythema and scaling after one week. Hydrocortisone cream was more effective than hamamelis cream.

Several clinical studies of witch hazel in the treatment of eczema have been reviewed.[G50] An uncontrolled study involving 37 patients treated with a witch hazel leaf cream twice daily for two weeks reported improvements in eczema and neurodermati-

tis. A double-blind, placebo-controlled trial of witch hazel salve (25% water distillate from leaf) involving 80 patients with toxic and degenerative eczema and 31 patients with endogenous eczema found that atopic dermatitis responded to the treatment, but that there was no significant effect on primary irritant contact dermatitis. An uncontrolled study involving 22 patients with atopic eczema who were treated with witch hazel (4 g leaf provided 25 mL distillate/100 g salve) applied to affected arms over a three-week period reported improvements symptoms, compared with baseline values.[G50]

Side-effects, Toxicity

The volatile oil contains safrole, a known carcinogen (*see* Sassafras), but in amounts too small to cause concern. Stomach irritation may occur in susceptible patients after oral treatment. Four of 1032 patients tested reacted to an ointment containing 25% witch hazel extract, but two of these patients were sensitive to wool fat in the ointment base.[G50]

Contra-indications, Warnings

None documented for witch hazel. In view of the tannin constituents, excessive ingestion of witch hazel is not recommended.

Pregnancy and lactation There are no known problems with the use of witch hazel during pregnancy, although excessive ingestion should be avoided in view of the tannin content.

Pharmaceutical Comment

Witch hazel is characterised by its tannin constituents and astringent properties. The documented herbal uses are related to these astringent properties. There is some evidence to indicate that witch hazel is effective in the treatment of haemorrhoids and venous tone, but its use in the treatment of eczema and dermatitis is more controversial.

References

See also General References G2, G3, G9, G12, G15, G16, G22, G28, G29, G31, G32, G36, G37, G41, G48, G43, G50, G52, G54, G56, G61 and G64.

1   Zeylstra H. *Hamamelis virginiana*. Br J Phytother 1998; 5: 23–28.
2   Duwiejua M *et al*. Anti-inflammatory activity of *Polygonum bistorta*, *Guaiacum officinale* and *Hamamelis virginiana* in rats. J Pharm Pharmacol 1994; 46: 286–290.

3 Erdelmeier CAJ *et al.* Antiviral and antiphlogistic activities of *Hamamelis virginiana*. *Planta Med* 1996; **62**: 241–245.

4 Hartisch C *et al.* Dual inhibitory activities of tannins from *Hamamelis virginiana* and related polyphenols on 5-lipoxygenase and lyso-PAF: acetyl-CoA acetyltransferase. *Planta Med* 1997;

63: 106–110.

5 Hughes-Formella BJ *et al.* Anti-inflammatory effect of hamamelis lotion in a UVB erythema test. *Dermatology* 1998; **196**: 316–322.

6 Korting HC *et al.* Comparative efficacy of hamamelis distillate and hydrocortisone cream in atopic eczema. *Eur J Clin Pharmacol* 1995; **48**: 461–465.

Yarrow

Species (Family)

Achillea millefolium L. (Asteraceae/Compositae)

Synonym(s)

Milfoil, Millefolium

Part(s) Used

Flowerhead

Pharmacopoeial and Other Monographs

BHC 1992[G6]
BHP 1996[G9]
BP 2001[G15]
Complete German Commission E[G3]
Martindale 32nd edition[G43]
PDR for Herbal Medicines 2nd edition[G36]
Ph Eur 2002[G28]

Legal Category (Licensed Products)

GSL[G37]

Constituents[G2,G6,G22,G41,G64]

Acids Amino acids (e.g. alanine, aspartic acid, glutamic acid, histidine, leucine, lysine, proline, valine),[1,2] fatty acids (e.g. linoleic, myristic, oleic, palmitic, stearic),[3,4] and others including ascorbic acid,[5] caffeic acid,[6] folic acid,[5] salicylic acid and succinic acid.[1]

Alkaloids/bases Betonicine and stachydrine (pyrrolidine),[1,7] trigonelline (pyridine),[1,7] betaine and choline (bases).[1,7] Uncharacterised alkaloids include achiceine, achilleine[8] (possible synonym for L-betonicine), which is stated to yield achilletine[7] on alkaline hydrolysis, and moscatine/moschatine[7], stated to be an ill-defined glucoalkaloid.

Flavonoids Predominantly flavone glycosides apigenin- and luteolin-7-glycosides,[9] with lesser quantities of artemetin, casticin, 5-hydroxy-3,6,7,4-tetramethoxyflavone and isorhamnetin.[6] Rutin (a flavonol glycoside).[5]

Tannins Condensed and hydrolysable,[3,10] with glucose as the carbohydrate component of the latter[2]

Volatile oils Numerous identified components include borneol, bornyl acetate (trace), camphor, 1,8-cineole, eucalyptol, limonene, sabinene, terpinen-4-ol, terpineol and α-thujone (monoterpenes), caryophyllene (a sesquiterpene), achillicin, achillin, millefin and millefolide (sesquiterpene lactones), azulene and chamazulene (sesquiterpene lactone-derived) and isoartemisia ketone. The relative composition of the components varies greatly between *Achillea* species, especially the azulene content. Azulene has been reported as the major component.[11] However, true yarrow (*A. millefolium*) is thought to be hexaploid and azulene-free, whereas closely related species, such as *Achillea lanulosa* Nutt. and *Achillea collina* Becker, are tetraploid and contain up to 50% azulene in their volatile oil.[5,10,11] The tetraploid species may be supplied for *A. millefolium*. The azulenes are not present in the fresh herb: they are formed as artefacts during steam distillation of the oil, from unstable precursors called proazulenes (e.g. achillin and achillicin), via equally unstable azulene–carboxylic acid intermediates.[12]

Other constituents Unknown cyanogenetic compound,[13] sugars including arabinose, galactose, dextrose, dulcitol, glucose, inositol, maltose, mannitol and sucrose.[1,2]

The constituents of yarrow have been reviewed in detail.[5]

Food Use

Yarrow is listed by the Council of Europe as a natural source of food flavouring (herb, flowers, essential oil and other preparations: category 4, with limits on camphor, eucalyptol and thujone) (*see* Appendix 23).[G17] In the USA, yarrow is only approved for use in alcoholic beverages, and the finished product must be thujone free.[G41]

Herbal Use

Yarrow is stated to possess diaphoretic, antipyretic, hypotensive, astringent, diuretic and urinary antiseptic properties. Traditionally, it has been used for bruises, swellings, strains, fevers, common cold, essential hypertension, amenorrhoea, dysentery, diarrhoea, and specifically for thrombotic conditions with hypertension, including cerebral and coronary thromboses. [G2,G6,G7,G8,G64]

Dosage

Dried herb 2–4 g or by infusion three times daily. [G6,G7]

Liquid extract 2–4 mL (1 : 1 in 25% alcohol) three times daily. [G6,G7]

Tincture 2–4 mL (1 : 5 in 45% alcohol) three times daily. [G6,G7]

Pharmacological Actions

Some activities documented for yarrow are associated with the azulene constituents, although it is now thought that azulene is absent from true yarrow (*see* Constituents). Presumably some of the documented pharmacological studies have used *Achillea* species other than *A. millefolium*.

In vitro and animal studies

Anti-inflammatory activity has been documented for an aqueous extract of yarrow using mouse[15] and rat[16] paw oedema models, with inflammation induced by yeast[15] and various inflammatory substances,[16] including histamine, carrageenan and prostaglandin. In mouse studies, the active fraction was reported as a series of protein–carbohydrate complexes. Topical anti-inflammatory activity in rabbits has also been documented for the aqueous extract.[15] In general, anti-inflammatory properties are associated with azulenes (*see* German Chamomile). Anti-inflammatory activity has been described for the azulene components documented for the volatile oil of yarrow.[5]

A diuretic effect was also noted in mice administered an aqueous extract of yarrow,[15] but only at a dose more than double that required for an anti-inflammatory effect.[15] Terpinen-4-ol, the diuretic principle in juniper, has been reported as a component of yarrow volatile oil.

CNS-depressant activity has been documented for the volatile oil: a dose of 300 mg/kg decreased the spontaneous activity of mice and lowered the body temperature of rats. In addition, 300–600 mg/kg doses inhibited pentetrazole-induced convulsions and prolonged sleep induced by a barbiturate preparation.[17]

Moderate antibacterial activity has been documented for an ethanolic extract of the herb against *Staphylococcus aureus*, *Bacillus subtilis*, *Mycobacterium smegmatis*, *Escherichia coli*, *Shigella sonnei* and *Shigella flexneri*.[18] Antimicrobial properties have been documented for the sesquiterpene lactone fraction.[5]

Achilleine 0.5 g/kg by intravenous injection has been noted to decrease the blood clotting time in rabbits by 32%.[8] The haemostatic action persisted for 45 minutes with no observable toxic effects.

Antispasmodic activity on the isolated rabbit intestine has been documented for a flavonoid-containing fraction of yarrow.[9] Antispasmodic activity is generally associated with azulene constituents (*see* German Chamomile).

Antipyretic and hypotensive actions have been reported for the basic fraction (alkaloid/base);[G41] the sesquiterpene lactone fraction is stated to possess cytotoxic activities,[5] although no further details were located. Tannins are known to possess astringent activity.

Side-effects, Toxicity

Allergic reactions to yarrow (e.g. dermatitis) have been documented, and positive patch tests have been produced in individuals sensitised to other plants.[5,G33,G51] An instance of yarrow tea causing a generalised eruption in a sensitised individual was reported in 1929. The allergenic properties of some sesquiterpene lactones are well documented, although none of those present in yarrow are recognised sensitisers.[G51] Yarrow has been suspected of being a photosensitiser, although extracts have been reported to lack phototoxicity and to be devoid of psoralens, compounds with known photosensitising properties.[G51]

Yarrow is considered to be non-toxic. In mice LD_{50} values have been reported of up to 3.65 g/kg (by mouth), 3.1 g/kg (by intraperitoneal injection), and greater than or equal to 1 g/kg (by subcutaneous injection).[15,17] In rats, an LD_{50} (subcutaneous injection) has been recorded as 16.86 g/kg, with corresponding LD_0 and LD_{100} values reported as 12 and 20 g/kg, respectively.[16] By comparison, an ED_{25} for anti-inflammatory activity has been estimated as about 0.43 g/kg.[16]

Terpenoid-rich volatile oils often possess irritant properties. Terpinen-4-ol, documented as a component of yarrow volatile oil, is thought to represent the diuretic principal of juniper as a result of its irritant action on the kidneys (*see* Juniper).[12] The known toxic principle thujone has been documented as a minor component of yarrow volatile oil, although concentrations present are probably too low to represent a risk to human health.

A single report of animal poisoning has been documented for yarrow in which a calf died following the ingestion of a single plant.[5] No additional reports of animal toxicity were located.

Contra-indications, Warnings

Yarrow may cause an allergic reaction in sensitive individuals, especially those with an existing hypersensitivity to other members of the Asteraceae/Compositae.[19] Individuals with such a known hypersensitivity should avoid drinking herbal teas containing yarrow.[G60] Excessive doses may interfere with existing anticoagulant and hypo- and hypertensive therapies, and may have sedative and diuretic effects.

Pregnancy and lactation Yarrow should not be taken during pregnancy. It is reputed to be an abortifacient and to affect the menstrual cycle,[G30] and the volatile oil contains trace amounts (0.3%) of the abortifacient principle thujone. Excessive use should be avoided during lactation.

Pharmaceutical Comment

The chemistry of yarrow is well documented although there has been some disagreement over the major component in the volatile oil. Various pharmacological actions have been reported in animal studies which support many of the reputed herbal uses although no human data were located. Yarrow is considered to be relatively non-toxic although allergic reactions in susceptible individuals have been documented. The volatile oil is contraindicated in pregnancy and yarrow should be used with caution in patients with epilepsy.[G58]

References

See also General References G2, G3, G6, G9, G15, G16, G22, G28, G30, G31, G32, G33, G36, G37, G41, G43, G51, G58, G60 and G64.

1 Ivanov Ch, Yankov L. Composition of *Achillea millefolium*. I. Preparation of the total extracts and composition of the part of the alcoholic extracts soluble in alcohol and water. *God Vissh Khimikotekhnol Inst Sofia* 1967; **14**: 195–222.

2 Ivanov Ch, Yankov L. Composition of *Achillea millefolium*. III. Composition of the parts soluble in water and insoluble in alcohol. *God Vissh Khimikotekhnol Inst Sofia* 1967; **14**: 223–241,

3 Ivanov Ch, Yankov L. Composition of *Achillea millefolium*. III. Composition of the acidic, water-insoluble part of the alcoholic extract. *God Vissh Khimikotekhnol Inst Sofia* 1967; **14**: 61–72.

4 Ivanov Ch, Yankov L. Composition of *Achillea millefolium*. V. Composition and structure of the components of neutral fraction insoluble in the aqueous part of the alcoholic extract. *God Vissh Khimikotekhnol Inst Sofia* 1967; **14**: 73–101.

5 Chandler RF *et al.* Ethnobotany and phytochemistry of yarrow, *Achillea millefolium*, Compositae. *Economic Bot* 1982; **36**: 203–223.

6 Falk AJ *et al.* Isolation and identification of three new flavones from *Achillea millefolium* L. *J Pharm Sci* 1975; **64**: 1838–1842.

7 Zirvi KA, Ikram M. Alkaloids of some of the plants of the Compositae. *Pakistan J Sci Ind Res* 1975; **18**: 93–101.

8 Miller FM, Chow LM. Alkaloids of *Achillea millefolium* L. I. Isolation and characterization of Achilleine. *J Am Chem Soc* 1954; **76**: 1353–1354.

9 Hoerhammer L. Flavone concentration of medical plants with regard to their spasmolytic action. *Congr Sci Farm Conf Commun 21st Pisa* 1961; 578–588.

10 Falk AJ *et al.* The constituents of the essential oil from *Achillea millefolium* L. *Lloydia* 1974; **37**: 598–602.

11 Haggag MY *et al.* Thin layer and gas-chromatographic studies on the essential oil from *Achillea millefolium*. *Planta Med* 1975; **27**: 361–366.

12 Sticher O. Plant mono-, di- and sesquiterpenoids with pharmacological and therapeutical activity. In: Wagner H, Wolff P, eds. *New Natural Products with Pharmacological Biological or Therapeutical Activity*. Berlin: Springer Verlag, 1977: 137–176.

13 Seigler DS. Plants of the Northeastern United States that produce cyanogenic compounds. *Economic Bot* 1976; **30**: 395–407.

14 Chandler F. Vindication of maritime Indian herbal remedies. *J Ethnopharmacol* 1983; **9**: 323–327.

15 Goldberg AS *et al.* Isolation of anti-inflammatory principles from *Achillea millefolium* (Compositae). *J Pharm Sci* 1969; **58**: 938–941.

16 Shipochliev T, Fournadjiev G. Spectrum of the antiinflammatory effect of *Arctostaphylos uva ursi* and *Achilea millefolium*, L. *Probl Vutr Med* 1984; **12**: 99–107.

17 Kudrzycka-Bieloszabska FW, Glowniak K. Pharmacodynamic properties of oleum chamomillae and oleum millefolii. *Diss Pharm Pharmacol* 1966; **18**: 449–454.

18 Moskalenko SA. Preliminary screening of far-Eastern ethnomedicinal plants for antibacterial activity. *J Ethnopharmacol* 1986; **15**: 231–259.

19 Mathias CGT *et al.* Plant dermatitis – patch test results (1975–78). Note on Juniperus extract. *Contact Dermatitis* 1979; **5**: 336.

Yellow Dock

Species (Family)

Rumex crispus L. (Polygonaceae)

Synonym(s)

Curled Dock

Part(s) Used

Root

Pharmacopoeial and Other Monographs

BHP 1983[G7]
PDR for Herbal Medicines 2nd edition[G36]

Legal Category (Licensed Products)

GSL[G37]

Constituents[G22,G48,G64]

Anthraquinones 2–4%. Chrysophanol, emodin, nepodin, physcion (aglycones).[1–3]

Tannins Catechol 5% (condensed-type).

Other plants parts The plant constituents documented include oxalic acid, oxalates, chrysophanic acid, emodin, tannin, and a complex volatile oil (more than 60 components identified).[4,G51]

Food Use

Yellow dock is not used in foods.

Herbal Use

Yellow dock is stated to possess gentle purgative and cholagogue properties. Traditionally, it has been used for chronic skin disease, obstructive jaundice, constipation, and specifically for psoriasis with constipation.[G7,G64]

Dosage

Dried root 2–4 g or by decoction three times daily.[G7]

Liquid extract 2–4 mL (1 : 1 in 25% alcohol) three times daily.[G7]

Tincture 1–2 mL (1 : 5 in 45% alcohol) three times daily.[G7]

Pharmacological Actions

In vitro and animal studies

None documented for the root. Slight antibacterial activity has been reported for herb extracts, which exhibited activity towards both Gram-positive (*Staphylococcus aureus*, *Mycobacterium smegmatis*) and Gram-negative (*Escherichia coli*, *Shigella sonnei*, *Shigella flexneri*) organisms.[4]

Side-effects, Toxicity

None documented for yellow dock. In view of the documented anthraquinone constituents, side-effects generally associated with laxatives are also applicable to yellow dock. Overuse may cause abdominal cramps and diarrhoea, and prolonged use may lead to intestinal atrophy and hypokalaemia.

Dermatitis has been reported in livestock following the ingestion of plant material in large quantities.[G51] Oxalic acid is known to be a toxic plant acid that forms insoluble calcium salts which cause a disturbance in calcium concentrations and hence affect the blood coagulation mechanism.[G33]

Contra-indications, Warnings

Warnings generally associated with stimulant laxatives are also applicable to yellow dock. Therefore, yellow dock should not be taken when there is existing intestinal obstruction, and excessive use should be avoided (*see* Side-effects, Toxicity).

Pregnancy and lactation In general, unstandardised stimulant laxatives are not recommended for use during pregnancy. The use of yellow dock should therefore be avoided in favour of a standardised preparation that is recommended for the treatment of constipation during pregnancy. The use of yellow dock by breastfeeding women should also be avoided, since it has been documened that anthraquinones can be secreted into the breast milk (*see* Senna).

Pharmaceutical Comment

Limited chemical, pharmacological, and toxicity information is available for yellow dock. Documented anthraquinone constituents justify the reputed purgative action. Although the purgative effect of yellow dock is reputed to be gentle, the use of unstandardised anthraquinone-containing preparations should be avoided since their pharmacological effect is unpredictable and may cause abdominal cramp and diarrhoea.

References

See also General References G7, G22, G31, G32, G33, G36, G37, G48, G51 and G64.

1   de Siqueira NCS *et al.* Hydroxyanthraquinones in *Rumex crispus* L. (of southern Rio Grande). *Rev Cent Cienc Biomed* 1977; **5**: 69–74.
2   Midiwo JO, Rukunga GM. Distribution of anthraquinone pigments in *Rumex* species of Kenya. *Phytochemistry* 1985; **24**: 1390–1391.
3   Fairbairn JW, El-Muhtadi FJ. Chemotaxonomy of anthraquinones in *Rumex*. *Phytochemistry* 1972; **11**: 263–268.
4   Miyazawa M, Kameoka H. Constituents of essential oil from *Rumex crispus*. *Yakagaku* 1983; **32**: 45–47.

Yucca

Species (Family)

Various *Yucca* species (Liliaceae/Agavaceae) including
(i) *Yucca schidigera* Roezl ex Ortgies
(ii) *Yucca brevifolia* Engelm.
(iii) *Yucca glauca*

Synonym(s)

(i) Mohave Yucca, *Yucca mohavensis* Sarg.
(ii) Joshua Tree, *Yucca arborescens* Trel.

Part(s) Used

Whole plant

Pharmacopoeial and Other Monographs

PDR for Herbal Medicines 2nd edition[G36]

Legal Category (Licensed Products)

Yucca is not listed in the GSL.

Constituents

Terpenoids Various saponins have been isolated from different *Yucca* species, including tigogenin and chlerogenin,[1] yuccagenin and kammogenin,[2] sarsaspogenin, markogenin, higogenin, neo-tigogenin, neo-gitogenin, hecogenin, gloriogenin, and diosgenin (trace)[3] and smilagenin.

Food Use

Yucca filamentosa L. (bear grass) is listed by the Council of Europe as a natural source of food flavouring (category N3). This category indicates that there is insufficient information available for an adequate assessment of potential toxicity.[G16] The yucca plant has been used traditionally as a major foodstuff by Indian tribes. In the USA, both *Y. schidigera* and *Y. brevifolia* are approved for food use.[G41]

Herbal Use

Yucca has been used for the treatment of arthritis, diabetes and stomach disorders. Concentrated plant juice has been used topically to soothe painful joints.

Dosage

None documented.

Pharmacological Actions

In vitro and animal studies

In the rat, anti-inflammatory activity against carrageenan-induced inflammation has been documented for a saponin-containing leaf extract from *Yucca schotti*.[2] Yucca saponin extract, from *Y. schidigera*, is reported to exhibit approximately half the haemolytic activity of commercial soap bark saponin.

Antitumour activity against B16 melanoma has been documented for a polysaccharide-containing extract of *Y. glauca*.[4] The extract was found to be inactive towards L1210 or P388 leukaemias.

Clinical studies

A saponin-containing yucca extract has been reported to reduce symptoms of swelling, pain and stiffness in approximately 75 of 150 arthritic patients given the extract in a double-blind study.[5] The onset of a positive response was found to vary from days to weeks or months. A saponin-containing yucca extract has also been documented to reduce blood pressure, abnormal triglyceride, and high cholesterol concentrations in a double-blind study involving 212 arthritic and hypertensive patients.[6] Optimum results were obtained in conjunction with diet and exercise. Yucca extracts have also been reported to provide relief from headaches and to improve circulation and gastrointestinal function.[5,6]

Side-effects, Toxicity

Limited toxicity data are available for yucca. A 12-week study in rats concluded that yucca was non-toxic. A saponin-containing yucca extract was given to more than 700 arthritic patients with no signs of toxicity documented. The yucca saponins are regarded to be a safe food supplement since they are not thought to be absorbed from the gastrointestinal tract, thereby reducing the dangers of systemic haemolytic activity.[5]

Contra-indications, Warnings

Pregnancy and lactation   There are no known problems with the use of yucca during pregnancy and lactation. However, it is advisable not to exceed amounts normally ingested as a food.

Pharmaceutical Comment

Limited phytochemical information is available for yucca, steroidal saponins being the only documented constituents. Human studies have reported a yucca saponin extract to have a beneficial effect on certain symptoms of arthritis such as pain and stiffness, and to reduce blood pressure and serum triglyceride and cholesterol concentrations. The traditional use of

yucca as a foodstuff would indicate it to be of low toxicity.

References

See also General References G16, G32, G36 and G41.

1   Dewidar AM, El-Munajjed D. The steroid sapogenin constituents of *Agave americana*, A. *variegata* and *Yucca gloriosa*. *Planta Med* 1970; **19**: 87–91.
2   Backer RC *et al.* A phytochemical investigation of *Yucca schotti* (Liliaceae). *J Pharm Sci* 1972; **61**: 1665–1666.
3   Stohs SJ *et al.* Steroidal sapogenins of *Yucca glauca* seeds. *Lloydia* 1973; **36**: 443.
4   Ali MS *et al.* Isolation of antitumor polysaccharide fractions from *Yucca glauca* Nutt. (Liliaceae). *Growth* 1978; **42**: 213–223.
5   Bingham R *et al.* Yucca plant saponin in the management of arthritis. *J Appl Nutr* 1975; **27**: 45–51.
6   Bingham R *et al.* Yucca plant saponin in the treatment of hypertension and hypercholesterolemia. *J Appl Nutr* 1978; **30**: 127–136.

Appendices

Appendix 1   Potential Drug–Herb Interactions

Until the emergence of reports of important inter-actions between St. John's wort (*Hypericum perfor-atum* L.) and certain conventional drugs (*see* St. John's Wort), very few interactions involving herbal products had been reported in the medical literature. Furthermore, there has been very little experimental and clinical research in this area.

The following list of *potential* drug–herb inter-actions has been compiled on the basis of known herbal constituents and their reported pharmacologi-cal actions. It should be emphasised that many drug interactions are harmless and many of those that are potentially harmful occur only in a small proportion of patients and may then vary in severity from patient to patient. Healthcare professionals should be alert to undeclared use of herbal medicines as a possible cause of unexplained toxicity or lack of effect of conven-tional medicines.

Suspected drug–herb interactions involving licensed or unlicensed herbal products should be reported to the regulatory authorities, as for any other suspected adverse reaction to drugs or herbs.

Drug/therapeutic category affected	Herbal ingredients interacting	Possible effects
Gastrointestinal system		
Antacids, ulcer-healing drugs	Herbal ingredients irritant to gastrointestinal tract. *See* Appendix 13	Exacerbation of symptoms Risk of systemic side-effects
Antidiarrhoeal drugs	Herbal ingredients with laxative activity. *See* Appendix 2	Antagonism
Laxatives	Herbal ingredients with laxative activity. *See* Appendix 2	Potentiation; increased risk of side-effects
Cardiovascular system		
Cardiac glycosides	Cardioactive herbal ingredients. *See* Appendix 3	Potentiation; increased risk of side-effects
	Herbal ingredients containing hydroxyanthracene laxatives. *See* Appendix 2	Potentiation; increased risk of side-effects
	St. John's wort	Risk of reduced therapeutic effect of digoxin
Diuretics	Herbal ingredients containing hydroxyanthracene laxatives. *See* Appendix 2	Potentiation; increased risk of hypokalaemia
	Herbal ingredients with diuretic activity. *See* Appendix 4	Potentiation; increased risk of hypokalaemia
	Herbal ingredients with hypotensive activity. *See* Appendix 5	Difficulty in controlling diuresis; hypotension
Anti-arrhythmic activity	Herbal ingredients containing hydroxyanthracene laxatives. *See* Appendix 2	Interference with existing therapy; increased risk of hypokalaemia
	Cardioactive herbal ingredients. *See* Appendix 3	Interference/antagonism with existing therapy
	Herbal ingredients with diuretic activity. *See* Appendix 4	Antagonism if hypokalaemia occurs
Beta-adrenoceptor blocking drugs	Cardioactive herbal ingredients. *See* Appendix 3	Potential antagonism

Appendix 1 (cont.)

Drug/therapeutic category affected	Herbal ingredients interacting	Possible effects
Beta-adrenoceptor blocking drugs (cont.)	Herbal ingredients with significant amine content or sympathomimetic activity. *See* Appendix 14	Potential risk of severe hypertension
Antihypertensive therapy	Herbal ingredients with hypertensive activity. *See* Appendix 5	Antagonism
	Herbal ingredients with mineralocorticoid activity, e.g. bayberry, liquorice. *See* Appendix 10	Antagonism
	Herbal ingredients with hypotensive activity. *See* Appendix 5	Potentiation
	Herbal ingredients with significant amine content or sympathomimetic activity. *See* Appendix 14	Antagonism
	Herbal ingredients with diuretic activity. *See* Appendix 4	Risk of potentiation/ interference with existing therapy
Lipid-lowering drugs	Herbal ingredients with hypolipidaemic activity. *See* Appendix 7	Additive effect
Nitrates and calcium-channel blockers	Cardioactive ingredients. *See* Appendix 3	Interference with therapy
	Cohosh, blue	Interference with therapy
	Herbal ingredients with hypertensive activity. *See* Appendix 5	Antagonism
	Herbal ingredients with anticholinergic activity	Reduced sublingual absorption of glyceryl trinitrate
Sympathomimetics	Herbal ingredients with significant sympathomimetic amine content. *See* Appendix 14	Potentiation; increased risk of hypertension
	Herbal ingredients with hypertensive activity. *See* Appendix 5	Increased risk of hypertension
	Herbal ingredients with hypotensive activity. *See* Appendix 5	Antagonism
Anticoagulants	Herbal ingredients with coagulant/ anticoagulant activity. *See* Appendix 6	Risk of antagonism or potentiation
	Herbal ingredients with coumarins. *See* Appendix 17	Risk of potentiation
	Herbal ingredients with significant salicylate concentrations. *See* Appendix 6	Risk of potentiation
	Garlic	Raised INR reported in two patients receiving warfarin
	Horse-chestnut	Plasma protein binding
	St. John's wort	Risk of reduced therapeutic effect of warfarin
Respiratory system		
	St. John's wort	Risk of reduced therapeutic effect of theophylline
	Herbal ingredients that are potentially allergenic. *See* Appendix 12	Risk of allergic reaction
Terfenadine	Cardioactive herbal ingredients. *See* Appendix 3	May increase arrhythmogenic potential of terfenadine
	Herbal ingredients with diuretic activity. *See* Appendix 4	Electrolyte imbalance may increase arrhythmogenic potential of terfenadine

Appendix 1 (cont.)

Drug/therapeutic category affected	Herbal ingredients interacting	Possible effects
Allergic disorders	Herbal ingredients claimed to have sedative activity. *See* Appendix 8	Potentiation of drowsiness associated with antihistamines
Central nervous system		
Hypnotics and anxiolytics	Herbal ingredients claimed to have sedative activity. *See* Appendix 8	Potentiation
Stimulants	Ginseng	Increased risk of ginseng side-effects
Antipsychotics	Herbal ingredients with diuretic activity. *See* Appendix 4	Potentiation of lithium therapy; increased risk of toxicity; diuretics reported to reduce lithium clearance
	Herbal ingredients with anticholinergic activity	Risk of interference with therapy; anticholinergic drug reported to reduce plasma phenothiazine concentrations
	Evening primrose	Potential risk of seizures
Antidepressants	Herbal ingredients containing sympathomimetic amines. *See* Appendix 14	Risk of hypertensive crisis with monoamine-oxidase inhibitors (MAOIs)
	Ginseng	Suspected phenelzine interaction
	Herbal ingredients containing tryptophan	Risk of CNS excitation and confusional states with MAOIs
	White horehound	Hydroxytryptamine antagonism, *in vivo*
	Herbal ingredients with sedative activity. *See* Appendix 8	May potentiate sedative side-effects
	Hops	Antagonism; contra-indicated in patients with depressive illness
	St. John's wort	Risk of increased serotonergic effects in patients taking selective serotonin reuptake inhibitors (SSRIs)
Drugs used in nausea and vertigo	Herbal ingredients with sedative activity. *See* Appendix 8	May potentiate sedative side-effects
	Herbal ingredients with anticholinergic activity	Antagonism
Analgesics	Herbal ingredients with diuretic activity. *See* Appendix 4	Increased risk of toxicity with anti-inflammatory analgesics
	Herbal ingredients with corticosteroid activity, e.g. bayberry, liquorice. *See* Appendix 10	Possible reduction in plasma-aspirin concentrations
	Herbal ingredients with sedative activity. *See* Appendix 8	May potentiate sedative side-effects
	St. John's wort	Risk of increased serotonergic effects, with possibility of increased risk of side-effects
Antiepileptics	Herbal ingredients with sedative activity. *See* Appendix 8	May potentiate sedative side-effects
	Borage	May increase risk of seizure
	Evening primrose oil	May increase risk of seizure
	Ground ivy	May increase risk of seizure
	Sage	May increase risk of seizure

Appendix 1 (cont.)

Drug/therapeutic category affected	Herbal ingredients interacting	Possible effects
Antiepileptics (cont.)	Herbal ingredients with significant salicylate content (meadowsweet, poplar, willow) See Appendix 6	Transient potentiation of phenytoin therapy may occur
	Herbal ingredients with significant folic acid content	Plasma phenytoin concentration may be reduced
	St. John's wort	Risk of reduced therapeutic effect of anticonvulsants (carbamazepine, phenobarbitone, phenytoin)
Drugs for parkinsonism	Herbal ingredients with anticholinergic activity	Potentiation; increased risk of side-effects
	Herbal ingredients with cholinergic activity	Antagonism
Infections		
Antifungal drugs	Herbal ingredients with anticholinergic activity	Risk of reduced absorption of ketoconazole
HIV protease inhibitors HIV non-nucleoside reverse transcriptase inhibitors	St. John's wort	Risk of reduced blood concentrations of anti-HIV drugs, with possible loss of HIV suppression
Endocrine system		
Antidiabetics	Herbal ingredients with hypo- or hyperglycaemic activity. See Appendix 7	Potentiation/antagonism of activity
	Herbal ingredients with diuretic activity. See Appendix 4	Antagonism
Drugs for hypo- and hyperthyroidism	Herbal ingredients with significant iodine content e.g. fucus	Interference with therapy
	Horseradish, myrrh	Interference with therapy
Corticosteroids	Herbal ingredients with diuretic activity. See Appendix 4	Risk of increased potassium loss
	Herbal ingredients with corticosteroid activity e.g. bayberry, liquorice. See Appendix 10	Increased risk of side-effects, e.g. water and sodium retention
Sex hormones	Herbal ingredients with hormonal activity. See Appendix 10	Possible interaction with existing therapy
Obstetrics and gynaecology		
Oral contraceptives	Herbal ingredients with hormonal activity. See Appendix 10	Possible interaction with existing therapy; may reduce effectiveness of oral contraceptive
	St. John's wort	Risk of reduced blood concentrations of oral contraceptives, breakthrough bleeding and unintended pregnancy
Malignant disease and immunosuppression		
Methotrexate	Herbal ingredients with significant salicylate content. See Appendix 6	Increased risk of toxicity
Drugs affecting immune response	Herbal ingredients with immunostimulant activity. See Appendix 11	Potentiation or antagonism
	St. John's wort	Risk of reduced therapeutic effect of ciclosporin

Appendix 1 (cont.)

Drug/therapeutic category affected	Herbal ingredients interacting	Possible effects
Musculoskeletal and joint diseases		
Systemic lupus erythematosus	Alfalfa	Antagonism; contra-indicated
Probenecid	Herbal ingredients with significant salicylate content. *See* Appendix 6	Risk of inhibition of probenecid
Eye		
Acetazolamide	Herbal ingredients with significant salicylate content. *See* Appendix 6	Increased risk of toxicity
Skin	Herbal ingredients with potential allergenic activity. *See* Appendix 12	Allergic reaction; exacerbation of existing symptoms
	Herbal ingredients with phototoxic activity. *See* Appendix 12	Phototoxic reaction; exacerbation of existing symptoms
Anaesthetics		
General anaesthetics	Herbal ingredients with hypotensive activity. *See* Appendix 5	Potentiation of hypotensive effect
Competitive muscle relaxants	Herbal ingredients with diuretic activity. *See* Appendix 4	Risk of potentiation if hypokalaemia occurs
Depolarising muscle relaxants	Cardioactive herbal ingredients. *See* Appendix 3	Risk of arrhythmias

Appendix 2 Laxative Herbal Ingredients

Drug	Effect
Aloes	Hydroxyanthracene constituents
Cascara	Hydroxyanthracene constituents
Eyebright	Iridoids, *in vivo*
Frangula	Hydroxyanthracene constituents
Horehound, White	Large doses
Ispaghula	Bulk laxative
Plantain	Iridoids, *in vivo* (much less than senna)
Rhubarb	Hydroxyanthracene constituents
Senna	Hydroxyanthracene constituents
Yellow Dock	Hydroxyanthracene constituents

Appendix 3 Cardioactive Herbal Ingredients

Drug	Effect
Broom	Alkaloid constituents: cardiac depressant activity
Calamus	Anti-arrhythmic activity
Cereus	Tyramine: cardiotonic amine
Cola	Caffeine
Coltsfoot	Cardiac calcium-channel blocking activity

Appendix 3 (cont.)

Drug	Effect
Devil's Claw	Activity *in vivo*
Fenugreek	Activity *in vitro*
Figwort	Cardioactive glycoside constituents, activity *in vitro*
Fumitory	Alkaloid constituent: cardioactive
Ginger	Activity *in vivo*
Ginseng, Panax	Activity *in vivo*
Golden Seal	Berberine: cardioactive alkaloid
Hawthorn	Tyramine: cardiotonic amine; activity *in vivo*
Horehound, White	Activity *in vivo*
Lime Flower	Activity reputed with excessive ingestion
Maté	Caffeine
Mistletoe	Viscotoxin, negative inotropic effect
Motherwort	Cardiac glycoside constituents; activity *in vitro*
Parsley	Apiole poisoning, high doses
Pleurisy Root	Cardenolides, active *in vitro* and *in vivo*
Prickly Ash, Northern	Interaction with Na^+K^+ ATPase
Prickly Ash, Southern	Interaction with Na^+K^+ ATPase
Quassia	Activity *in vitro*

Appendix 3 (cont.)

Drug	Effect
Shepherd's Purse	Activity *in vitro*
Squill	Cardiac glycoside constituents
Wild Carrot	Depressant activity *in vivo*

Appendix 4   Diuretic Herbal Ingredients

Drug	Effect
Agrimony	Activity *in vivo*
Artichoke	Reputed action
Boldo	Irritant oil
Broom	Reputed action
Buchu	Reputed action
Burdock	Reputed action
Celery	Reputed action
Cornsilk	Activity in humans
Couchgrass	Activity *in vivo*
Dandelion	Activity *in vivo*
Devil's Claw	Reputed action
Elder	Activity *in vivo*
Guaiacum	Reputed action
Java Tea	Activity *in vivo*
Juniper	Reputed action; terpinen-4-ol
Nettle	Activity in humans
Pokeroot	Activity *in vivo*
Shepherd's Purse	Activity *in vivo*
Squill	Activity *in vivo*
Uva-Ursi	Reputed action
Yarrow	Activity *in vivo*

Appendix 5   Hypotensive and Hypertensive Herbal Ingredients

Drug	Effect
Hypotensive	
Agrimony	Hypotensive, *in vivo*
Asafoetida	Hypotensive, *in vivo*
Avens	Hypotensive, *in vivo*
Calamus	Hypotensive, *in vivo*
Cat's Claw	Hypotensive, *in vivo*
Celery	Hypotensive, human and *in vivo*
Cohosh, Black	Hypotensive, *in vivo*
Cornsilk	Hypotensive, *in vivo*
Cowslip	Hypotensive, then hypertensive *in vivo*
Devil's Claw	Hypotensive, *in vivo*
Elecampane	Hypotensive, *in vivo*
Fenugreek	Hypotensive

Appendix 5 (cont.)

Drug	Effect
Fucus	Hypotensive
Fumitory	Hypotensive, *in vivo*
Garlic	Hypotensive, human and *in vivo*
Ginger	Hypotensive
Ginseng, Panax	Hypotensive, human and *in vivo*
Golden Seal	Hypotensive, alkaloid effect
Hawthorn	Hypotensive, *in vivo*
Horehound, White	Vasodilator (volatile oil)
Horse-chestnut	Hypotensive, *in vivo*
Horseradish	Hypotensive, *in vivo*
Java Tea	Hypotensive, *in vivo*
Juniper	Hypotensive, *in vivo*
Mistletoe	Hypotensive, *in vivo*
Nettle	Hypotensive, *in vivo*
Parsley	Hypotensive, *in vivo*
Plantain	Hypotensive, *in vivo*
Pokeroot	Hypotensive, *in vivo*
Prickly Ash, Northern	Hypotensive, *in vivo*
Prickly Ash, Southern	Hypotensive, *in vivo*
Sage	Hypotensive
Shepherd's Purse	Hypotensive
Squill	Vasodilator, *in vivo*
St. John's Wort	Hypotensive, *in vivo*
Thyme	Hypotensive, *in vivo*
Vervain	Hypotensive
Wild Carrot	Hypotensive, *in vivo*
Yarrow	Hypotensive, *in vivo*
Hypertensive	
Bayberry	Hypertensive, myricitrin mineralocorticoid side-effect
Broom	Hypertensive, alkaloid effect, stated to be contra-indicated in hypertensive individuals
Capsicum	Hypertensive, increased catecholamine secretion
Cohosh, Blue	Hypertensive, methylcytisine has nicotinic action, alkaloid effect
Cola	Hypertensive, caffeine
Coltsfoot	Hypertensive, pressor activity
Ephedra	Hypertensive, human and *in vivo*
Gentian	Stated to be contra-indicated in hypertensive individuals
Ginger	Hypertensive
Ginseng, Panax	Hypertensive, human and *in vivo*
Liquorice	Hypertensive, mineralocorticoid side-effect
Maté	Hypertensive, caffeine
Vervain	Hypertensive

Appendix 6   Anticoagulant and Coagulant Herbal Ingredients

Drug	Effect
Anticoagulants	
Alfalfa	Coumarin constituents
Angelica	Coumarin constituents
Aniseed	Coumarin constituents
Arnica	Coumarin constituents
Asafoetida	Coumarin constituents, anticoagulant *in vivo*
Bilberry	Inhibits platelet aggregation, human, *in vivo*, *in vitro*
Boldo	Coumarin constituents
Capsicum	Coumarin constituents
Cat's Claw	Inhibits platelet aggregation, *in vitro*
Celery	Coumarin constituents
Chamomile, German	Coumarin constituents
Chamomile, Roman	Coumarin constituents
Clove	Eugenol inhibitor of platelet activity
Dandelion	Coumarin constituents
Fenugreek	Coumarin constituents
Feverfew	Inhibits platelet aggregation
Fucus	Anticoagulant action
Garlic	Interaction with warfarin reported
Ginger	Inhibition of platelet activity
Ginkgo	Inhibition of platelet activity
Ginseng, Panax	Reduction of blood coagulation
Horse-chestnut	Coumarin constituents
Horseradish	Peroxidase stimulates synthesis of arachidonic acid metabolites
Liquorice	Inhibition of platelet activity
Meadowsweet	Salicylate constituents
Nettle	Coumarin constituents
Passionflower	Coumarin constituents
Poplar	Salicylate constituents
Prickly Ash, Northern	Coumarin constituents
Prickly Ash, Southern	Coumarin constituents
Quassia	Coumarin constituents
Red Clover	Coumarin constituents
Willow	Salicylate constituents
Coagulants	
Agrimony	Coagulant, human
Golden Seal	Heparin antagonist
Mistletoe	Lectins, agglutinating activity
Yarrow	Coagulant, *in vivo*

Appendix 7   Hypolipidaemic and Hyperlipidaemic Herbal Ingredients

Drug	Effect
Hypocholesterolaemic	
Alfalfa	Hypocholesterolaemic, *in vivo*
Artichoke	Hypocholesterolaemic, *in vivo*, human
Bilberry	Hypocholesterolaemic, *in vivo*
Capsicum	Hypocholesterolaemic, *in vivo*
Cohosh, Black	Hypocholesterolaemic, *in vivo*
Fenugreek	Hypocholesterolaemic, *in vivo*, human
Garlic	Hypocholesterolaemic, *in vivo*, human
Ginger	Hypocholesterolaemic, *in vivo*
Ispaghula	Hypocholesterolaemic, human
Milk thistle	Hypocholesterolaemic, *in vivo*
Myrrh	Hypolipidaemic, *in vivo*, human
Plantain	Hypocholesterolaemic, *in vivo*
Scullcap	Hypocholesterolaemic, *in vivo*
Senega	Hypolipidaemic, *in vivo*
Tansy	Hypocholesterolaemic, *in vivo*
Hypercholesterolaemic	
Hydrocotyle	Hypercholesterolaemic, *in vivo*

Appendix 8   Sedative Herbal Ingredients

Drug	Effect
Calamus	Potentiates barbiturate sleeping time
Celery	*In vivo*
Centaury	Reputed action
Chamomile, German	Human
Couchgrass	*In vivo*
Elecampane	*In vivo*
Ginsengs	CNS depressant and stimulant
Golden Seal	*In vivo*
Hawthorn	CNS depressant; potentiates barbiturate sleeping time
Hops	*In vivo*
Hydrocotyle	*In vivo*
Jamaica Dogwood	*In vivo*
Nettle	CNS depression, *in vivo*
Passionflower	*In vivo*
Sage	*In vivo*
Scullcap	Reputed action
Senega	CNS depressant, *in vivo*

Appendix 8 (cont.)

Drug	Effect
Shepherd's Purse	Potentiates barbiturate sleeping time
St. John's Wort	Traditional use, biflavonoids
Valerian	Human, *in vivo*
Wild Carrot	*In vivo*
Wild Lettuce	*In vivo*, related species

Appendix 9 Hypoglycaemic and Hyperglycaemic Herbal Ingredients

Drug	Effect
Hypoglycaemic	
Agrimony	Hypoglycaemic, *in vivo*
Alfalfa	Hypoglycaemic, manganese, human
Aloes/Aloe vera	Hypoglycaemic, *in vivo*
Burdock	Hypoglycaemic, *in vivo*
Celery	Hypoglycaemic, *in vivo*
Cornsilk	Hypoglycaemic, *in vivo*
Damiana	Hypoglycaemic
Dandelion	Hypoglycaemic, *in vivo*
Elecampane	Hypoglycaemic
Eucalyptus	Hypoglycaemic, *in vivo*
Fenugreek	Hypoglycaemic, human
Garlic	Hypoglycaemic, *in vivo*, human
Ginger	Hypoglycaemic, *in vivo*
Ginseng, Panax	Hypoglycaemic
Ispaghula	Hypoglycaemic, humans
Java Tea	Hypoglycaemic *in vivo*
Juniper	Hypoglycaemic *in vivo*
Marshmallow	Hypoglycaemic, *in vivo*, human
Myrrh	Hypoglycaemic, *in vivo*
Nettle	Hypoglycaemic, *in vivo*
Sage	Hypoglycaemic, *in vivo*
Senega	Hypoglycaemic, *in vivo*
Tansy	Hypoglycaemic, *in vivo*
Hyperglycaemic	
Elecampane	Hyperglycaemic
Ginseng, Panax	Hyperglycaemic
Hydrocotyle	Hyperglycaemic, human
Liquorice	Reduced K⁺ aggravates glucose tolerance
Rosemary	Hyperglycaemic, *in vivo*

Appendix 10 Hormonally Active Herbal Ingredients

Drug	Effect
Agnus Castus	Many uses in hormonal imbalance disorders
Agrimony	Oestrogenic
Alfalfa	Oestrogenic, *in vivo*
Aniseed	Oestrogenic
Bayberry	Mineralocorticoid
Cohosh, Black	Oestrogenic
Fucus	Hyper-/hypothyroidism reported
Ginsengs	Oestrogenic, human
Horseradish	May depress thyroid activity
Liquorice	Mineralocorticoid activity, human; oestrogenic *in vivo*, *in vitro*
Motherwort	Oxytocic
Pleurisy Root	Oestrogenic
Red Clover	Oestrogenic *in vivo*
Saw Palmetto	Oestrogenic and anti-androgenic *in vivo*; human use in prostate cancer
Vervain	Inhibition of gonadotrophic activity
Wild Carrot	Oestrogenic

Appendix 11 Immunomodulating Herbal Ingredients

Drug	Effects
Alfalfa	Stimulant, *in vitro*
Boneset	Stimulant, *in vitro*
Calendula	Stimulant, *in vitro*
Cat's Claw	Stimulant, *in vitro*
Chamomile, German	Stimulant, *in vitro*
Drosera	Stimulant and depressant (*in vitro*)
Echinacea	Stimulant, *in vitro*, *in vivo*
Ephedra	Inhibits complement pathway, *in vitro*
Ginseng, Eleutherococcus	Stimulant, *in vivo*, human
Mistletoe	Stimulant, *in vivo*, human; suppressant (high doses), human
Saw Palmetto	Stimulant, *in vivo*

Appendix 12 Allergenic Herbal Ingredients

Drug	Effect
Agnus Castus	Allergic effects reported
Angelica	Furanocoumarins, photosensitivity, contact allergy
Aniseed	Furanocoumarins, photosensitivity, contact allergy
Apricot	Contact allergy, kernels
Arnica	Contact allergy
Artichoke	Sesquiterpene lactone constituents
Asafoetida	Irritant gum, contact allergy
Boneset	Sesquiterpene lactone constituents
Calendula	Individuals sensitive to plants from the Compositae/ Asteraceae families
Cassia	Allergic reactions, mainly contact
Celery	Furanocoumarins, photosensitivity
Chamomile, German	Sesquiterpene lactone constituents
Chamomile, Roman	Sesquiterpene lactone constituents
Cinnamon	Contact allergy
Cornsilk	Allergic reactions
Cowslip	Allergic reactions
Dandelion	Sesquiterpene lactone constituents
Elecampane	Sesquiterpene lactone constituents
Euphorbia	Histamine potentiating properties
Feverfew	Sesquiterpene lactone constituents
Fucus	Iodine may aggravate/trigger acne
Garlic	Sulfur-containing compounds, allergic reaction
Ginger	Dermatitis in sensitive individuals
Ginkgo	Fruit pulp and seeds: severe allergic reactions
Gravel Root	Sesquiterpene lactone constituents
Guaiacum	Irritant resin
Holy Thistle	Sesquiterpene lactone constituents
Hops	Contact allergy
Hydrangea	Contact allergy
Hydrocotyle	Photosensitivity
Ispaghula	Rare cases of allergy
Juniper	Contact allergy

Appendix 12 (cont.)

Drug	Effect
Lady's Slipper	Contact allergy
Meadowsweet	Potentiation of histamine bronchospastic properties
Motherwort	Dermatitis, photosensitisation
Parsley	Furanocoumarins, photosensitivity
Pilewort	Contact allergy, protanemonin
Plantain	Contact allergy
Pleurisy Root	Contact allergy
Pulsatilla	Contact allergy, protoanemonin
Rosemary	Dermatitis, photosensitisation
St. John's Wort	Photodermatitis, hypericin
Tansy	Sesquiterpene lactone constituents
Wild Carrot	Furanocoumarins, photosensitivity
Yarrow	Sesquiterpene lactone constituents

Appendix 13 Irritant Herbal Ingredients

Drug	Effects
Alfalfa	Irritant, canavanine in seeds
Arnica	Irritant to mucous membranes
Asafoetida	Irritant gum
Blue Flag	Irritant gum and oil
Bogbean	Irritant to GI tract
Boldo	Irritant oil
Buchu	Irritant oil
Capsicum	Capsaicinoids, mucosal irritants
Cassia	Irritant to mucous membranes, oil
Cinnamon	Irritant to mucous membranes, oil
Cohosh, Blue	Irritant to mucous membranes; spasmogenic in vitro
Cowslip	Irritant saponins
Drosera	Plumbagin, irritant
Eucalyptus	Irritant oil
False Unicorn	Large doses may cause vomiting
Figwort	Purgative effect
Garlic	Raw clove
Ground Ivy	Irritant oil
Guaiacum	Avoid if inflammatory condition
Horse-chestnut	Saponin constituents, contraindicated in existing renal disease
Horseradish	Irritant oil
Hydrangea	May cause gastro-enteritis, hydrangin

Appendix 13 (cont.)

Drug	Effects
Jamaica Dogwood	Irritant to humans
Juniper	Irritant oil
Lemon Verbena	Irritant oil
Lime Flower	Irritant to kidney, oil
Nettle	Tea irritant to stomach
Parsley	Irritant oil
Pennyroyal	Toxic and irritant oil
Pilewort	Irritant sap
Pleurisy Root	Gastrointestinal irritant
Pokeroot	Irritant saponins
Pulsatilla	Irritant to mucous membranes
Queen's Delight	Diterpene constituents
Sage	Irritant oil
Sarsaparilla	Saponins
Senega	Saponins
Skunk Cabbage	Inflammatory and blistering to skin
Squill	Saponins
Thyme	Irritant oil
Willow	Salicylates
Witch Hazel	Irritant to stomach

Appendix 14 Herbal Ingredients containing Amines or Alkaloids, or with Sympathomimetic Action

Drug	Effects
Agnus Castus	Alkaloids
Alfalfa	Alkaloids
Aniseed	Anethole, sympathomimetic
Arnica	Betaines, choline
Bloodroot	Alkaloids
Bogbean	Alkaloids
Boldo	Alkaloids
Borage	Alkaloids
Broom	Alkaloids, amines
Calamus	Amines
Capsicum	Sympathomimetic
Cat's Claw	Alkaloids
Centaury	Alkaloids
Cereus	Tyramine
Cohosh, Black	Alkaloids
Cohosh, Blue	Alkaloids
Cola	Alkaloids
Coltsfoot	Alkaloids
Comfrey	Alkaloids
Cornsilk	Amines
Echinacea	Alkaloids

Appendix 14 (cont.)

Drug	Effects
Ephedra	Alkaloids
Eyebright	Alkaloids
Fenugreek	Choline, trigonelline
Fumitory	Alkaloids
Gentian	Alkaloids
Ginkgo	Seed: alkaloids Leaf: MAOI activity
Ginseng, Panax	MAOI potentiation, suspected phenelzine interaction
Golden Seal	Alkaloids
Gravel Root	Alkaloids
Hawthorn	Tyramine
Horehound, White	Alkaloids
Hydrocotyle	Alkaloids
Ispaghula	Alkaloids
Jamaica Dogwood	Alkaloids
Liferoot	Alkaloids
Lobelia	Alkaloids
Maté	Alkaloids, amines
Mistletoe	Histamine release
Motherwort	Alkaloids
Nettle	Choline
Parsley	Myristicin, sympathomimetic
Passionflower	Alkaloids (traces or absent)
Plantain	Alkaloids
Pleurisy Root	Sympathomimetic
Pokeroot	Betalains
Prickly Ash, Northern	Alkaloids
Prickly Ash, Southern	Alkaloids
Quassia	Alkaloids
Sassafras	Alkaloids
Shepherd's Purse	Choline, tyramine
Skunk Cabbage	Alkaloids
St. John's Wort	MAOI activity, *in vitro*
Stone Root	Alkaloids
Valerian	Alkaloids
Vervain	Sympathomimetic
Yarrow	Betonicine, stachydrine, betaine

Appendix 15 Anti-inflammatory Herbal Ingredients

Aloe Vera, Angelica, Arnica, Bilberry, Black Cohosh, Bloodroot, Blue Flag, Boldo, Boneset, Borage, Buchu, Calendula, Cassia, Cat's Claw, Centaury, Coltsfoot, Comfrey, Cowslip, Dandelion, Devil's Claw, Echinacea, Elder, Ephedra, Evening Primrose, Feverfew,

Figwort, Gentian, German Chamomile, Ginger, Ground Ivy, Horse-chestnut, Hydrocotyle, Juniper, Liquorice, Milk Thistle, Myrrh, Nettle, Plantain, Pokeroot, Prickly Ash (Southern), Roman Chamomile, Rosemary, Sarsaparilla, Shepherd's Purse, Uva-Ursi, Willow, Yarrow, Yucca

Appendix 16 Antispasmodic Herbal Ingredients

Angelica, Aniseed, Asafoetida, Blue Cohosh, Calendula, Capsicum, Cassia, Celery, Cinnamon, Clove, Cowslip, Echinacea, Elecampane, Euphorbia, Chamomile (German), Hops, Jamaica Dogwood, Lime Flower, Raspberry, Chamomile (Roman), Rosemary, Sage, Scullcap, Tansy, Thyme, Valerian

Appendix 17 Herbal Ingredients containing Coumarins

Alfalfa, Angelica, Aniseed, Arnica, Asafoetida, Bogbean, Boldo, Buchu, Capsicum, Cassia, Celery, Chamomile (German), Chamomile (Roman), Dandelion, Fenugreek, Horse-chestnut, Horseradish, Liquorice, Meadowsweet, Nettle, Parsley, Passionflower, Prickly Ash (Northern), Quassia, Wild Carrot, Wild Lettuce

Appendix 18 Herbal Ingredients containing Flavonoids

Agnus Castus, Agrimony, Angelica, Aniseed, Apricot, Arnica, Artichoke, Bayberry, Bilberry, Bogbean, Boldo, Boneset, Broom, Buchu, Burdock, Burnet, Calendula, Celery, Cereus, Chamomile (German), Chamomile (Roman), Chaparral, Clivers, Coltsfoot, Cornsilk, Couchgrass, Cowslip, Damiana, Dandelion, Devil's Claw, Drosera, Elder, Ephedra, Eucalyptus, Euphorbia, Eyebright, Fenugreek, Feverfew, Figwort, Frangula, Fumitory, Ginkgo, Gravel Root, Ground Ivy, Hawthorn, Hops, Horehound (Black), Horehound (White), Horse-chestnut, Hydrangea, Hydrocotyle, Java Tea, Juniper, Lemon Verbena, Lime Flower, Liquorice, Marshmallow, Maté, Meadowsweet, Melissa, Milk thistle, Mistletoe, Motherwort, Nettle, Parsley, Passionflower, Plantain, Pulsatilla, Raspberry, Red Clover, Rhubarb, Rosemary, Sage, Sarsaparilla, Saw Palmetto, Scullcap, Senna, Shepherd's Purse, Squill, St. John's Wort, Thyme, Uva-Ursi, Wild Carrot, Wild Lettuce, Willow, Witch Hazel, Yarrow

Appendix 19 Herbal Ingredients containing Iridoids

Agnus Castus, Bilberry, Bogbean, Centaury, Clivers, Devil's Claw, Eyebright, Figwort, Gentian, Ispa-

ghula, Motherwort, Plantain, Scullcap, Uva-Ursi, Valerian, Vervain

Appendix 20 Herbal Ingredients containing Saponins

Alfalfa, Aloe Vera, Bogbean, Burnet, Calendula, Chaparral, Cohosh (Blue), Cornsilk, Cowslip, False Unicorn, Fenugreek, Ginseng (Eleutherococcus), Ginseng (Panax), Hawthorn, Horehound (White), Horse-chestnut, Hydrangea, Hydrocotyle, Jamaica Dogwood, Lime Flower, Milk Thistle, Pokeroot, Pulsatilla, Red Clover, Sarsaparilla, Senega, Senna, Stone Root, Thyme, Witch Hazel, Yucca

Appendix 21 Herbal Ingredients containing Tannins

Agrimony, Apricot, Arnica, Artichoke, Avens, Bayberry, Bilberry, Blue Flag, Boldo, Borage, Burnet, Calamus, Cascara, Cassia, Chamomile (German), Cinnamon, Clivers, Cohosh (Black), Cola, Coltsfoot, Comfrey, Cornsilk, Cowslip, Damiana, Drosera, Elder, Ephedra, Eucalyptus, Eyebright, Feverfew, Frangula, Gentian, Ground Ivy, Hawthorn, Holy Thistle, Hops, Horse-chestnut, Ispaghula, Juniper, Lady's Slipper, Lime Flower, Marshmallow, Meadowsweet, Mistletoe, Motherwort, Nettle, Pilewort, Plantain, Poplar, Prickly Ash (Northern), Prickly Ash (Southern), Queen's Delight, Raspberry, Rhubarb, Sage, Sassafras, Saw Palmetto, Scullcap, Slippery Elm, Squill, St. John's Wort, Stone Root, Tansy, Thyme, Uva-Ursi, Valerian, Vervain, Willow, Witch Hazel, Yarrow, Yellow Dock

Appendix 22 Herbal Ingredients containing Volatile Oils

Agnus Castus, Agrimony, Angelica, Aniseed, Arnica, Artichoke, Asafoetida, Avens, Blue Flag, Boldo, Boneset, Buchu, Burdock, Burnet, Calamus, Calendula, Capsicum, Cassia, Celery, Chamomile (German), Chamomile (Roman), Chaparral, Cinnamon, Cloves, Cohosh (Black), Coltsfoot, Couchgrass, Damiana, Ephedra, Elder, Elecampane, Eucalyptus, Eyebright, Feverfew, Garlic, Gentian, Ginger, Ginseng (Eleutherococcus), Ginseng (Panax), Golden Seal, Ground Ivy, Holy Thistle, Hops, Horehound (Black), Horseradish, Hydrocotyle, Java Tea, Juniper, Lemon Verbena, Lime Flower, Liquorice, Lobelia, Meadowsweet, Melissa, Motherwort, Myrrh, Parsley, Pennyroyal, Prickly Ash (Northern), Queen's Delight, Red Clover, Rosemary, Sage, Sassafras, Saw Palmetto, Senna (trace), Skunk Cabbage,

Squill, St. John's Wort, Stone Root, Tansy, Thyme, Uva-Ursi, Valerian, Wild Carrot, Witch Hazel, Yarrow

Appendix 23 Council of Europe. Categories for Natural Sources of Flavourings (Report No. 1. Strasbourg: Council of Europe, 2000)

Category	Natural source of flavouring
1	Plants, animals and other organisms, and parts of these or products thereof, normally consumed as food items, herbs or spices in Europe for which it is considered that there should be no restrictions on use. Flavouring preparations, which are not themselves consumed as food but which are derived from plants, animals and other organisms, and parts of these or products thereof, normally consumed as food items, herbs or spices in Europe. These preparations, on the basis of the information available, are not considered a risk to health in the quantities used.
2	Plants, animals and other organisms, and parts of these or products thereof, and preparations derived therefrom, not normally consumed as food items, herbs or spices in Europe. These source materials and preparations, on the basis of the information available, are not considered to constitute a risk to health in the quantities used.
3	Plants, animals and other organisms, and parts of these or products thereof, normally consumed as food items, herbs or spices in Europe which contain defined 'active principles' or 'other chemical components' requiring limits on use levels. Flavouring preparations, which are not themselves consumed as food but which are derived from plants, animals and other organisms, and parts

Appendix 23 (cont.)

Category	Natural source of flavouring
	of these or products thereof, normally consumed as food items, herbs or spices in Europe which contain defined 'active principles' or 'other chemical components' requiring limits on use levels. These source materials and preparations are not considered to constitute a risk to health in the quantities used provided that the limits set for the 'active principles' or 'other chemical components' are not exceeded.
4	Plants, animals and other organisms, and parts of these or products thereof, and preparations derived therefrom, not normally consumed as food items, herbs or spices in Europe which contain defined 'active principles' or 'other chemical components' requiring limits on use levels. These source materials and preparations are not considered to constitute a risk to health in the quantities used provided that the limits set for the 'active principles' or 'other chemical components' are not exceeded.
5	Plants, animals and other organisms, and parts of these or products thereof, and preparations derived therefrom, for which additional toxicological and/or chemical information is required. These could temporarily be acceptable provided that any limits set for the 'active principles' or the 'other chemical components' are not exceeded.
6	Plants, animals and other organisms, and parts of these or products thereof, and preparations derived therefrom, which are considered to be unfit for human consumption in any amount.

Index

Page numbers in **bold** refer to monographs.